# Clinical Cases in Hepatology

Nora V. Bergasa

Editor

# Clinical Cases in Hepatology

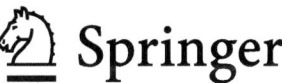 Springer

*Editor*
Nora V. Bergasa
Department of Medicine, H+H/Metropolitan
Physician Affiliate Group of New York
New York, NY
USA

New York Medical College
New York, NY
USA

Hepatology
H+H/Woodhull
Brooklyn, NY
USA

The author(s) has/have asserted their right(s) to be identified as the author(s) of this work in accordance with the Copyright, Designs and Patents Act 1988.
ISBN 978-1-4471-4714-5        ISBN 978-1-4471-4715-2   (eBook)
https://doi.org/10.1007/978-1-4471-4715-2

This Springer imprint is published by the registered company Springer-Verlag London Ltd. part of Springer Nature.
The registered company address is: The Campus, 4 Crinan Street, London, N1 9XW, United Kingdom

*I dedicate this book to my mother, Delia, who showed her bravery and love for me: she let me go as an adolescent to live free from the oppressive communist Cuban regimen.*

# Preface

This book is the beginning of clinical hepatology. As such, it concerns some of the most common conditions seen in the hepatology clinics of two community hospitals where I have worked for several years. The book is intended for residents, gastroenterology and hepatology fellows, nurse practitioners, and physician assistants who want to become familiar with the approach to patients with liver disease.

I have worked on this book for several years with long breaks in between, which has resulted in a product that includes dramatic changes in the discipline of hepatology and which include the development of drugs that cure chronic hepatitis C, clinical trials on primary biliary cholangitis, and the approval of a new medication to treat this disease, the name of which changed from primary biliary cirrhosis during the writing of this book, and the expansion in the study of nonalcoholic fatty liver disease. I am indebted to Springer for having waited for the completion of this book.

New York, NY                                                    Nora V. Bergasa, MD, MACP

# Acknowledgements

I thank the colleagues who contributed to this book.

Dr. Barbara S. Koppel, MD, FAAN, Professor of Clinical Neurology at New York Medical College, Valhalla, New York, was my academic editor. I am very grateful for her important contribution to this book.

From New York City, Health + Hospitals/Woodhull, Brooklyn, Dr. Anatole Sladen, Department of Radiology, provided the radiographic images. Dr. Cesar del Rosario, Chief of Pathology, provided most of the pictures of liver histology. From the Icahn School of Medicine at Mount Sinai, New York, Dr. Maria Isabel Fiel, Professor of Pathology, contributed the liver histology picture in Chap. 10.

Martha M. Dao from GRAPHIC (+WEB) DESIGN **MMD** for the illustrations.

I am grateful to the patients for their trust; it has been my greatest privilege to provide their medical care. I am thankful for the medical residents, gastroenterology fellows, physician assistants, and a dedicated Doctor in Pharmacy who have worked with me in the hepatology clinic over the years.

I thank God every day for my life, for the opportunities I have had, and for opening doors for me when others closed.

# Contents

# Chapter 1
# The Liver

**Nora V. Bergasa**

The liver is a gland surrounded by Glisson's capsule. It is located in the right upper quadrant of the abdomen, triangular in shape, and comprised of the right and left lobes, also known as the right and left livers, divided by the round and falciform ligaments. The quadrate lobe is in the liver's inferior surface, limited by the umbilical fissure, the gallbladder bed, and the hilus. The caudate lobe is in the liver's posterior surface; it is limited to the right by the inferior vena cava and to the left by the fissure of the ligamentum venosum [1].

The right, middle, and hepatic veins divide the liver into four sectors, each receiving a portal pedicle. Each part of the liver that gets a portal pedicle is called a segment, of which there are eight. The right liver is comprised of two sectors, divided themselves into two segments. The anterior sector is comprised of segment V, inferiorly, and segment VIII, superiorly. The posterior sector is divided into segment VI inferiorly and segment VII superiorly [1].

The left liver has two sectors; the anterior sector is comprised of segment IV, medially, and segment III laterally. The posterior sector of the left liver contains segment II [1].

The caudate lobe is segment I, which receives its blood flow from the right and left branches of the portal veins and hepatic artery, and its veins drain directly into the inferior vena cava [1].

N. V. Bergasa (✉)
Department of Medicine, H+H/Metropolitan, New York, NY, USA

New York Medical College, Valhalla, NY, USA

Hepatology, H+H/Woodhull, Brooklyn, NY, USA

## Hepatic Blood Flow

The portal vein, formed by the splenic and superior mesenteric veins, provides two-thirds of the hepatic blood flow, with the hepatic artery providing the rest [2]. Mixed arterial and venous blood circulate through the sinusoids [3], which converge into the hepatic veins to drain into the superior vena cava, except as noted above for the caudate lobe [1].

## Liver Lymphatics

The initial lymphatic vessels arise in the portal tracts. There is a capsular lymph network; it is unclear whether these two networks communicate with each other. Lymphatics drain lymph from interstitial spaces within the liver, most notably, the space of Disse. The liver provides 25–50% of the lymph that enters the thoracic duct [4]. The increase in venous pressure results in increased capillary filtration and hence, increased lymph flow, as it happens in portal hypertension. There are large lymphatic vessels in the hepatic hilum through which lymph circulates toward the cisterna chyli [4].

## Liver Histology

The hepatocyte is the parenchymal cell that carries the liver function and comprises 70% of the liver mass.

The nonparenchymal liver cells include liver sinusoidal endothelial cells that comprise 50% of the population; Kupffer cells, 20%; lymphocytes, 25%; biliary epithelial cells, 5%; and hepatic stellate cells, 1%.

The hepatic sinusoids are channels throughout the liver through which blood flows. Sinusoidal endothelial cells form the walls of the hepatic sinusoids, which characteristically lack a basement membrane, i.e., they have fenestrae to allow for an intimate contact with the space of Disse [5]. The space of Disse is located between the endothelial cells and the sinusoidal surface of the hepatocyte. Projections from the hepatocytes lie in the space of Disse, through which substances circulating in the sinusoidal stream are taken up by the parenchymal cells for metabolism.

The Kupffer cells are liver macrophages that clear circulating endotoxin and other exogenous substances perceived as foreign or injurious to the body [6]. They promote regulatory T cells to inhibit cytotoxic T cells in physiological conditions [7].

The lymphocyte component of the liver is comprised of natural killer and natural killer T cells, which are pivotal in the immune response and lymphocyte recruitment [8].

Biliary epithelial cells line the intrahepatic and extrahepatic bile ducts and modify the composition and flow of the bile formed by the hepatocyte [9]. Biliary epithelial cells can also participate in liver regeneration and immune-mediated processes [10].

The hepatic stellate cells are perisinusoidal cells that store vitamin A in the normal liver. In response to liver injury, they are activated and turn into alpha-smooth muscle actin-expressing contractile myofibroblasts increasing portal pressure by their effect on the vasculature. In addition, when activated, they participate in mitogen-mediated proliferation, increased fibrogenesis, and abnormal matrix degradation [11].

Afferent and efferent nerve fibers innervate the liver. The portal tract contains parasympathetic and sympathetic fibers; the latter coursing into the liver sinusoids. Hepatic afferent fibers are considered to participate in osmosensation and metabolic sensing. Hepatic efferents are believed to regulate hepatic vasculature tone, metabolism, and liver regeneration. Neuropeptides and neurotransmitters regulate the function of the biliary epithelium. A role for the autonomic nervous system in the activation of hepatic stellate cells has been suggested [12].

## Liver Organization

The liver is organized in hexagonal, one cell thick plates of 15–25 hepatocytes, known as hepatic lobules [13]. The portal triads, comprised of a vein, artery, bile duct, and nerve, are located at the apices of the hexagon. Between cell plates, mixed arterial and venous blood circulates through the hepatic sinusoids from the portal tract to the central vein through which a functional gradient, known as metabolic zonation, regulated by Wnt/β-catenin signaling [14] exists. Zone 1 is periportal, followed by zone 2 and zone 3, which is pericentral [15]. The acinus is a term used to describe the smallest functional liver unit, with acinar zones 1, 2, and 3 being located in the same area as those of the lobule.

Oxygenation, beta-oxidation, gluconeogenesis, glycogen synthesis from lactate, and ureagenesis predominantly occur in zone 1. Triglyceride synthesis, lipogenesis and ketogenesis, glycolysis, and glycogen synthesis from glucose occur in zone 3. However, cells from the three zones have the flexibility to provide functions that may be impaired by injury or fasting, for example, in other zones [15].

## Liver Function

The liver is a generous organ. It processes substances from the splanchnic circulation prior to their availability to the systemic circulation. The function of the liver includes the synthesis and secretion of proteins, transport and biotransformation of drugs, production of bile, bile acids and heme, metabolism of carbohydrates, lipids and lipoproteins, amino acids, and metals and trace elements, in addition to urea production, pH regulation, and excretion of porphyrins [15, 16].

# References

1. Bismuth H, Aldridge MC, Kunstlinger F. Structure of the liver. In: McIntyre N, Benhamou J-P, Birher J, Rizzetto M, Rodes J, editors. Oxford textbook of clinical hepatology, vol. 1. Oxford: Oxford University Press; 1991. p. 3–11.
2. Tystrup N, Winkler K, Mellemgaard K. Determination of arterial blood flow and oxygen supply in man by clamping the hepatic artery during surgery. J Clin Invest. 1962;41:447–54.
3. Wake K, Sato T. "The sinusoid" in the liver: lessons learned from the original definition by Charles Sedgwick Minot (1900). Anat Rec. 2015;298:2071–80.
4. Ohtani O, Ohtani Y. Lymph circulation in the liver. Anat Rec. 2008;291(6):643–52.
5. Elvevold K, Smedsrød B, Martinez I. The liver sinusoidal endothelial cell: a cell type of controversial and confusing identity. Am J Physiol Gastrointest Liver Physiol. 2008;294(2):G391–400.
6. Krenkel O, Tacke F. Liver macrophages in tissue homeostasis and disease. Nat Rev Immunol. 2017;17(5):306–21.
7. Heymann F, Peusquens J, Ludwig-Portugall I, Kohlhepp M, Ergen C, Niemietz P, Martin C, van Rooijen N, Ochando JC, Randolph GJ, Luedde T, Ginhoux T, Kurts C, Trautwein C, Tacke F. Liver inflammation abrogates immunological tolerance induced by Kupffer cells. Hepatology. 2015;62(1):279–91.
8. Racanelli V, Rehermann B. The liver as an immunological organ. Hepatology. 2006;43(2 Suppl 1):S54–62.
9. Boyer JL. Bile formation and secretion. Compr Physiol. 2013;3(3):1035–78.
10. Banales JM, Huebert RC, Karlsen T, Strazzabosco M, LaRusso NF, Gores GJ. Cholangiocyte pathobiology. Nat Rev Gastroenterol Hepatol. 2019;16(5):269–81.
11. Puche JE, Saiman S, Friedman SL. Hepatic stellate cells and liver fibrosis. Compr Physiol. 2013;3(4):1473–92.
12. Jense KJ, Alpini G, Glaser S. Hepatic nervous system and neurobiology of the liver. Compr Physiol. 2013;3(2):655–65.
13. Rappaport AM, Borowy ZJ, Lougheed WM, Lotto WN. Subdivision of hexagonal liver lobules into a structural and functional unit: role in hepatic physiology and pathology. Anat Rec. 1954;119:11–33.
14. Gebhardt R, Matz-Soja M. Liver zonation: novel aspects of its regulation and its impact on homeostasis. World J Gastroenterol. 2014;20(26):8491–504.
15. Trefts E, Gannon M, Wasserman DH. The liver. Curr Biol. 2017;27(21):R1147–R51.
16. McIntyre N, Benhamou J-P, Birher J, Rizzetto M, Rodes J. Function of the liver. In: Oxford of clinical hepatology, vol. 1. Oxford: Oxford University Press; 1991. p. 31–227.

# Chapter 2
# Approach to the Patient with Liver Disease

**Nora V. Bergasa**

The approach to a patient with liver disease should be guided by an inquisitive mind, judicious yet bold use of diagnostic blood tests, and a prudent choice of invasive procedures. The identification of a chief complaint, a complete medical history, and a thorough physical examination form the basis of the approach to a patient with liver disease. The identification of risk factors for liver disease is particularly important.

Patients with liver disease may present with subtle symptoms, the recognition of which will alert the clinician to hepatic pathology. Other times, the quality of life of the patients may be markedly impaired [1]. It is implicit in the title of this chapter that the clinician knows that the patient has liver disease, e.g., a referral made to the hepatology clinic. However, a suggestion of liver disease is often laboratory data derived from health maintenance efforts or obtained for other medical reasons. Thus, it is the prepared mind that will recognize a connection between symptom(s) or abnormal laboratory tests and liver disease.

The range of liver injury varies from inflammation to fibrosis and cirrhosis, characterized by a disruption of the liver architecture by regenerating nodules. Liver failure is characterized by impaired liver function, which can be the presentation of advanced liver disease, or it can be acute and fulminant. The majority of liver conditions that lead to long-term complications, however, tend to be chronic and some progress slowly; a detailed investigation is necessary to arrive at the correct diagnosis and treatment.

N. V. Bergasa (✉)
Department of Medicine, H+H/Metropolitan, New York, NY, USA

New York Medical College, Valhalla, NY, USA

Hepatology, H+H/Woodhull, Brooklyn, NY, USA

N. V. Bergasa (ed.), *Clinical Cases in Hepatology*,
https://doi.org/10.1007/978-1-4471-4715-2_2

## Symptoms of Liver Disease

The identification of a chief complaint and the exploration of its onset, duration, and characteristics are necessary.

### *Jaundice*

Recognized as a sign of liver disease, jaundice may be identified by the patient and hence be part of the chief complaint as "yellow eyes" (Fig. 2.1). In general, it is a good indication that some aspect of bilirubin metabolism is altered (e.g., bilirubin availability, uptake, conjugation, or excretion).

### *Fatigue*

Fatigue is a manifestation of liver disease; its cause is unknown. It is a prevalent symptom of patients with primary biliary cholangitis (PBC), reported to occur in 80% [2, 3]. Like pruritus, fatigue can precede the diagnosis of PBC. In an internet-based survey of patients with PBC who were members of the PBCers organization, fatigue was experienced by 85% of the patients, and it preceded the diagnosis of PBC in 83% of patients [4]. Fatigue does not correlate with the degree of liver disease in PBC. Hypothyroidism and depression, which manifest themselves with decreased energy levels, can coexist in patients with PBC; accordingly, a full workup to exclude such comorbidities is necessary for the approach to patients with suspected or documented PBC.

### *Pruritus*

Pruritus or itch can be a manifestation of liver disease, in particular of those characterized by cholestasis (i.e., impaired secretion of bile). It is inferred that pruritus results from the accumulation of substances normally excreted in bile and that, as a result of cholestasis, accumulate in tissues. The nature of the pruritogen(s) is

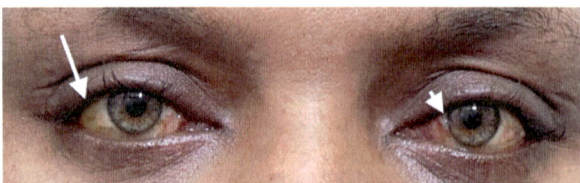

**Fig. 2.1** Icteric conjunctivae (arrow) and pterigum (arrow head) in a patient with decompensated liver disease in association with alcohol use disorder

unknown. It has been hypothesized that the pruritus of cholestasis is mediated, at least in part, by increased opioidergic neurotransmission; the amelioration of this type of pruritus by opiate antagonists supports this hypothesis [5, 6]. It is important to appreciate that pruritus (and fatigue) can precede the diagnosis of liver disease by years [4].

## Poor Appetite and Weight Loss

Poor appetite may accompany the presentation of acute liver disease. Patients with advanced liver disease may also present with a chronic history of poor appetite [7] and either weight loss or muscle wasting [8]. In advanced liver disease, weight loss may not be a reliable indicator of liver disease as fluid retention may compensate for the loss of muscle, giving an equivocated weight.

## Abdominal Pain

A questionnaire-based study reported that abdominal pain was experienced more frequently by patients with liver disease than by the control group over 1 month [9]. The pain was worse after meals. It has been written that stretching of Glisson's capsule from "liver inflammation" results in pain in the liver area; this statement is difficult to confirm in a controlled fashion. In contrast, right upper quadrant pain secondary to biliary colic and acute cholecystitis must be considered in patients with liver disease. The prevalence of gallstones is higher in patients with cirrhosis than in non-cirrhotic subjects.

## Alterations in the Senses of Taste and Smell

Taste abnormalities (e.g., hypogeusia and dysgeusia) are recognized complications of liver disease [10]. An interesting observation, initially reported in patients with acute hepatitis B, is the loss of appetite for cigarettes in smokers; this finding is not specific for hepatitis B, and it may be due to a perverted sense of taste from liver inflammation [11]. Impaired gustatory function with decreased sensitivity for detection of salt, sweet, and sour and for recognition of bitter, salt, sweet, and sour, and a decrease in the mean value of a gustatory score have been reported in patients with cirrhosis [12].

The serum concentrations of certain elements, including magnesium, zinc, and vitamin A have been reported to be decreased in patients with liver disease and an altered sense of taste [12]. A central mediation of taste abnormalities in patients with liver disease has been proposed [13]. A report by a patient with acute drug-induced hepatitis equating the taste of chocolate to that of lard should tell the reader how inconvenient this symptom can be, especially to a chocolate lover (NVBergasa, 2004, unpublished). Hyposmia can be associated with cirrhosis and was reported in association with hepatic encephalopathy [14]. In a study that included nine patients, hyposmia resolved after liver transplantation [15].

## Personality Changes and Sleep Disturbances

One of the most dramatic manifestations of decompensated liver disease is hepatic encephalopathy, characterized by inhibitory neurotransmission [16, 17]. Its presentation can be subtle or florid [18]. The reversal of the sleep pattern is well recognized, with patients reporting insomnia and inability to stay awake during the day, confusion, and cognitive deficiencies [16, 19]. Family members may report personality changes, including combativeness.

## Dyspnea

Decreased exercise tolerance and shortness of breath in patients with liver disease may be secondary to hepatopulmonary syndrome, porto-pulmonary hypertension, and cardiomyopathy [20, 21], the latter traditionally associated with alcohol abuse [22] and recently being inconsistently documented as a complication of chronic hepatitis C infection [23, 24]. A recent study that addresses specifically dyspnea in patients attending a pretransplant clinic did not find a correlation between the Medical Research Council scale of dyspnea (mMRC) and the MELD score, or duration of disease and MELD score or mMRC [25]. Dyspnea can also result from impaired diaphragmatic excursion due to ascites [26] or hepatic hydrothorax [27].

## Bleeding

A history of gastrointestinal bleeding, including hematemesis, melena, or hematochezia, may identify patients with portal hypertension [28].

## Stool Characteristics

Jaundice associated with acholic stools (e.g., pale), resulting from decreased bile pigments in feces, suggests biliary obstruction. In liver diseases characterized by profound cholestasis, the critical micellar concentration of bile acids is reduced in the small intestine [29]; hence, diarrhea from fat malabsorption and, in some cases, from maldigestion may ensue. Diarrhea is a manifestation of inflammatory bowel disease, which can be associated with primary sclerosing cholangitis and cholestasis.

## Vision Disturbance

Deficiency in vitamin A usually manifests itself as an impaired visual adaptation to darkness, of which patients may not be aware. Patients with liver disease may be deficient in vitamin A because of malabsorption and decreased availability of retinol-binding protein. In addition, there may be impaired release of vitamin A from liver stores [30].

## Bone Pain and Fractures

Pain in the long bones (e.g., tibia) and joints, sometimes associated with clubbing, is suggestive of hypertrophic osteoarthropathy, a complication of cirrhosis [31]. A dramatic presentation of liver disease of the cholestatic type can be bone fractures from osteoporosis, the etiology of which is unknown.

## Pain

Peripheral neuropathy manifested by numbness, weakness, and neuropathic pain can be a symptom of liver disease due to cholestasis; in adults, this manifestation is rare. Xanthomatous neuropathy from lipid deposition on peripheral nerves associated with hyperlipidemia from profound cholestasis is well described [32, 33].

## Hyperpigmentation

Patients may note skin darkening. Hyperpigmentation is a complication of liver disease, mainly of the cholestatic type; its pathogenesis is unknown. Increased availability of a melanocyte-stimulating hormone has been proposed as a contributing factor [34].

## *Vascular Ulcers*

Leg ulcers can occur in patients with liver disease and are usually considered secondary to venous insufficiency. However, the healing of leg ulcers in association with a transjugular intrahepatic portosystemic shunt, i.e., a decrease in portal pressure, in patients with decompensated cirrhosis has been reported [35], and in association with treatment of portal hypertension from thrombotic disease [36]; the existence of a hepatodermal syndrome was proposed [35].

## *Chills and Rigors*

Chills and rigors are manifestations of infection, which can complicate the course of liver disease as spontaneous bacterial peritonitis in patients with ascites, an infected biliary tree in patients with primary sclerosing cholangitis, and meningitis [37, 38].

## *Dark Urine*

Dark brown urine suggests bilirubinuria and it indicates hyperbilirubinemia and suggests the presence of liver damage; the finding can precede jaundice.

## *Sexual Dysfunction and Disinterest*

Decreased libido and impotence in men is a manifestation of cirrhosis. Men with cirrhosis secondary to alcohol have been reported to have lower serum concentrations of testosterone and higher serum concentrations of gonadotrophins than patients without a history of alcohol abuse. In these patients, hypogonadism may result from the toxic effect of alcohol and its metabolites on the gonads and estrogens' systemic effect on the hypothalamic–pituitary–gonadal axis [39]. Cure of chronic HCV infection was associated with improved sexual health [40].

In women, important contributors to lack of interest in sexual activities have been reported to be depression and fatigue.

## *Muscle Cramps*

Mostly nocturnal, muscle cramps affecting the calves, toes, and fingers can complicate cirrhosis and have a marked negative impact on the quality of life [41, 42]. The pathogenesis is unknown.

# Identification of Risks for Liver Disease

Activities that involve contact with blood and body fluids are risks for acquiring viral hepatitides [43–46]. Subjects at risk for having contracted viral hepatitides (e.g., hepatitis C, B, and delta hepatitis) include those with a history of blood transfusions prior to 1992, intravenous injections of illicit drugs, even in the distant past, subjects on chronic hemodialysis, and individuals who received other blood products (e.g., clotting factors) prior to 1987. Body piercing and tattoos may be risk factors for viral hepatitis if the tools used, including the ink, are contaminated. Multiple sexual partners are a risk factor for viral hepatitis.

Alcohol abuse is an important cause of cirrhosis of the liver [47]. Information on the use of medications or dietary supplements, acutely or chronically, by prescription, over the counter, or from health food stores is fundamental in cases of drug-induced liver injury [48]. The drinking of "bush tea," a practice carried out in some countries, has been associated with Budd–Chiari syndrome, which can present dramatically with ascites and hepatic insufficiency [49]. Contraceptive pills can be associated with hepatic adenomata and vascular thrombosis [50].

Malignant liver tumors have been associated with exposure to certain compounds used in industry (e.g., vinyl chloride [51], inorganic arsenical [52], and to aflatoxin B1 [53], which can result from the ingestion of contaminated food products (e.g., grains) with the mold Aspergillus flavus.

Inquiring about travel to geographic areas where certain conditions are endemic may reveal diagnostic possibilities. Examples of infectious diseases that may involve the liver include leptospirosis, malaria, Q fever, amebiasis, and schistosomiasis [54].

# Recognizing Hepatic Manifestations of Comorbidities

Chronic conditions can be associated with liver involvement, clinical or subclinical. Heart and liver disease can coexist [55]. Jaundice is not uncommon in patients with decompensated heart failure [56] and patients with sepsis [57, 58]. Obesity can be associated with an abnormal serum liver profile, as can diabetes mellitus [59], usually associated with fatty liver. A patient with amyloidosis may have the liver infiltrated by amyloid manifested as hepatomegaly [60], and an immunosuppressed patient may have the liver infiltrated by mycobacteria, for example [61]. Patients with renal insufficiency from polycystic kidney disease may have liver cysts as part of the syndrome [62]. Stauffer's syndrome, characterized by hepatomegaly and cholestasis in the absence of liver metastases, can be a manifestation of patients with renal cell carcinoma; the syndrome resolves when the tumor is resected [63]. Cystic fibrosis can be associated with cholestasis [64]. Subtle changes in the liver profile, including increased activity of transaminases, can be seen in hypothyroidism and hyperthyroidism. Basedowiana-Haban cirrhosis, characterized by hepatomegaly and episodes of jaundice, was originally described in patients with thyrotoxicosis by the German physician Karl Basedow [65, 66]. In the context of interpreting thyroid function tests, it is important to recognize that an increase in thyroid binding globulin, and not hyperthyroidism, appears to be the most common cause of increased serum levels of thyroxine (T4) in patients with liver disease [67]. Free T4 concentrations are necessary to confirm hyperthyroidism [68].

## Past Medical and Surgical History

A history of jaundice or abnormal liver profile may suggest previous hepatitis or the passage of a gallstone, sometimes accompanied by pain. History of gallbladder surgery, including laparoscopic cholecystectomy, in a patient with cholestasis, should trigger the search for post-surgical biliary strictures, which need to be repaired to prevent biliary cirrhosis [69]. Biliary strictures can also be a complication of chronic pancreatitis [70].

## Family History

A history of liver disease in family members is relevant as it may be lead to the diagnosis of hereditary diseases, including primary hemochromatosis [71], Wilson's disease [71], and alpha-1-antitrypsin deficiency [72]. History of viral hepatitis B in the mother may suggest perinatally acquired hepatitis in the patient under evaluation.

## Review of Systems

A florid presentation of hemochromatosis may include arthralgias and glucose intolerance, hypogonadism, and cardiomyopathy. Psychiatric and neurological alterations may suggest Wilson's disease. Classically, emphysema and liver disease suggest alpha-1-antitrypsin deficiency; liver disease may present without pulmonary complications in this condition. Easy bruising in a patient with infiltrative liver disease suggests amyloidosis, and in a patient with "red eyes," silvery skin nodules, and pulmonary complaints, it suggests sarcoidosis [73]. Dyspnea may suggest hepatopulmonary syndrome. CREST (calcinosis, Raynaud's phenomenon, esophageal dysmotility, sclerodactyly, and telangiectasias) syndrome can be associated with PBC [74].

## The Physical Examination

Signs of liver disease may be overt or absent. Fever in a patient with liver disease should trigger the exclusion of infections. In patients with decompensated liver disease, the blood pressure tends to be low, secondary to systemic vasodilatation.

### Fetor Hepaticus

A sweet odor emanating from the patient's breath can be perceived in patients with advanced liver disease, including those with extensive portosystemic shunting [75].

### The Skin, Mucous Membranes, and Nails

Jaundice is the yellow discoloration of the skin, conjunctivae, and mucous membranes. It jumps out at the examiner (Fig. 2.1) [76, 77]. It is a manifestation of liver disease, secondary to intra- or extrahepatic cholestasis, i.e., from acute hepatitis, hepatocellular failure, or biliary tract obstruction. Excess in bilirubin production from hemolysis is also a cause of jaundice. Kayser–Fleischer rings, a brown rim on the cornea's periphery, secondary to copper accumulation in Descemet's membrane, is a classic finding of Wilson's disease [78, 79]; it is necessary to examine the cornea with a slit lamp for adequate visualization most of the times. In cases of prolonged cholestasis and not related to Wilson's disease, Kayser–Fleischer rings may also be present.

The skin of patients with liver disease and pruritus does not display pruritic skin lesions, but excoriations complicated by prurigo nodularis may abound, especially in patients with severe pruritus (Fig. 2.2); they are evidence of how devastating this symptom can be. The skin is warm from the hyperdynamic circulation of patients with portal hypertension. Spider angiomata are characterized by vascular arborizations that blanch on pressure (Fig. 2.3); they are found on the face and upper back, thorax, and upper arms [80]. The pathogenesis of spider angiomata has been

**Fig. 2.2** Prurigo lesions in a patient with chronic pruritus from cholestasis

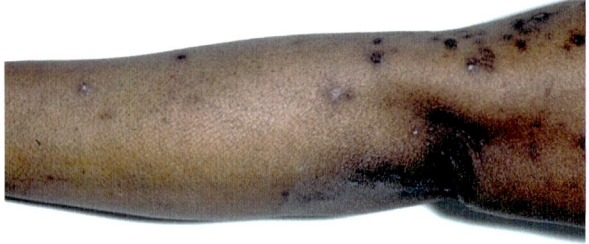

**Fig. 2.3** Spider angiomata on the right side of the neck in a woman with decompensated liver disease in association with alcohol use disorder

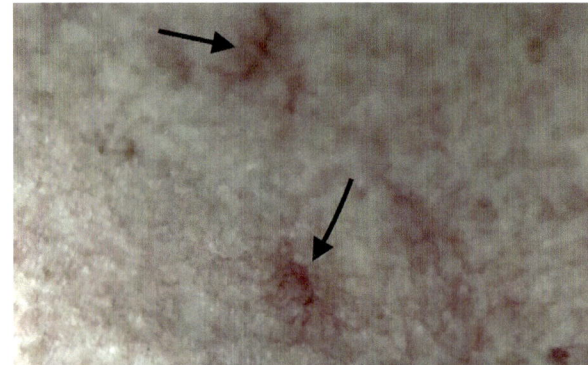

**Fig. 2.4** Butterfly sign on the back of a patient with primary biliary cholangitis

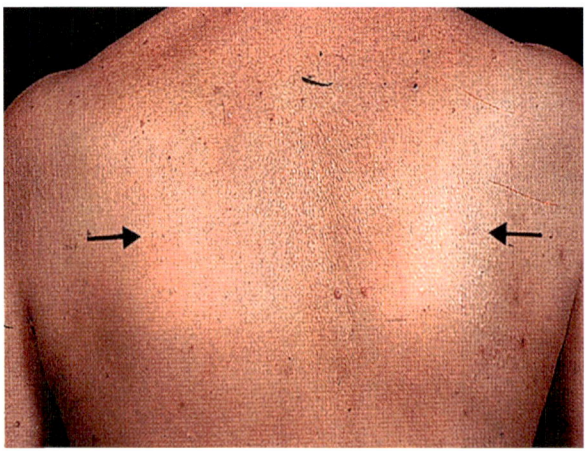

considered to be systemic excess of estrogen and portosystemic shunting from cirrhosis. Skin hyperpigmentation is common in patients with cholestasis, in particular, that secondary to PBC. Patients with PBC may display what has been named the "butterfly sign," an area of relative hypopigmentation between the scapulae in relationship to the surrounding skin (Fig. 2.4). A gray to brown discoloration of the skin and mucous membranes due to the accumulation of hemosiderin and hemofuscin (gray hue) and melanin (brown hue) suggests hereditary hemochromatosis [81].

**Fig. 2.5** *Paper money* appearance in a patient with decompensated liver disease from alcohol abuse disorder

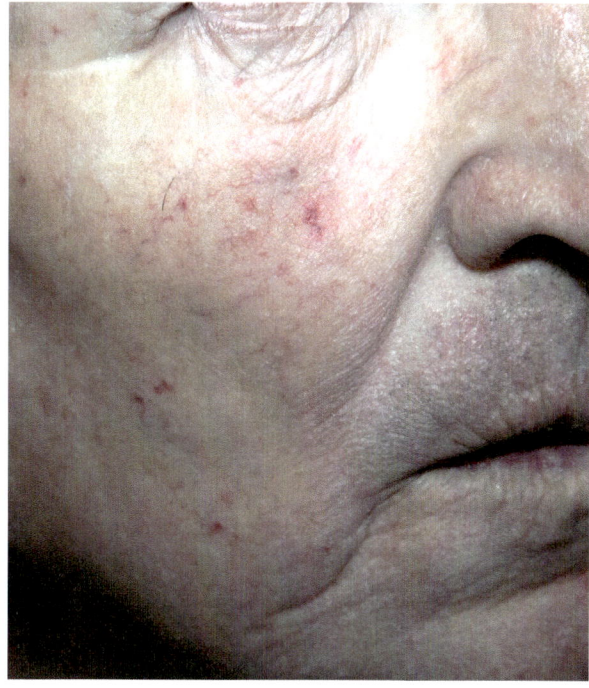

Xanthomatosis, accumulation of lipids in the skin, is a manifestation of hyperlipidemia in cholestasis (e.g., PBC); it presents as plane xanthomata on the palms, soles, trunk, and flexor surfaces, as tuberous xanthomata over the joints, and as xanthelasmas on the eyelids and under the eyes [33, 82]. Lichen planus is also associated with PBC. "Paper money" skin, characterized by telangiectasias on the cheeks, can be a sign of cirrhosis (Fig. 2.5) [83]. Purpura is a manifestation of vasculitis, which can be associated with chronic hepatitis C and B infections [84]. Telangiectasias on lips suggest CREST syndrome or hereditary hemorrhagic telangiectasia, in which vascular malformations can occur in the liver [85]. The distribution of body hair of men with cirrhosis is feminine. Nails can display white horizontal lines, Muerhcke's lines, indicative of hypoalbuminemia. Azure lunulae (sky blue moon) discoloration of the nails [86] and a green hue on the skin from the accumulation of copper are described in Wilson's disease.

## Glands and Lymph Nodes

Parotid gland enlargement can be detected in 20% of patients with cirrhosis secondary to alcohol abuse [87] (Fig. 2.6). Testicular atrophy and feminization [88], including gynecomastia [89], is a classic finding of men with cirrhosis, which may result from increased peripheral conversion of androgens; tender gynecomastia is also a side effect of spironolactone, a diuretic used to treat ascites [90].

**Fig. 2.6** Parotid glad enlargement in a patient with cirrhosis in association with alcohol use disorder

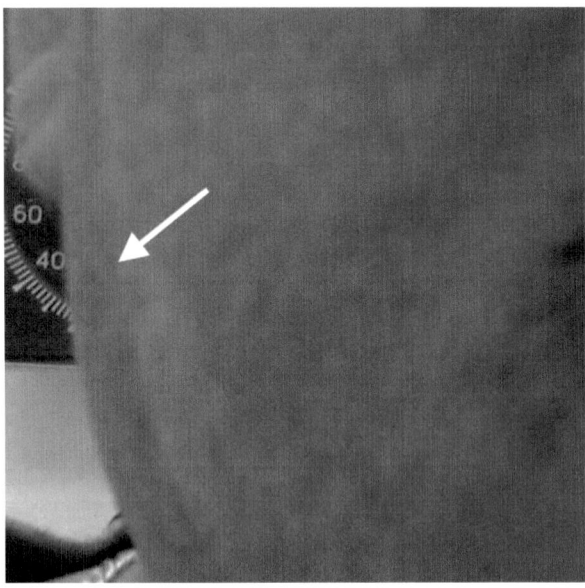

## Cardiovascular System

Findings suggesting pericardial (e.g., constrictive pericarditis) or cardiac disease, including cardiomegaly, gallops, and distended neck veins, may explain hepatomegaly and ascites [91]. Pulmonary hypertension associated with portal hypertension or liver disease (i.e., portopulmonary hypertension) is suggested by an accentuated pulmonary component of the second heart sound at cardiac auscultation and the presence of a systolic murmur consistent with tricuspid insufficiency [92]. Pounding pulses from systemic vasodilatation and increased cardiac output are characteristic of patients with decompensated liver disease [93].

## Respiratory System

Decreased breath sounds at the lung bases, usually at the right base, suggest hydrothorax in a patient with decompensated liver disease and ascites. Hepatopulmonary syndrome, which is associated with intrapulmonary vascular dilatation, is characterized by orthodeoxia (i.e., arterial deoxygenation from the supine to the upright position) and platypnea (i.e., dyspnea from the supine to the upright position) [94]. These phenomena result from increases in intrapulmonary shunting due to perfusion of the lower lobes [94].

## *Abdomen*

Dilated veins on the abdominal wall may be a sign of intrahepatic portal hypertension (Fig. 2.7). This phenomenon results from the recanalization of the paraumbilical or umbilical veins to decompress the portal system. Veins that radiate away from the umbilicus become prominent and are described as the "caput Medusa," after the gorgon of Greek mythology with snakes entwined in her hair. Dilated abdominal veins can also be seen high up in the abdomen.

In patients with liver disease, abdominal auscultation may reveal a venous hum, suggesting portal hypertension; a bruit over the liver area, in synchrony with the pulse, suggests a vascular tumor with arterial blood supply (e.g., hepatocellular carcinoma) or florid alcoholic hepatitis. A hepatic friction rub has been described in tumors eroding the liver capsule, hepatic syphilis, and liver abscesses. Distended abdomen and bulging flanks suggest ascites (Fig. 2.8), a defining complication in the natural history of liver disease, as it correlates with morbidity and mortality. Ascites can be detected by palpation and percussion, seeking a fluid wave and shifting dullness. Abdominal tenderness in a patient with ascites suggests peritonitis (e.g., spontaneous bacterial peritonitis), which is an ominous complication of liver disease.

The liver is dull to percussion. To feel the liver, the abdomen is examined with the patient in the supine position, arms parallel to the sides of the body, and the knees bent, to relax the abdominal muscles. It is useful to start palpating from the right lower quadrant of the abdomen toward the ribcage, to encounter the liver edge on the way up. The liver edge is smooth, and sometimes a little tender when pressed. In general, feeling the edge up to 2 cm below the right costal margin is considered normal. The liver can be displaced downwards by emphysematous lungs. In thin

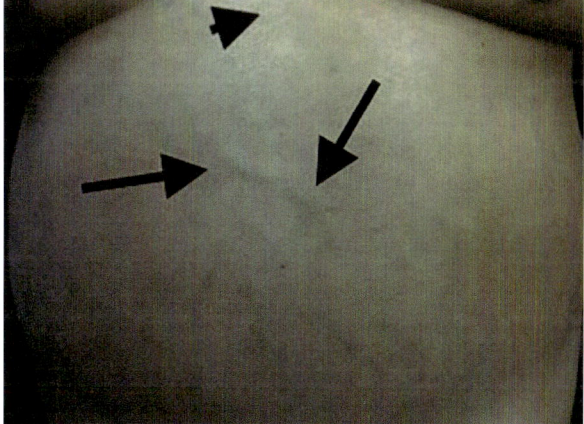

**Fig. 2.7** Dilated veins (arrows) in the abdominal wall in a patient with portal hypertension and decompensated liver disease as evidenced by ascites (arrow head: epigastrium)

**Fig. 2.8** Abdominal
distension from ascites in a
patient with
decompensated liver
disease from alcohol abuse
disorder

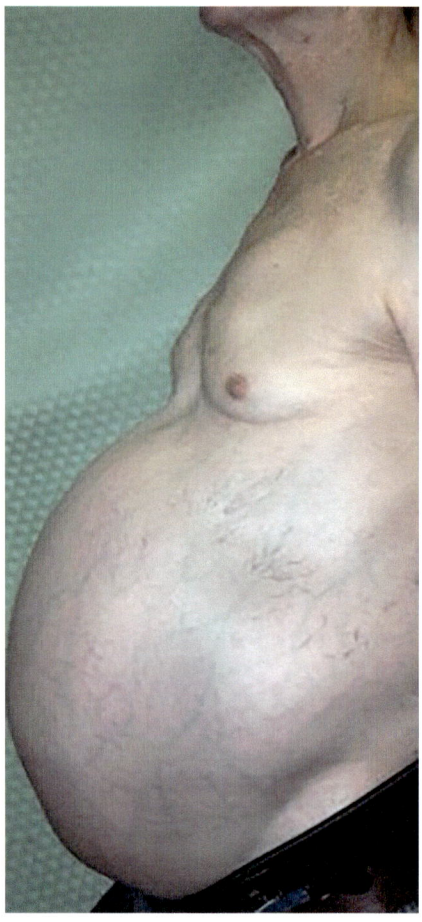

subjects, the liver can be felt on deep inspiration, not necessarily suggesting hepatic pathology. Hepatomegaly may indicate cirrhosis, infiltrative disease, or space-occupying lesions (e.g., tumors). A hard consistency of the liver is consistent with cirrhosis [95]. In disease, the liver can extend over the midline, and the left lobe can be felt in the epigastrium. When hepatomegaly is uncertain, the scratch test may be useful. This maneuver is conducted by placing the bell of the stethoscope on the right upper quadrant over the ribcage and scratching the abdominal wall's surface from the mid-abdomen toward the liver. When the scratch is done on an area under which the liver lays, the sound is amplified. When there is ascites, the liver edge can be made to bounce by exerting a quick pressure with the fingertips below the ribcage. Splenomegaly suggests portal hypertension.

## *Extremities*

Red palms, especially on the thenar and hypothenar eminences, can be seen in patients with cirrhosis (Fig. 2.9). Retraction of the palmar fascia with subsequent contracture of palms and fingers is known as Dupuytren's contracture (Fig. 2.10), with increased prevalence in patients with liver disease. Acquired finger clubbing can be seen in patients with cirrhosis and patients with hepatopulmonary syndrome (Fig. 2.11) [96].

**Fig. 2.9** Palmar erythema in the thenar and hypothenar eminences in a patient with cirrhosis from chronic hepatitis C

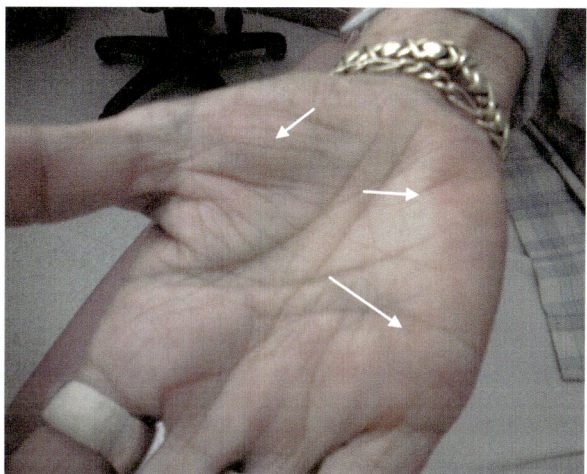

**Fig. 2.10** Incipient Dupotryen's contracture (arrow) and palmar erythema (short arrow) in a man with cirrhosis from alcohol abuse disorder

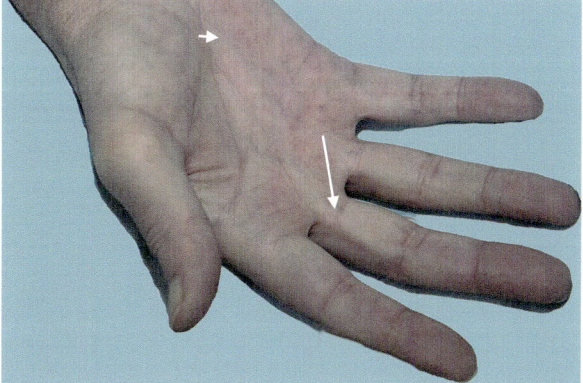

**Fig. 2.11** Finger clubbing in a patient with hepatopulmonary syndrome associated with cirrhosis secondary to alcohol use disorder

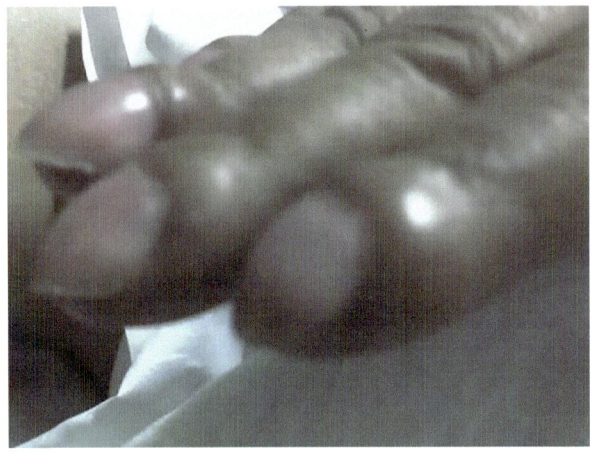

Lower extremity edema complicates fluid retention in liver disease. The edema is usually pitting unless it is chronic or complicated by venous insufficiency, in which the appearance can be reminiscent of elephantiasis.

## Neuropsychiatric Alterations

Family members can report subtle alterations in personality. Constructional apraxia (e.g., inability to draw a five-point star or to write legibly) in fully conscious patients is a finding of hepatic encephalopathy. The Reitan number connection test can be used to diagnose and follow the response to treatment of hepatic encephalopathy. Asterixis, a sign of encephalopathy, can be appreciated by having the patient extend the arms, palms down, and dorsiflex the wrists while separating the fingers for at least 15 s. It is characterized by a series of extension and flexion movements at the level of the wrist. Electromyography of the contracted muscles has revealed lapses of electrical input that coincide with asterixis [97]. Tremors can also be noted.

## Investigation of Liver Disease

An impression of liver disease can be confirmed by laboratory exams, radiographic tests, or a combination, which should be analyzed in concert. A liver profile suggestive of cholestasis, including that resulting from infiltrative disease, is characterized by an increase in alkaline phosphatase serum activity and, in the majority of cases, gamma-glutamyl transpeptidase. Transaminases are reportedly released by injury to the hepatocytes, such as that occurring in acute or chronic hepatitis. A prolonged prothrombin time (or high International Normalized Ratio) suggests synthetic hepatic dysfunction, as does a decreased concentration of serum albumin. A complete blood count may reveal pancytopenia secondary to bone marrow suppression and hypersplenism due to portal hypertension, which tends to be associated with thrombocytopenia.

The review of the urine analysis and renal function tests in patients with liver disease is very relevant. Bilirubinuria is a sign of liver damage and usually precedes jaundice. In the absence of bilirubinuria, jaundice is from unconjugated hyperbilirubinemia (e.g., from hemolysis) [98]. Microscopic hematuria and proteinuria suggest glomerulopathies (e.g., associated with cryoglobulinemia, deposition of immune complexes, most commonly IgA). An alkaline urine pH suggests renal tubular acidosis, which can complicate Wilson's disease and PBC. Renal insufficiency, oliguria, and marked reduction of urine sodium are consistent with hepatorenal syndrome, a dreadful complication of liver disease.

A liver sonogram with Doppler studies is an important tool in the investigation of liver disease. This test gives information on liver architecture, vascular flow, biliary obstruction or bile duct dilation, gallbladder disease, and echogenicity that may suggest liver disease, fat, and space-occupying lesions, including livers cysts, and masses [99]. A sonographic study of the liver can also suggest parenchymal liver disease (e.g., increased echogenicity, nodularity) and the opportunity to identify space-occupying lesions, including tumors and cysts. Other radiological modalities include computed tomography, usually with contrast, if the renal function allows it, multiphasic, or magnetic resonance imaging, especially for the characterization of liver masses, including hepatocellular carcinoma [100, 101].

## Liver Biopsy

To examine the liver histology provides the opportunity to diagnose or confirm a particular disease, determine the degree of liver injury (e.g., presence of cirrhosis) and assess the response to treatment. The decision to perform a liver biopsy is always individualized, and the risks versus benefits are considered.

Noninvasive methods to determine liver fibrosis are available, including Fibrosure, Fibrotest-Actitest, and the aspartate transaminase to platelets ratio index (APRI). They combine the analysis of certain blood components including serum proteins and enzyme activities and for the APRI, platelet count, to generate a score that provides information regarding inflammatory activity and fibrosis. Transient elastography assesses the liver's stiffness by measuring the velocity of a vibration wave, i.e., shear wave, generated through an intercostal space over the liver area. Shear wave velocity is determined by measuring the time the vibration wave takes to travel to a particular depth inside the liver. In contrast to the normal liver, the fibrotic liver is hard; thus, the degree of fibrosis can be inferred from liver stiffness. The results are expressed in kilopascals (kPa) [102–104]. Concerns about the reliability of these tests exist; however, the wish to develop reliable noninvasive exams to assess the degree of liver disease continues to stimulate the development of novel investigational procedures.

The exclusion of hereditary diseases (e.g., primary hemochromatosis, Wilson's disease, alpha-1-antitrypsin deficiency) in a patient with an acquired disease (e.g., viral hepatitis) is part of a liver disease workup. By the same reasoning, a patient with a hereditary or autoimmune disease in whom risk factors for viral hepatitides have been identified should have these excluded.

In evaluating a patient with suspected liver disease, the author excludes treatable causes, with a basic liver disease workup, as done in clinical trials of liver disease. In addition to a hemogram, serum electrolytes, blood urea nitrogen, and creatinine, and hepatic panel, including gamma-glutamyl transpeptidase, the basic workup includes hepatitis B serology, i.e., surface antigen, anti-core, and anti-HBs, and IgG hepatitis A antibodies, with IgM in cases of acute hepatitis, hepatitis C antibody with reflex to HCV RNA quantitation, iron studies, alpha-1 antitrypsin, and ceruloplasmin concentrations, autoantibodies (i.e., antinuclear antibodies and anti-smooth muscle antibodies), and glycosylated hemoglobin, if appropriate, e.g., in patients at risk for nonalcoholic fatty liver disease. If PBC is in the differential diagnosis, anti-mitochondrial antibodies and IgM are added at the start. If primary sclerosing cholangitis is being considered, perinuclear anti-neutrophil cytoplasmic antibodies are also requested. Specific tests to exclude specific diseases are discussed in the relevant chapters.

Judicious but liberal use of noninvasive diagnostic tests guided by an inquisitive mind will identify the etiology of liver disease in most patients.

## References

1. Younossi ZM. Chronic liver disease and health-related quality of life. Gastroenterology. 2001 Jan;120(1):305–7.
2. Heathcote J. The clinical expression of primary biliary cirrhosis. Semin Liver Dis. 1997;17(1):23–33.
3. Goldblatt J, Taylor PJ, Lipman T, Prince MI, Baragiotta A, Bassendine MF, et al. The true impact of fatigue in primary biliary cirrhosis: a population study. Gastroenterology. 2002 May;122(5):1235–41.
4. Rishe E, Azarm A, Bergasa NV. Itch in primary biliary cirrhosis: a patients' perspective. Acta Derm Venereol. 2008;88(1):34–7.
5. Jones EA, Bergasa NV. The pruritus of cholestasis: from bile acids to opiate agonists. Hepatology. 1990 May;11(5):884–7.
6. Bergasa NV. The pruritus of cholestasis: from bile acids to opiate agonists: relevant after all these years. Med Hypotheses. 2018 Jan;110:86–9.
7. Chapman B, Sinclair M, Gow PJ, Testro AG. Malnutrition in cirrhosis: more food for thought. World J Hepatol. 2020;12(11):883–96.
8. Aby ES, Saab S. Frailty, sarcopenia, and malnutrition in cirrhotic patients. Clin Liver Dis. 2019 Nov;23(4):589–605. https://doi.org/10.1016/j.cld.2019.06.001. Epub 2019 Aug 21.
9. Riley TR, 3rd, Koch K. Characteristics of upper abdominal pain in those with chronic liver disease. Digest Dis Sci. 2003;48(10):1914–8.
10. Burch RE, Sackin DA, Ursick JA, Jetton MM, Sullivan JF. Decreased taste and smell acuity in cirrhosis. Arch Intern Med. 1978;138(5):743–6.

11. Smith FR, Henkin RI, Dell RB. Disordered gustatory acuity in liver disease. Gastroenterology. 1976;70(4):568–71.
12. Madden AM, Bradbury W, Morgan MY. Taste perception in cirrhosis: its relationship to circulating micronutrients and food preferences. Hepatology. 1997;26(1):40–8.
13. Bergasa NV. Hypothesis: taste disorders in patients with liver disease may be mediated in the brain: potential mechanisms for a central phenomenon. Am J Gastroenterol. 1998;93(8):1209–10.
14. Heiser C, Haller B, Sohn M, Hofauer B, Knopf A, Muhling T, et al. Olfactory function is affected in patients with cirrhosis depending on the severity of hepatic encephalopathy. Ann Hepatol. 2018;17(5):822–9.
15. Bloomfeld RS, Graham BG, Schiffman SS, Killenberg PG. Alterations of chemosensory function in end-stage liver disease. Physiol Behav. 1999;66(2):203–7.
16. Jones EA. Ammonia, the GABA neurotransmitter system, and hepatic encephalopathy. Metab Brain Dis. 2002;17(4):275–81.
17. Wijdicks EF. Hepatic Encephalopathy. N Engl J Med. 2016;375(17):1660–70.
18. Hadjihambi A, Arias N, Sheikh M, Jalan R. Hepatic encephalopathy: a critical current review. Hepatol Int. 2018;12(Suppl 1):135–47.
19. Singh J, Sharma BC, Puri V, Sachdeva S, Srivastava S. Sleep disturbances in patients of liver cirrhosis with minimal hepatic encephalopathy before and after lactulose therapy. Metab Brain Dis. 2017;32(2):595–605.
20. Ramalingam VS, Ansari S, Fisher M. Respiratory complication in liver disease. Crit Care Clin. 2016 Jul;32(3):357–69.
21. Milic S, Lulic D, Stimac D, Ruzic A, Zaputovic L. Cardiac manifestations in alcoholic liver disease. Postgrad Med J. 2016 Apr;92(1086):235–9.
22. Maisch B. Alcoholic cardiomyopathy: the result of dosage and individual predisposition. Herz. 2016 Sep;41(6):484–93.
23. Matsumori A. Hepatitis C virus and cardiomyopathy. Herz. 2000 May;25(3):249–54.
24. Boyella V, Onyebueke I, Farraj N, Graham-Hill S, El Younis C, Bergasa NV. Prevalence of hepatitis C virus infection in patients with cardiomyopathy. Ann Hepatol. 2009 Apr–June;8(2):113–5.
25. Monte da Silva AG, de ARAB, Chiavegato LD. Association between dyspnea and severity of liver disease in patients in the pre-transplantation period-a pilot study. Transplant Proc. 2016;48(7):2328–32.
26. Kwo PY. Shortness of breath in the patient with chronic liver disease. Clin Liver Dis. 2012 May;16(2):321–9.
27. Lv Y, Han G, Fan D. Hepatic hydrothorax. Ann Hepatol. 2018 January–February;17(1):33–46.
28. Bosch J, Iwakiri Y. The portal hypertension syndrome: etiology, classification, relevance, and animal models. Hepatol Int. 2018 Feb;12(Suppl 1):1–10.
29. Badley BW, Murphy GM, Bouchier IA, Sherlock S. Diminished micellar phase lipid in patients with chronic nonalcoholic liver disease and steatorrhea. Gastroenterology. 1970 June;58(6):781–9.
30. Saeed A, Hoekstra M, Hoeke MO, Heegsma J, Faber KN. The interrelationship between bile acid and vitamin A homeostasis. Biochim Biophys Acta Mol Cell Biol Lipids. 2017 May;1862(5):496–512.
31. Moran LM, Ariza A. Hypertrophic osteoarthropathy associated to liver cirrhosis. Reumatol Clin. 2013 July–Aug;9(4):248–9.
32. Zak A, Zeman M, Slaby A, Vecka M. Xanthomas: clinical and pathophysiological relations. Biomed Pap Med Fac Univ Palacky Olomouc Czech Repub. 2014 June;158(2):181–8.
33. Peters MG, Hoffnagle JH, McGarvey C, Fox I, Gregg RE, Jones EA. Primary biliary cirrhosis: management of an unusual case with severe xanthomata by hepatic transplantation. J Clin Gastroenterol. 1989 Dec;11(6):694–7.
34. Bergasa NV, Vergalla J, Turner ML, Loh PY, Jones EA. Alpha-melanocyte-stimulating hormone in primary biliary cirrhosis. Ann N Y Acad Sci. 1993;680:454–8.

35. El Younis CM, Bergasa NV. Healing of leg ulcers associated with transjugular intrahepatic portosystemic shunt in decompensated cirrhosis: case series of a possible hepatodermal syndrome. Gastroenterol Hepatol (N Y). 2008 Mar;4(3):211–4.
36. Zhu W, Song H. A rare case of recurrent lower extremity ulcer. Int J Low Extrem Wounds. 2019 Dec;18(4):389–92.
37. Pagliano P, Boccia G, De Caro F, Esposito S. Bacterial meningitis complicating the course of liver cirrhosis. Infection. 2017 Dec;45(6):795–800.
38. Piano S, Brocca A, Mareso S, Angeli P. Infections complicating cirrhosis. Liver Int. 2018 Feb;38(Suppl 1):126–33.
39. Neong SF, Billington EO, Congly SE. Sexual dysfunction and sex hormone abnormalities in patients with cirrhosis: review of pathogenesis and management. Hepatology. 2019 June;69(6):2683–95.
40. Bonkovsky HL, Snow KK, Malet PF, Back-Madruga C, Fontana RJ, Sterling RK, et al. Health-related quality of life in patients with chronic hepatitis C and advanced fibrosis. J Hepatol. 2007 Mar;46(3):420–31.
41. Vidot H, Carey S, Allman-Farinelli M, Shackel N. Systematic review: the treatment of muscle cramps in patients with cirrhosis. Aliment Pharmacol Ther. 2014 Aug;40(3):221–32.
42. Corbani A, Manousou P, Calvaruso V, Xirouchakis I, Burroughs AK. Muscle cramps in cirrhosis: the therapeutic value of quinine. Is it underused? Digest Liver Dis. 2008 Sep;40(9): 794–9.
43. Sayed IM, Vercouter AS, Abdelwahab SF, Vercauteren K, Meuleman P. Is hepatitis E virus an emerging problem in industrialized countries? Hepatology. 2015 Dec;62(6):1883–92.
44. Nelson NP, Link-Gelles R, Hofmeister MG, Romero JR, Moore KL, Ward JW, et al. Update: recommendations of the advisory committee on immunization practices for use of hepatitis a vaccine for postexposure prophylaxis and for preexposure prophylaxis for international travel. MMWR. 2018 Nov 2;67(43):1216–20.
45. Mysore KR, Leung DH. Hepatitis B and C. Clin Liver Dis. 2018 Nov;22(4):703–22.
46. CDC. Surveillance for viral hepatitis – United States, 2017. 2019.
47. CDC. CDC - alcohol and public health home page - Alcohol.
48. Fisher K, Vuppalanchi R, Saxena R. Drug-induced liver injury. Arch Pathol Lab Med. 2015 July;139(7):876–87.
49. Valla DC, Cazals-Hatem D. Sinusoidal obstruction syndrome. Clin Res Hepatol Gastroenterol. 2016;40(4):378–85.
50. Ponnatapura J, Kielar A, Burke LMB, Lockhart ME, Abualruz AR, Tappouni R, et al. Hepatic complications of oral contraceptive pills and estrogen on MRI: controversies and update - adenoma and beyond. Magn Reson Imaging. 2019;60:110–21.
51. Mastrangelo G, Fedeli U, Fadda E, Valentini F, Agnesi R, Magarotto G, et al. Increased risk of hepatocellular carcinoma and liver cirrhosis in vinyl chloride workers: synergistic effect of occupational exposure with alcohol intake. Environ Health Perspect. 2004 Aug;112(11):1188–92.
52. Wang W, Cheng S, Zhang D. Association of inorganic arsenic exposure with liver cancer mortality: a meta-analysis. Environ Res. 2014 Nov;135:120–5.
53. Nugraha A, Khotimah K, Rietjens I. Risk assessment of aflatoxin B1 exposure from maize and peanut consumption in Indonesia using the margin of exposure and liver cancer risk estimation approaches. Food Chem Toxicol. 2018 Mar;113:134–44.
54. Talwani R, Gilliam BL, Howell C. Infectious diseases and the liver. Clin Liver Dis. 2011 Feb;15(1):111–30.
55. Hilscher MB, Kamath PS. The liver in circulatory disturbances. Clin Liver Dis. 2019 May;23(2):209–20.
56. Giallourakis CC, Rosenberg PM, Friedman LS. The liver in heart failure. Clin Liver Dis. 2002 Nov;6(4):947–67.
57. Gilroy RK, Mailliard ME, Gollan JL. Gastrointestinal disorders of the critically ill. Cholestasis of sepsis. Best Pract Res Clin Gastroenterol. 2003 Jun;17(3):357–67.
58. Chand N, Sanyal AJ. Sepsis-induced cholestasis. Hepatology. 2007 Jan;45(1):230–41.

59. Rinella ME. Nonalcoholic fatty liver disease: a systematic review. JAMA. 2015 June 9;313(22):2263–73.
60. Ebert EC, Nagar M. Gastrointestinal manifestations of amyloidosis. Am J Gastroenterol. 2008 Mar;103(3):776–87.
61. Hickey AJ, Gounder L, Moosa MY, Drain PK. A systematic review of hepatic tuberculosis with considerations in human immunodeficiency virus co-infection. BMC Infect Dis. 2015 May 6;15:209.
62. Cornec-Le Gall E, Torres VE, Harris PC. Genetic complexity of autosomal dominant polycystic kidney and liver diseases. J Am Soc Nephrol. 2018 Jan;29(1):13–23.
63. Fontes-Sousa M, Magalhaes H, da Silva FC, Mauricio MJ. Stauffer's syndrome: a comprehensive review and proposed updated diagnostic criteria. Urol Oncol. 2018 July;36(7):321–6.
64. Elborn JS. Cystic fibrosis. Lancet. 2016 Nov 19;388(10059):2519–31.
65. Cameron GR, Karunaratne WAE. Liver changes in exophthalmic goitre. J Pathol Bacteriol. 1935;41(2):267–82.
66. Nicol AaS G. Histological changes in the thyroid in cirrhosis of the liver. J Clin Pathol. 1962;15:26–30.
67. Kyriacou A, McLaughlin J, Syed AA. Thyroid disorders and gastrointestinal and liver dysfunction: a state of the art review. Eur J Intern Med. 2015 Oct;26(8):563–71.
68. De Leo S, Lee SY, Braverman LE. Hyperthyroidism. Lancet. 2016 Aug 27;388(10047):906–18.
69. Ferreira R, Loureiro R, Nunes N, Santos AA, Maio R, Cravo M, et al. Role of endoscopic retrograde cholangiopancreatography in the management of benign biliary strictures: what's new? World J Gastrointest Endosc. 2016 Feb 25;8(4):220–31.
70. Kwek AB, Ang TL, Maydeo A. Current status of endotherapy for chronic pancreatitis. Singap Med J. 2014 Dec;55(12):613–20.
71. Neimark E, Schilsky ML, Shneider BL. Wilson's disease and hemochromatosis. Adolesc Med Clin. 2004;15(1):175-94, xi.
72. Hersh CP. Diagnosing alpha-1 antitrypsin deficiency: the first step in precision medicine. F1000Res. 2017;6:2049.
73. Prasse A. The diagnosis, differential diagnosis, and treatment of sarcoidosis. Deutsches Arzteblatt Int. 2016 Aug 22;113(33–34):565–74.
74. Chalifoux SL, Konyn PG, Choi G, Saab S. Extrahepatic manifestations of primary biliary cholangitis. Gut Liver. 2017 Nov 15;11(6):771–80.
75. Calenic B, Amann A. Detection of volatile malodorous compounds in breath: current analytical techniques and implications in human disease. Bioanalysis. 2014 Feb;6(3):357–76.
76. Tripathi RC, Sidrys LA. 'Conjunctival icterus,' not 'scleral icterus'. JAMA. 1979 Dec 7;242(23):2558.
77. Azzuqa A, Watchko JF. Conjunctival icterus - an important but neglected sign of clinically relevant hyperbilirubinemia in jaundiced neonates. Curr Pediatr Rev. 2017;13(3):169–75.
78. Johnson RE, Campbell RJ. Wilson's disease. Electron microscopic, x-ray energy spectroscopic, and atomic absorption spectroscopic studies of corneal copper deposition and distribution. Lab Investig. 1982 June;46(6):564–9.
79. Pandey N, John S. Kayser-Fleischer Ring. Treasure Island, FL: StatPearls; 2019.
80. Li H, Wang R, Mendez-Sanchez N, Peng Y, Guo X, Qi X. Impact of spider nevus and subcutaneous collateral vessel of chest/abdominal wall on outcomes of liver cirrhosis. Arch Med Sci. 2019 Mar;15(2):434–48.
81. Chevrant-Breton J, Simon M, Bourel M, Ferrand B. Cutaneous manifestations of idiopathic hemochromatosis. Study of 100 cases. Arch Dermatol. 1977 Feb;113(2):161–5.
82. Ahrens EH Jr, Kunkel HG. The relationship between serum lipids and skin xanthomata in eighteen patients with primary biliary cirrhosis. J Clin Invest. 1949;28(6):1565–74.
83. Koulaouzidis A, Bhat S, Moschos J. Skin manifestations of liver diseases. Ann Hepatol. 2007 July–Sep;6(3):181–4.
84. Choudhury BN, Jain A, Baruah UD. Dermatological manifestations of chronic liver disease. Int J Res Dermatol. 2018;4(2):224–9.

85. Garcia-Tsao G, Korzenik JR, Young L, Henderson KJ, Jain D, Byrd B, et al. Liver disease in patients with hereditary hemorrhagic telangiectasia. N Engl J Med. 2000 Sep 28;343(13):931–6.
86. Bearn AG, Mc KV. Azure lunulae; an unusual change in the fingernails in two patients with hepatolenticular degeneration (Wilson's disease). J Am Med Assoc. 1958 Feb 22;166(8):904–6.
87. Dutta SK, Dukehart M, Narang A, Latham PS. Functional and structural changes in parotid glands of alcoholic cirrhotic patients. Gastroenterology. 1989 Feb;96(2 Pt 1):510–8.
88. Gluud C. Testosterone and alcoholic cirrhosis. Epidemiologic, pathophysiologic and therapeutic studies in men. Dan Med Bull. 1988 Dec;35(6):564–75.
89. Cavanaugh J, Niewoehner CB, Nuttall FQ. Gynecomastia and cirrhosis of the liver. Arch Intern Med. 1990 Mar;150(3):563–5.
90. Lainscak M, Pelliccia F, Rosano G, Vitale C, Schiariti M, Greco C, et al. Safety profile of mineralocorticoid receptor antagonists: spironolactone and eplerenone. Int J Cardiol. 2015 Dec 1;200:25–9.
91. Alvarez AM, Mukherjee D. Liver abnormalities in cardiac diseases and heart failure. Int J Angiol. 2011 Sep;20(3):135–42.
92. Colman R, Whittingham H, Tomlinson G, Granton J. Utility of the physical examination in detecting pulmonary hypertension. A mixed methods study. PLoS One. 2014;9(10):e108499.
93. Moller S, Henriksen JH, Bendtsen F. Extrahepatic complications to cirrhosis and portal hypertension: haemodynamic and homeostatic aspects. World J Gastroenterol. 2014 Nov 14;20(42):15499–517.
94. Gomez FP, Martinez-Palli G, Barbera JA, Roca J, Navasa M, Rodriguez-Roisin R. Gas exchange mechanism of orthodeoxia in hepatopulmonary syndrome. Hepatology. 2004 Sep;40(3):660–6.
95. Oberti F, Valsesia E, Pilette C, Rousselet MC, Bedossa P, Aube C, et al. Noninvasive diagnosis of hepatic fibrosis or cirrhosis. Gastroenterology. 1997 Nov;113(5):1609–16.
96. Yap FY, Skalski MR, Patel DB, Schein AJ, White EA, Tomasian A, et al. Hypertrophic osteoarthropathy: clinical and imaging features. Radiographics. 2017 Jan–Feb;37(1):157–95.
97. Ugawa Y, Shimpo T, Mannen T. Physiological analysis of asterixis: silent period locked averaging. J Neurol Neurosurg Psychiatry. 1989 Jan;52(1):89–93.
98. McIntyre N, Rosalki S. Biochemical investigations in the management of liver disease. In: Bircher J, Benhamou JP, McIntyre N, Rizzetto M, Rodes J, editors. Oxford textbook of clinical hepatology, vol. 1. Oxford: Oxford University Press; 1993. p. 293–309.
99. Gaiani S, Gramantieri L, Venturoli N, Piscaglia F, Siringo S, D'Errico A, et al. What is the criterion for differentiating chronic hepatitis from compensated cirrhosis? A prospective study comparing ultrasonography and percutaneous liver biopsy. J Hepatol. 1997 Dec;27(6):979–85.
100. Jiang HY, Chen J, Xia CC, Cao LK, Duan T, Song B. Noninvasive imaging of hepatocellular carcinoma: from diagnosis to prognosis. World J Gastroenterol. 2018 June 14;24(22):2348–62.
101. Marrero JA, Kulik LM, Sirlin CB, Zhu AX, Finn RS, Abecassis MM, et al. Diagnosis, staging, and management of hepatocellular carcinoma: 2018 practice guidance by the American Association for the Study of Liver Diseases. Hepatology. 2018 Aug;68(2):723–50.
102. Castera L, Forns X, Alberti A. Non-invasive evaluation of liver fibrosis using transient elastography. J Hepatol. 2008 May;48(5):835–47.
103. Afdhal NH. Fibroscan (transient elastography) for the measurement of liver fibrosis. Gastroenterol Hepatol (N Y). 2012 Sep;8(9):605–7.
104. Jung KS, Kim SU. Clinical applications of transient elastography. Clin Mol Hepatol. 2012 Jun;18(2):163–73.

# Chapter 3
# Primary Biliary Cholangitis

**Nora V. Bergasa**

A 57-year-old woman was referred to the hepatology clinic because of increased serum activity of alkaline phosphatase (AP). She felt well and did not report pruritus or fatigue. On physical exam, she did not exhibit any findings suggestive of liver disease. Her liver disease workup was significant for + antimitochondrial antibodies (AMA), 1:160 titer, and high serum IgM. These findings were consistent with primary biliary cholangitis (PBC). The patient opted to have a liver biopsy, which revealed stage II PBC. She was started on ursodeoxycholic acid (UDCA) at a dose of 13–15 mg/kg of body weight in divided doses with meals. In association with UDCA, the serum activity of AP normalized itself. She has remained asymptomatic for 12 years.

The salient features that suggest a diagnosis of PBC in this patient are female gender and a liver profile suggestive of cholestasis. The presence of AMA in serum and increased serum IgM concentration are classic findings of PBC and substantiate the diagnosis. At the time of her presentation, the patient met the criteria for the diagnosis of probable PBC as previously defined [1, 2], i.e., increased serum activity of AP for at least 6 months and presence of AMA in serum, with typical histological features, as a definitive diagnosis. As per current guidelines, a diagnosis of PBC is based on meeting two of the following criteria: (1) biochemical evidence of cholestasis with an elevation of AP activity, (2) the presence of AMA, and (3) histopathologic evidence of nonsuppurative cholangitis and destruction of small or medium-sized bile ducts [3].

N. V. Bergasa (✉)
Department of Medicine, H+H/Metropolitan, New York, NY, USA

New York Medical College, Valhalla, NY, USA

Hepatology, H+H/Woodhull, Brooklyn, NY, USA

The serological hallmark of PBC is the presence of AMA [4–7]. However, a condition known as AMA-negative PBC exists; the clinical features and its natural history are the same as that of classic PBC [8]. The 2 oxoacid dehydrogenase family of enzymes is comprised of pyruvate dehydrogenase complex (PDC), 2 oxo-glutarate dehydrogenase complex (OGDC), and the branched-chain 2 oxoacid dehydrogenase complex (BCOADC) [9]. These complexes play a key role in the oxidative metabolism in the mitochondria. AMA react with the E2 components of PDC, OGDC, and BCOADC, and with protein X and with the E1a and E1b subunits of PDC. The inner lipoyl domain is the dominant B cell autoepitope, with lipoic acid, which plays a crucial role in these complexes' enzymatic activity, as a cofactor [6, 10–14]. A definitive diagnosis is considered when liver histology reveals the classic bile duct injury of chronic nonsuppurative destructive cholangitis (CNSDC) [2] (Fig. 3.1).

PBC is a liver disease initially described in 1851 [15] and subsequently as a series of cases in 1950 [16] when patients tended to present with hyperbilirubinemia in advanced stages. The disease is characterized by chronic nonsuppurative destructive cholangitis that affects septal and interlobular intrahepatic bile ducts [17] (Fig. 3.1); it tends to progress and to lead to biliary cirrhosis and liver failure [18, 19]. A cure for PBC has not been identified; the administration of UDCA is approved for the treatment of PBC [3, 20, 21], and it has been associated with a prolonged period free of the need for liver transplantation [22], indicated for patients who develop liver failure [23]. Obeticholic acid was approved for the treatment of PBC in combination with UDCA for the use in patients whose AP activity has not decreased to less than 1.67 times the upper limit of normal after 1 year of treatment, or alone for patients who do not tolerate UDCA. The drug is contraindicated in patients with decompensated liver disease, i.e., Child's B and C [3], with a history of a decompensation event, and with portal hypertension in association with compensated cirrhosis.

**Fig. 3.1** The florid bile duct lesion, i.e. nonsuppurative destructive cholangitis, in a patient with primary biliary cholangitis.
The inflammatory infiltrate is comprised of mononuclear cells, some plasma cells and, characteristically, eosinophils

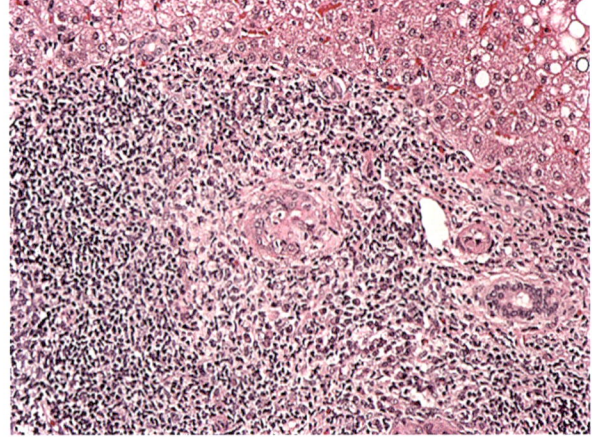

# Etiology

The trigger of the inflammatory destruction of the intrahepatic bile ducts is unknown. PBC is considered an autoimmune disease, an idea supported by the immunological alterations reported in association with this condition. Infectious agents, or infection related processes, as a cause of the CNSDC of PBC have been proposed; in this context, lipopolysaccharide, secreted by Gram negative organisms [24], and lipoteichoic acid, a component of the cellular wall of Gram positive organisms including *Staphylococcus aureus* [25, 26], have been reported to accumulate in the inflammatory infiltrate of the CNSDC of PBC, and *Propionibacterium acnes* 16 ribosomal RNA was extracted from granulomata from the liver of patients with PBC. These proteins and organisms function as pathogen-associated molecular patterns (PAMPS) [27]. PAMPS can elicit inflammatory reactions, which, around bile ducts, may contribute to the pathogenesis of the CNSDC of PBC. Biliary epithelial cells (BECs), like other epithelial cells, exhibit pattern recognition receptors (PRRs) [28], including Toll-like receptors (TLRs), the most prevalent type on this type of cell. In human beings, responses to LPS, for example, are mediated by TLR4, which culminates with the stimulation of nuclear factor kappa-B (NFkB) and production of antimicrobial peptides and proinflammatory cytokines [29, 30]. Accordingly, if not causally related to the disease, a potential effect of PAMPS in the biliary epithelial cell milieu has been interpreted to suggest a role of defense mechanisms against infections, and hence, the innate immune system, in the pathogenesis of the CNSDC of PBC [31]. Bacteriuria [32] and urinary tract infections [33] have been reported, although inconsistently [34, 35], to be significantly more prevalent in patients with PBC than in disease control groups. In this context, AMA were reported in the serum of subjects with recurrent urinary tract infections without a diagnosis of PBC [36]. As mitochondrial antigens are well conserved among species, an antibody response against bacterial mitochondrial antigens may trigger antibody formation (i.e., AMA) against endogenous antigens in a susceptible individual, defining the hypothetical process of molecular mimicry in the pathogenesis of autoimmune diseases [37], potentially including PBC [36].

*Novosphingobium aromaticivorans* is an organism that metabolizes organic compounds; some of its proteins have homology with the E2 component of the pyruvate dehydrogenase complex, the lipoyl domain of which seems critical in the production of AMA, the serological hallmark of PBC [4–7]. *Novosphingobium aromaticivorans* has been identified in the feces of human beings, including patients with PBC. It was reported that serum samples that contained antibodies against various components of the PDC-E2 group of enzymes from patients with PBC, and some serum samples from patients with PBC without AMA, reacted against proteins of *Novosphingobium aromaticivorans*, in contrast to the absence of reactivity from the control serum samples. These results have been interpreted to suggest that this organism may contribute to the induction of PBC [38].

The cloning of a human betaretrovirus from isolates from perihepatic lymph nodes from patients with PBC has been reported [39]. The viral sequence of the isolated provirus is homologous to the mouse mammary tumor virus, and viral sequences derived from human breast cancer tissue [40, 41] in 95–99% of its genetic makeup. By the use of reversed transcriptase-polymerase chain reaction, viremia has been reported in patients with PBC; immunohistochemistry studies indicate that the human betaretrovirus can be detected in lymphoid tissue in an important percentage of patients with the disease [39]. These findings have advanced further the idea that PBC results, in part, from an infectious agent [39].

Estrogen containing medications, e.g., contraceptives, can be associated with cholestasis [42, 43]. In this regard, the use of estrogen containing contraceptive medications in women with PBC is not rare; this observation may be a reflection of the use of oral contraceptives by subjects who might have developed PBC anyway, and not indicative of causation by estrogen, which interestingly, as an oral contraceptive, was found to be associated with a decrease in the risk of developing PBC [44]. However, the use of hormone replacement therapy was found in association with the disease [45]. Other factors that have been identified in association with PBC include smoking and certain cosmetic practices (e.g., use of hair dye and nail polish) [44–46].

Environmental factors have also been considered as a cause of PBC, perhaps in a genetically predisposed individual. In a study comprised of patients from New York City, the prevalence ratio of patients with PBC who had been listed for liver transplantation was significantly higher in proximity to Superfund toxic waste sites than in the control group composed of patients with primary sclerosing cholangitis [47]. Studies that used population-based data from northeast England from 1987 to 2003 have found space-time clustering [48]; space-time clustering is observed when an increased number of cases of the disease are located within a specific geographic area over a limited period, and it is usually associated with environmental factors, especially infections, as potential causes of disease [48]. In addition, a seasonal pattern of diagnoses for PBC has been reported with the highest number of diagnoses made in June, and a sinusoidal pattern in the rate of diagnoses also peaking in June [49]. These findings may suggest that a seasonal factor contributes to the cause of PBC [49].

Regarding environmental exposure, it has been suggested that xenobiotics may contribute to the pathogenesis of PBC, as they are metabolized in the liver and may form reactive metabolites that can induce changes in cellular proteins to create neoantigens. Structures mimicking a lipoyl hapten as modified by xenobiotics were used to replace the lipoic acid of the E2 component of synthetic pyruvate dehydrogenase; some of these synthetic compounds reacted with AMA containing serum from patients with PBC. It was reported that the presence of halogenated compounds correlated with antibody binding. As halogenated products can result from the metabolism of chemicals to which human beings are exposed, it was proposed that these compounds may function as mimeotopes for a self antigen, thus identifying environmental exposure as a potential cause of PBC [50].

Interestingly, a study that explored the metabolomic signature of PBC in comparison with that of celiac disease, which has been reported in association with the former [51], documented a unique metabolomic fingerprint, different from celiac disease, that was interpreted as suggestive of impaired energy metabolism possibly associated with altered gut microbiota, the study of which, as suggested by the authors, may provide some insight into the pathogenesis of PBC [52].

# Genetics

Susceptibility to the development of PBC is considered to be genetically determined, in part. This idea is supported by the high risk of developing PBC in first degree relatives of patients with the disease, reported to be 1–2% [53, 54] and by the concordance, albeit incomplete, of the disease in monozygotic twins, reported at 63% [55]. The loss of one X chromosome is a process of aging of cells [56]; an increase in the number of peripheral lymphocytes with only one X chromosome (i.e., monosomy) has been reported to occur in PBC [57], suggesting that epigenetic activities associated with gene silencing [58] may contribute to the susceptibility to develop PBC.

The human leukocyte antigen genes, located in the major compatibility complex (MHC) region in chromosome 6 21p, have been associated with diseases considered to be of autoimmune origin [59, 60]. Ethnic and geographic groupings are likely to define the results of these types of studies. They have revealed a complex relationship with alleles grouping towards protection from and vulnerability to develop PBC. Various alleles within the HLA class II genes have been reported to be associated with PBC, including the HLA DRB1*08 allele in patients from Europe, North America, Japan, and Italy [61–65]. Genome wide associated studies (GWAS) in PBC have confirmed previously reported HLA II associations. They have identified new gene loci of interest [66–69] including: (i) several single nucleotide polymorphisms (SNP) over the HLA region, and other SNP in non-HLA regions identified as the IL12A locus and the IL12RB2 locus, which encode IL-12alpha and IL-12 receptor beta 2, respectively [66, 68], (ii) variants at IRF5-TNPO3, various genes in chromosome17q12.21, and MMEL1 [67], and (iii) (a) the STAT4 gene, a downstream participant of the IL-12 signaling pathway, a process involved in the regulation of innate resistance and adaptive immunity, (b) the NF-kB gene itself, and genes that concern its activation including TAB1, TNFRSF1A, CD80, and RPS6KA4, and (c) RPS6KA4, which suppresses the production of cytokines dependent on the activation of TLRs, and genes in the signaling pathway of TNF-alpha including TNFRSF1A, DENND1B, and TNFA1P2 [69]. In this regard, NK function is related to the IL-12/STAT4 pathway. It was documented that peripheral NK cells were constitutively activated, intensively expressing CD49a and the liver-homing marker, CXCR6, in patients with PBC versus disease and healthy control subjects. NK cells from patients with PBC were activated by minuscule amounts of IL-12, which resulted in the upregulation of CXCR6 and significantly increased the production of IFNγ in contrast to the control groups. These results were interpreted as evidence for the regulation of the IL12/STAT4 pathway. In addition, resting cells from the PBC group exhibited markers of activated transcriptional profile and upregulation of genes related to the IL-12/STAT axis, suggesting that they exist in a stage of activation gravitating towards the liver by the expression of homing factors, thus, contributing to the pathogenesis of PBC [70]. These findings have supported an important role of immune mediated processes in the pathogenesis of PBC and have suggested that the IL- 12 pathway may be relevant in the predisposition to develop this disease.

## Epigenetics

Epigenetic differences have been documented in studies of monozygotic female twins and sisters discordant for PBC [71]. Aberrant demethylation on CXCR3 promoter in PBC was identified in a study of DNA methylation profile of the X chromosome in patients with PBC [72]; specifically, 20, 15, and 19 distinct gene promoters reflected differences in DNA methylation in CD4+ T, CD8+ T, and CD14+ cells, with hypermethylation of FUNDC2 in CD8+ T cells, demethylation of CXCR3 in CD4+ T cells found to correlate inversely with the expression of CXCR3 in CD4+ T cells from patients defined as having early-stage PBC patients, findings interpreted to suggest that the genes with epigenetic alterations were likely to be indicators of autoimmunity [72]. In this regard, CXCR3 has been documented in the development of autoimmune diseases by "creating local amplification loops of inflammation in target organs...", thus, the identification of aberrant demethylation of CXCR3 has suggested its involvement in the natural history of PBC [72].

A significant increase in CpG methylation was documented in the *AE2/SLC4A2* gene in patients with PBC; methylation rates of *AE2* promoter regions were correlated inversely with the levels of AE2 mRNAs in the liver and peripheral blood mononuclear cells (PBMCs) of patients with PBC [73]. As the *AE2* encodes a $Cl^-/HCO_3^-$ exchanger involved in biliary secretion and intracellular pH regulation, a decrease in the concentration of this transporter increases the vulnerability of the biliary epithelium to injury; in addition, hypermethylation in PBMCs was interpreted as a potential disturbance to immunological homeostasis [74].

T cell survival is regulated, in part, by beta arrestins (Barr1). It was documented that the expression of Barr1 was significantly increased in T cells from patients with PBC, and was associated with T cell proliferation, interferon production, decreased nuclear factor κB and AP-1 activity, stimulation of histone H4 acetylation in the promoter regions of CD40L, LIGHT, IL-17 and interferon-γ, and decreased acetylation of histone H4 in the promoter regions of TRAIL, Apo2, and HDAC7A; these results were interpreted to suggest that Barr1 regulates the expression of those genes and they may contribute to the pathogenesis of PBC [75].

# Epidemiology

Estimating from a publication from the USA in 2005 [76], which reported the prevalence of PBC as being 40.2 per 100,000 inhabitants in 1995, PBC meets the definition of a rare disease, according to the Rare Disease Act of 2002 of the US Government [77], which defines a rare disease as one that affects less than 200,000 persons [77]. The incidence and prevalence of PBC differ among geographic areas. It has varied over the past 40 years with a trend towards an increase (Table 3.1);

**Table 3.1**  Selected studies on the prevalence and incidence of PBC

| | Study period | Methodology | Prevalence (per inhabitants) | Incidence | References |
|---|---|---|---|---|---|
| Sheffield, England | 1977–1979 | Diagnosed cases | 54/million | NR | [78] |
| Northern England | 1965–1987 | Case finding | Increased from 18/million in 1976 to 125.5/million in 1987 | NR | [79] |
| Northern Sweden | 1973–1982 | Case finding | 151 per million | 13.3 per million | [80] |
| Newcastle upon Tyne, England | 1987–1994 | Case finding | 14–32 per million | Increased from 180 per million in 1987 to 240 in 1994 | [1] |
| Northern England | | Cases identification | Increased from 201.9 per million in 1987 to 334.6 per million in 1994 | Increased from 23 per million in 1987 and 32.2 per million in 1994 | [81] |
| Olmstead County, Minnesota, United States | 1975–1995 | Retrospective chart review from database | 2.7 (95% CI, 1.9–3.5) | NR | [76] |
| Alaska, United States (native population) | 1984–2000 | Retrospective chart review | 16 per 100,000 (95% CI = 12.9–25.4) | NR | [82] |
| Victoria, Australia | | Case finding | 51 per million | NR | [83] |
| Calgary, Canada | 1996 and 2002 | Population based administrative database | Increased from 100 per million in 1996 to 227 per million in 2002 | 30.3 cases per million | [84] |
| The Netherland | 2008 | Identification of patients in databases from 44 hospitals | 0.1 per 100,000, 0.3 in men and 1.9 in women, with a point prevalence of 13.2 per 100,000 | NR | [85] |

*CI* confidence interval; *NR* not reported

this change may be due to improved diagnostic abilities. A review of the word literature reported an incidence rate ranging from 0.33 to 5.8 per 100,000 inhabitants per year and a prevalence ranging from 1.91 to 40.2 per 100,000 inhabitants [86]. PBC is more prevalent in women than in men [76, 84]; from a nationwide study from the USA for which data were collected from surveys, it was reported that the disease was more common in women than in men at a ratio of eight to one [45].

## Clinical Manifestations

PBC must be considered in asymptomatic patients with or without stigmata of liver disease and a liver profile suggestive of cholestasis. The classical presentation of PBC is in a middle age woman, who may report pruritus and or fatigue, and who has a serum liver profile suggestive of cholestasis. Patients can present with jaundice at the time of diagnosis. Male patients present similarly.

In symptomatic patients, the earliest and sometimes the only manifestations are pruritus and fatigue. The pruritus of PBC is from cholestasis, defined as impaired secretion of bile [87]. The reason patients with cholestasis experience pruritus is not known; it has been inferred that the pruritus results from substances that accumulate in the body and that cannot be excreted normally as a result of cholestasis. Increased opioidergic neurotransmission has been hypothesized to mediate, at least in part, the pruritus of cholestasis [88]; results of controlled clinical trials that have documented a decrease in the perception of pruritus and its behavioral manifestation, scratching activity, support this hypothesis [89–92]. Other neurotransmitter systems may be involved [93]. Patients with PBC often report having experienced pruritus for several years prior to the diagnosis of the disease. In this context, a study that consisted of an internet survey via the organization PBCers revealed that in 75% of the patients, the pruritus preceded the diagnosis of PBC by 2–5 years [94]; this finding underscores the importance of considering internal medicine causes of pruritus, e.g., liver disease, when this symptom presents in the absence of rash. Indeed, the skin of patients with PBC is devoid of primary pruritic skin lesions; in contrast, excoriations and prurigo nodularis secondary to scratching abound. Pruritus is experienced by most patients with PBC, with a reported frequency of 70% [95] to 73.5% [96]. Of interest, in the recent study from the UK that used survey methodology, 11.7% of subjects reported severe pruritus [96], similar to the 11% of subjects who reported that nothing relieved their pruritus in a study conducted almost 20 years ago [94]. The reason some patients with PBC do not experience pruritus is unknown. It was suggested that genetic predisposition might protect or facilitate the sensation of pruritus in patients with PBC because in a series of 101 patients with PBC from Italy and from the USA, a novel mutation (t3563a) in codon 1188 in exon 25, the region most frequently associated with mutations, of the MRP2 gene was identified. This mutation resulted from the substitution of valine by glutamate (V1188E). V1188E was identified in heterozygosity, in 19.5% of the patients who reported pruritus, and in 7.8% of the patients who did not ($p = 0.02$, RR = 2.51, 95% CI: 1.13–5.69) [97]. MRP2 (ABCC2) is a member of the family of ATP binding cassette (ABC) transporters expressed in various organs, including the liver and the blood brain barrier [98–100]. In the hepatocyte, MRP2 mediates the transport of several organic anions, especially conjugated compounds, including dianionic conjugated bile salts into the bile [98] and endogenous opioids [99, 100]. The presence of SNP in the MRP2 gene may be associated with a decrease in the in vivo function of the transporter [101]; thus, it was hypothesized that the novel V1188E mutation might alter the ability of the protein to transport substrates. Alterations in the transport of pruritogen(s) or its cofactors from the hepatocyte into bile or the central nervous system may be a way by which V1188E has an impact on whether patients with PBC perceive pruritus.

Whether the pruritus from PBC specifically relates to immunological abnormalities that may mediate the NSDC lesion of PBC is unknown. However, a recent study reported a serum profile in peripheral blood cell populations related to pruritus. Specifically, the study documented a significant decrease in the $CD4^+CD3^+$ and $CD3^+CD25^+$ counts, and in NKT-like cells $CD3^+/CD16^+CD56^+$, and ($CD3^+$) T lymphocytes in patients with pruritus than in those without pruritus. At present, this finding cannot be explained in the context of pruritus, but it merits further investigation [102].

Xerostomia and xerophthalmia are manifestations of PBC, suggesting an inflammatory process that affects bile flow and affects the secretory functions of the salivary and lacrimal glands. Indeed, the term dry gland syndrome has been used to describe PBC [103]. The assessment of patients with PBC includes information regarding the function of lacrimal and salivary glands, which can be addressed by asking about the ability to cry normally and to be able to eat a cracker, for example, without drinking any liquids.

Fatigue was reported by 50% of patients with PBC, with 20% experiencing substantial changes in the quality of life [104]. The cause of fatigue in PBC is unknown; a central component, as in pruritus, has been suggested [104, 105]. Fatigue can be subtle, and, in general, patients state that they have to push themselves to do what they easily did in the past. Because PBC can be associated with thyroid disease, specifically, hypothyroidism, which is often subclinical, exclusion of thyroid abnormalities is part of the approach to patients with possible PBC.

Patients with PBC can report dull, right upper quadrant pain. Upper endoscopy revealed some diagnoses interpreted to be associated with abdominal pain in a small series [106]; the pain tends to resolve itself spontaneously. It does not relate to the use of UDCA [106]. Bone pain secondary to osteoporosis is another symptom of patients with PBC, and it can be debilitating.

# Natural History

The natural history of PBC seems to have changed over the years and may differ among different countries. A study conducted in North England included 770 patients followed from 1987 to 1994. The prevalence of pruritus at presentation was 18.9% and that of fatigue 21%. Over 60% of the patients were asymptomatic at diagnosis; however, 62% had pruritus or fatigue within 5 years with only 5% of patients remaining asymptomatic after 20 years of follow-up. Over 10 years, 26% of patients had developed liver failure. Seventy percent of the patients underwent liver transplantation during follow-up; in 77%, 30 patients, the transplant was performed because of complication of liver failure and worsening prognosis, and nine were transplanted because of symptoms, which can be devastating in PBC [107]. Four hundred and seventeen (54.1%) patients died during the follow-up period, with a median calculated survival of 9.3 years. The mortality was calculated as three times over that of the general population suggesting that PBC impairs survival even in association with what was considered "milder disease" [107]. A study examined the development of esophageal varices over a period of 5.6 years in 265 patients with PBC [108]. Eighty-three (31%) of the patients developed esophageal varices with 48% of those experiencing at least one bleeding episode. Survival decreased after the development of esophageal varices, with 83% and 59% surviving at one and 3 years, respectively. The survival was strongly impaired by the index bleed with estimated calculations of 65% and 46% at 1 and 3 years, respectively. Patients with early stages of PBC may also have variceal bleeding from portal hypertension associated with hepatic granulomata; thus, this peculiarity must be remembered when facing such patients who, although bleeding, may not have advanced liver disease [108].

Patients can be diagnosed years prior to manifestations of symptoms as routine laboratory testing may be conducted. In a study from the northeast of the USA, 33% of a group of 247 patients from whom data were available for follow-up remained asymptomatic for a median of 12 years [109]. The median predicted survival for patients who did not have symptoms at presentation was 16 years, in contrast to seven and a half for those with symptoms. Once patients experienced symptoms, their survival was the same as that of those who presented with symptoms; however, the survival for asymptomatic patients was shorter than what was predicted for a properly matched control group [109]. This observation was consistent with that from a prior publication [110], which reported that from a group of 36 asymptomatic patients, the majority (89%) developed symptoms after 2–4 years [110]; however, asymptomatic patients had a decreased survival time, as compared to the matched control group. These observations support the idea of treating patients with PBC without symptoms attributed to the disease.

## Associated Conditions

PBC can be associated with other diseases, particularly those considered of autoimmune etiology [111]. Non-hepatic disorders in patients with PBC have been reported in close to 70% of patients. The inability to produce tears, difficulties in wearing contact lenses, inability to eat a cracker without drinking fluids, and recent onset of dental caries suggest Sjogren's syndrome, one of the most common syndromes associated with PBC. Joint pains, dysphagia, and pyrosis are among the symptoms experienced by patients with PBC as CREST syndrome (calcinosis, rheumatoid nodules, scleroderma, esophageal dysmotility, and telangiectasias) can also be associated with the disease [111]. There are case reports and/or small series reporting the association between PBC and multiple myeloma [112], celiac disease [113], autoimmune thrombocytopenia [114], lichen planus [115], systemic lupus erythematosus [116], pernicious anemia [117], ulcerative colitis [118], pulmonary disease [119], cardiomyopathy [120], Graves' disease [121], and retroperitoneal fibrosis [122]. Patients sometimes report a generalized, insidious progression of hyperpigmentation, which may come to their attention after the suntan obtained during the summer seasons persists.

The incidence of cholelithiasis is increased in patients with PBC. The incidence of hepatocellular carcinoma is also increased in patients with PBC, calling for screening efforts for early diagnosis [21].

The lipid metabolism in PBC is complex, and it is altered in relation to the stages of the disease [123]. As a result of cholestasis, the secretion of biliary bile acids and biliary lipids decreases; as the disease progresses, the production of bile acids, the total and neutral excretion of sterols, and the cholesterol synthesis decrease [124]. High-density lipoprotein (HDL) concentration is high, decreasing at the end stages of the disease. Characteristically, the serum of patients with PBC has structurally abnormal lipoproteins that fall within the density range of low density lipoproteins (LDL) and HDL. These lipoproteins are discoidal LP-X lacking the core lipids and apoprotein (apo) B, large triglyceride-rich LP-Y, and discoidal, apo E-enriched HDL. Oxidized LDL facilitates apoptosis and has antiangiogenic effects; LP-X is reported to be antiatherogenic by preventing oxidation of LDL [125]. The relatively low risk for cardiovascular complications in PBC, in spite of its characteristic hypercholesterolemia, has been interpreted to result from the presence of LP-X in the lipid compartment of patients with this disease [125]; however, the antioxidant properties of the LDL fraction of patients with PBC decrease after liver transplantation [125]. Serum adiponectin, reported as high in patients with PBC, correlated negatively with body mass index and positively with the disease stage, and it was suggested that it might have protective effects against atherosclerosis [126]. Apolipoproteins facilitate the absorption and secretion of fat from the intestine, act as activators of enzymes of lipoprotein metabolism, and are ligands for lipoprotein receptors on cell surfaces; in this regard, an increase in the mean plasma apolipoprotein B and C-II concentrations [127], a decrease in apolipoprotein A-I, low in advanced disease, and high in pre-cirrhotic disease have been reported [128]. Mean postheparin hepatic lipase activity was documented as decreased in all stages of the disease [128, 129], possibly due to the presence of an inhibitor in plasma, impaired cholesterol esterification was noted in advanced disease only; these findings were interpreted as contributors to the lipoprotein abnormalities exhibited by patients with PBC [128]. A study of cholesterol absorption and synthesis related to lipoprotein levels and kinetics in PBC indicated that the LDL B receptor activity was low in advanced disease, and the transport rate of apo-A-I was reduced [123]. Although the absorption of cholesterol is low in advanced stages, the LDL uptake was reported to be upregulated, and total very low density lipoprotein and LDL cholesterol and LDL triglyceride levels were found to be increased, and HDL concentration decreased [123]. The relationship between LDL apo B levels, cholesterol absorption, and synthesis, and LDL apo B kinetics documented in control subjects was absent in PBC, likely secondary to cholestasis and hepatic synthetic dysfunction [123], as it is likely to be the case for LP-X [125].

The limited epidemiological data available from retrospective studies have not suggested that patients with PBC have a high risk of complications due to atherosclerosis [130, 131]. In conjunction with the characteristic lipid profile of PBC, these reported observations have not supported the specific treatment of hypercholesterolemia in these patients. Marked hypercholesterolemia was not associated with increased risk for cardiovascular complications, whereas moderate hypercholesterolemia was, in a study from Italy [132]; this finding suggested the existence of protective factors in the former group [132]. It is possible that patients with PBC and who have risk factors for adverse cardiovascular events, in addition to high cholesterol, may benefit from treatment with lipid lowering drugs. In fact, myocardial infarction was reported in patients with PBC in one published series [133]. Recommendations for specific treatment of hypercholesterolemia in patients with PBC are not available at present [3, 21] but, referral of patients who have hypercholesterolemia and who are at risk for cardiovascular events according to current guidelines to lipid experts seems reasonable. In support of this position are the study results that concerned measurements of intima media thickness in patients with PBC. It was reported that control subjects with hypercholesterolemia had greater intima-media thickness and prevalence of carotid stenosis than patients with PBC and hypercholesterolemia, whose intima-media thickness was similar to that of patients with normal serum cholesterol levels; the risk of increased intima-media thickness increased and associated with age and hypertension, but not with hypercholesterolemia [134]. In the context of treatment, the use of statins and fibrates, standard drugs for hyperlipidemia has been reported to be associated with decreased serum activity of liver-derived enzymes in patients who have not responded to therapy with UDCA [135, 136], suggesting salutary effects of these types of drugs on the disease process.

The reported prevalence of osteoporosis in patients with PBC by densitometry, which should be performed in patients according to international guidelines [137], is approximately 30% [138–140]. The pathogenesis of osteoporosis in patients with PBC is unknown [141]. Low bone formation and some components of high bone resorption have been reported [142, 143]. Specific genetic polymorphisms have not been identified as susceptibility factors for bone disease [144]. Osteoporosis and osteopenia in women with PBC were reported in associations with age, and duration and stage of the disease [140, 145], and osteopenia, in association with disease stage [140]. However, the risk factors identified to predispose patients to fractures were age, menopause, height, and falls, for which they were documented to be at risk, but not liver disease stage [146].

A study reported that the resting metabolic rate of patients with PBC was significantly higher than in patients who had undergone liver transplantation for complications from this disease and than in control subjects [147]; indeed, high resting metabolic rate is increased in PBC [147] and was one of the first metabolic abnormalities described in this condition.

## Physical Exam

Physical findings vary and include some typical signs such as xanthoma and xanthelasma, paper-money skin on the malar area [148], labial telangiectasia, usually in association with CREST syndrome, spider angiomata, palmar erythema, excoriations secondary to scratching, hepatomegaly, and splenomegaly. Jaundice and ascites are features of advanced and or decompensated liver disease. Hyperpigmentation is characteristic of PBC; the sparing of the skin in the interscapular area is a classical finding, and it has been named the butterfly sign [149] (Fig. 3.2).

**Fig. 3.2** Back of a patient with primary biliary cholangitis displaying the butterfly sign. Arrows point to the skin color lighter than the color of the surrounding skin, relatively hyperpigmented

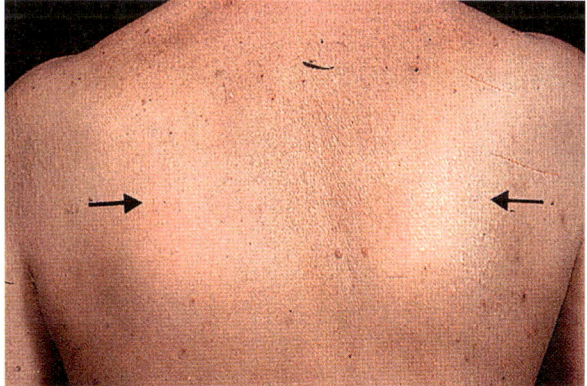

## Laboratory Exams

The characteristic laboratory features in patients with PBC are elevated serum activity of liver associated enzymes specifically, increased activity of AP (and gamma glutamyl transpeptidase (GGTP) and 5′-nucleotidase), reflective of cholestasis, and positive AMA. The activity of alanine and aspartate transaminases (ALT and AST, respectively) is usually modestly elevated. Characteristically, the serum concentration of IgM is increased although the disease can occur in patients with IgM deficiency. Thrombocytopenia secondary to hypersplenism or immune complex abnormalities may also be present. Anemia and neutropenia may be a finding in patients with advanced disease. Urine analysis may reveal an alkaline pH suggestive of renal tubular acidosis believed to be secondary to copper deposits in the distal renal tubules; also, bacteriuria, asymptomatic in many cases, is reported as common in PBC. Serum levels of bile acids may be elevated (fasting and 2 h post-prandially), reflecting the degree of cholestasis.

The differential diagnosis of PBC includes conditions associated with cholestasis, including drug induced liver injury, granulomatous diseases, e.g., sarcoidosis, and post-cholecystectomy syndrome with secondary biliary strictures. Hepatitis A can be complicated by prolonged cholestasis, but its serology is diagnostic. A form of cholangitis associated with ductopenia has also been described; the terms immunocholangitis and AMA negative PBC have been used to refer to this condition, the natural history of which is similar to that of PBC, and it is considered a variant form of the disease [8, 150, 151]. However, a recommendation against the interchangeable use of autoimmune cholangitis and AMA negative PBC was published in the last published guidance from the American Association for the Study of Liver Disease (AASLD). It has been documented that AMA negative PBC tends to be associated with serum anti-sp100, gp210, anti-kelch-like 12, and anti-hexokinase 1 antibodies more commonly than in AMA positive PBC [152–154], making a liver biopsy a necessary diagnostic test in the absence of this type of serology.

## Radiographic Studies

Evaluation of gross liver architecture (and vascularity) is recommended with a sonogram, which will exclude biliary obstruction, and to rule out the presence of cysts (often benign) and hepatic hemangiomata, which may represent a problem when a blind procedure such as percutaneous liver biopsy is being considered.

Endoscopic retrograde cholangio-pancreatography (ERCP) is not recommended to evaluate patients with suspected PBC. A magnetic resonance cholangiopancreatography (MRCP) is the first radiographic test used when the diagnosis of PBC is questionable (e.g., negative AMA, non-diagnostic liver biopsy). When the patients are male, particularly when AMA is negative, primary sclerosing cholangitis (PSC) has to be considered, and in those cases, an MRCP is in order.

## Serology and Immunological Features

An AMA titer of 1:40 in the right clinical context is a diagnostic criterion for PBC and, thus, should be requested when evaluating a patient for possible PBC. The 2 oxoacid dehydrogenase family of enzymes is comprised of pyruvate dehydrogenase complex (PDC), 2 oxo-glutarate dehydrogenase complex (OGDC), and the branched chain 2 oxoacid dehydrogenase complex (BCOADC). These complexes play a key role in the oxidative metabolism in the mitochondria. AMA react with the E2 components of PDC, OGDC, and BCOADC, and with protein X, and with the E1alpha and E1beta subunits of PDC. The inner lipoyl domain has been considered to be the dominant B cell autoepitope, with lipoic acid, which plays a pivotal role in the enzymatic activity of these complexes, as a cofactor [7, 11]; however, some studies have suggested that AMA are a group of heterogeneous antibodies that differ in specificity but that, in general, react with a relatively well-defined part of PDC-E2 that includes the lipoyl domain [155]. T cell clones developed specifically to recognize the PDC-E2 complex identified the main epitope of the mitochondrial antigens to be the amino acid sequence 163–176, which corresponds to the inner lipoyl domain [156]; T cells also recognized the sequence 36–49, which corresponds to the outer lipoyl domain. In addition, the recognition of PDC-E2 from *Escherichia coli* by some T cells has been reported; this finding has been interpreted by some to support the theory of molecular mimicry [37] in developing AMA in PBC [156]. This hypothesis proposes that a break of tolerance is triggered by the mimic, leading to the development of antibodies against PDC-E2 and other antigens of the 2 oxo acid dehydrogenase family of enzymes. Loss of tolerance is implicated in the pathogenesis of autoimmune diseases [157], including systemic lupus erythematosus, through activation of Toll-like receptor 9 on hyperreactive B cells [158].

In vitro experiments have shown that in patients with PBC, the frequency of T cells restricted to HLA DRB4 0101 that recognize the sequence 163–176 of the PDC-E2 complex was significantly higher from hilar lymph nodes and liver than from the peripheral blood pool [159]. It was also reported that there was cross reactivity between the T cells identifying the 163–176 sequence with the 36–49 sequence also from PDC-E2, and with the peptide sequence 100–113 from the 2 oxo-glutarate dehydrogenase complex [159]. These results have been interpreted as evidence supporting the ExETDK sequence as a common T cell epitope recognized by T cells hence contributing to the pathogenesis of PBC [159]. Patients with AMA negative PBC have a cholestatic disease that behaves like PBC, in the absence of the characteristic presence of AMA in serum (see above) [151, 160, 161]. In this regard, experiments done with peripheral autologous mononuclear cells from patients with AMA negative and AMA positive PBC have been reported to reveal similar PDC-E2 CD4+ T cell frequency and cytokine production on stimulation, suggesting that the absence of AMA in serum does not mean a lack of response of T cells to the major epitope PDC-E2 163–176 of PBC [162].

BEC from patients with PBC in culture were reported to express E2 on their membrane [163], and monoclonal antibodies designed to react with PDC-E2 were reported to have strong localization on the apical surface of BEC from patients with PBC [155]. It was proposed that this surface stain was comprised of a modified form of PDC-E2 or a molecule that cross reacted with the antibody, acting as a molecular mimic [164], and generating a self-perpetuating attraction of inflammatory cells that result in the CNSDC of PBC [155]. The epitope specificity of several anti-PDC-E2 monoclonal antibodies that recognize a certain protein in BEC of patients with PBC and not in control liver tissue has been shown to differ; however, this finding has been interpreted to suggest that the recognized epitopes form part of PDC-E2 and include the lipoyl domain, which, localized at the apical domain of the BEC itself, contributes to the pathogenesis of the CNSDC of PBC [155]. In this regard, immune complexes were reported to exist within the bile ducts; as the dimeric form of immunoglobulin A (IgA) can traverse from the basal to the apical domain of the BEC by transcytosis [165], it has been proposed that IgA may bind a relevant antigen in the lumen prior to transcytosis and take it into the cell. In this context, IgA from serum in patients with PBC was reported to colocalize with PDC-E2 within the cytoplasm and on the apical side of the BEC [166], which may contribute to the staining in the luminal domain of BEC, as described above [155]. These findings have been interpreted to suggest that the IgG binding of a complex formed by IgA bound to its epitope may exert an inflammatory response around the bile duct area, in spite of the noninflammatory regulatory role of IgA [167, 168].

Non-protein and protein antigens can generate antibody production; however, antibodies to protein antigens require that the antigen be internalized by B cells and be presented to T cells of the CD4+ type of helper T cells [169]. The humoral immune response is initiated by the recognition of antigens that bind to IgM (and to IgD) on the surface of mature, naïve B cells; this recognition results in activation of B cells with the proliferation of antigen-specific cells, which differentiate and generate memory B cells and plasma cells that secrete antibodies in large quantities to keep up with the rapidity with which microbes multiply themselves [169]. The first antibody response to a specific protein or non-protein antigen is mostly of the IgM class; the second response is induced by the stimulation of memory B cells by a formerly encountered protein antigen, mainly of the IgG class. Characteristically, patients with PBC have high levels of serum IgM [19]. In the context of the humoral response, it has been recognized that the lack of methylation of CpG dinucleotides in bacterial DNA, in contrast to the mammalian methylated form, allows its recognition by toll-like receptor (TLR) 9, which is associated with a robust immunogenic response CD27+ memory B cells were reported to produce IgM via the stimulation of the TLR9 receptor signaling in studies of peripheral mononuclear cells from patients with PBC in vitro, in contrast to the absence of a response from cells from control subjects [170]. In addition, the stimulation of peripheral mononuclear cells from patients with PBC with CpG-B was reported to be associated with phenotypical changes that include an increased expression of TLR9, and of CD86, a co-stimulator of T cells, on B cells, and also with enhanced production of AMA [171]. These findings have been interpreted to suggest that CpG-B [170] may be a potential endogenous trigger of B cells to produce IgM and AMA and have further suggested an involvement of the innate immune system in the pathogenesis of PBC. In this regard, BEC express IL-17 receptors; in response to IL-17, they secrete chemokines and cytokines, including IL-6, IL-1B, and IL-23p19, which are associated with responses to PAMPs (see above) [172].

The genesis of AMA and their potential role in the pathogenesis of the CNSDC of PBC may be associated with the characteristic response to apoptosis by bile ducts [173–175]. In addition to PDC-E2, which can be recognized by T cells, apoptotic bile ducts retain the three 2-oxoacid dehydrogenase enzymes immunologically intact [176] within apoptotic bodies, termed apotopes [177, 178]. In a controlled in vitro system, macrophages from patients with PBC co-cultured with apoptotic bodies from intrahepatic BEC and AMA were reported to produce robust amounts of cytokines [178]. Macrophage stimulation was through the classic (M1) pathway, as suggested by decreased cytokine production in association with the addition of anti-CD16 to the system. Anti-CD16 blocks the fragment crystallizable receptor for immunoglobulin (FcgR). FcgR is expressed on macrophages' surface and is activated by microbial products and cytokines, especially interferon gamma. FcgR recognizes antibody coated cells, which are subsequently killed by macrophages [179]. Stimulated macrophages in the presence of apoptotic bodies from intrahepatic BEC and AMA demonstrated the ability to phagocytize apoptotic bodies, as studied by confocal microscopy methodology; however, the calculated index of phagocytosis by activated mononuclear cells from patients with PBC was significantly lower than that of control stimulated mononuclear cells [178]. Phagocytosis was not blocked by anti-CD16 [178], suggesting that, as measured in an in vitro system, phagocytosis and cytokine secretion by activated macrophages are conducted via independent pathways. In addition, the expression of the messenger RNA of tumor necrosis factor-related apoptosis-inducing ligand (TRAIL) in macrophages from patients with PBC that had been cocultured with apoptotic bodies from intrahepatic BEC and AMA was reported as markedly increased, suggesting a role of TRAIL in the inflammatory injury of BEC.

These findings add to the developing consensus of an active role of the innate immune system and apoptosis of BEC in the pathogenesis of the CNSDC of PBC, and it may shed light on the question of the remarkable selection of small intrahepatic bile ducts as targets of the inflammatory destruction in this disease [178]. The term dry gland syndrome has been used in reference to PBC because of its association with the decreased flow of tears, saliva, and pancreatic juice [103, 180–183], in addition to impaired bile secretion, as a result of the CNSDC, and ductopenia. Histological studies have confirmed inflammatory changes in the ducts of glandular structures other than BEC [103, 180–183], as well as the immunoreactivity against PDC-E2 monoclonal antibody [184]; however, studies of apoptosis of the epithelium of those glandular ducts in the context of PBC have not been published.

Antinuclear antibodies (ANAs) with various patterns of expression including speckled, multiple nuclear dots, rim-like and membranous, centromeric, and homogeneous are detected in approximately half of the patients with PBC, their presence reported to be more common in patients in whom serum AMA are not detected than in patients with AMA [185]. ANAs displaying multiple nuclear dots and rim-like/membranous are infrequently found (1.3%). When found, they are highly

**Table 3.2** Features of the most common types of antinuclear antibodies in the serum of patients with PBC

| ANA patterns on immunofluorescence | Recognized cellular element | Nature of antigen | References |
|---|---|---|---|
| Multiple nuclear dots | SP 100 proteins | Transcription activating proteins | [187] |
| Multiple nuclear dots | PML | Transformation and cell growth suppressing protein aberrantly expressed in promyelocytic leukemia cells | [188] |
| | sp 140 | Promyelocytic leukemia protein nuclear body | [186] |
| Rim like/membranous | gp 210 | Integral glycoprotein of the nuclear envelope pore membrane | [189] |
| Rim like/membranous | np62 | A functional protein of the nuclear pore complex | [190] |
| Rim like/membranous | LBR | Integral membrane protein of the nuclear envelope | [191] |
| Granules in cells in mitosis (i.e. interphase) | CENP-B | Polyprotein that interacts with centromeric heterochromatin in human chromosomes | [192] |

*ANA* antinuclear antibodies; *sp* speckled protein; *PML* promyelocytic leukemia protein; *gp* glycoprotein; *np* nucleoporin; *LBR* lamin B receptor; *CENP-B* centromere protein B

suggestive of the diagnosis of PBC, independent of the AMA status of the patients [186]. The elements recognized by the ANAs of patients with PBC are reported in Table 3.2 [187–190, 193–197]. The presence of antibodies against the nuclear pore protein gp210 was reported in association with severe cholestasis and impaired liver function [185, 198] and anticentromere antibody with the development of portal hypertension [198].

As described previously in this chapter, other autoantibodies can also be detected in the serum of patients with PBC. Still, their presence does not contribute significantly to diagnosing and managing a patient with this disease.

# Histology

The Scheuer's histological classification of PBC is comprised of four stages; the characterization of which are I: chronic nonsuppurative destructive cholangitis (CNSDC) or florid bile duct lesion, II: bile ductular proliferation, III: biliary fibrosis, IV: biliary cirrhosis [17]. The florid bile duct lesion, i.e., nonsuppurative destructive cholangitis, is considered the primordial lesion of PBC [17] (Fig. 3.1). Cholangiolitis, comprised of polymorphonuclear leukocytes in the inflammatory infiltrate and pseudoxanthomatous changes, a "bubbly" appearance of periportal hepatocytes resulting from cholate stasis (accumulation of bile acids), characterize the histological findings of nonsuppurative destructive cholangitis, leading to ductopenia, a decrease in the number of intrahepatic bile ducts [17]. Granulomata tend to be appreciated in early disease. As a result of cholestasis, there is an accumulation of copper in the liver and other organs.

The cellular infiltrate of the CNSDC of PBC is composed of plasma cells, eosinophils, B and natural killer cells, and T lymphocytes, the latter being the majority [199–206]. The Ludwig classification consists of stage 1, characterized by portal hepatitis, stage 2 by periportal hepatitis, stage 3 by bridging fibrosis or necrosis, and stage 4 by cirrhosis [207].

## Cellular Immunology

Studies to identify cellular immunological phenotypes have characterized the lymphocytes of the CNSDC as being of the CD4+ and CD8+ types [177, 208, 209]. It may be that the predominance of a particular phenotype may depend on the stage of the disease [159]. A marked increase in PDC-E2 specific CD4+ cells in the periportal lymph nodes, and the liver of patients with PBC compared with peripheral mononuclear cells was reported [159]. In addition, compared to the blood compartment, there is an important increase in the frequency of PDC-E2 specific CD8+ in the liver of patients with PBC [210], particularly in the inflammatory infiltrate in the portal areas [211]. The predominance of interferon gamma mRNA in the inflammatory infiltrate of livers of patients with PBC suggests that the most prominent T cell subset in the CNSDC lesion is the Th1 [212].

The presence of autoreactive T cells in the CNSDC of PBC suggests that this type of cell is attracted to the biliary epithelium, where they participate in the genesis of the lesion. Most of the T lymphocytes found in the CNSDC of PBC are TCRalpha beta, which are MCH restricted, meaning that they can only recognize antigens in association with MHC molecules [199, 213, 214]. A small proportion of gamma delta T cells has also been reported in the CNSDC lesion of PBC [215].

Loss of self tolerance is considered to be a fundamental pathophysiological process in autoimmunity [216]. CD4 + CD25high regulatory T cells (Tregs) are considered to play an important role in self-tolerance. Studies of this population of cells in PBC have revealed Tregs' normal function; however, alterations in the proportion of Tregs in the CD4 + TCR-alpha-beta and FoxP3+ T cell pool in the periphery and liver tissue have been reported [217, 218]. These data have been interpreted to suggest that Tregs are involved in the pathogenesis of PBC [217, 218]. In this regard, the proportion of CD4 + CD25+ and CD8+ and CD28− T cell subpopulations in the circulation is not significantly different between patients with PBC and control subjects; however, the characteristic surface features of CD8 Tregs, including increased expression of CD127 and decreased expression of CD39, and the reduced induction of CD8 Tregs in response to stimulation of IL10 in vitro, have suggested resistance from CD8Treg cells to commit to their regulatory functions [219], which has been interpreted to suggest substantial alterations in this cell compartment in patients with PBC, as reported in other autoimmune diseases [219].

Antigen presentation is a fundamental process in recognition of antigens by T cell receptors (TCRs). Antigen presenting cells (APCs) present antigenic peptides associated with major histocompatibility complex (MHC) class II to T cells; they must also express on their surface B 7, a co-stimulatory protein that interacts with the CD28 molecule expressed on the TCRs, to generate signals for T cell activation. Professional APCs constitutively express MHC class II and include dendritic cells, macrophages, and B cells [220]; immunological studies have reported markers for dendritic cells in the cellular component of this histological findings, including dendritic cell CD11c. A role of double-negative (DN)-T cells as contributors to the break of tolerance in PBC was suggested by a study that documented a significantly decreased number of cells in the periphery and the liver of patients with PBC, with their presence negatively correlating with advanced disease stages and positively correlating with response to treatment with UDCA. DN-T cells demonstrated decreased capacity to stimulate proliferation of CD4, effectors, and CD8 cytotoxic cells, finding interpreted to suggest that the DN-T cells' impaired function may contribute to the pathogenesis of PBC [221].

B cells and plasma cells expressing IgM were reported to abound in the liver's granulomata of PBC [222]. Langerhans cells (LCs), which mature into dendritic cells in the lymph nodes, have been found infiltrating the bile ducts in the lesion of CNSDC [223]. BEC in culture produce LC-attracting chemokines in response to certain cytokines and pathogen associated molecular patterns; thus, the presence of LC in the lesion of CNSDC has been interpreted to suggest that the cytokine milieu of the liver in PBC perpetuates the inflammatory process by the production of chemokines that attract APC, and also, that innate immunity processes inherent to bile ducts contribute to the pathogenesis of the CNSDC of PBC [223, 224]. Innate immunity is an endogenous defense mechanism against bacterial and viral infections that consistently reacts rapidly to microbes upon reexposure. The innate immune system is comprised of epithelial barriers, natural killer (NK) cells, phagocytic cells (neutrophils and macrophages), cytokines, and the complement system [224]. BEC are reported to secrete antimicrobial agents, including immunoglobulin A, cytokines, and chemokines that recognize pathogen associated molecular patterns (PAMP), to fight infection. PAMPs induce inflammatory reactions; as they have been found in BEC overtaken by CNSDC, they have been proposed to contribute to this cholangiopathy [31].

A contribution of the biliary epithelial cell itself to the lesion of CNSDC by its possible ability to express class II MHC antigen when activated by inflammatory processes, consistent with features of antigen presenting cells, has been proposed in PBC; however, BEC do not express the co-stimulatory CD28 ligands B7-1 or B7-2 suggesting that BEC alone cannot activate T cells [225]. In spite of the absence of B7 in BEC, aberrant expression of MHC II has been reported, likely mediated by the production of interferon gamma stimulated by the inflammatory process, finding that has led to the proposition that the incomplete ability to present antigens by BEC renders the exposed T cell anergic. T cell anergy is defined as a state of long-lasting, partial, or total unresponsiveness induced by partial activation [226]; anergic T cells operate like suppressor cells by interfering with the maturation and function of dendritic cells, interfering with the inflammatory process [226]; thus, the ability of the biliary epithelial cell to present antigen seems to contribute, at least in part, to the prevention of further inflammatory destruction in the complex CNSDC lesion of PBC. Vulnerability to a T cell-mediated inflammatory destruction of BEC, however, is increased by the expression of functional adhesion molecules by BEC, which attract cytotoxic T cells that can adhere to the biliary epithelium, susceptible to its inflammatory destruction [225]. Chemokines are cytokines that stimulate leukocytes movement and regulate their migration from blood to tissues [224]. A reason for T lymphocytes to be attracted to the biliary epithelium may also relate to the chemokine environment of the intrahepatic bile ducts in PBC. In this regard, BEC from patients with PBC and control subjects produce similar amounts of chemokines in response to appropriate challenges in vitro; however, chemokines expressed by BEC from patients with PBC have been reported to trigger enhanced transmigration of liver lymphocytes from patients with PBC, as compared to controls, in vitro [227]. Furthermore, the addition of autologous liver mononuclear cells to the experimental system has been associated with increased production of chemokines, suggesting that the BEC's inflammatory destruction in the CNSDC lesion of PBC is facilitated by local mononuclear cells [227]. Fractalkine (CX3C) is a chemokine that participates in controlling leukocyte trafficking in the endothelium; it has a soluble form and a membrane-bound form. Soluble fractalkine is a potent chemoattractant for T cells and monocytes. The membrane anchored form, induced on activated primary endothelial cells, promotes adhesion of the cells it attracts [228]. The receptor for fractalkine is CX3CR1, and it is expressed in mononuclear cells, including NK cells [229]. The soluble form of fractalkine (CX3CL1) was increased in the serum of patients with PBC and its receptor expressed in liver mononuclear cells [230]. Isolated BEC can produce CX3CL1 in response to Toll receptor ligands and at contact with autologous liver mononuclear cells, and in the presence of tumor necrosis factor (TNF) alpha in greater amounts than BEC from disease control livers [231]. In addition, the adherence of liver mononuclear cells from PBC livers to endothelial cells and BEC is stronger than that of mononuclear cells from disease control. Furthermore, activated T cells (CD 154+) and monocytes (CD 68+) have been found in the periportal inflammatory infiltrate, and the latter, infiltrating the biliary epithelium of bile ducts affected by the CNSDC of PBC, in contrast to their random presence in disease control liver samples [231]. Considering the limitations of in vitro studies, as they may not reproduce the disease state in vivo, and the anticipated differences in the hepatic inflammatory milieu in different stages of the disease (e.g., pre cirrhosis vs. cirrhosis), these reported findings suggest that there is a robust chemotactic milieu in the CNSDC of PBC that probably perpetuates the inflammatory destruction of BEC by attracting monocytes that have been stimulated by Toll receptor ligands, and that are transported into the liver by the portal blood flow, as has been proposed [231].

The presence of plasma cells expressing CD38 [232, 233] and intracellular IgM, IgG, or both, has been reported around bile ducts in the lesion of CNSDC of PBC, and not in disease control liver tissue; the presence of CD + 38 cells correlated with high serum AMA titers [220]. The existence of B cells in the lesion of CNSDC has suggested that immunological mechanisms related to this type of cell and humoral immunity [31, 179], including AMA, may be involved in the pathogenesis of the CNSDC of PBC [199, 201, 220]. Natural killer (NK) T cells express alpha beta TCRs that are restricted to cells expressing CD1. NKT cells recognize lipid antigens presented by CD1 molecules, including those associated with endocytosed microbes, which may give NK T cells a role in defense against pathogens, especially those rich in lipid components, including mycobacteria. The role of these cells in human disease is not clear; interestingly, however, is the report of an increase in the proportion of NK T cells in the blood and the liver of patients with PBC [205].

Natural killer (NK) cells are important components of the innate immune response. NK cells respond against intracellular viruses and bacteria. They are characterized by their membrane expression of CD 56 and have also been reported as increased in the blood and liver of patients with PBC and to have increased cytotoxic activity in vitro [234]. Toll like receptors (TLRs) are members of a family of pattern recognition receptors expressed on certain cell types and recognized microbe products [224]. In vitro and under specific stimulation paradigms that involved TLR 3 and 4, NK cells' cytotoxic activity from patients with PBC was reported to be higher than that of control cells [235]. These findings have been interpreted to support innate immunity mechanisms in the genesis of the CNSDC of PBC.

Processes inherent to cellular longevity have also been reported to contribute to the lesion of CNSDC of PBC, including apoptosis and autophagy, and senescence. Autophagy is a cellular process by which the cell balances energy and nutrients for basic cell functions, including the removal of misfolded proteins resulting from mutation or other pathological conditions, and the turnover of intracellular organelles including mitochondria, endoplasmic reticulum, and peroxisomes, under physiologic and pathological conditions [236, 237]. Autophagy is activated under stress, leading to autophagosomes, where organelles are sequestered and delivered to lysosomes by fusion, where they are digested to produce energy. Experiments performed in cultured epithelial cells have suggested that autophagy mediates the process of senescence of BEC [237]. Senescent BEC express senescent-associated secretory phenotypes (SASP) (e.g., chemokines (CCL2 and CX3CL1), which, in vitro, were reported to attract macrophages (i.e., RAW264.7 cells), suggesting that senescent cells may alter the microenvironment in which they exist [238]. Thus, autophagy, by increasing senescence and senescent epithelial cells, by attracting inflammatory cells through chemokines, may contribute to the CNSDC of PBC. In addition, endoplasmic reticulum stress may contribute to dysregulated biliary autophagy and subsequent senescence, as suggested by the enhanced expression of glucose-regulated protein 78 (GRP78) and protein disulfide isomerases (PDI), markers of ER stress, on BEC from patients with PBC versus control cells [239]. The anion exchanger 2 (AE2) protects the biliary epithelium from deleterious effects of minuscule concentrations of toxic bile acids by secreting bicarbonate into the bile duct lumen; it was reported that the expression of AE2 in the biliary epithelium of patients with PBC was decreased in association with dysregulated autophagy, abnormal expression of PDC-E2, and cellular senescence markers p16INK4a and p21WAF1/Cip1, which has suggested that lack of protection due to an impaired AE2 may result in dysregulated autophagy contributing to the pathogenesis of PBC [240]. It was recently reported that senescent BECs were significantly increased in small bile ducts in PBC, as suggested by the expression of senescent markers (p21$^{WAF1/Cip1}$, p16$^{INK4a}$) and B-cell lymphoma-extra large (Bcl-xL), an important regulator of senescent cell anti-apoptotic pathway, as compared to control hepatic tissue. Senescent BECs were notable in ductular reactions and stages 3 and 4 disease, versus stages 1 and 2 and control liver tissue. In addition, there was a correlation between the number of senescent BEDs in bile ductules with the stage of the disease and necroinflammatory activity, with the expression of p16 being correlated with suboptimal response to UDCA. These results tend to support a pathogenetic role of senescence of BECs in PBC, and that high degree of senescence impairs the response to UDCA [241].

An increased number of apoptotic BEC has been recognized in the lesion of CNSDC of PBC. Glutathionylation is a process through which the lysine-lipoic acid moiety is changed with glutathione during apoptosis. Glutathionylation prevents the accumulation of potentially autoreactive PDC-E2 and it is absent in BECs and in salivary gland epithelial cells, which may also be affected in PBC [242]. Lack of glutathionylation interferes with the process of apoptosis of BEC [173, 242], allowing PDC-E2 to remain intact; it is hypothesized that intact PDC-E2 is recognized by AMA, suggesting that apoptotic BECs can be a source of immunogenic PDC-E2 in PBC [173]. In a culture system where apoptosis was induced in BECs, intact PDC-E 2 within apoptotic blebs without permeabilization of the cell membrane was recognized by AMA from various sources, including sera from patients with PBC, suggesting that intracellular immunogenic PDC-E2 is accessible to immunological recognition [177]. Furthermore, it has been reported that BECs can themselves phagocytize apoptotic BEC [174] and present them to immunologically primed cells that recognize immunogenic intracellular components (e.g., PDC-E2) [174]. In this regard, the presence of CD4 and CD8 T cells that specifically react to the major antigen of AMA in PBC, PDC E2 163–176 suggests that T cells have been primed to react with this particular amino acid sequence, contributing importantly to the CNSDC of PBC. Additional phenotypic studies of peripheral CD 8+ cells in the blood of patients with PBC were reported to identify an increase in the number of CD45ROhighCD57+ CD8high T cells that expressed alpha4beta7, a gut homing integrin, supporting a role of adhesion in the inflammatory process of the CNSDC of PBC [243]. The expression of CD28 on the CD45ROhighCD57 + CD8high was decreased, suggesting a strong effector function [243, 244]. The CD45ROhigh subset of CD57 + CD8high group of cells was less susceptible to apoptosis [243]. The cells produced more IL-5 than the control cells; the relevance of IL-5 in PBC may relate, in part, to eosinophils, which can be increased in the serum of patients with PBC, and which are found in the lesion of CNSDC [202], a finding that provides confidence to the histological diagnosis of PBC. The presence of major basic protein in the lesion of CNSDC of PBC is consistent with eosinophils' activation and degranulation. Major basic protein also contributes to the differentiation of activated B cells into immunoglobulin producing cells [245], a relevant PBC finding. In this regard, serum concentrations of IL-5 have also been found to be increased in patients with PBC [246]. Immunohistochemistry studies of CD8+ cells from a small number of tissue samples from patients with PBC were reported to express CD57+, compared to control tissue; the cells from the diseased livers responded to stimulation with PDC-E2 with the secretion of interferon gamma, in contrast to the control cells [243]. These studies were interpreted to support a role of CD45ROhighCD57+ CD8high T cells, as terminally differentiated cytotoxic T effector memory T cells, in the pathogenesis of the CNSDC of PBC [243].

The maintenance of tolerance to self antigens depends on a balance between mechanisms that prevent the maturation of lymphocytes that have been sensitized to self antigens and those that prevent the destruction of self-reactive lymphocytes that have matured [216]. T cells play an important role in autoimmunity because they are involved in the regulation of immune responses to proteins, which comprise the majority of self antigens implicated in autoimmunity, and because of the integral role of the major histocompatibility complex (MHC), human lymphocyte antigen (HLA), which presents peptide antigens to T cells [216]. Breakdown of tolerance against self-antigens in T lymphocytes may be central in autoimmune mediated inflammatory tissular processes. In addition, abnormalities in helper T cells may be associated with autoantibody production, as helper T cells are required to produce antibodies against protein antigens [216]. Autoimmunity is considered to play a role in the pathogenesis of PBC [14].

In summary, PBC was described as a dry gland syndrome [247], as it can be associated with a reduction of tear and saliva production, presumably from inflammatory involvement of the epithelial structures of salivary and lacrimal glands, limited pancreatic secretions, and biliary cirrhosis from ductopenia due to specific injury of intrahepatic bile ducts. The latter is the fundamental pathogenetic process in PBC; thus, two central processes are the focus of research in PBC: the vulnerability of intrahepatic bile ducts to destruction and the development and potential role of AMA in the pathogenesis of the CNSDC of PBC. In this regard, the manner in which PDC-E2 is accessible to T cells may be related to the peculiar defect in glutathionylation of BEC, which, in the process of apoptosis, allows for PDC-E2 to remain intact in apoptotic blebs, or apotopes, and presumably, exposed for recognition by T cells [14, 173, 177]. The combined effect of macrophages from patients with PBC, biliary apotopes, and AMA can be associated with an important secretion of inflammatory cytokines [178], perpetuating inflammation.

# Treatment

The drugs approved for the treatment of PBC are ursodeoxycholic acid (URSO) and obeticholic acid (Ocaliva®). Although there is no cure, several drugs are being developed to treat PBC, including agonists at nuclear receptors and ileal bile acid transporter inhibitors.

The first drug approved for the treatment of PBC was ursodeoxycholic acid (URSO), the chemical name of which is 3α, 7ß-dihydroxy-5-cholan-24-oic acid. UDCA is a hydrophilic bile acid that comprises approximately 2% of the endogenous bile acid pool. The administration of UDCA changes the proportion of the bile acid pool from the hydrophobic profile of cholestasis to a hydrophilic one, thus decreasing the exposure of the hepatic cells to the toxic bile acid milieu. UDCA stimulates the insertion of bile salt export pump (BSEP) and multidrug resistance associated protein 2 (MRP2) in the canalicular side of the hepatocyte thus, stimulating the export of bile acids by the former and organic anions by the latter, giving it choleretic properties; also, UDCA has been reported to prevent hepatocyte apoptosis induced by bile acids [248]. Perisinusoidal fibrosis and degree of apoptosis were lower in liver tissues from patients with PBC in association with UDCA treatment for 2 years than in the liver tissue from the group of patients treated with placebo, in which the number of apoptotic cells increased [249]. The dose recommended for the treatment of PBC is 13–15 mg/kg of body weight, in divided doses, taken with meals. It is generally well tolerated. In some patients, the use of UDCA is associated with pruritus, which is a major inconvenience to those patients who already have pruritus from the disease. Another matter is an average of 3.6 kg weight gain over the first year of treatment that remained stable for the 4 years reported in the study [250]. UDCA may be injurious in patients with decompensated liver disease, i.e., Child's B and C, in regard to liver injury, a likelihood score of D, i.e., a possible rare cause of acute decompensation of preexisting liver disease. The mechanism of liver injury is described as possibly related to choleresis and not intrinsic or idiosyncratic reaction to the drug itself [251]. The guidelines from the American Association for the Study of Liver Disease report that UDCA should be used in all stages of the disease; however, its use in decompensation is not addressed [3]. Vigilance is required if UDCA is used in patients with advanced disease by providing close follow-up.

A combined analysis of three controlled clinical trials of UDCA for the treatment of PBC revealed that the use of the drug had been associated with an increase in the time free of liver transplantation in patients with stages III and IV disease, as compared to the patients who had been randomized to placebo at the time of initiation of the study; it was inferred that a survival advantage was not demonstrated in the group of patients with stages I and II because the duration of the studies was limited to 4 years, which would not allow for the natural history of the disease to reveal itself [20]. Combined analysis of available paired liver biopsies from participants, 200 randomized to UDCA and 167 to placebo, from four clinical trials, revealed a lack of difference in the progression of the histological stage between the two groups; however, in the group of patients with disease stages I and II, there was a significant decrease in the progression of the disease, as compared to the group of patients that had taken the placebo. There was a substantial halt in the progression of periportal inflammation and bile ductular proliferation in the UDCA group relative to the placebo group. These results were interpreted to support the use of UDCA for patients with stages I and II of PBC [252]. In contrast, the review of paired liver biopsies from patients with PBC who participated in a placebo controlled study of

UDCA revealed that the prevalence of the florid bile duct lesion that characterizes PBC was 36%; on treatment, the prevalence of the florid duct lesion decreased by 16.6% in the group that had been assigned to placebo, and by 14.5% in the group that had been assigned to UDCA, after 2 years of treatment [253]. These results were interpreted to suggest that the salutary effect of UDCA in patients with PBC is related to the consequences of cholestasis and not on the primary bile duct injury that characterizes this disease [253]. Although the serum activity of liver associated enzymes is not an accurate reflection of disease activity, UDCA treatment is associated with a decrease in the activity of AP in two-thirds of the patients but not with the prevention of the CNSDC of PBC. Immunosuppressants (e.g., azathioprine, cyclosporine, steroids, methotrexate), anti-inflammatory drugs (e.g., colchicine, sulindac), cuprouretic (e.g., D-penicillamine), and fibrates [254, 255] have been studied in the treatment of PBC. Most drugs have been associated with a decrease in the serum activity of AP but no impact on the natural history of the disease, as measured by time to referral for liver transplantation. It can be argued that time to liver transplantation, or liver death, is a final endpoint that does not address the effect that a drug may have on the CNSDC of PBC or the effects of cholestasis resulting from ductopenia. This might have been the case of methotrexate, which was found to decrease the inflammatory infiltrate of the CNSDC of PBC in patients with early disease but no effect on disease progression in a pilot study [256]. However, these results contrast to those of another pilot study that tested the combination of methotrexate and UDCA and compared its effect with results from a historical placebo controlled study of UDCA; in their analysis, there was no evidence of increased fibrosis or differences in portal inflammation with combination therapy, as compared with the results from the placebo controlled study of UDCA [257]. The use of methotrexate in combination with UDCA versus placebo and UDCA studied in the multicenter trial for 7.6 years did not demonstrate a therapeutic advantage, defined as time to referral to liver transplantation, and complications from liver disease. The effects of the combination therapy on the liver histology have not been published; this information would still be helpful, as it would reveal the impact of the drug on the CNSDC lesion and other histological features of PBC, especially in a stratified analysis of patients with stages I and II versus stages III and IV PBC [258]. In this regard, a publication of the long-term follow-up of patients who had been treated with the combination of UDCA and methotrexate in a randomized controlled trial that had lasted 10 years reported that 9 of the 11 patients who had taken methotrexate and UDCA were well and that the two deaths that had occurred were not related to liver disease [259]. Thus, the effect of combination therapy with UDCA and methotrexate on the CNSDC, which is what drives the disease, remains unknown.

Analyses of clinical trial data on the effect of various drugs including azathioprine [260–262], D-penicillamine [263–265], colchicine [266–268], cyclosporine [269–271], chlorambucil [272], prednisolone [273, 274], and methotrexate [256, 275] have provided limited, encouraging results, or insufficient therapeutic advantage for the disease, as evidenced by the lack of approval for or standard use in the treatment of PBC. In a controlled study, prednisolone was associated with a better outcome in regards to liver disease than the placebo after three years of treatment, with no strong evidence of increased bone loss, which had been a concern at the one year mark; thus, the use of prednisolone, perhaps at small doses, in pre-cirrhotic disease, may remain a treatment option [273, 274].

Reports of individual studies of variable sample sizes have reported beneficial effects of UDCA on PBC, including a lower predicted risk of death, as per the Mayo model, as compared to a group treated with placebo for comparable periods [276], halting the progression of the disease [277], and exerting delay in the development of esophageal varices [278]. Analysis of 262 patients who received UDCA for 8 years was reported to reveal an overall survival rate of 92% at 10 years and 82% and 20 years. The survival rate without liver transplantation was 84% at 10 years and 66% at 20 years, both of which were lower than a control group matched for gender and age. However, the use of UDCA was associated with improved survival over what was predicted by the Mayo score. The probability of death or liver transplantation was increased in patients with advanced disease. However, survival in patients with disease stages I and II was similar to that of the control population [279]. Patients who responded to treatment of UDCA with a decrease in the serum activity of AP by 40%, defined as a response in the analysis, as compared to baseline, or normal activity after 1 year of treatment, had higher survival than that predicted by the Mayo score, and similar to the estimated survival of the control population; these findings were in contrast to that of the group of patients who had not responded to UDCA, which had lower survival than that of the control population, but higher than that estimated by the Mayo model. It was suggested that patients who do not respond to UDCA, as defined in this analysis, constitute a group for which alternate therapies should be developed and studied [280]. A stable or a decrease in the portohepatic pressure gradient after 2 years on UDCA and a normalization in AST activity predicted improved survival free of liver transplantation, survival being similar to a control population at 15 years [281]. The role of UDCA in the prolongation of survival without liver transplantation in patients with PBC seems equivocal [22, 280, 282]; the report of the analysis of 16 studies that evaluated the effect of UDCA versus placebo or no intervention did not document a therapeutic advantage of the drug on the disease. UDCA did not have an impact on mortality or liver transplantation; in addition, the analysis did not report an ameliorating effect on pruritus or fatigue, or histology [283]. Combination therapies that include UDCA have also been studied in patients with PBC. UDCA and budesonide, a glucocorticoid preparation, was reported as favorable, including a decrease in the histological score [284, 285]. UDCA with prednisone and azathioprine was reported in association with improvement, including disease stage and fibrosis [286]. UDCA with colchicine or methotrexate was reported to be associated with sustained clinical remission [259], or significant reduction of disease progression in a study that enrolled patients with advanced disease and pruritus [287]. In regard to the latter, however, a large randomized placebo controlled study of methotrexate and UDCA was stopped for reasons of futility [258]; in addition, an analysis of a large database reported increased mortality in patients who took methotrexate alone or in combination with other drugs [288].

Obeticholic acid (OCA) is a derivative of chenodeoxycholic acid with marked agonist activity at the farnesoid X receptor. It is approved for the treatment of patients with PBC alone if UDCA is not well tolerated, which is uncommon and related mostly to diarrhea and pruritus in some patients [3] or in combination with UDCA for patients who have not achieved an optimal response to the latter. It has been associated with liver failure and death in patients with decompensated liver disease; thus, the drug is contraindicated in patients with decompensated decompensated cirrhosis (e.g., Child-Pugh Class B or C) or history of a decompensating event, and in patients with esophageal varices and thrombocytopenia, because of portal hypertension [289].

In a randomized, placebo controlled study of 1 year duration that included 217 patients with suboptimal response to UDCA or intolerability to the drug, OCA at doses of 10 mg and 5 to be escalated to 10 mg versus placebo was studied in patients with PBC. The majority of the patients received UDCA concomitantly with the study drug. OCA was associated with a decrease in serum activity of AP to less than 1.67 the upper limit of normal, the primary endpoint of the trial, in 46% (5 to 10 mg dose) and 47% of patients (10 mg dose) versus the response to placebo, which was observed in 10%, a significantly different finding, as well as total serum bilirubin concentrations, which decreased significantly more by fractions of deciliters in association with the drug versus placebo. Indirect measures of fibrosis, including kilopascals by transient elastography and enhanced liver fibrosis score, did not change significantly in any of the groups. Consistent with the expected effect of the drug, there was a reported dose-dependent increase of FGF-19 and a decrease in serum bile acid levels not observed in the placebo treated group. Pruritus, as previously stated, was reported by 56% and 68% of the patients in association with OCA at doses of 5 mg to escalate to 10 mg and at doses of 10 mg per day, respectively, in contrast to the 38% in association with placebo [290]. A follow-up randomized, double blind, placebo controlled study that included 165 patients with PBC who had not responded adequately to UDCA reported that at daily doses of 10 mg, 25 mg, or 50 mg in combination with UDCA versus placebo, OCA was associated with a decrease in serum AP activity that ranged from 21% to 25% in association with the drug, versus a reduction of 3% in the placebo group for the duration of the study, which was 85 days; the activities of GGTP, AST, and ALT decreased concomitantly also in association with the drug. Pruritus was reported by 47%, 87%, and 80% of the subjects randomized to each of OCA doses, respectively, and by 50% of the subjects randomized to placebo. At the time of the publication, it was reported that serum AP continued to decrease over the extension part of the study that went on for 1 year [291]. A study that explored the effects of OCA as monotherapy reported that at daily doses of 10 mg in 20 patients, and 50 mg in 16, versus placebo in 23 for 3 months documented a significant decreased activity of AP by 53.9%, 37.2%, and 0.8%, respectively, which was sustained in an open label phase over 6 years. The concentration of direct bilirubin, serum IgM, and the serum activities of GGTP, AST, and ALT also decreased over time in association with OCA [292]. After 3 years of treatment, liver histology in the 17 patients who had had a baseline biopsy was reported to show a decrease or stabilization of fibrosis, ductular reaction, interface hepatitis, and lobular hepatitis, and a reduction in the fibrosis composite score, and collagen features assessed by morphometry [52, 293]. OCA is not recommended in decompensated liver disease. OCA was associated with further decompensation of liver disease and several deaths reported in association with inappropriate dosing; a likelihood score of C was given to this occurrence, i.e. "a suspected rare cause of clinically apparent liver injury occurring mostly in patients with preexisting cirrhosis" [251, 289]. The marked pruritus in association with OCA may reveal clues to the pathogenesis of the pruritus of cholestasis.

The treatment of hypercholesterolemia with clofibrate was associated with a marked increase in serum cholesterol and the novo formation of cholesterol stones several months after discontinuation of therapy [294]; this observation, reported in 1975, led to the recommendation not to use this drug to treat hypercholesterolemia in patients with PBC [295]. Clofibrate was discontinued from the market in 2002 because of side effects, including deaths from noncardiovascular conditions during treatment, in spite of a decrease in coronary heart disease [296, 297]. Drugs that decrease triglycerides and increase HDL–cholesterol without decreasing LDL concentrations, including the PPAR receptor activators bezafibrate, fenofibrate, and gemfibrozil, are associated with a decrease in coronary artery disease [298]. The potential effect of stimulation of the PPAR-alpha activator by bezafibrate, a receptor pan agonist [299] in PBC, alone in four patients, and in combination with UDCA in seven, was explored in an open label study that documented a decrease in symptoms (i.e., fatigue and pruritus), a decrease in serum activity of AP activity in all the patients, and a reduction in the serum concentration of IgM in some [300]. Several clinical trials on the use of fibrates for the treatment of PBC have been conducted [301–305], including a double blind randomized placebo controlled study of 2-year duration that evaluated the effect of bezafibrate at a dose of 400 mg/day, versus placebo in patients who had not responded optimally to UDCA, which continued to be administered during the study. Bezafibrate, in combination with UDCA, was associated with normalization of liver associated enzymes, bilirubin, albumin, and a measure of prothrombin time, which was the primary endpoint, in 31% of patients in contrast to those in the placebo arm, none of whom had that response. It was reported that serum AP became normal in 67% of patients randomized to the study drug, and only in 2% of those randomized to placebo. Pruritus, fatigue, and fibrosis markers improved and decreased, respectively, in the study group [306]. Seladelpar, a selective PPAR-δ agonist, was studied at two doses in patients with PBC with inadequate response to UDCA in a double-blind, randomized, placebo-controlled study, qualified as proof of concept [307]; the study was terminated because of hepatitis in association with the drug in some patients, however, the five patients who completed 5 weeks of treatment exhibited normalization of serum AP activity. Pruritus was reported as a side effect more frequently in association with the drug than with placebo. It was concluded that seladelpar should be studied at lower doses than those tested in the proof of concept trial [307]. Indeed, preliminary results on the use of seladelpar at doses lower than those from the prior study [307, 308] and elafibranor [309], a PPAR alpha/delta agonist, have suggested that both drugs are associated with decreased serum activity of AP and no major side effects in controlled studies. The reader is referred to clinicaltrials.com to view studies on PBC.

Fifteen studies from North America and long-term follow-up studies from Europe of patients with PBC were used as the data source for a meta-analysis to identify predictors of survival. Of 4845 participants, 1118 met a study endpoint, i.e., death or need for liver transplantation, with a median follow-up of 7.3 years. Seventy percent of patients survived for 10 years. The serum activity of AP two times the upper limit of normal was the best predictor of survival. Patients with serum activity of AP equal or less than two times the upper limit of normal (ULN) was the best predictor of survival, with 84% surviving at 10 years, versus 62% for those whose AP activity was greater than two times the ULN ($p < 0.0001$). A serum bilirubin one time the ULN was the best predictor of survival free from liver transplantation at 1 year. 86% of patients with serum bilirubin of less than one time the ULN survived 10 years from the time of entry into the studies versus 41% of those with serum bilirubin greater than one time the ULN, which was significantly different. The combination of serum AP activity and serum bilirubin was the best predictor of survival. It was concluded from this meta-analysis that serum activity of AP and bilirubin can predict liver transplantation or death in patients with PBC and suggested that these factors be used in clinical trials as surrogate endpoints [310]. Most clinical trials published in peer-reviewed journals or in abstract form use serum activity of AP as endpoints; little information is available on liver histology in association with experimental drugs for the treatment of PBC.

In an international collaboration, a scoring system termed the GLOBE score was developed to predict transplant free survival in patients with PBC treated with UDCA [311]. The score includes age at which UDCA was started and the following variables after 1 year of UDCA treatment, AP, total bilirubin, albumin, and platelet count. The GLOBE score uses age-specific thresholds beyond which survival significantly deviates from an age- and sex matched general population. In subgroups of patients aged less than 45 years and from 45–52, 52–58, 58–66, and at least 66 years, age-specific GLOBE-score thresholds beyond which survival significantly deviates from matched individuals are 0.52, 0.01, 0.60, 1.01, and 1.69, respectively. The UK-PBC score uses baseline albumin platelet count, bilirubin, transaminases, and AP after 12 months of UDCA to calculate survival [312]. The reader is referred to. UK-PBC. com for information on this study group and to calculate the UK-PBC score. A recent study documented that the GLOBE and the UK-scores were also good predictors of complications from cirrhosis in patients with PBC on UDCA [313].

# Treatment of Complications of PBC

## *Pruritus*

The approach to a patient with PBC and pruritus requires the exclusion of conditions associated with pruritus (e.g., skin diseases, malignancies), which can contribute to the pruritus of cholestasis or be the cause of the pruritus. Once it has been established that the patient is experiencing the pruritus of cholestasis, several therapeutic interventions to treat the pruritus specifically can be implemented.

The treatment of the pruritus of cholestasis can be divided into two types of interventions: (i) those that treat the disease itself, i.e., if cholestasis decreases as a result of a salutary effect of a given medication or transplant, in cases of intractable pruritus, and (ii) those that treat the sensation of pruritus. The subject of pruritus is covered in Chap. 15 of this book.

UDCA has not been studied in controlled clinical trials specifically to assess its effect on the pruritus. The choleretic effect of UDCA [248] may have some beneficial impact on the pruritus by the presumed enhanced biliary excretion of pruritogen(s); however, evidence from controlled studies of UDCA for the treatment of PBC does not support an antipruritic effect of UDCA in this disease [314]; thus, specific antipruritic interventions need to be prescribed. OCA does not ameliorate the pruritus; in fact, it is one of its side effects.

## Fatigue

Central [315] and peripheral [316] mechanisms have been considered to contribute to the pathophysiology of fatigue in PBC. Treatment with UDCA has not been reported to have an impact on the degree of fatigue in patients with PBC. Specific treatments for fatigue have to be developed [283]. The reader is referred to Chap. 15, where fatigue is addressed.

## Sicca Symptoms

The treatment of sicca symptoms is the humidification of mucous and ocular membranes to halt the damage caused by decreased exocrine secretion of the respective glands. Components of artificial tears, the initial treatment of dry eyes, include hydroxypropyl methylcellulose and carboxymethylcellulose and can be used as needed over the day. Tear hyperosmolarity is a common characteristic among all the forms of dry eyes [317]. In this context, the use of hyposmolar (150 mOsm/L) 0.4% sodium hyaluronate eye drops was associated with significant improvement in the global discomfort index for ocular symptoms, tear production, and epithelial healing sooner than that associated with isotonic preparation [318]. Evolving evidence suggests that the pathophysiology of dry eye concerns local inflammation, in addition to a decrease in tear production; in this context, anti-inflammatory and immunosuppressant agents have been used to treat dry eyes [319]. Cyclosporine ophthalmic emulsion, a prescription product approved for the treatment of dry eyes [319], was associated with a significant increase in tear production compared to placebo in controlled clinical trials [319]. In cases refractory to drugs, blocking the puncta to prevent draining of tears can be performed in combination with artificial tears [320]. General measures to improve eye care include frequent blinking, protection of the eyes from air currents, humidification of the household environment, and avoidance of smoking and smoky rooms [321, 322]. Referral to ophthalmology is recommended.

The dramatic presentation of PBC with rampant dental caries has been reported in a patient with severe symptoms of Sjogren's syndrome [323]. General measures to improve oral health in patients with sicca symptoms include regular visits to the dentist, mouth rinsing with water, the use of fluoride containing toothpaste, daily flossing, and avoidance of sugar between meals. Chewing sugar-free gum and hard candy can stimulate saliva production, and the use of oil or petroleum based lip balm or lipstick can decrease oral dryness [324]. Saliva substitutes are recommended for patients with xerostomia [325]. Irrigation of parotid glands with prednisolone solution of 2 mg/ml over several sessions was associated with a significant increase in salivary flow rate compared to saline irrigation in patients with primary and secondary Sjogren's syndrome in an open label study [326]. Cholinergic agents, such as pilocarpine and cevimeline, are the cornerstone of current therapy in Sjogren's syndrome [327, 328]. Dysphagia can be associated with xerostomia in patients with PBC [329]; interventions to increase saliva production and improve the process of mastication can be recommended [329].

Oral candidiasis can be a complication of dry mouth, and it requires specific antifungal medications.

Vaginal dryness can contribute to the sicca symptom complex. Vaginal moisturizers are helpful, but vaginal lubricants are not recommended for routine use because they are not moisturizers; a review on the management of complications of Sjogren's syndrome, including vaginal dryness, is referenced [330]. Estrogen creams have specific indications and should only be used under the direction of a gynecologist.

Itching from dry skin may complicate the sicca symptom complex, which can worsen the quality of life of patients already suffering from pruritus. Dry skin can be treated with heavy moisturizing creams and ointments.

## *Osteoporosis*

The development of osteoporosis in patients with PBC seems to be related to the degree of cholestasis and end-stage liver disease [331, 332]. The National Osteoporosis Foundation has provided guidelines for daily vitamin D and calcium supplements, as necessary.

Several pharmacological interventions have been studied in clinical trials of various designs in patients with PBC, including fluoride [333], calcitonin [334], UDCA [257], the bisphosphonates etidronate [335], alendronate [335, 336], and clodronate [337], vitamin K2 [338], and estrogens [339, 340]. UDCA was not associated with improvement in bone mineral density in a randomized controlled study [341], and in two studies of different designs, calcitonin was associated with no effect on bone mass in one [334] and with the stability of bone mass in another one [342]. All other interventions have been associated with either improvement or stability in bone mass density; however, the trials have few patients, and the results do not allow for strong recommendations on the use of most of the drugs studied. The use of estrogens alone or in combination with progestin, and with or without vitamin D and calcium, has been reported in a few publications to be associated with protection from bone loss in patients with PBC. In one of the studies, which was placebo controlled, that included 31 postmenopausal women with PBC and low bone mass as measured by T scores at the lumbar and femoral sites, it was reported that two new fractures were diagnosed in the placebo group, which comprised of 15 patients, in contrast to none in the treatment group, which comprised of 16 [343]. The studies on estrogen replacement therapy provided temporary encouragement on the use of this type of medication to treat osteoporosis in patients with PBC albeit the small number of patients studied and the limited duration of the studies [340, 343, 344]; however, the results from the Heart and Estrogen/Progestin Replacement Study (II) [345] and subsequently from the Women's Health Initiative Randomized Controlled Trial [346] revealed that estrogen replacement was not associated with salutary effects [345]. Estrogens, therefore, cannot be recommended to prevent bone loss in patients at risk, including those with PBC [345]. In this context, an alternative mechanism in estrogen therapy, estrogen receptor modulation [347] with the drug raloxifene has been explored [348]. Raloxifene was evaluated in an open label pilot study of nine patients with PBC, seven of whom completed the 1 year study [348]. In this trial, raloxifene was associated with a nonsignificant increase in the median value of lumbosacral spine bone density compared to baseline values, in contrast to stable values for the control group. No side effects were reported at short term [348].

Bisphosphonates, including alendronate and risedronate, are derivatives of pyrophosphate that bind to the bone surface and inhibit bone resorption by osteoclasts [349]. These drugs have a significant antifracture effect at several sites, including the spine and hip. Bisphosphonates have also been studied in patients with bone disease and PBC. Etidronate was not associated with a significant improvement in bone density in patients with PBC and bone disease [350]. Alendronate, in contrast, was reported to be associated with an increase in bone mass and to have greater antiresorptive activity than etidronate, another bisphosphonate, in patients with PBC and osteopenia [335]; however, alendronate was not associated with the prevention of new bone fractures [335]. An increase in bone mass density was also associated with alendronate 70 mg per orally per week for 1 year, in a placebo-controlled study in patients with PBC, all of whom were maintained on 1000 mg of calcium and 5000 units of vitamin D supplementation per week, and most of whom were also taking estrogen replacement therapy [336]. The use of sodium clodronate, a bisphosphonate derivative, at doses of 100 mg every 10 days intramuscularly, in combination with 1000 mg calcium carbonate and 880 IU of vitamin D3 daily by mouth did not improve bone disease, but it was associated with a decrease in bone loss in patients who were not receiving estrogen replacement therapy [351]. These results may suggest that bisphosphonates or their derivatives may have a role in the prevention of bone disease in postmenopausal women with PBC [351]; however, a publication that reported on what was defined as a comprehensive database search from inception to early 2017 reported that none of the studies demonstrated a significant improvement in bone health, including reduction of fractures [352]; the small number of patients per study was reported as a limiting factor. Thus, the development of medications to treat bone disease in PBC has not been met; in this regard, from a pilot study that included six post-menopausal patients with PBC, all on UDCA therapy (and four with autoimmune hepatitis) with osteoporosis, aged between 59 and 79 years who had not been exposed to bisphosphonates, it was reported that the use of subcutaneous denosumab at a dose of 60 mg every 6 months for at least 36 months for the treatment of osteoporosis was associated with increased bone mineral density, in the absence of side effects, in association with a reduction of serum concentration of TRACP-5b, a bone resorption marker, and ALP3, suggesting that the drug decreased bone turnover [353]. Denosumab is a human monoclonal antibody against the receptor activator of nuclear factor-dB ligand (RANKL), which increases bone mineral density (BMD) by inhibiting the development and activity of osteoclasts, thus decreasing bone resorption [353]. The investigators concluded that long-term controlled studies were warranted to confirm these results [353]. A letter to the editor that referenced this publication stated that denosumab could exert effects on PBC beyond bone health. In this context, SNP analyses have identified the RANKL gene near a novel locus associated with a genetic predisposition to PBC; in addition, the RANK-RANKL axis was proposed to contribute to the pathogenesis of PBC as BEC express RANK and the inflammatory infiltrate associated with bile duct injury is rich in cells expressing RANKL, which correlated with disease severity. It was suggested that RANK attracts RANKL, exacerbating the inflammatory process; thus, the authors hypothesized that the use of denosumab might offer a beneficial therapeutic effect in PBC beyond that reported for osteoporosis by preventing the action of RANKL [354]. This interesting hypothesis is likely to be tested in clinical studies.

The participation of men with PBC in studies addressing the effect of medications on bone disease has been very limited [336]; it is necessary, however, to consider that osteoporosis can be a complication of cirrhosis in men, thus encouraging their participation would be important.

## Complications Secondary to Chronic Scratching

Excoriations and prurigo nodularis may result from chronic scratching in patients with chronic pruritus. Any of the lesions that result from chronic scratching can get secondarily infected, in which case specific antibiotic treatment is indicated.

## Cholelithiasis

The prevalence of cholelithiasis in patients with cirrhosis is higher than that of the general population [355]. In a series that included 23 patients with PBC, 39% were found to have gallstones [356]. The effect of UDCA, a treatment approved for PBC, specifically on the incidence of gallstones in this disease, has not been published.

## Xanthomata and Xanthelasmata

PBC is associated with hyperlipidemia of unique features (see above). Patients with PBC can have xanthomata and xanthelasmata, which consist of foam cells laden with lipids that appear as circumscribed lesions in the skin's connective tissue, tendons, or fasciae [357]. They are termed xanthelasmata when their location is in the periorbital area. Xanthomata tend to result from relatively extreme and chronic hyperlipidemia and were described in the publications related to PBC in the 1940s when it was hypothesized that in association with a decrease in "biliary obstruction," the xanthomata would disappear. In addition, xanthomatous neuropathy can be a complication of PBC. A series comprised of 18 patients reported that 15 had xanthomata (83%), and of these, eight had them on the face (i.e., xanthelasmata) [358]. Plasmapheresis was associated with decreased xanthomata and neuropathic pain (and pruritus) in association with plasmapheresis [359]. Severe symptoms from xanthomata resolved after liver transplantation in a patient with generalized painful xanthomata [360].

## Complications from Liver Disease from PBC

The complications of cirrhosis from PBC include those secondary to cirrhosis from any etiology, including complications of portal hypertension, and hepatic synthetic dysfunction. Two complications, portal hypertension and hepatocellular carcinoma (HCC), merit discussion here, as they have certain peculiarities in PBC.

## Portal Hypertension

Patients with PBC may develop portal hypertension as a result of biliary cirrhosis, or in the pre-cirrhotic stage of the disease [361–363], in association with focal nodular hyperplasia [361–363], and a postulated obstruction to portal venous flow at a presinusoidal level possibly from portal inflammation [363]. The approach to gastroesophageal varices and variceal hemorrhage in cirrhosis in patients with PBC follows the guidelines published by the American Association for the Study of Liver Disease (AASLD) [364]. Salient points of those recommendations include a screening upper endoscopy when the diagnosis of cirrhosis is made [364]. The published report from the Single Topic conference of portal hypertension sponsored by the AASLD [365] stated that a platelet count of 140,000/mm$^3$ correlated with the presence of varices hence, an indication of upper endoscopy; this number has been changed to 150,000/mm$^3$ in the most recent guidance [364]. However, a published retrospective review of data from 236 patients, 79 of whom had PBC suggested that a platelet count of less than 200,000/mm$^3$, a serum albumin concentration of less than 4.0 g/dl, or serum bilirubin greater than 1.7 mg/dl predicted the presence of esophageal varices on upper endoscopy [366] in patients with PBC, suggesting that screening upper endoscopies may need to be done earlier in these patients than in patients with liver disease from other etiologies. If no varices are documented at the index endoscopy, it is recommended in the guidelines that the procedure be repeated in 2 years [364]. The management of variceal bleeding in patients with cirrhosis secondary to PBC also follows the gastroesophageal varices and variceal hemorrhage in cirrhosis guidelines published by the AASLD [364]. Variceal bleeding that does not respond to pharmacological and endoscopic therapy in patients with PBC in the pre-cirrhotic stage poses a specific challenge, as orthotopic liver transplantation is not desirable in patients with good synthetic liver function [367]. In this context, a transjugular intrahepatic portosystemic shunt (TIPS) or a distal splenorenal shunt, which does not deprive the liver of its blood supply, can be therapeutic alternative [368]. This type of shunt was not associated with accelerated liver failure in patients with PBC who underwent surgery to treat variceal bleeding [368].

Bleeding from esophageal varices in patients with PBC whose bilirubin was less than 2 mg/dl had better survival than patients with advanced disease, especially those of a certain age, who had ascites and hepatic encephalopathy, as expected [369]. The general approach to patients with portal hypertension is described in Chap. 15 of this book.

## *Hepatocellular Carcinoma*

The incidence of hepatocellular carcinoma (HHC) was reported to range from 0.7 to 3.8% in patients with PBC, and more commonly in patients who did not respond to treatment with UDCA, from a total of 375 after a median follow-up of 9.7 years [370]; advanced stage was associated with an increase in the risk for HCC, with an odds ratio of 5.8, with a confidence interval of 2.34–14.38 in an analysis from patients from Italy and Spain [371]. Portal hypertension and history of blood transfusions were identified as risk factors for the development of hepatocellular carcinoma in patients with PBC, in a retrospective study, identifying these features as potentially useful in developing some scoring system to develop screening guidelines specifically for PBC [372]. For now, all cirrhotic patients should be surveyed for HCC every 6 months with a liver sonogram and alpha fetoprotein.

## *Hepatic Synthetic Dysfunction*

Liver failure from PBC is an indication for liver transplantation. As reported in 2007, analysis from the United Network for Organ Sharing database throughout 1995 to 2006 indicated that there is a decrease in the number of liver transplants done in the USA because of PBC, with a reported decrease by five per year [373]; also, the indication for liver transplantation for PBC in 2008 according to the United Network for Organ Sharing database was 5%. According to the European Liver Transplant Registry report from 2008, liver transplantation for PBC comprised 10% of those operations, in contrast to over 50% in the initial years of implementing this practice. The experience from Europe is similar with a reported decrease in liver transplantation for PBC over the years of 1988 to 2006; this is likely a reflection of the reported change in the natural history of the disease in association with UDCA or the fact that patients are being diagnosed earlier than in the past, and, as years go by before patients meet transplantation criteria, there will be a lag between the need for transplant to the procedure itself. In regards to the timing for transplantation, bilirubin is the most important prognostic factor in PBC. In a landmark publication, it was reported that serum bilirubin over 2 mg/dl 6 months apart defined the late phase of the disease, which was characterized by a period of a rapid increase in this marker [374]. If the serum bilirubin reached 6 mg/dl, the survival time was calculated to be 25 months, and if it was 10 g/dl in two successive 6 month periods, the survival time was 17 months. The rapidity with which the bilirubin increases was identified as prognostic, with a rise of 2.5 mg/dl/year in the patients who died [374]. The importance of serum bilirubin was confirmed in the era of UCDA [375], and it should continue to be interpreted as an invaluable prognostic factor. In an analysis from a group of over 500 patients who had participated in clinical trials, survival without liver transplantation was estimated to be increased in association with normalization of serum bilirubin in the group of patients that took UDCA for at least 6 months, as compared to the group that took the placebo. Survival without liver transplantation was estimated to be not significantly different in the group that took UDCA, and that normalized the serum bilirubin versus the group that took the placebo and that had had normal serum bilirubin at baseline. The relative risk of death or liver transplantation was 6 for the group of patients that had taken UDCA and 5.7 for the group that had taken the placebo [375]. Various models have been developed to predict survival and the need for liver transplantation, including that of patients with PBC [376–378]. The Mayo Model predicts survival [379–381]. The variables are the patient's age, total serum bilirubin and serum albumin concentrations, prothrombin time, and severity of edema. The prognostic index R is calculated by the following equation: $R = 0.871 \times \log e$ (bilirubin[mg/dl] $- 2.53 \times \log e$ (albumin[g/

dl]) + 0.039 × age (years) + 2.38 × log e (prothrombin time[s]) + 0.859 edema (0 = no edema, no diuretic therapy, 0.5 = edema, no diuretic therapy or no edema, diuretic therapy; 1 = edema and diuretic therapy); the application of this model predicted survival intra and extramurally from the developing institution [379–381]. The initial experience with the Mayo Model suggested that the risk of death after liver transplantation was high when the score reached 7.8 and suggested this number to be the optimal time for the operation. In association with the development of the Mayo score, patients were transplanted at an earlier stage than prior to the availability of the model; post transplantation, the probability of survival was 93, 90, and 88 percentages at 1, 2, and 5 years. At present, the Model for End Stage Liver Disease (MELD) score is used to determine priority for liver transplantation, including patients with PBC [382, 383]. A MELD score of 15 is an indication for referral to liver transplantation; however, the referral can be made when the score is greater than 10 to allow for relationships to develop with the transplant team. For PBC, in general, recommendations to refer to liver transplantation are [383]:

1. plasma bilirubin concentration is greater than 5 mg/dL and is increasing
2. the serum albumin concentration is below 2.8 g/dL (28 g/L) and is decreasing
3. signs of decompensation or portal hypertension develop, such as ascites, variceal bleeding, coagulopathy malnutrition, or encephalopathy
4. the patient has intractable pruritus
5. the patient has recurrent, debilitating, nontraumatic bone fractures

Survival after liver transplantation for PBC has been reported to be 88% at 5 years in a large center from the USA [384] and 80% from a comparable large experience in England [385]. Death after liver transplantation was reported to be 25.5%; 60% of patients died within 6 months from sepsis and multisystem organ failure [385]. The number of liver transplantations for PBC has declined over the past 30 years, with the proportion of liver transplantations significantly decreasing from 20% in 1986 to 4% in 2015 from a study conducted in Europe [383].

Acute rejection occurs in 46% to 50% of patients with PBC post liver transplantation; it usually responds to immunosuppression. Chronic rejection has been reported to occur in 2–9% of patients, being more common when cyclosporine was used instead of tacrolimus [386].

Liver transplantation is associated with significant improvement in the quality of life in patients with PBC, although aspects of physical activity remain impaired as compared to control subjects [387].

PBC recurs in the graft at a reported rate from 9% to 35% [388, 389]. The diagnosis is made by histology, as AMA persist in the serum after transplantation, and liver profile may not be normal after liver transplantation, making it difficult to use the criteria for probable disease [2]. HLA mismatches do not seem to be associated with recurrence [390]. The use of cyclosporine and azathioprine has been reported to be associated with protection from recurrence of disease in the graft [391]. Disease recurrence has been reported to increase in association with a graft with fibrosis and fat [392]. The natural history of recurrent PBC seems to be characterized by slow progression and infrequent loss of graft [391].

In summary, PBC is a rare disease; however, clinicians evaluating patients with a liver profile suggestive of cholestasis must generate a liver disease workup to exclude this disease, to identify it early. The treatment of PBC is UDCA, and obeticholic acid as an added treatment, in patients who have not responded optimally to the former, if the patient has compensated disease; however, other options must be explored as there is no cure for the disease. The frequency of follow-up depends on the severity of the disease. Referral for liver transplantation when the bilirubin is 2 mg/dl on two occasions, 6 months apart, is a good practice. A MELD score of 15 is an indication for referral to liver transplantation.

# References

1. Metcalf JV, Bhopal RS, Gray J, Howel D, James OF. Incidence and prevalence of primary biliary cirrhosis in the city of Newcastle upon Tyne, England. Int J Epidemiol. 1997;26:830–6.
2. Prince MI, Chetwynd A, Craig WL, Metcalf JV, James OF. Asymptomatic primary biliary cirrhosis: clinical features, prognosis, and symptom progression in a large population based cohort. Gut. 2004;53:865–70.
3. Lindor KD, Bowlus CL, Boyer J, Levy C, Mayo M. Primary biliary cholangitis: 2018 practice guidance from the American Association for the Study of Liver Diseases. Hepatology. 2019;69:394–419.
4. Doniach D, Walker G. Mitochondrial antibodies (AMA). Gut. 1974;15:664–8.
5. Sherlock S, Dooley J. Primary biliary cirrhosis. In: Diseases of the liver and biliary system. London: Blackwell; 1991. p. 236–48.
6. Fussey SP, Guest JR, James OF, Bassendine MF, Yeaman SJ. Identification and analysis of the major M2 autoantigens in primary biliary cirrhosis. Proc Natl Acad Sci U S A. 1988;85:8654–8.
7. Quinn J, Diamond AG, Palmer JM, Bassendine MF, James OF, Yeaman SJ. Lipoylated and unlipoylated domains of human PDC-E2 as autoantigens in primary biliary cirrhosis: significance of lipoate attachment. Hepatology. 1993;18:1384–91.
8. Hirschfield GM, Heathcote EJ. Antimitochondrial antibody-negative primary biliary cirrhosis. Clin Liver Dis. 2008;12:323–31.
9. Reed LJ, Hackert ML. Structure-function relationships in dihydrolipoamide acyltransferases. J Biol Chem. 1990;265:8971–4.
10. Van de Water J, Ansari AA, Surh CD, Coppel R, Roche T, Bonkovsky H, Kaplan M, et al. Evidence for the targeting by 2-oxo-dehydrogenase enzymes in the T cell response of primary biliary cirrhosis. J Immunol. 1991;146:89–94.
11. Bassendine MF, Jones DE, Yeaman SJ. Biochemistry and autoimmune response to the 2-oxoacid dehydrogenase complexes in primary biliary cirrhosis. Semin Liver Dis. 1997;17:49–60.
12. Ichiki Y, Shimoda S, Hara H, Shigematsu H, Nakamura M, Hayashida K, Ishibashi H, et al. Analysis of T-cell receptor beta of the T-cell clones reactive to the human PDC-E2 163-176 peptide in the context of HLA-DR53 in patients with primary biliary cirrhosis. Hepatology. 1997;26:728–33.
13. Howard MJ, Fuller C, Broadhurst RW, Perham RN, Tang JG, Quinn J, Diamond AG, et al. Three-dimensional structure of the major autoantigen in primary biliary cirrhosis. Gastroenterology. 1998;115:139–46.
14. Bruggraber SF, Leung PS, Amano K, Quan C, Kurth MJ, Nantz MH, Benson GD, et al. Autoreactivity to lipoate and a conjugated form of lipoate in primary biliary cirrhosis. Gastroenterology. 2003;125:1705–13.

15. Addison T, Gull W. On certain affection of the skin, vitiligoidea: (α) plana, (β) tuberosa. Guys Hosp Rep. 1851;7:265–76.
16. Ahrens EH Jr, Payne MA, Kunkel HG, Eisenmenger WJ, Blondheim SH. Primary biliary cirrhosis. Medicine (Baltimore). 1950;29:299–364.
17. Scheuer P. Primary biliary cirrhosis. Proc R Soc Med. 1967;60:1257–60.
18. Long RG, Scheuer PJ, Sherlock S. Presentation and course of asymptomatic primary biliary cirrhosis. Gastroenterology. 1977;72:1204–7.
19. Sherlock S, Scheuer PJ. The presentation and diagnosis of 100 patients with primary biliary cirrhosis. N Engl J Med. 1973;289:674–8.
20. Poupon RE, Lindor KD, Cauch-Dudek K, Dickson ER, Poupon R, Heathcote EJ. Combined analysis of randomized controlled trials of ursodeoxycholic acid in primary biliary cirrhosis. Gastroenterology. 1997;113:884–90.
21. Lindor KD, Gershwin ME, Poupon R, Kaplan M, Bergasa NV, Heathcote EJ. Primary biliary cirrhosis. Hepatology. 2009;50:291–308.
22. Poupon R. Treatment of primary biliary cirrhosis with ursodeoxycholic acid, budesonide and fibrates. Dig Dis. 2011;29:85–8.
23. Carithers RL Jr. Liver transplantation. American Association for the Study of Liver Diseases. Liver Transpl. 2000;6:122–35.
24. Sasatomi K, Noguchi K, Sakisaka S, Sata M, Tanikawa K. Abnormal accumulation of endo-toxin in biliary epithelial cells in primary biliary cirrhosis and primary sclerosing cholangitis. J Hepatol. 1998;29:409–16.
25. Harada K, Tsuneyama K, Sudo Y, Masuda S, Nakanuma Y. Molecular identification of bacte-rial 16S ribosomal RNA gene in liver tissue of primary biliary cirrhosis: is *Propionibacterium acnes* involved in granuloma formation? Hepatology. 2001;33:530–6.
26. Haruta I, Hashimoto E, Kato Y, Kikuchi K, Kato H, Yagi J, Uchiyama T, et al. Lipoteichoic acid may affect the pathogenesis of bile duct damage in primary biliary cirrhosis. Autoimmunity. 2006;39:129–35.
27. Vance RE, Isberg RR, Portnoy DA. Patterns of pathogenesis: discrimination of pathogenic and nonpathogenic microbes by the innate immune system. Cell Host Microbe. 2009;6:10–21.
28. Chen XM, O'Hara SP, Nelson JB, Splinter PL, Small AJ, Tietz PS, Limper AH, et al. Multiple TLRs are expressed in human *cholangiocytes and mediate host epithelial defense responses to Cryptosporidium parvum* via activation of NF-kappaB. J Immunol. 2005;175:7447–56.
29. Hayashi T, Suzuki K. LPS-toll-like receptor-mediated signaling on expression of protein S and C4b-binding protein in the liver. Gastroenterol Res Pract. 2010;2010:189561.
30. Palsson-McDermott EM, O'Neill LA. Signal transduction by the lipopolysaccharide recep-tor, toll-like receptor-4. Immunology. 2004;113:153–62.
31. Harada K, Nakanuma Y. Biliary innate immunity: function and modulation. Mediat Inflamm. 2010;2010:373878.
32. Burroughs AK, Rosenstein IJ, Epstein O, Hamilton-Miller JM, Brumfitt W, Sherlock S. Bacteriuria and primary biliary cirrhosis. Gut. 1984;25:133–7.
33. Parikh-Patel A, Gold EB, Worman H, Krivy KE, Gershwin ME. Risk factors for primary bili-ary cirrhosis in a cohort of patients from the United States. Hepatology. 2001;33:16–21.
34. Floreani A, Bassendine MF, Mitchison H, Freeman R, James OF. No specific association between primary biliary cirrhosis and bacteriuria? J Hepatol. 1989;8:201–7.
35. O'Donohue J, Workman MR, Rolando N, Yates M, Philpott-Howard J, Williams R. Urinary tract infections in primary biliary cirrhosis and other chronic liver diseases. Eur J Clin Microbiol Infect Dis. 1997;16:743–6.
36. Butler P, Hamilton-Miller J, Baum H, Burroughs AK. Detection of M2 antibodies in patients with recurrent urinary tract infection using an ELISA and purified PBC specific antigens. Evidence for a molecular mimicry mechanism in the pathogenesis of primary biliary cirrho-sis? Biochem Mol Biol Int. 1995;35:473–85.
37. Fourneau JM, Bach JM, van Endert PM, Bach JF. The elusive case for a role of mimicry in autoimmune diseases. Mol Immunol. 2004;40:1095–102.

38. Selmi C, Balkwill DL, Invernizzi P, Ansari AA, Coppel RL, Podda M, Leung PS, et al. Patients with primary biliary cirrhosis react against a ubiquitous xenobiotic-metabolizing bacterium. Hepatology. 2003;38:1250–7.
39. Xu L, Shen Z, Guo L, Fodera B, Keogh A, Joplin R, O'Donnell B, et al. Does a betaretrovirus infection trigger primary biliary cirrhosis? Proc Natl Acad Sci U S A. 2003;100:8454–9.
40. Xu L, Sakalian M, Shen Z, Loss G, Neuberger J, Mason A. Cloning the human betaretrovirus proviral genome from patients with primary biliary cirrhosis. Hepatology. 2004;39:151–6.
41. Liu B, Wang Y, Melana SM, Pelisson I, Najfeld V, Holland JF, Pogo BG. Identification of a proviral structure in human breast cancer. Cancer Res. 2001;61:1754–9.
42. Kaplowitz N, Aw TY, Simon FR, Stolz A. Drug-induced hepatotoxicity. Ann Intern Med. 1986;104:826–39.
43. Alvaro D, Mancino MG, Onori P, Franchitto A, Alpini G, Francis H, Glaser S, et al. Estrogens and the pathophysiology of the biliary tree. World J Gastroenterol. 2006;12:3537–45.
44. Corpechot C, Chretien Y, Chazouilleres O, Poupon R. Demographic, lifestyle, medical and familial factors associated with primary biliary cirrhosis. J Hepatol. 2010;53:162–9.
45. Gershwin ME, Selmi C, Worman HJ, Gold EB, Watnik M, Utts J, Lindor KD, et al. Risk factors and comorbidities in primary biliary cirrhosis: a controlled interview-based study of 1032 patients. Hepatology. 2005;42:1194–202.
46. Prince MI, Ducker SJ, James OF. Case-control studies of risk factors for primary biliary cirrhosis in two United Kingdom populations. Gut. 2010;59:508–12.
47. Ala A, Stanca CM, Bu-Ghanim M, Ahmado I, Branch AD, Schiano TD, Odin JA, et al. Increased prevalence of primary biliary cirrhosis near superfund toxic waste sites. Hepatology. 2006;43:525–31.
48. McNally RJ, Ducker S, James OF. Are transient environmental agents involved in the cause of primary biliary cirrhosis? Evidence from space-time clustering analysis. Hepatology. 2009;50:1169–74.
49. McNally RJ, James PW, Ducker S, James OF. Seasonal variation in the patient diagnosis of primary biliary cirrhosis: further evidence for an environmental component to etiology. Hepatology. 2011;54:2099–103.
50. Long SA, Quan C, Van de Water J, Nantz MH, Kurth MJ, Barsky D, Colvin ME, et al. Immunoreactivity of organic mimeotopes of the E2 component of pyruvate dehydrogenase: connecting xenobiotics with primary biliary cirrhosis. J Immunol. 2001;167:2956–63.
51. Volta U, Caio G, Tovoli F, De Giorgio R. Gut-liver axis: an immune link between celiac disease and primary biliary cirrhosis. Expert review of gastroenterology & hepatology. 2013;7(3):253–61.
52. Vignoli A, Orlandini B, Tenori L, Biagini MR, Milani S, Renzi D, et al. Metabolic Signature of Primary Biliary Cholangitis and Its Comparison with Celiac Disease. Journal of proteome research. 2019;18(3):1228–36.
53. Jones DE, Watt FE, Metcalf JV, Bassendine MF, James OF. Familial primary biliary cirrhosis reassessed: a geographically-based population study. J Hepatol. 1999;30:402–7.
54. Lazaridis KN, Juran BD, Boe GM, Slusser JP, de Andrade M, Homburger HA, Ghosh K, et al. Increased prevalence of antimitochondrial antibodies in first-degree relatives of patients with primary biliary cirrhosis. Hepatology. 2007;46:785–92.
55. Selmi C, Mayo MJ, Bach N, Ishibashi H, Invernizzi P, Gish RG, Gordon SC, et al. Primary biliary cirrhosis in monozygotic and dizygotic twins: genetics, epigenetics, and environment. Gastroenterology. 2004;127:485–92.
56. Guttenbach M, Koschorz B, Bernthaler U, Grimm T, Schmid M. Sex chromosome loss and aging: in situ hybridization studies on human interphase nuclei. Am J Hum Genet. 1995;57:1143–50.
57. Invernizzi P, Miozzo M, Battezzati PM, Bianchi I, Grati FR, Simoni G, Selmi C, et al. Frequency of monosomy X in women with primary biliary cirrhosis. Lancet. 2004;363:533–5.
58. Bird A. Perceptions of epigenetics. Nature. 2007;447:396–8.

59. Rioux JD, Abbas AK. Paths to understanding the genetic basis of autoimmune disease. Nature. 2005;435:584–9.
60. Gregersen PK, Olsson LM. Recent advances in the genetics of autoimmune disease. Annu Rev Immunol. 2009;27:363–91.
61. Onishi S, Sakamaki T, Maeda T, Iwamura S, Tomita A, Saibara T, Yamamoto Y. DNA typing of HLA class II genes; DRB1*0803 increases the susceptibility of Japanese to primary biliary cirrhosis. J Hepatol. 1994;21:1053–60.
62. Mullarkey ME, Stevens AM, McDonnell WM, Loubiere LS, Brackensick JA, Pang JM, Porter AJ, et al. Human leukocyte antigen class II alleles in Caucasian women with primary biliary cirrhosis. Tissue Antigens. 2005;65:199–205.
63. Donaldson PT, Baragiotta A, Heneghan MA, Floreani A, Venturi C, Underhill JA, Jones DE, et al. HLA class II alleles, genotypes, haplotypes, and amino acids in primary biliary cirrhosis: a large-scale study. Hepatology. 2006;44:667–74.
64. Invernizzi P, Selmi C, Poli F, Frison S, Floreani A, Alvaro D, Almasio P, et al. Human leukocyte antigen polymorphisms in Italian primary biliary cirrhosis: a multicenter study of 664 patients and 1992 healthy controls. Hepatology. 2008;48:1906–12.
65. Invernizzi P, Ransom M, Raychaudhuri S, Kosoy R, Lleo A, Shigeta R, Franke A, et al. Classical HLA-DRB1 and DPB1 alleles account for HLA associations with primary biliary cirrhosis. Genes Immun. 2012;13(6):461–8.
66. Hirschfield GM, Liu X, Xu C, Lu Y, Xie G, Lu Y, Gu X, et al. Primary biliary cirrhosis associated with HLA, IL12A, and IL12RB2 variants. N Engl J Med. 2009;360:2544–55.
67. Hirschfield GM, Liu X, Han Y, Gorlov IP, Lu Y, Xu C, Lu Y, et al. Variants at IRF5-TNPO3, 17q12-21 and MMEL1 are associated with primary biliary cirrhosis. Nat Genet. 2010;42:655–7.
68. Liu X, Invernizzi P, Lu Y, Kosoy R, Lu Y, Bianchi I, Podda M, et al. Genome-wide meta-analyses identify three loci associated with primary biliary cirrhosis. Nat Genet. 2010;42:658–60.
69. Mells GF, Floyd JA, Morley KI, Cordell HJ, Franklin CS, Shin SY, Heneghan MA, et al. Genome-wide association study identifies 12 new susceptibility loci for primary biliary cirrhosis. Nat Genet. 2011;43:329–32.
70. Hydes TJ, Blunt MD, Naftel J, Vallejo AF, Seumois G, Wang A, Vijayanand P, et al. Constitutive activation of natural killer cells in primary biliary cholangitis. Front Immunol. 2019;10:2633.
71. Selmi C, Cavaciocchi F, Lleo A, Cheroni C, De Francesco R, Lombardi SA, De Santis M, et al. Genome-wide analysis of DNA methylation, copy number variation, and gene expression in monozygotic twins discordant for primary biliary cirrhosis. Front Immunol. 2014;5:128.
72. Lleo A, Zhang W, Zhao M, Tan Y, Bernuzzi F, Zhu B, Liu Q, et al. DNA methylation profiling of the X chromosome reveals an aberrant demethylation on CXCR3 promoter in primary biliary cirrhosis. Clin Epigenetics. 2015;7:61.
73. Arenas F, Hervías I, Sáez E, Melero S, Prieto J, Pares A, Medina JF. Promoter hypermethylation of the AE2/SLC4A2 gene in PBC. JHEP Rep. 2019;1:145–53.
74. Concepcion AR, Salas JT, Sarvide S, Saez E, Ferrer A, Lopez M, Portu A, et al. Anion exchanger 2 is critical for CD8(+) T cells to maintain pHi homeostasis and modulate immune responses. Eur J Immunol. 2014;44:1341–51.
75. Hu Z, Huang Y, Liu Y, Sun Y, Zhou Y, Gu M, Chen Y, et al. β-Arrestin 1 modulates functions of autoimmune T cells from primary biliary cirrhosis patients. J Clin Immunol. 2011;31:346–55.
76. Kim WR, Lindor KD, Locke GR 3rd, Therneau TM, Homburger HA, Batts KP, Yawn BP, et al. Epidemiology and natural history of primary biliary cirrhosis in a US community. Gastroenterology. 2000;119:1631–6.
77. Governement U.S. Rare disease act, 2002.
78. Triger DR. Primary biliary cirrhosis: an epidemiological study. Br Med J. 1980;281:772–5.

79. Myszor M, James OF. The epidemiology of primary biliary cirrhosis in north-east England: an increasingly common disease? Q J Med. 1990;75:377–85.
80. Danielsson A, Boqvist L, Uddenfeldt P. Epidemiology of primary biliary cirrhosis in a defined rural population in the northern part of Sweden. Hepatology. 1990;11:458–64.
81. James OF, Bhopal R, Howel D, Gray J, Burt AD, Metcalf JV. Primary biliary cirrhosis once rare, now common in the United Kingdom? Hepatology. 1999;30:390–4.
82. Hurlburt KJ, McMahon BJ, Deubner H, Hsu-Trawinski B, Williams JL, Kowdley KV. Prevalence of autoimmune liver disease in Alaska natives. Am J Gastroenterol. 2002;97:2402–7.
83. Sood S, Gow PJ, Christie JM, Angus PW. Epidemiology of primary biliary cirrhosis in Victoria, Australia: high prevalence in migrant populations. Gastroenterology. 2004;127:470–5.
84. Myers RP, Shaheen AA, Fong A, Burak KW, Wan A, Swain MG, Hilsden RJ, et al. Epidemiology and natural history of primary biliary cirrhosis in a Canadian health region: a population-based study. Hepatology. 2009;50:1884–92.
85. Boonstra K, Kunst AE, Stadhouders PH, Tuynman HA, Poen AC, van Nieuwkerk KM, Witteman EM, et al. Rising incidence and prevalence of primary biliary cirrhosis: a large population-based study. Liver Int. 2014;34:e31–8.
86. Boonstra K, Beuers U, Ponsioen CY. Epidemiology of primary sclerosing cholangitis and primary biliary cirrhosis: a systematic review. J Hepatol. 2012;56:1181–8.
87. Reichen J, Simon F. Cholestasis. In: Arias IMJW, Popper H, Schachter D, Schafritz DA, editors. The liver: biology and pathobiology. 2nd ed. New York: Raven Press; 1988. p. 1105–24.
88. Jones EA, Bergasa NV. The pruritus of cholestasis: from bile acids to opiate agonists. Hepatology. 1990;11:884–7.
89. Bergasa NV, Talbot TL, Alling DW, Schmitt JM, Walker EC, Baker BL, Korenman JC, et al. A controlled trial of naloxone infusions for the pruritus of chronic cholestasis. Gastroenterology. 1992;102:544–9.
90. Bergasa NV, Alling DW, Talbot TL, Swain MG, Yurdaydin C, Turner ML, Schmitt JM, et al. Effects of naloxone infusions in patients with the pruritus of cholestasis. A double-blind, randomized, controlled trial. Ann Intern Med. 1995;123:161–7.
91. Bergasa NV, Schmitt JM, Talbot TL, Alling DW, Swain MG, Turner ML, et al. Open-label trial of oral nalmefene therapy for the pruritus of cholestasis. Hepatology. 1998;27(3):679–84.
92. Bergasa NV, Alling DW, Talbot TL, Wells MC, Jones EA. Oral nalmefene therapy reduces scratching activity due to the pruritus of cholestasis: a controlled study. J Am Acad Dermatol. 1999;41:431–4.
93. Bergasa NV. Pruritus of cholestasis. In: Carstens E, Akiyama T, editors. Itch: mechanisms and treatment. Boca Raton, FL: CRC Press; 2014.
94. Rishe E, Azarm A, Bergasa NV. Itch in primary biliary cirrhosis: a patients' perspective. Acta Derm Venereol. 2008;88:34–7.
95. Heathcote J. The clinical expression of primary biliary cirrhosis. Semin Liver Dis. 1997;17:23–33.
96. Hegade VS, Mells GF, Fisher H, Kendrick S, DiBello J, Gilchrist K, Alexander GJ, et al. Pruritus is common and undertreated in patients with primary biliary cholangitis in the United Kingdom. Clin Gastroenterol Hepatol. 2019;17:1379–87.
97. Floreani A, Carderi I, Variola A, Rizzotto ER, Nicol J, Bergasa NV. A novel multidrug-resistance protein 2 gene mutation identifies a subgroup of patients with primary biliary cirrhosis and pruritus. Hepatology. 2006;43:1152–4.
98. Keppler D, Leier I, Jedlitschky G. Transport of glutathione conjugates and glucuronides by the multidrug resistance proteins MRP1 and MRP2. Biol Chem. 1997;378:787–91.
99. Dombrowski SM, Desai SY, Marroni M, Cucullo L, Goodrich K, Bingaman W, Mayberg MR, et al. Overexpression of multiple drug resistance genes in endothelial cells from patients with refractory epilepsy. Epilepsia. 2001;42:1501–6.

100. Hoffmaster KA, Zamek-Gliszczynski MJ, Pollack GM, Brouwer KL. Multiple transport systems mediate the hepatic uptake and biliary excretion of the metabolically stable opioid peptide [D-penicillamine2,5]enkephalin. Drug Metab Dispos. 2005;33:287–93.

101. Hirouchi M, Suzuki H, Itoda M, Ozawa S, Sawada J, Ieiri I, Ohtsubo K, et al. Characterization of the cellular localization, expression level, and function of SNP variants of MRP2/ABCC2. Pharm Res. 2004;21:742–8.

102. Cichoz-Lach H, Grywalska E, Michalak A, Kowalik A, Mielnik M, Rolinski J. Deviations in peripheral blood cell populations are associated with the stage of primary biliary cholangitis and presence of itching. Arch Immunol Ther Exp. 2018;66:443–52.

103. Epstein O, Thomas HC, Sherlock S. Primary biliary cirrhosis is a dry gland syndrome with features of chronic graft-versus-host disease. Lancet. 1980;1:1166–8.

104. Jopson L, Jones DE. Fatigue in primary biliary cirrhosis: prevalence, pathogenesis and management. Dig Dis. 2015;33(Suppl 2):109–14.

105. Jones EA, Bergasa NV. The pathogenesis and treatment of pruritus and fatigue in patients with PBC. Eur J Gastroenterol Hepatol. 1999;11:623–31.

106. Laurin JM, DeSotel CK, Jorgensen RA, Dickson ER, Lindor KD. The natural history of abdominal pain associated with primary biliary cirrhosis. Am J Gastroenterol. 1994;89:1840–3.

107. Prince M, Chetwynd A, Newman W, Metcalf JV, James OF. Survival and symptom progression in a geographically based cohort of patients with primary biliary cirrhosis: follow-up for up to 28 years. Gastroenterology. 2002;123:1044–51.

108. Gores GJ, Wiesner RH, Dickson ER, Zinsmeister AR, Jorgensen RA, Langworthy A. Prospective evaluation of esophageal varices in primary biliary cirrhosis: development, natural history, and influence on survival. Gastroenterology. 1989;96:1552–9.

109. Mahl TC, Shockcor W, Boyer JL. Primary biliary cirrhosis: survival of a large cohort of symptomatic and asymptomatic patients followed for 24 years. J Hepatol. 1994;20:707–13.

110. Balasubramaniam K, Grambsch PM, Wiesner RH, Lindor KD, Dickson ER. Diminished survival in asymptomatic primary biliary cirrhosis. A prospective study. Gastroenterology. 1990;98:1567–71.

111. Floreani A, Franceschet I, Cazzagon N, Spinazze A, Buja A, Furlan P, Baldo V, et al. Extrahepatic autoimmune conditions associated with primary biliary cirrhosis. Clin Rev Allergy Immunol. 2015;48:192–7.

112. Kaneko H, Endo T, Saitoh H, Katsuta Y, Aramaki T, Hayakawa H. Primary biliary cirrhosis associated with multiple myeloma. Intern Med. 1993;32(10):802–5.

113. Logan RF, Ferguson A, Finlayson ND, Weir DG. Primary biliary cirrhosis and coeliac disease: an association? Lancet. 1978;1(8058):230–3.

114. Toshikuni N, Yamato R, Kobashi H, Nishino K, Inada N, Sakanoue R, Suehiro M, et al. Association of primary biliary cirrhosis with idiopathic thrombocytopenic purpura. World J Gastroenterol. 2008;14:2451–3.

115. Terzioli Beretta-Piccoli B, Guillod C, Marsteller I, Blum R, Mazzucchelli L, Mondino C, Invernizzi P, et al. Primary biliary cholangitis associated with skin disorders: a case report and review of the literature. Arch Immunol Ther Exp. 2017;65:299–309.

116. Shizuma T. Clinical characteristics of concomitant systemic lupus erythematosus and primary biliary cirrhosis: a literature review. J Immunol Res. 2015;2015:713728.

117. Aoyama H, Sakugawa H, Nakasone H, Nakayoshi T, Kinjo A, Tamayose M, Higa H, et al. A rare association of primary biliary cirrhosis and pernicious anemia. J Gastroenterol. 2002;37:560–3.

118. Polychronopoulou E, Lygoura V, Gatselis NK, Dalekos GN. Increased cholestatic enzymes in two patients with long-term history of ulcerative colitis: consider primary biliary cholangitis not always primary sclerosing cholangitis. BMJ Case Rep. 2017;2017:bcr2017220824.

119. Koksal D, Koksal AS, Gurakar A. Pulmonary manifestations among patients with primary biliary cirrhosis. J Clin Transl Hepatol. 2016;4:258–62.

120. Bian S, Chen H, Wang L, Fei Y, Yang Y, Peng L, Li Y, et al. Cardiac involvement in patients with primary biliary cholangitis: a 14-year longitudinal survey-based study. PLoS One. 2018;13:e0194397.
121. Suzuki Y, Ishida K, Takahashi H, Koeda N, Kakisaka K, Miyamoto Y, Suzuki A, et al. Primary biliary cirrhosis associated with graves' disease in a male patient. Clin J Gastroenterol. 2016;9:99–103.
122. Tang KH, Schofield JB, Powell-Jackson PR. Primary biliary cirrhosis and idiopathic retroperitoneal fibrosis: a rare association. Eur J Gastroenterol Hepatol. 2002;14:783–6.
123. Gylling H, Farkkila M, Vuoristo M, Miettinen TA. Metabolism of cholesterol and low- and high-density lipoproteins in primary biliary cirrhosis: cholesterol absorption and synthesis related to lipoprotein levels and their kinetics. Hepatology. 1995;21:89–95.
124. Li T, Apte U. Bile acid metabolism and signaling in cholestasis, inflammation, and cancer. Adv Pharmacol. 2015;74:263–302.
125. Chang PY, Lu SC, Su TC, Chou SF, Huang WH, Morrisett JD, Chen CH, et al. Lipoprotein-X reduces LDL atherogenicity in primary biliary cirrhosis by preventing LDL oxidation. J Lipid Res. 2004;45:2116–22.
126. Floreani A, Variola A, Niro G, Premoli A, Baldo V, Gambino R, Musso G, et al. Plasma adiponectin levels in primary biliary cirrhosis: a novel perspective for link between hypercholesterolemia and protection against atherosclerosis. Am J Gastroenterol. 2008;103:1959–65.
127. Frohlich JJ, Seccombe DW, Pritchard PH. The role of apoproteins in disorders of lipoprotein metabolism. Clin Biochem. 1989;22:51–6.
128. Jahn CE, Schaefer EJ, Taam LA, Hoofnagle JH, Lindgren FT, Albers JJ, Jones EA, et al. Lipoprotein abnormalities in primary biliary cirrhosis. Association with hepatic lipase inhibition as well as altered cholesterol esterification. Gastroenterology. 1985;89:1266–78.
129. Baldo-Enzi G, Baiocchi MR, Grotto M, Floreani AR, Zagolin M, Chiaramonte M, Cera F, et al. Lipoprotein pattern and plasma lipoprotein lipase activities in patients with primary biliary cirrhosis. Relationship with increase of HDL2 fraction in Lp-X-positive and Lp-X-negative subjects. Dig Dis Sci. 1988;33:1201–7.
130. Crippin JS, Lindor KD, Jorgensen R, Kottke BA, Harrison JM, Murtaugh PA, Dickson ER. Hypercholesterolemia and atherosclerosis in primary biliary cirrhosis: what is the risk? Hepatology. 1992;15:858–62.
131. Van Dam GM, Gips CH. Primary biliary cirrhosis in the Netherlands. An analysis of associated diseases, cardiovascular risk, and malignancies on the basis of mortality figures. Scand J Gastroenterol. 1997;32:77–83.
132. Longo M, Crosignani A, Battezzati PM, Squarcia Giussani C, Invernizzi P, Zuin M, Podda M. Hyperlipidaemic state and cardiovascular risk in primary biliary cirrhosis. Gut. 2002;51:265–9.
133. Schaffner F. Treatment of primary biliary cirrhosis. Mod Treat. 1969;6:205–14.
134. Allocca M, Crosignani A, Gritti A, Ghilardi G, Gobatti D, Caruso D, Zuin M, et al. Hypercholesterolaemia is not associated with early atherosclerotic lesions in primary biliary cirrhosis. Gut. 2006;55:1795–800.
135. Kurihara T, Niimi A, Maeda A, Shigemoto M, YAMAhita K. Bezafibrate in the treatment of primary biliary cirrhosis: comparison with ursodeoxycholic acid. Am J Gastroenterol. 2000;95:2990–2.
136. Nakai S, Masaki T, Kurokohchi K, Deguchi A, Nishioka M. Combination therapy of bezafibrate and ursodeoxycholic acid in primary biliary cirrhosis: a preliminary study. Am J Gastroenterol. 2000;95:326–7.
137. Leib ES, Lewiecki EM, Binkley N, Hamdy RC. Official positions of the International Society for Clinical Densitometry. J Clin Densitom. 2004;7:1–6.
138. Solerio E, Isaia G, Innarella R, Di Stefano M, Farina M, Borghesio E, Framarin L, et al. Osteoporosis: still a typical complication of primary biliary cirrhosis? Dig Liver Dis. 2003;35:339–46.

139. Guanabens N, Pares A, Ros I, Caballeria L, Pons F, Vidal S, Monegal A, et al. Severity of cholestasis and advanced histological stage but not menopausal status are the major risk factors for osteoporosis in primary biliary cirrhosis. J Hepatol. 2005;42:573–7.

140. Guanabens N, Cerda D, Monegal A, Pons F, Caballeria L, Peris P, Pares A. Low bone mass and severity of cholestasis affect fracture risk in patients with primary biliary cirrhosis. Gastroenterology. 2010;138:2348–56.

141. McCaughan GW, Feller RB. Osteoporosis in chronic liver disease: pathogenesis, risk factors, and management. Dig Dis. 1994;12:223–31.

142. Herlong HF, Recker RR, Maddrey WC. Bone disease in primary biliary cirrhosis: histologic features and response to 25-hydroxyvitamin D. Gastroenterology. 1982;83:103–8.

143. Hodgson SF, Dickson ER, Eastell R, Eriksen EF, Bryant SC, Riggs BL. Rates of cancellous bone remodeling and turnover in osteopenia associated with primary biliary cirrhosis. Bone. 1993;14:819–27.

144. Pares A, Guanabens N, Rodes J. Gene polymorphisms as predictors of decreased bone mineral density and osteoporosis in primary biliary cirrhosis. Eur J Gastroenterol Hepatol. 2005;17:311–5.

145. Menon KV, Angulo P, Weston S, Dickson ER, Lindor KD. Bone disease in primary biliary cirrhosis: independent indicators and rate of progression. J Hepatol. 2001;35:316–23.

146. Frith J, Kerr S, Robinson L, Elliott C, Ghazala C, Wilton K, Pairman J, et al. Primary biliary cirrhosis is associated with falls and significant fall related injury. QJM. 2010;103:153–61.

147. Green JH, Bramley PN, Losowsky MS. Are patients with primary biliary cirrhosis hypermetabolic? A comparison between patients before and after liver transplantation and controls. Hepatology. 1991;14:464–72.

148. Koulaouzidis A, Bhat S, Moschos J. Skin manifestations of liver diseases. Ann Hepatol. 2007;6:181–4.

149. Reynolds TB. The "butterfly" sign in patients with chronic jaundice and pruritus. Ann Intern Med. 1973;78:545–6.

150. Heathcote J. Autoimmune cholangitis. Gut. 1997;40:440–2.

151. Heathcote J. Primary biliary cirrhosis with features of autoimmune hepatitis. Curr Gastroenterol Rep. 2001;3:60–4.

152. Michieletti P, Wanless IR, Katz A, Scheuer PJ, Yeaman SJ, Bassendine MF, Palmer JM, et al. Antimitochondrial antibody negative primary biliary cirrhosis: a distinct syndrome of autoimmune cholangitis. Gut. 1994;35:260–5.

153. Lacerda MA, Ludwig J, Dickson ER, Jorgensen RA, Lindor KD. Antimitochondrial antibody-negative primary biliary cirrhosis. Am J Gastroenterol. 1995;90:247–9.

154. Invernizzi P, Crosignani A, Battezzati PM, Covini G, De Valle G, Larghi A, Zuin M, et al. Comparison of the clinical features and clinical course of antimitochondrial antibody-positive and -negative primary biliary cirrhosis. Hepatology. 1997;25:1090–5.

155. Migliaccio C, Van de Water J, Ansari AA, Kaplan MM, Coppel RL, Lam KS, Thompson RK, et al. Heterogeneous response of antimitochondrial autoantibodies and bile duct apical staining monoclonal antibodies to pyruvate dehydrogenase complex E2: the molecule versus the mimic. Hepatology. 2001;33:792–801.

156. Shimoda S, Nakamura M, Ishibashi H, Hayashida K, Niho Y. HLA DRB4 0101-restricted immunodominant T cell autoepitope of pyruvate dehydrogenase complex in primary biliary cirrhosis: evidence of molecular mimicry in human autoimmune diseases. J Exp Med. 1995;181:1835–45.

157. Wing K, Sakaguchi S. Regulatory T cells exert checks and balances on self tolerance and autoimmunity. Nat Immunol. 2010;11:7–13.

158. Marshak-Rothstein A. Toll-like receptors in systemic autoimmune disease. Nat Rev Immunol. 2006;6:823–35.

159. Shimoda S, Van de Water J, Ansari A, Nakamura M, Ishibashi H, Coppel R, Lake J, et al. Identification and precursor frequency analysis of a common T cell epitope motif in mitochondrial autoantigens in primary biliary cirrhosis. J Clin Invest. 1998;102:1831–40.

160. Joshi S, Cauch-Dudek K, Wanless IR, Lindor KD, Jorgensen R, Batts K, Heathcote EJ. Primary biliary cirrhosis with additional features of autoimmune hepatitis: response to therapy with ursodeoxycholic acid. Hepatology. 2002;35:409–13.
161. Su CW, Hung HH, Huo TI, Huang YH, Li CP, Lin HC, Lee PC, et al. Natural history and prognostic factors of primary biliary cirrhosis in Taiwan: a follow-up study up to 18 years. Liver Int. 2008;28:1305–13.
162. Shimoda S, Miyakawa H, Nakamura M, Ishibashi H, Kikuchi K, Kita H, Niiro H, et al. CD4 T-cell autoreactivity to the mitochondrial autoantigen PDC-E2 in AMA-negative primary biliary cirrhosis. J Autoimmun. 2008;31:110–5.
163. Joplin R, Lindsay JG, Johnson GD, Strain A, Neuberger J. Membrane dihydrolipoamide acetyltransferase (E2) on human biliary epithelial cells in primary biliary cirrhosis. Lancet. 1992;339:93–4.
164. Van de Water J, Turchany J, Leung PS, Lake J, Munoz S, Surh CD, Coppel R, et al. Molecular mimicry in primary biliary cirrhosis. Evidence for biliary epithelial expression of a molecule cross-reactive with pyruvate dehydrogenase complex-E2. J Clin Invest. 1993;91:2653–64.
165. Brown WR, Kloppel TM. The liver and IgA: immunological, cell biological and clinical implications. Hepatology. 1989;9:763–84.
166. Malmborg AC, Shultz DB, Luton F, Mostov KE, Richly E, Leung PS, Benson GD, et al. Penetration and co-localization in MDCK cell mitochondria of IgA derived from patients with primary biliary cirrhosis. J Autoimmun. 1998;11:573–80.
167. Russell MW, Sibley DA, Nikolova EB, Tomana M, Mestecky J. IgA antibody as a non-inflammatory regulator of immunity. Biochem Soc Trans. 1997;25:466–70.
168. Hexham JM, Carayannopoulos L, Capra JD. Structure and function in IgA. Chem Immunol. 1997;65:73–87.
169. Abbas A, Lichtman A, Pillai S. B cell activation and antibody production. Cellular and Molecular Immunology. New York: Elsevier, W. B. Saunders; 2012. p. 243–68.
170. Kikuchi K, Lian ZX, Yang GX, Ansari AA, Ikehara S, Kaplan M, Miyakawa H, et al. Bacterial CpG induces hyper-IgM production in CD27(+) memory B cells in primary biliary cirrhosis. Gastroenterology. 2005;128:304–12.
171. Moritoki Y, Lian ZX, Wulff H, Yang GX, Chuang YH, Lan RY, Ueno Y, et al. AMA production in primary biliary cirrhosis is promoted by the TLR9 ligand CpG and suppressed by potassium channel blockers. Hepatology. 2007;45:314–22.
172. Harada K, Shimoda S, Sato Y, Isse K, Ikeda H, Nakanuma Y. Periductal interleukin-17 production in association with biliary innate immunity contributes to the pathogenesis of cholangiopathy in primary biliary cirrhosis. Clin Exp Immunol. 2009;157:261–70.
173. Odin JA, Huebert RC, Casciola-Rosen L, LaRusso NF, Rosen A. Bcl-2-dependent oxidation of pyruvate dehydrogenase-E2, a primary biliary cirrhosis autoantigen, during apoptosis. J Clin Invest. 2001;108:223–32.
174. Allina J, Hu B, Sullivan DM, Fiel MI, Thung SN, Bronk SF, Huebert RC, et al. T cell targeting and phagocytosis of apoptotic biliary epithelial cells in primary biliary cirrhosis. J Autoimmun. 2006;27:232–41.
175. Allina J, Stanca CM, Garber J, Hu B, Sautes-Fridman C, Bach N, Odin JA. Anti-CD16 autoantibodies and delayed phagocytosis of apoptotic cells in primary biliary cirrhosis. J Autoimmun. 2008;30:238–45.
176. Rong G, Zhong R, Lleo A, Leung PS, Bowlus CL, Yang GX, Yang CY, et al. Epithelial cell specificity and apotope recognition by serum autoantibodies in primary biliary cirrhosis. Hepatology. 2011;54:196–203.
177. Lleo A, Selmi C, Invernizzi P, Podda M, Coppel RL, Mackay IR, Gores GJ, et al. Apotopes and the biliary specificity of primary biliary cirrhosis. Hepatology. 2009;49:871–9.
178. Lleo A, Bowlus CL, Yang GX, Invernizzi P, Podda M, Van de Water J, Ansari AA, et al. Biliary apotopes and anti-mitochondrial antibodies activate innate immune responses in primary biliary cirrhosis. Hepatology. 2010;52:987–98.

179. Abbas A, Lichtman A, Pillai S. Effector mechanisms of humoral immunity. In: Cellular and molecular immunology. New York: Elsevier, W. B. Saunders; 2012. p. 269–92.

180. Prieto J, Qian C, Garcia N, Diez J, Medina JF. Abnormal expression of anion exchanger genes in primary biliary cirrhosis. Gastroenterology. 1993;105:572–8.

181. Ros E, Garcia-Puges A, Reixach M, Cuso E, Rodes J. Fat digestion and exocrine pancreatic function in primary biliary cirrhosis. Gastroenterology. 1984;87:180–7.

182. Epstein O, Chapman RW, Lake-Bakaar G, Foo AY, Rosalki SB, Sherlock S. The pancreas in primary biliary cirrhosis and primary sclerosing cholangitis. Gastroenterology. 1982;83:1177–82.

183. Lake-Bakaar G, McKavanagh S, Rubio CE, Epstein O, Summerfield JA. Measurement of trypsin in duodenal juice by radioimmunoassay. Gut. 1980;21:402–7.

184. Tsuneyama K, Van De Water J, Yamazaki K, Suzuki K, Sato S, Takeda Y, Ruebner B, et al. Primary biliary cirrhosis an epithelitis: evidence of abnormal salivary gland immunohistochemistry. Autoimmunity. 1997;26:23–31.

185. Muratori P, Muratori L, Ferrari R, Cassani F, Bianchi G, Lenzi M, Rodrigo L, et al. Characterization and clinical impact of antinuclear antibodies in primary biliary cirrhosis. Am J Gastroenterol. 2003;98:431–7.

186. Granito A, Muratori P, Muratori L, Pappas G, Cassani F, Worthington J, Guidi M, et al. Antinuclear antibodies giving the 'multiple nuclear dots' or the 'rim-like/membranous' patterns: diagnostic accuracy for primary biliary cirrhosis. Aliment Pharmacol Ther. 2006;24:1575–83.

187. Szostecki C, Guldner HH, Netter HJ, Will H. Isolation and characterization of cDNA encoding a human nuclear antigen predominantly recognized by autoantibodies from patients with primary biliary cirrhosis. J Immunol. 1990;145:4338–47.

188. Sternsdorf T, Guldner HH, Szostecki C, Grotzinger T, Will H. Two nuclear dot-associated proteins, PML and Sp100, are often co-autoimmunogenic in patients with primary biliary cirrhosis. Scand J Immunol. 1995;42:257–68.

189. Lassoued K, Brenard R, Degos F, Courvalin JC, Andre C, Danon F, Brouet JC, et al. Antinuclear antibodies directed to a 200-kilodalton polypeptide of the nuclear envelope in primary biliary cirrhosis. A clinical and immunological study of a series of 150 patients with primary biliary cirrhosis. Gastroenterology. 1990;99:181–6.

190. Wesierska-Gadek J, Hohenuer H, Hitchman E, Penner E. Autoantibodies against nucleoporin p62 constitute a novel marker of primary biliary cirrhosis. Gastroenterology. 1996;110:840–7.

191. Courvalin JC, Lassoued K, Worman HJ, Blobel G. Identification and characterization of autoantibodies against the nuclear envelope Lamin B receptor from patients with primary biliary cirrhosis. J Exp Med. 1990;172:961–7.

192. Parveen S, Morshed SA, Nishioka M. High prevalence of antibodies to recombinant CENP-B in primary biliary cirrhosis: nuclear immunofluorescence patterns and ELISA reactivities. J Gastroenterol Hepatol. 1995;10:438–45.

193. Szostecki C, Will H, Netter HJ, Guldner HH. Autoantibodies to the nuclear Sp100 protein in primary biliary cirrhosis and associated diseases: epitope specificity and immunoglobulin class distribution. Scand J Immunol. 1992;36:555–64.

194. Zuchner D, Sternsdorf T, Szostecki C, Heathcote EJ, Cauch-Dudek K, Will H. Prevalence, kinetics, and therapeutic modulation of autoantibodies against Sp100 and promyelocytic leukemia protein in a large cohort of patients with primary biliary cirrhosis. Hepatology. 1997;26:1123–30.

195. Granito A, Yang WH, Muratori L, Lim MJ, Nakajima A, Ferri S, Pappas G, et al. PML nuclear body component Sp140 is a novel autoantigen in primary biliary cirrhosis. Am J Gastroenterol. 2010;105:125–31.

196. Lassoued K, Guilly MN, Andre C, Paintrand M, Dhumeaux D, Danon F, Brouet JC, et al. Autoantibodies to 200 kD polypeptide(s) of the nuclear envelope: a new serologic marker of primary biliary cirrhosis. Clin Exp Immunol. 1988;74:283–8.

197. Nickowitz RE, Worman HJ. Autoantibodies from patients with primary biliary cirrhosis recognize a restricted region within the cytoplasmic tail of nuclear pore membrane glycoprotein Gp210. J Exp Med. 1993;178:2237–42.
198. Nakamura M, Kondo H, Mori T, Komori A, Matsuyama M, Ito M, Takii Y, et al. Anti-gp210 and anti-centromere antibodies are different risk factors for the progression of primary biliary cirrhosis. Hepatology. 2007;45:118–27.
199. Krams SM, Van de Water J, Coppel RL, Esquivel C, Roberts J, Ansari A, Gershwin ME. Analysis of hepatic T lymphocyte and immunoglobulin deposits in patients with primary biliary cirrhosis. Hepatology. 1990;12:306–13.
200. Bjorkland A, Festin R, Mendel-Hartvig I, Nyberg A, Loof L, Totterman TH. Blood and liver-infiltrating lymphocytes in primary biliary cirrhosis: increase in activated T and natural killer cells and recruitment of primed memory T cells. Hepatology. 1991;13:1106–11.
201. Nakanuma Y. Distribution of B lymphocytes in nonsuppurative cholangitis in primary biliary cirrhosis. Hepatology. 1993;18:570–5.
202. Terasaki S, Nakanuma Y, Yamazaki M, Unoura M. Eosinophilic infiltration of the liver in primary biliary cirrhosis: a morphological study. Hepatology. 1993;17:206–12.
203. Bjorkland A, Loof L, Mendel-Hartvig I, Totterman TH. Primary biliary cirrhosis. High proportions of B cells in blood and liver tissue produce anti-mitochondrial antibodies of several Ig classes. J Immunol. 1994;153:2750–7.
204. Goldstein NS, Soman A, Gordon SC. Portal tract eosinophils and hepatocyte cytokeratin 7 immunoreactivity helps distinguish early-stage, mildly active primary biliary cirrhosis and autoimmune hepatitis. Am J Clin Pathol. 2001;116:846–53.
205. Kita H, Naidenko OV, Kronenberg M, Ansari AA, Rogers P, He XS, Koning F, et al. Quantitation and phenotypic analysis of natural killer T cells in primary biliary cirrhosis using a human CD1d tetramer. Gastroenterology. 2002;123:1031–43.
206. Daniels JA, Torbenson M, Anders RA, Boitnott JK. Immunostaining of plasma cells in primary biliary cirrhosis. Am J Clin Pathol. 2009;131:243–9.
207. Ludwig J, Dickson ER, McDonald GS. Staging of chronic nonsuppurative destructive cholangitis (syndrome of primary biliary cirrhosis). Virchows Arch A Pathol Anat Histol. 1978;379:103–12.
208. Gershwin ME, Ansari AA, Mackay IR, Nakanuma Y, Nishio A, Rowley MJ, Coppel RL. Primary biliary cirrhosis: an orchestrated immune response against epithelial cells. Immunol Rev. 2000;174:210–25.
209. Kaplan MM, Gershwin ME. Primary biliary cirrhosis. N Engl J Med. 2005;353:1261–73.
210. Kita H, Matsumura S, He XS, Ansari AA, Lian ZX, Van de Water J, Coppel RL, et al. Quantitative and functional analysis of PDC-E2-specific autoreactive cytotoxic T lymphocytes in primary biliary cirrhosis. J Clin Invest. 2002;109:1231–40.
211. Hashimoto E, Lindor KD, Homburger HA, Dickson ER, Czaja AJ, Wiesner RH, Ludwig J. Immunohistochemical characterization of hepatic lymphocytes in primary biliary cirrhosis in comparison with primary sclerosing cholangitis and autoimmune chronic active hepatitis. Mayo Clin Proc. 1993;68:1049–55.
212. Harada K. In situ nucleic acid hybridization of cytokines in primary biliary cirrhosis: predominance of the Th1 subset. Hepatology. 1997;25:791–6.
213. Lohr HF, Schlaak JF, Gerken G, Fleischer B, Dienes HP, Meyer zum Buschenfelde KH. Phenotypical analysis and cytokine release of liver-infiltrating and peripheral blood T lymphocytes from patients with chronic hepatitis of different etiology. Liver. 1994;14:161–6.
214. Diu A, Moebius U, Ferradini L, Genevee C, Roman-Roman S, Claudon M, Delorme D, et al. Limited T-cell receptor diversity in liver-infiltrating lymphocytes from patients with primary biliary cirrhosis. J Autoimmun. 1993;6:611–9.
215. Martins EB, Graham AK, Chapman RW, Fleming KA. Elevation of gamma delta T lymphocytes in peripheral blood and livers of patients with primary sclerosing cholangitis and other autoimmune liver diseases. Hepatology. 1996;23:988–93.

216. Abbas A, Lichtman A, Pillai S. Immunologic tolerance and autoimmunity. In: Abbas A, Lichtman A, Pillai S, editors. Cellular and molecular immunology. New York: Elsevier, W. B. Saunders; 2012. p. 319–43.

217. Lan RY, Cheng C, Lian ZX, Tsuneyama K, Yang GX, Moritoki Y, Chuang YH, et al. Liver-targeted and peripheral blood alterations of regulatory T cells in primary biliary cirrhosis. Hepatology. 2006;43:729–37.

218. Wang D, Zhang H, Liang J, Gu Z, Zhou Q, Fan X, Hou Y, et al. CD4+ CD25+ but not CD4+ Foxp3+ T cells as a regulatory subset in primary biliary cirrhosis. Cell Mol Immunol. 2010;7:485–90.

219. Bernuzzi F, Fenoglio D, Battaglia F, Fravega M, Gershwin ME, Indiveri F, Ansari AA, et al. Phenotypical and functional alterations of CD8 regulatory T cells in primary biliary cirrhosis. J Autoimmun. 2010;35:176–80.

220. Takahashi T, Miura T, Nakamura J, Yamada S, Miura T, Yanagi M, Matsuda Y, et al. Plasma cells and the chronic nonsuppurative destructive cholangitis of primary biliary cirrhosis. Hepatology. 2012;55:846–55.

221. Li SX, Lv TT, Zhang CP, Wang TQ, Tian D, Sun GY, Wang Y, et al. Alteration of liver-infiltrated and peripheral blood double-negative T-cells in primary biliary cholangitis. Liver Int. 2019;39:1755–67.

222. You Z, Wang Q, Bian Z, Liu Y, Han X, Peng Y, Shen L, et al. The immunopathology of liver granulomas in primary biliary cirrhosis. J Autoimmun. 2012;39:216–21.

223. Harada K, Shimoda S, Ikeda H, Chiba M, Hsu M, Sato Y, Kobayashi M, et al. Significance of periductal Langerhans cells and biliary epithelial cell-derived macrophage inflammatory protein-3alpha in the pathogenesis of primary biliary cirrhosis. Liver Int. 2010;31:245–53.

224. Abbas A, Lichtman A, Pillai S. Innate immunity. In: Abbas A, Lichtman A, Pillai S, editors. Cellular and molecular immunology. New York: Elsevier, W. B. Saunders; 2012. p. 55–88.

225. Leon MP, Bassendine MF, Gibbs P, Thick M, Kirby JA. Immunogenicity of biliary epithelium: study of the adhesive interaction with lymphocytes. Gastroenterology. 1997;112:968–77.

226. Lechler R, Chai JG, Marelli-Berg F, Lombardi G. The contributions of T-cell anergy to peripheral T-cell tolerance. Immunology. 2001;103:262–9.

227. Shimoda S, Harada K, Niiro H, Yoshizumi T, Soejima Y, Taketomi A, Maehara Y, et al. Biliary epithelial cells and primary biliary cirrhosis: the role of liver-infiltrating mononuclear cells. Hepatology. 2008;47:958–65.

228. Bazan JF, Bacon KB, Hardiman G, Wang W, Soo K, Rossi D, Greaves DR, et al. A new class of membrane-bound chemokine with a CX3C motif. Nature. 1997;385:640–4.

229. Imai T, Hieshima K, Haskell C, Baba M, Nagira M, Nishimura M, Kakizaki M, et al. Identification and molecular characterization of fractalkine receptor CX3CR1, which mediates both leukocyte migration and adhesion. Cell. 1997;91:521–30.

230. Isse K, Harada K, Zen Y, Kamihira T, Shimoda S, Harada M, Nakanuma Y. Fractalkine and CX3CR1 are involved in the recruitment of intraepithelial lymphocytes of intrahepatic bile ducts. Hepatology. 2005;41:506–16.

231. Shimoda S, Harada K, Niiro H, Taketomi A, Maehara Y, Tsuneyama K, Kikuchi K, et al. CX3CL1 (fractalkine): a signpost for biliary inflammation in primary biliary cirrhosis. Hepatology. 2010;51:567–75.

232. Funaro A, Malavasi F. Human CD38, a surface receptor, an enzyme, an adhesion molecule and not a simple marker. J Biol Regul Homeost Agents. 1999;13:54–61.

233. Rawstron AC, Orfao A, Beksac M, Bezdickova L, Brooimans RA, Bumbea H, Dalva K, et al. Report of the European myeloma network on multiparametric flow cytometry in multiple myeloma and related disorders. Haematologica. 2008;93:431–8.

234. Chuang YH, Lian ZX, Tsuneyama K, Chiang BL, Ansari AA, Coppel RL, Gershwin ME. Increased killing activity and decreased cytokine production in NK cells in patients with primary biliary cirrhosis. J Autoimmun. 2006;26:232–40.

235. Shimoda S, Harada K, Niiro H, Shirabe K, Taketomi A, Maehara Y, Tsuneyama K, et al. Interaction between toll-like receptors and natural killer cells in the destruction of bile ducts in primary biliary cirrhosis. Hepatology. 2011;53:1270–81.
236. Yin XM, Ding WX, Gao W. Autophagy in the liver. Hepatology. 2008;47:1773–85.
237. Sasaki M, Miyakoshi M, Sato Y, Nakanuma Y. Autophagy mediates the process of cellular senescence characterizing bile duct damages in primary biliary cirrhosis. Lab Investig. 2010;90:835–43.
238. Sasaki M, Miyakoshi M, Sato Y, Nakanuma Y. Modulation of the microenvironment by senescent biliary epithelial cells may be involved in the pathogenesis of primary biliary cirrhosis. J Hepatol. 2010;53:318–25.
239. Sasaki M, Yoshimura-Miyakoshi M, Sato Y, Nakanuma Y. A possible involvement of endoplasmic reticulum stress in biliary epithelial autophagy and senescence in primary biliary cirrhosis. J Gastroenterol. 2015;50:984–95.
240. Sasaki M, Sato Y, Nakanuma Y. An impaired biliary bicarbonate umbrella may be involved in dysregulated autophagy in primary biliary cholangitis. Lab Investig. 2018;98:745–54.
241. Sasaki M, Sato Y, Nakanuma Y. Increased p16(INK4a)-expressing senescent bile ductular cells are associated with inadequate response to ursodeoxycholic acid in primary biliary cholangitis. J Autoimmun. 2019;107:102377.
242. Mao TK, Davis PA, Odin JA, Coppel RL, Gershwin ME. Sidechain biology and the immunogenicity of PDC-E2, the major autoantigen of primary biliary cirrhosis. Hepatology. 2004;40:1241–8.
243. Tsuda M, Ambrosini YM, Zhang W, Yang GX, Ando Y, Rong G, Tsuneyama K, et al. Fine phenotypic and functional characterization of effector cluster of differentiation 8 positive T cells in human patients with primary biliary cirrhosis. Hepatology. 2011;54:1293–302.
244. Tomiyama H, Matsuda T, Takiguchi M. Differentiation of human CD8(+) T cells from a memory to memory/effector phenotype. J Immunol. 2002;168:5538–50.
245. Morikawa K, Oseko F, Morikawa S, Imai K, Sawada M. Recombinant human IL-5 augments immunoglobulin generation by human B lymphocytes in the presence of IL-2. Cell Immunol. 1993;149:390–401.
246. Krams SM, Cao S, Hayashi M, Villanueva JC, Martinez OM. Elevations in IFN-gamma, IL-5, and IL-10 in patients with the autoimmune disease primary biliary cirrhosis: association with autoantibodies and soluble CD30. Clin Immunol Immunopathol. 1996;80:311–20.
247. MacGregor GA. Primary biliary cirrhosis is a dry-gland syndrome. Lancet. 1980;2:535.
248. Paumgartner G, Beuers U. Ursodeoxycholic acid in cholestatic liver disease: mechanisms of action and therapeutic use revisited. Hepatology. 2002;36:525–31.
249. Neuman MG, Cameron RG, Haber JA, Katz GG, Blendis LM. An electron microscopic and morphometric study of ursodeoxycholic effect in primary biliary cirrhosis. Liver. 2002;22:235–44.
250. Siegel J, Jorgensen R, Angulo P, Lindor K. Treatment with ursodeoxycholic acid is associated with weight gain in patients with primary biliary cirrhosis. J Clin Gastgroenterol. 2003;37:185.
251. LiverTox: clinical and research information on drug-induced liver injury [Internet]. Review; 2012.
252. Poupon RE, Lindor KD, Pares A, Chazouilleres O, Poupon R, Heathcote EJ. Combined analysis of the effect of treatment with ursodeoxycholic acid on histologic progression in primary biliary cirrhosis. J Hepatol. 2003;39:12–6.
253. Combes B, Markin RS, Wheeler DE, Rubin R, West AB, Mills AS, Eigenbrodt EH, et al. The effect of ursodeoxycholic acid on the florid duct lesion of primary biliary cirrhosis. Hepatology. 1999;30:602–5.
254. Miyaguchi S, Ebinuma H, Imaeda H, Nitta Y, Watanabe T, Saito H, Ishii H. A novel treatment for refractory primary biliary cirrhosis? Hepato-Gastroenterology. 2000;47:1518–21.
255. Dohmen K, Mizuta T, Nakamuta M, Shimohashi N, Ishibashi H, Yamamoto K. Fenofibrate for patients with asymptomatic primary biliary cirrhosis. World J Gastroenterol. 2004;10:894–8.

256. Bergasa NV, Jones A, Kleiner DE, Rabin L, Park Y, Wells MC, Hoofnagle JH. Pilot study of low dose oral methotrexate treatment for primary biliary cirrhosis. Am J Gastroenterol. 1996;91:295–9.

257. Lindor KD, Dickson ER, Jorgensen RA, Anderson ML, Wiesner RH, Gores GJ, Lange SM, et al. The combination of ursodeoxycholic acid and methotrexate for patients with primary biliary cirrhosis: the results of a pilot study. Hepatology. 1995;22:1158–62.

258. Combes B, Emerson SS, Flye NL, Munoz SJ, Luketic VA, Mayo MJ, McCashland TM, et al. Methotrexate (MTX) plus ursodeoxycholic acid (UDCA) in the treatment of primary biliary cirrhosis. Hepatology. 2005;42:1184–93.

259. Leung J, Bonis PA, Kaplan MM. Colchicine or methotrexate, with ursodiol, are effective after 20 years in a subset of patients with primary biliary cirrhosis. Clin Gastroenterol Hepatol. 2011;9:776–80.

260. Heathcote J, Ross A, Sherlock S. A prospective controlled trial of azathioprine in primary biliary cirrhosis. Gastroenterology. 1976;70:656–60.

261. Christensen E, Neuberger J, Crowe J, Altman DG, Popper H, Portmann B, Doniach D, et al. Beneficial effect of azathioprine and prediction of prognosis in primary biliary cirrhosis. Final results of an international trial. Gastroenterology. 1985;89:1084–91.

262. Gong Y, Christensen E, Gluud C. Azathioprine for primary biliary cirrhosis. Cochrane Database Syst Rev. 2007;18:CD006000.

263. Neuberger J, Christensen E, Portmann B, Caballeria J, Rodes J, Ranek L, Tygstrup N, et al. Double blind controlled trial of d-penicillamine in patients with primary biliary cirrhosis. Gut. 1985;26:114–9.

264. Gong Y, Frederiksen SL, Gluud C. D-penicillamine for primary biliary cirrhosis. Cochrane Database Syst Rev. 2004;18:CD004789.

265. Gong Y, Klingenberg SL, Gluud C. Systematic review and meta-analysis: D-Penicillamine vs. placebo/no intervention in patients with primary biliary cirrhosis – Cochrane Hepato-biliary group. Aliment Pharmacol Ther. 2006;24:1535–44.

266. Kaplan MM, Alling DW, Zimmerman HJ, Wolfe HJ, Sepersky RA, Hirsch GS, Elta GH, et al. A prospective trial of colchicine for primary biliary cirrhosis. N Engl J Med. 1986;315:1448–54.

267. Gong Y, Gluud C. Colchicine for primary biliary cirrhosis. Cochrane Database Syst Rev. 2004;2:CD004481.

268. Gong Y, Gluud C. Colchicine for primary biliary cirrhosis: a Cochrane Hepato-biliary group systematic review of randomized clinical trials. Am J Gastroenterol. 2005;100:1876–85.

269. Minuk GY, Bohme CE, Burgess E, Hershfield NB, Kelly JK, Shaffer EA, Sutherland LR, et al. Pilot study of cyclosporin a in patients with symptomatic primary biliary cirrhosis. Gastroenterology. 1988;95:1356–63.

270. Wiesner RH, Ludwig J, Lindor KD, Jorgensen RA, Baldus WP, Homburger HA, Dickson ER. A controlled trial of cyclosporine in the treatment of primary biliary cirrhosis [see comments]. N Engl J Med. 1990;322:1419–24.

271. Gong Y, Christensen E, Gluud C. Cyclosporin a for primary biliary cirrhosis. Cochrane Database Syst Rev. 2007;3:CD005526.

272. Hoofnagle JH, Davis GL, Schafer DF, Peters M, Avigan MI, Pappas SC, Hanson RG, et al. Randomized trial of chlorambucil for primary biliary cirrhosis. Gastroenterology. 1986;91:1327–34.

273. Mitchison HC, Palmer JM, Bassendine MF, Watson AJ, Record CO, James OF. A controlled trial of prednisolone treatment in primary biliary cirrhosis. Three-year results. J Hepatol. 1992;15:336–44.

274. Mitchison HC, Bassendine MF, Malcolm AJ, Watson AJ, Record CO, James OF. A pilot, double-blind, controlled 1-year trial of prednisolone treatment in primary biliary cirrhosis: hepatic improvement but greater bone loss. Hepatology. 1989;10:420–9.

275. Kaplan MM, Knox TA. Treatment of primary biliary cirrhosis with low-dose weekly methotrexate [see comments]. Gastroenterology. 1991;101:1332–8.

276. Lindor KD, Therneau TM, Jorgensen RA, Malinchoc M, Dickson ER. Effects of ursode-oxycholic acid on survival in patients with primary biliary cirrhosis. Gastroenterology. 1996;110:1515–8.

277. Corpechot C, Carrat F, Bonnand AM, Poupon RE, Poupon R. The effect of ursodeoxy-cholic acid therapy on liver fibrosis progression in primary biliary cirrhosis. Hepatology. 2000;32:1196–9.

278. Lindor KD, Jorgensen RA, Therneau TM, Malinchoc M, Dickson ER. Ursodeoxycholic acid delays the onset of esophageal varices in primary biliary cirrhosis. Mayo Clin Proc. 1997;72:1137–40.

279. Corpechot C, Carrat F, Bahr A, Chretien Y, Poupon RE, Poupon R. The effect of ursode-oxycholic acid therapy on the natural course of primary biliary cirrhosis. Gastroenterology. 2005;128:297–303.

280. Pares A, Caballeria L, Rodes J. Excellent long-term survival in patients with primary biliary cirrhosis and biochemical response to ursodeoxycholic acid. Gastroenterology. 2006;130:715–20.

281. Huet PM, Vincent C, Deslaurier J, Cote J, Matsutami S, Boileau R, Huet-van KJ. Portal hypertension and primary biliary cirrhosis: effect of long-term ursodeoxycholic acid treat-ment. Gastroenterology. 2008;135:1552–60.

282. Combes B, Luketic VA, Peters MG, Zetterman RK, Garcia-Tsao G, Munoz SJ, Lin D, et al. Prolonged follow-up of patients in the U.S. multicenter trial of ursodeoxycholic acid for primary biliary cirrhosis. Am J Gastroenterol. 2004;99:264–8.

283. Gong Y, Huang ZB, Christensen E, Gluud C. Ursodeoxycholic acid for primary biliary cir-rhosis. Cochrane Database Syst Rev. 2008;3:CD000551.

284. Leuschner M, Maier KP, Schlichting J, Strahl S, Herrmann G, Dahm HH, Ackermann H, et al. Oral budesonide and ursodeoxycholic acid for treatment of primary biliary cirrhosis: results of a prospective double-blind trial. Gastroenterology. 1999;117:918–25.

285. Rautiainen H, Karkkainen P, Karvonen AL, Nurmi H, Pikkarainen P, Nuutinen H, Farkkila M. Budesonide combined with UDCA to improve liver histology in primary biliary cirrhosis: a three-year randomized trial. Hepatology. 2005;41:747–52.

286. Wolfhagen FH, van Hoogstraten HJ, van Buuren HR, van Berge-Henegouwen GP, ten Kate FJ, Hop WC, van der Hoek EW, et al. Triple therapy with ursodeoxycholic acid, prednisone and azathioprine in primary biliary cirrhosis: a 1-year randomized, placebo-controlled study. J Hepatol. 1998;29:736–42.

287. Almasio PL, Floreani A, Chiaramonte M, Provenzano G, Battezzati P, Crosignani A, Podda M, et al. Multicentre randomized placebo-controlled trial of ursodeoxycholic acid with or without colchicine in symptomatic primary biliary cirrhosis. Aliment Pharmacol Ther. 2000;14:1645–52.

288. Gong Y, Gluud C. Methotrexate for primary biliary cirrhosis. Cochrane Database Syst Rev. 2005;3:CD004385.

289. https://www.accessdata.fda.gov Ocaliva - Accessdata.fda.gov

290. Nevens F, Andreone P, Mazzella G, Strasser SI, Bowlus C, Invernizzi P, Drenth JP, et al. A placebo-controlled trial of obeticholic acid in primary biliary cholangitis. N Engl J Med. 2016;375:631–43.

291. Hirschfield GM, Mason A, Luketic V, Lindor K, Gordon SC, Mayo M, Kowdley KV, et al. Efficacy of obeticholic acid in patients with primary biliary cirrhosis and inadequate response to ursodeoxycholic acid. Gastroenterology. 2015;148:751–61.

292. Kowdley KV, Luketic V, Chapman R, Hirschfield GM, Poupon R, Schramm C, Vincent C, et al. A randomized trial of obeticholic acid monotherapy in patients with primary biliary cholangitis. Hepatology. 2018;67:1890–902.

293. Bowlus CL, Pockros PJ, Kremer AE, Pares A, Forman LM, JPH D, Ryder SD, et al. Long-term obeticholic acid therapy improves histological endpoints in patients with primary biliary cholangitis. Clin Gastroenterol Hepatol. 2019;18(5):1170–1178.e6.

294. Summerfield JA, Elias E, Sherlock S. Effects of clofibrate in primary biliary cirrhosis hyper-cholesterolemia and gallstones. Gastroenterology. 1975;69:998–1000.

295. Sherlock S. Cholestasis. In: Diseases of the liver and biliary system. Oxford: Blackwell Scientific Publications; 1981. p. 209–43.

296. WHO cooperative trial on primary prevention of ischaemic heart disease with clofibrate to lower serum cholesterol: final mortality follow-up. Report of the Committee of Principal Investigators. Lancet. 1984;2:600–4.

297. Oliver M. The clofibrate saga: a retrospective commentary. Br J Clin Pharmacol. 2012;74:907–10.

298. Fruchart JC, Duriez P. Mode of action of fibrates in the regulation of triglyceride and HDL-cholesterol metabolism. Drugs Today (Barc). 2006;42:39–64.

299. Tenenbaum A, Motro M, Fisman EZ. Dual and pan-peroxisome proliferator-activated receptors (PPAR) co-agonism: the bezafibrate lessons. Cardiovasc Diabetol. 2005;4:14.

300. Iwasaki S, Tsuda K, Ueta H, Aono R, Ono M, Saibara T, Maeda T, Onishi S. Bezafibrate may have a beneficial effect in pre-cirrhotic primary biliary cirrhosis. Hepatol Res. 1999;16:12–8.

301. Kanda T, Yokosuka O, Imazeki F, Saisho H. Bezafibrate treatment: a new medical approach for PBC patients? J Gastroenterol. 2003;38:573–8.

302. Nakamuta M, Fujino T, Yada R, Yasutake K, Yoshimoto T, Harada N, Yada M, et al. Therapeutic effect of bezafibrate against biliary damage: a study of phospholipid secretion via the PPARalpha-MDR3 pathway. Int J Clin Pharmacol Ther. 2010;48:22–8.

303. Hazzan R, Tur-Kaspa R. Bezafibrate treatment of primary biliary cirrhosis following incomplete response to ursodeoxycholic acid. J Clin Gastroenterol. 2010;44:371–3.

304. Honda A, Ikegami T, Nakamuta M, Miyazaki T, Iwamoto J, Hirayama T, Saito Y, et al. Anticholestatic effects of bezafibrate in patients with primary biliary cirrhosis treated with ursodeoxycholic acid. Hepatology. 2013;57:1931–41.

305. Hosonuma K, Sato K, Yamazaki Y, Yanagisawa M, Hashizume H, Horiguchi N, Kakizaki S, et al. A prospective randomized controlled study of long-term combination therapy using ursodeoxycholic acid and bezafibrate in patients with primary biliary cirrhosis and dyslipidemia. Am J Gastroenterol. 2015;110:423–31.

306. Corpechot C, Chazouilleres O, Rousseau A, Le Gruyer A, Habersetzer F, Mathurin P, Goria O, et al. A placebo-controlled trial of bezafibrate in primary biliary cholangitis. N Engl J Med. 2018;378:2171–81.

307. Jones D, Boudes PF, Swain MG, Bowlus CL, Galambos MR, Bacon BR, Doerffel Y, et al. Seladelpar (MBX-8025), a selective PPAR-delta agonist, in patients with primary biliary cholangitis with an inadequate response to ursodeoxycholic acid: a double-blind, randomised, placebo-controlled, phase 2, proof-of-concept study. Lancet Gastroenterol Hepatol. 2017;2:716–26.

308. Bowlus CA, Hirschfield G, Bacon B, Galambos M, Harrison S, Odin J, Amato G, Steinberg S, Rosenbusch S, Bergheanu S, Boudes P. Safety and efficacy of seladelpar in patients with primary biliary cholangitis with cirrhosis. Hepatology. 2019;70:1898.

309. Schattenberg JM, Pares A, Kowdley KV, Heneghan MA, Caldwell S, Pratt D, et al. A randomized placebo-controlled trial of elafibranor in patients with primary biliary cholangitis and incomplete response to UDCA. J Hepatol. 2021;74(6):1344–54.

310. Lammers WJ, van Buuren HR, Hirschfield GM, Janssen HL, Invernizzi P, Mason AL, Ponsioen CY, et al. Levels of alkaline phosphatase and bilirubin are surrogate end points of outcomes of patients with primary biliary cirrhosis: an international follow-up study. Gastroenterology. 2014;147:1338–1349 e1335.

311. Lammers WJ, Hirschfield GM, Corpechot C, Nevens F, Lindor KD, Janssen HL, Floreani A, et al. Development and validation of a scoring system to predict outcomes of patients with primary biliary cirrhosis receiving ursodeoxycholic acid therapy. Gastroenterology. 2015;149:1804–12.

312. Carbone M, Sharp SJ, Flack S, Paximadas D, Spiess K, Adgey C, Griffiths L, et al. The UK-PBC risk scores: derivation and validation of a scoring system for long-term prediction of end-stage liver disease in primary biliary cholangitis. Hepatology. 2016;63:930–50.
313. Efe C, Tascilar K, Henriksson I, Lytvyak E, Alalkim F, Trivedi H, Eren F, et al. Validation of risk scoring systems in ursodeoxycholic acid-treated patients with primary biliary cholangitis. Am J Gastroenterol. 2019;114:1101–8.
314. Gluud C, Brok J, Gong Y, Koretz RL. Hepatology may have problems with putative surrogate outcome measures. J Hepatol. 2007;46:734–42.
315. Cauch-Dudek K, Abbey S, Stewart DE, Heathcote EJ. Fatigue in primary biliary cirrhosis. Gut. 1998;43:705–10.
316. Goldblatt J, James OF, Jones DE. Grip strength and subjective fatigue in patients with primary biliary cirrhosis. JAMA. 2001;285:2196–7.
317. Lemp MA. Report of the National Eye Institute/industry workshop on clinical trials in dry eyes. CLAO J. 1995;21:221–32.
318. Aragona P, Papa V, Micali A, Santocono M, Milazzo G. Long term treatment with sodium hyaluronate-containing artificial tears reduces ocular surface damage in patients with dry eye. Br J Ophthalmol. 2002;86:181–4.
319. Tatlipinar S, Akpek EK. Topical ciclosporin in the treatment of ocular surface disorders. Br J Ophthalmol. 2005;89:1363–7.
320. Hamano T. Lacrimal duct occlusion for the treatment of dry eye. Semin Ophthalmol. 2005;20:71–4.
321. Alves M, Novaes P, Morraye Mde A, Reinach PS, Rocha EM. Is dry eye an environmental disease? Arq Bras Oftalmol. 2014;77:193–200.
322. Wolkoff P. The mystery of dry indoor air - an overview. Environ Int. 2018;121:1058–65.
323. Richards A, Rooney J, Prime S, Scully C. Primary biliary cirrhosis. Sole presentation with rampant dental caries. Oral Surg Oral Med Oral Pathol. 1994;77:16–8.
324. Olsson H, Spak CJ, Axell T. The effect of a chewing gum on salivary secretion, oral mucosal friction, and the feeling of dry mouth in xerostomic patients. Acta Odontol Scand. 1991;49:273–9.
325. Alsakran AM. Update knowledge of dry mouth - a guideline for dentists. Afr Health Sci. 2014;14:736–42.
326. Izumi M, Eguchi K, Nakamura H, Takagi Y, Kawabe Y, Nakamura T. Corticosteroid irrigation of parotid gland for treatment of xerostomia in patients with Sjogren's syndrome. Ann Rheum Dis. 1998;57:464–9.
327. Mavragani CP, Moutsopoulos HM. Conventional therapy of Sjogren's syndrome. Clin Rev Allergy Immunol. 2007;32:284–91.
328. Mavragani CP. Mechanisms and new strategies for primary Sjogren's syndrome. Annu Rev Med. 2017;68:331–43.
329. Mang FW, Michieletti P, O'Rourke K, Cauch-Dudek K, Diamant N, Bookman A, Heathcote J. Primary biliary cirrhosis, sicca complex, and dysphagia. Dysphagia. 1997;12:167–70.
330. Romao VC, Talarico R, Scire CA, Vieira A, Alexander T, Baldini C, Gottenberg JE, et al. Sjogren's syndrome: state of the art on clinical practice guidelines. RMD Open. 2018;4:e000789.
331. Floreani A, Mega A, Camozzi V, Baldo V, Plebani M, Burra P, Luisetto G. Is osteoporosis a peculiar association with primary biliary cirrhosis? World J Gastroenterol. 2005;11:5347–50.
332. Boulton-Jones JR, Fenn RM, West J, Logan RF, Ryder SD. Fracture risk of women with primary biliary cirrhosis: no increase compared with general population controls. Aliment Pharmacol Ther. 2004;20:551–7.
333. Guanabens N, Pares A, del Rio L, Roca M, Gomez R, Munoz J, Rodes J. Sodium fluoride prevents bone loss in primary biliary cirrhosis. J Hepatol. 1992;15:345–9.
334. Camisasca M, Crosignani A, Battezzati PM, Albisetti W, Grandinetti G, Pietrogrande L, Biffi A, et al. Parenteral calcitonin for metabolic bone disease associated with primary biliary cirrhosis. Hepatology. 1994;20:633–7.

335. Guanabens N, Pares A, Ros I, Alvarez L, Pons F, Caballeria L, Monegal A, et al. Alendronate is more effective than etidronate for increasing bone mass in osteopenic patients with primary biliary cirrhosis. Am J Gastroenterol. 2003;98:2268–74.
336. Zein CO, Jorgensen RA, Clarke B, Wenger DE, Keach JC, Angulo P, Lindor KD. Alendronate improves bone mineral density in primary biliary cirrhosis: a randomized placebo-controlled trial. Hepatology. 2005;42:762–71.
337. Floreani A, Carderi I, Ferrara F, Rizzotto ER, Luisetto G, Camozzi V, Baldo V. A 4-year treatment with clodronate plus calcium and vitamin D supplements does not improve bone mass in primary biliary cirrhosis. Dig Liver Dis. 2007;39:544–8.
338. Nishiguchi S, Shimoi S, Kurooka H, Tamori A, Habu D, Takeda T, Kubo S. Randomized pilot trial of vitamin K2 for bone loss in patients with primary biliary cirrhosis. J Hepatol. 2001;35:543–5.
339. Pereira SP, O'Donohue J, Moniz C, Phillips MG, Abraha H, Buxton-Thomas M, Williams R. Transdermal hormone replacement therapy improves vertebral bone density in primary biliary cirrhosis: results of a 1-year controlled trial. Aliment Pharmacol Ther. 2004;19:563–70.
340. Ormarsdottir S, Mallmin H, Naessen T, Petren-Mallmin M, Broome U, Hultcrantz R, Loof L. An open, randomized, controlled study of transdermal hormone replacement therapy on the rate of bone loss in primary biliary cirrhosis. J Intern Med. 2004;256:63–9.
341. Lindor KD, Janes CH, Crippin JS, Jorgensen RA, Dickson ER. Bone disease in primary biliary cirrhosis: does ursodeoxycholic acid make a difference? Hepatology. 1995;21:389–92.
342. Floreani A, Zappala F, Fries W, Naccarato R, Plebani M, D'Angelo A, Chiaramonte M. A 3-year pilot study with 1,25-dihydroxyvitamin D, calcium, and calcitonin for severe osteodystrophy in primary biliary cirrhosis. J Clin Gastroenterol. 1997;24:239–44.
343. Boone RH, Cheung AM, Girlan LM, Heathcote EJ. Osteoporosis in primary biliary cirrhosis: a randomized trial of the efficacy and feasibility of estrogen/progestin. Dig Dis Sci. 2006;51:1103–12.
344. Crippin JS, Jorgensen RA, Dickson ER, Lindor KD. Hepatic osteodystrophy in primary biliary cirrhosis: effects of medical treatment. Am J Gastroenterol. 1994;89:47–50.
345. Hulley S, Grady D, Bush T, Furberg C, Herrington D, Riggs B, et al. Randomized trial of estrogen plus progestin for secondary prevention of coronary heart disease in postmenopausal women. Heart and Estrogen/progestin Replacement Study (HERS) Research Group. JAMA. 1998;280(7):605–13.
346. Rossouw JE, Anderson GL, Prentice RL, LaCroix AZ, Kooperberg C, Stefanick ML, et al. Risks and benefits of estrogen plus progestin in healthy postmenopausal women: principal results From the Women's Health Initiative randomized controlled trial. JAMA. 2002;288(3):321–33.
347. Seeman E. Raloxifene. J Bone Miner Metab. 2001;19(2):65–75.
348. Levy C, Harnois DM, Angulo P, Jorgensen R, Lindor KD. Raloxifene improves bone mass in osteopenic women with primary biliary cirrhosis: results of a pilot study. Liver international: official journal of the International Association for the Study of the Liver. 2005;25(1):117–21.
349. Cremers S, Drake MT, Ebetino FH, Bilezikian JP, Russell RGG. Pharmacology of bisphosphonates. British journal of clinical pharmacology. 2019;85(6):1052–62.
350. Lindor KD, Jorgensen RA, Tiegs RD, Khosla S, Dickson ER. Etidronate for osteoporosis in primary biliary cirrhosis: a randomized trial. J Hepatol. 2000;33(6):878–82.
351. Floreani A, Carderi I, Ferrara F, Rizzotto ER, Luisetto G, Camozzi V, et al. A 4-year treatment with clodronate plus calcium and vitamin D supplements does not improve bone mass in primary biliary cirrhosis. Digestive and liver disease: official journal of the Italian Society of Gastroenterology and the Italian Association for the Study of the Liver. 2007;39(6):544–8.
352. Danford CJ, Ezaz G, Trivedi HD, Tapper EB, Bonder A. The pharmacologic management of osteoporosis in primary biliary cholangitis: a systematic review and meta-analysis. J Clin Densitom. 2019;23(2):223–36.
353. Arase Y, Tsuruya K, Hirose S, Ogiwara N, Yokota M, Anzai K, Deguchi R, et al. Efficacy and safety of 3-year Denosumab therapy for osteoporosis in patients with autoimmune liver diseases. Hepatology. 2019;71(2):757–9.

354. Lleo A, Ma X, Gershwin ME, Invernizzi P. Letter to the editor: might Denosumab fit in PBC treatment? Hepatology. 2019;72(1):359–60.
355. Acalovschi M. Gallstones in patients with liver cirrhosis: incidence, etiology, clinical and therapeutical aspects. World J Gastroenterol. 2014;20(23):7277–85.
356. Summerfield JA, Elias E, Hungerford GD, Nikapota VL, Dick R, Sherlock S. The biliary system in primary biliary cirrhosis. A study by endoscopic retrograde cholangiopancreatography. Gastroenterology. 1976;70(2):240–3.
357. Zak A, Zeman M, Slaby A, Vecka M. Xanthomas: clinical and pathophysiological relations. Biomedical papers of the Medical Faculty of the University Palacky, Olomouc, Czechoslovakia. 2014;158(2):181–8.
358. Ahrens EH, Jr., Kunkel HG. The relationship between serum lipids and skin xanthomata in 18 patients with primary biliary cirrhosis. The Journal of clinical investigation. 1949;28(6 Pt 2):1565–74.
359. Turnberg LA, Mahoney MP, Gleeson MH, Freeman CB, Gowenlock AH. Plasmaphoresis and plasma exchange in the treatment of hyperlipaemia and xanthomatous neuropathy in patients with primary biliary cirrhosis. Gut. 1972;13(12):976–81.
360. Peters MG, Hoffnagle JH, McGarvey C, Fox I, Gregg RE, Jones EA. Primary biliary cirrhosis: management of an unusual case with severe xanthomata by hepatic transplantation. Journal of clinical gastroenterology. 1989;11(6):694–7.
361. Kew MC, Varma RR, Dos Santos HA, Scheuer PJ, Sherlock S. Portal hypertension in primary biliary cirrhosis. Gut. 1971;12(10):830–4.
362. Lebrec D, Sicot C, Degott C, Benhamou JP. Portal hypertension and primary biliary cirrhosis. Digestion. 1976;14(3):220–6.
363. Abraham SC, Kamath PS, Eghtesad B, Demetris AJ, Krasinskas AM. Liver transplantation in precirrhotic biliary tract disease: portal hypertension is frequently associated with nodular regenerative hyperplasia and obliterative portal venopathy. Am J Surg Pathol. 2006;30:1454–61.
364. Garcia-Tsao G, Abraldes JG, Berzigotti A, Bosch J. Portal hypertensive bleeding in cirrhosis: risk stratification, diagnosis, and management: 2016 practice guidance by the American Association for the Study of Liver Diseases. Hepatology. 2017;65:310–35.
365. Grace ND, Groszmann RJ, Garcia-Tsao G, Burroughs AK, Pagliaro L, Makuch RW, et al. Portal hypertension and variceal bleeding: an AASLD single topic symposium. Hepatology. 1998;28(3):868–80.
366. Bressler B, Pinto R, El-Ashry D, Heathcote EJ. Which patients with primary biliary cirrhosis or primary sclerosing cholangitis should undergo endoscopic screening for oesophageal varices detection? Gut. 2005;54:407–10.
367. Lindor KD, Gershwin ME, Poupon R, Kaplan M, Bergasa NV, Heathcote EJ, et al. Primary biliary cirrhosis. Hepatology. 2009;50(1):291–308.
368. Boyer TD, Kokenes DD, Hertzler G, Kutner MH, Henderson JM. Effect of distal splenorenal shunt on survival of patients with primary biliary cirrhosis. Hepatology. 1994;20:1482–6.
369. Vlachogiannakos J, Carpenter J, Goulis J, Triantos C, Patch D, Burroughs AK. Variceal bleeding in primary biliary cirrhosis patients: a subgroup with improved prognosis and a model to predict survival after first bleeding. Eur J Gastroenterol Hepatol. 2009;21: 701–7.
370. Kuiper EM, Hansen BE, Adang RP, van Nieuwkerk CM, Timmer R, Drenth JP, et al. Relatively high risk for hepatocellular carcinoma in patients with primary biliary cirrhosis not responding to ursodeoxycholic acid. Eur J Gastroenterol Hepatol. 2010;22(12):1495–502.
371. Cavazza A, Caballeria L, Floreani A, Farinati F, Bruguera M, Caroli D, Pares A. Incidence, risk factors, and survival of hepatocellular carcinoma in primary biliary cirrhosis: comparative analysis from two centers. Hepatology. 2009;50:1162–8.
372. Silveira MG, Suzuki A, Lindor KD. Surveillance for hepatocellular carcinoma in patients with primary biliary cirrhosis. Hepatology. 2008;48(4):1149–56.
373. Lee J, Belanger A, Doucette JT, Stanca C, Friedman S, Bach N. Transplantation trends in primary biliary cirrhosis. Clin Gastroenterol Hepatol. 2007;5(11):1313–5.

374. Shapiro JM, Smith H, Schaffner F. Serum bilirubin: a prognostic factor in primary biliary cirrhosis. Gut. 1979;20(2):137–40.
375. Bonnand AM, Heathcote EJ, Lindor KD, Poupon RE. Clinical significance of serum bilirubin levels under ursodeoxycholic acid therapy in patients with primary biliary cirrhosis. Hepatology. 1999;29(1):39–43.
376. Neuberger J, Altman DG, Christensen E, Tygstrup N, Williams R. Use of a prognostic index in evaluation of liver transplantation for primary biliary cirrhosis. Transplantation. 1986;41:713–6.
377. Christensen E, Altman DG, Neuberger J, De Stavola BL, Tygstrup N, Williams R. Updating prognosis in primary biliary cirrhosis using a time-dependent cox regression model. PBC1 and PBC2 trial groups. Gastroenterology. 1993;105:1865–76.
378. Christensen E, Gunson B, Neuberger J. Optimal timing of liver transplantation for patients with primary biliary cirrhosis: use of prognostic modelling. J Hepatol. 1999;30:285–92.
379. Dickson ER, Grambsch PM, Fleming TR, Fisher LD, Langworthy A. Prognosis in primary biliary cirrhosis: model for decision making. Hepatology. 1989;10:1–7.
380. Grambsch PM, Dickson ER, Kaplan M, LeSage G, Fleming TR, Langworthy AL. Extramural cross-validation of the Mayo primary biliary cirrhosis survival model establishes its generalizability. Hepatology. 1989;10:846–50.
381. Grambsch PM, Dickson ER, Wiesner RH, Langworthy A. Application of the Mayo primary biliary cirrhosis survival model to Mayo liver transplant patients. Mayo Clin Proc. 1989;64:699–704.
382. Cholongitas E, Burroughs AK. The evolution in the prioritization for liver transplantation. Ann Gastroenterol. 2012;25(1):6–13.
383. Harms MH, Janssen QP, Adam R, Duvoux C, Mirza D, Hidalgo E, Watson C, et al. Trends in liver transplantation for primary biliary cholangitis in Europe over the past three decades. Aliment Pharmacol Ther. 2019;49:285–95.
384. Kim WR, Wiesner RH, Therneau TM, Poterucha JJ, Porayko MK, Evans RW, et al. Optimal timing of liver transplantation for primary biliary cirrhosis. Hepatology. 1998;28(1):33–8.
385. Liermann Garcia RF, Evangelista Garcia C, McMaster P, Neuberger J. Transplantation for primary biliary cirrhosis: retrospective analysis of 400 patients in a single center. Hepatology. 2001;33(1):22–7.
386. Neuberger J. Incidence, timing, and risk factors for acute and chronic rejection. Liver Transpl Surg. 1999;5(4 Suppl 1):S30–6.
387. Krawczyk M, Kozma M, Szymanska A, Leszko K, Przedniczek M, Mucha K, Foroncewicz B, et al. Effects of liver transplantation on health-related quality of life in patients with primary biliary cholangitis. Clin Transpl. 2018;32:e13434.
388. Silveira MG, Talwalkar JA, Lindor KD, Wiesner RH. Recurrent primary biliary cirrhosis after liver transplantation. Am J Transplant. 2010;10:720–6.
389. Neuberger J, Gunson B, Hubscher S, Nightingale P. Immunosuppression affects the rate of recurrent primary biliary cirrhosis after liver transplantation. Liver Transpl. 2004;10:488–91.
390. Manousou P, Arvaniti V, Tsochatzis E, Isgro G, Jones K, Shirling G, et al. Primary biliary cirrhosis after liver transplantation: influence of immunosuppression and human leukocyte antigen locus disparity. Liver Transpl. 2010;16(1):64–73.
391. Montano-Loza AJ, Wasilenko S, Bintner J, Mason AL. Cyclosporine A protects against primary biliary cirrhosis recurrence after liver transplantation. Am J Transplant. 2010;10:852–8.
392. Jacob DA, Haase E, Klein F, Pratschke J, Neumann UP, Neuhaus P, Bahra M. Donor influence on outcome in patients undergoing liver transplant for primary biliary cirrhosis. Exp Clin Transplant. 2010;8:104–10.

# Chapter 4
# Autoimmune Hepatitis

**Nora V. Bergasa**

A 39-year-old woman presented to the emergency room because of jaundice. She did not have any symptoms. Her serum activity of AST and ALT was ten times the upper limit of normal, and bilirubin was 6 mg/dl. She was admitted to the hospital where a liver disease workup was notable for positive antinuclear antibodies, and high serum concentrations of immunoglobulin G (IgG). A liver biopsy revealed moderate to severe interface hepatitis with marked lymphoplasmacytic infiltrate, focal lobular necrosis, ballooning degeneration, and giant cell transformation of hepatocytes with Mallory bodies and focal regenerative rosette formation consistent with autoimmune hepatitis (AIH); trichrome stain showed mild periportal fibrosis. The patient was started on prednisone 60 mg/day and referred to the hepatology clinic. On follow up, she was feeling well. The liver profile was notable for a decrease in the serum activity of AST and ALT and bilirubin concentration as compared to the pre treatment values. Prednisone was tapered to 30 mg/day over 2 weeks, at which time azathioprine at 50 mg/day was added, after confirming normal TMPT phenotype. Prednisone was gradually tapered, and the patient was maintained on azathioprine 50 mg/day in association with normalization of liver profile and serum IgG. After 3 years of treatment, including 2 years of normal liver tests, azathioprine was discontinued. She remained well and with a normal liver profile for 2 years, at which time her AST and ALT increased beyond the normal range. Over a short period of observation, a liver biopsy was performed to rule out

N. V. Bergasa (✉)
Department of Medicine, H+H/Metropolitan, New York, NY, USA

New York Medical College, Valhalla, NY, USA

Hepatology, H+H/Woodhull, Brooklyn, NY, USA

recurrence of disease versus fatty liver for which she was at risk. Liver histology revealed a relapse of AIH. The patient was restarted on treatment as initially. At present, prednisone has been discontinued; her liver profile is normal. She is on azathioprine 50 mg/day, doing well.

## Autoimmune Hepatitis

The patient described in this chapter presented with acute hepatitis. The liver disease workup at presentation excluded viral causes of acute hepatitis, and drug-induced hepatitis, including that caused by over the counter medications and supplements. The autoantibodies panel suggested an autoimmune etiology of liver disease, as did the high serum concentration of immunoglobulin G. A liver biopsy (Fig. 4.1) supported the diagnosis. She responded to immunosuppressant medications also in support of a diagnosis of autoimmune hepatitis but subsequently relapsed off treatment, as it happens in this disease.

## Etiology

Autoimmune hepatitis (AIH) is defined as hepatitis associated with markers of autoimmunity and typical histological findings. The etiology of autoimmune hepatitis is unknown.

**Fig. 4.1** Liver histology of autoimmune hepatitis. The interface (arrows) between inflamed portal tract and parenchyma is irregular and blurred by inflammatory infiltration and hepatocyte loss. Hematoxylin and Eosin, original magnification, 20×

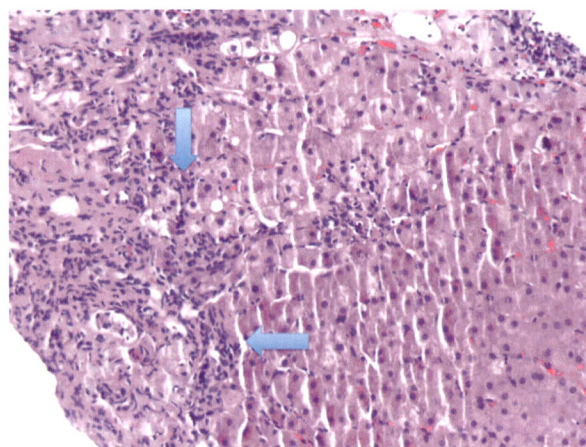

## Pathogenetics

Regulatory T cells, Tregs, mediate immune tolerance by suppressing lymphocytes that react to self-antigens [1]. Studies of this type of cells in autoimmune hepatitis have suggested alterations in their number and function, although not consistently. Serum CD4+ CD 25+ Tregs cells were reported as decreased in patients with AIH compared to those in the control group at the time of diagnosis and in remission. In vitro, their ability to expand was decreased; however, their capacity to suppress effector function, tested in vitro by assessing interferon gamma production by the CD4(+)CD25(−) T-cells, was preserved. The decrease in number and ability to expand CD4(+)CD25(+) T cells was interpreted as possible causes for the development of cellular responses that contribute to AIH [2]. Although the ability of Tregs in AIH to suppress interferon gamma production by CD4+CD25- T-cells has been reported to be intact, CD4+CD25+ (Tregs) were also reported not to be able to regulate the proliferation of CD8 T-cells and cytokine production in patients at the time of diagnosis of AIH, however, they were able to suppress CD8 T-cell proliferation and trigger an increase in the CD8 T cells that produce IL-4 in remission after pharmacological therapy, which was interpreted as indicating that treatment of AIH with immunosuppressant medications restore proper function of CD4+CD25+ (Tregs) [3]. In an ex vivo study, regulatory CD4+CD25+ T cells (Tregs) from patients with AIH and control subjects required direct contact with CD4+CD25− and CD8+ T cells to suppress proliferation and production of interferon gamma, a proinflammatory cytokine. Direct contact with Tregs was also required for an increase in the production of IL-10, TGF-β, and IL-4, all regulatory cytokines. It has been documented that serum levels of IL-33, sST2, IL-17A, IFN gamma and alpha, and IL-4 were significantly elevated in patients with AIH and that IL-33 correlated positively with hypergammaglobulinemia, and serum activity of alkaline phosphatase (AP) and gamma glutamyl transpeptidase (GGTP), interpreted as markers of liver injury, findings that have suggested a role of the IL-33/sST2 axis in the progression of AIH [4]. IL-17 has been reported to correlate with histology [5].

Serum levels of M2BPGi were increased in patients with untreated AIH and were decreased following steroid treatment that resulted in clinical improvement. This marker might reflect liver fibrosis and autoimmune-mediated hepatic inflammation in parallel to the induction of hepatitis-related inflammatory cytokines [6].

Co-culture of Tregs with CD4+CD25− T cells was associated with increased interferon gamma and interleukin (IL)-10 production by cells from patients with AIH and by those from control subjects; however, the production of TGF-beta, involved in innate immunity, was significantly lower from cells from the AIH group than from the control group. The expression of FOXP3, a key transcription factor in Tregs' regulation, was documented as decreased in the cells from the patients compared to those from control subjects. In addition, it was reported that spontaneous apoptosis of CD4(+)CD25(−) T cells was reduced in the patients. These results have suggested that in AIH, Tregs do interact with their target cells to produce specific cytokines; however, they do not make interferon beta, a cytokine relevant in innate immunity, and that they have a decrease in their apoptotic process, which may contribute to the development of autoimmunity [7]. In these experiments, patients had been treated with immunosuppressant drugs; thus, the results of these ex vivo experiments might have been influenced by pharmacotherapy [7].

From a study that used peripheral mononuclear cells from control and subjects with AIH with active disease and in remission, it was reported that the regulatory T cells (Tregs) compartment had fewer CD4(+)CD25(hi) T cells, particularly during active disease, expressed lower levels of FOXP3 and inhibited cellular proliferation in an in vitro assay to a lesser degree than cells from control subjects. The number of natural killer (NK) cells was reduced, and the production of IL-4 was less in patients with autoimmune hepatitis than in control subjects. In regard to gamma delta T cells, they were documented as being more numerous in patients than in the control subjects; the Vdelta1/V delta2 ratio changed to a predominance of Vdelta 1 cells, which have an increased ability to produce proinflammatory cytokines, and their production of interferon gamma and granzyme B was raised, which was reported to correlate with serum markers of liver inflammation. The portal tracts of patients with AIH had few FOXP3(+), which was interpreted to suggest that, in this disease, the effector cells are gamma delta T cells [8].

The idea of the role of CD4+CD25+FOXP3+ regulatory T cells (Treg) in the pathogenesis of AIH has been further explored by the use of more specific identifiers of this compartment of T cells, i.e. CD4+CD25(high)CD127(low)FOXP3+. The frequency of CD4+CD25(high)CD127(low)FOXP3+ was not different in patients with AIH as compared with those of control subjects, and the function, tested by an in vitro suppression assay, was normal. The frequency of Treg in patients with active disease was, however, higher than in patients in remission; these results were interpreted to suggest that the number of Treg T cells may parallel the degree of inflammation. In this regard, it was documented that the population of FOXP3+ Treg in the liver of patients with AIH correlated with the liver's inflammatory activity. These results have not confirmed an impaired compartment of Treg cells in AIH [9]. T cell immunoglobulin mucin-3 (TIM-3) is a T helper type 1 specific cell surface molecule that is reported to regulate T helper cell responses and the induction of peripheral tolerance whose ligand is galectin-9 [10]; in AIH, the levels of Tim-3 on CD4posCD25neg effector cells and Gal 9 + cells are decreased in Tregs, which is associated with impaired Tregs control and with a reduced ability of Tregs to suppress proliferative activity. These results have suggested that the characteristics of Tregs in AIH contribute to the pathogenesis of this disease [11].

Molecular mimicry may contribute to the pathogenesis of AIH, as suggested for other autoimmune diseases [12]. In this regard, anti-LKM1 antibodies, prevalent in the AHI type 2, which affects mostly children, bind to liver and kidney endoplasmic reticulum and recognize cytochrome P450 2D6 (CYP2D6) [13]. Of interest, a study documented similarity and cross-reactivity between CYP2D6, sequence 193–212, and a sequence from the cytomegalovirus and the hepatitis C virus with similarities to self, which may constitute a triggering factor to autoimmune disease, e.g. AIH [14]; indeed, a case of autoimmune hepatitis type 2 induced by HCV has been reported [15].

The serum of patients with AIH was reported to recognize the IL-4 receptor fibronectin type III domain of the IL-4 receptor (CD124), which has an expression on hepatocyte and lymphocyte surfaces, with documented inhibition of STAT6 phosphorylation induced by the binding of IL-4 to CD124; these results have suggested that neutralization of IL-4 contributes to the pathogenesis of AIH [16].

Certain environmental factors are considered contributory to the development of an autoimmune disease, including AIH. Exposure to antibiotics within 1 year prior to the diagnosis of AIH was an independent significant risk factor in developing the disease. In contrast, alcohol consumption and history of a childhood home with wood heating were independently associated with reduced risks for its development in a study from New Zealand [17]. Intestinal dysbiosis, which can result from antibiotic use [18], has been reported in patients with AIH; specifically, it was documented in a group of 24 patients with AIH who had increased intestinal permeability, a deranged microbiome, and bacterial translocation [19].

There is a developing interest in the role of chemokines in the pathogenesis of AIH. Chemokines are small heparin-binding molecules secreted by hepatocytes and other liver resident cells and cells that infiltrate the liver, including neutrophils and platelets [20].

An expert summary of the potential role of chemokines in AIH suggested that T helper type 17 lymphocytes that express CXCR3 and CCR6 are attracted to the liver by the chemokines CXCL9, CXCL10, and CXCL11, and they themselves recruit proinflammatory T helper type 1 lymphocytes that express CXCR3 and CCR5 by secreting CXCL10. The local secretion of CXCL16 stimulates the movement of NK cells, which contribute to the inflammatory process. A decrease in the inflammatory process is mediated by chemokines CCL17 and CCL22, which attract the T helper type 2 lymphocytes that express CCR4; in addition, Tregs that express CXCR3 are attracted by the secretion of CXCL9, which also decreases the inflammatory response. Fibrosis is promoted by CCL2, CCL3, CCL5, CXCL4, CXCL10, and CXCL16 by the activation or attraction of hepatic stellate cells, whereas CX3CL1 may prevent fibrosis by altering apoptosis of monocytes [20]. It is suggested that the development of drugs that interfere with the proinflammatory action of some chemokines will improve the management of AIH [20].

Additional studies have reported that the C-C receptor 7 programmed cell death 1 (CCR7 PD-1) chemokine, a subset of follicular helper T cells (Tfh), was significantly increased in the blood of patients with AIH versus that from patients from viral hepatitis and normal controls, with correlation with serum IgG concentrations and markers of liver function, and associated with a decrease after treatment with steroids; in addition, the number of activated Tfh cells was significantly increased in the liver of patients with AIH, correlated with their number in blood, and produced more IL-21 and Il-17 than those from control subjects, findings interpreted to suggest an involvement of this type of cells and their cytokines in the pathogenesis of AIH [21]. In this regard, the frequency of CCR7 PD-1 Tfh was reported as significantly higher in patients with AIH versus those with viral hepatitis and from control subjects and was found to correlate with the International Autoimmune Hepatitis Group scoring system, suggesting an involvement in the inflammatory activity associated with AIH [21].

# Genetics

Genetic susceptibility is presumed to contribute to the pathogenesis of AIH in association with genes on the human leukocyte antigen (HLA) class I. In children, HLA-DRB1*1301 was reported as a susceptibility allele and HLA-DRB1*1302 as protective; in contrast, in adult subjects from the same country, Argentina, HLA-DRB1*0405 was identified in association with a risk for AIH, but not with markers found in children. These findings suggested that the triggering factors of AIH in children and adults differ, at least in that part of the world [22]. In Brazil, in close geographic proximity to Argentina, but with a different ethnic and racial population, HLA DR13 and DRB1*1301 were found more frequently in the patients than in the control group [23]. DRB1*0301 was identified as a risk for autoimmune hepatitis in patients from North America, in which a secondary association with DRB1*0401 was also identified. This association was not detected in Italy, where the prevalent phenotype was B8-DR3-DQ2, and HLA DR11 appeared to be protective against the disease [24]; in a study from North America, the DRB5*0101-DRB1*1501 haplotype was identified as protective from the disease [25]. A relatively large genome-wide association study (GWAS) from the Netherlands documented a significant association between AIH and a variant in the MHC region at rs2187668; in the discovery cohort, HLA-DRB1*0301 was identified as a primary susceptibility genotype and HLA-DRB1*0401 as a secondary, with HLA-DRB1*03:01 having been reported as the strongest modifier of disease severity [26]. Variants of SH2B3, rs3184504, 12q24, and of CARD10, rs6000782, 22q13.1 were also associated with the disease, in addition to some single nucleotide polymorphisms (SPN)s already identified in other autoimmune liver diseases, which suggested a genetic overlap [26].

In association with AIH, genetic polymorphisms in genes outside the major histocompatibility complex (MHC) that code for proteins that participate in the regulation of the immune response have been identified including: (i) Fas [27, 28], coding for a member of the tumor necrosis factor (TNF) receptor superfamily that contains a death domain, which plays a fundamental role in the regulation of programmed cell death [29], (ii) TNF-alpha [30], coding for TNF [31], a cytokine that is an acute phase reactant, and that is produced by cells of the immune system mostly, activated macrophages, but also natural killer cells (NK), and T lymphocytes [32], (iii) TGF-beta1 [33], coding for TGF-beta1, a polypeptide that mediates immune suppression in innate and adaptive immunity [34], (iv) TBX21 [35], coding TBX21, a Th1-specific T box transcription factor that controls the expression of IFN gamma, a Th1 cytokine [36], (v) VDR [37], coding for the nuclear vitamin D receptor, which modulates adaptive immunity by direct activation of T cells, and which has effects on the phenotype and function of antigen-presenting cells, including dendritic cells. Vitamin D modulates the adaptive immune system by direct effects on T cell activation and the phenotype and function of antigen-presenting cells (APCs), particularly of dendritic cells [38], and also, acts as a receptor for the secondary bile acid lithocholic acid; 1,25(OH)2D3-induced changes in their phenotype and function ultimately affect T lymphocytes, and inconsistently, CTLA-4 [39–41], coding for CTLA-4 (Cytotoxic T-Lymphocyte Antigen 4) [42], a receptor localized on the surface of T cells that downregulates the immune response [42], (vi) the SH2B3 T and the PTPN22 A allele, with protection being given by the presence of the CC and GG genotypes; no significant associations were documented in polymorphisms detected in TGFβ1 and STAT4 [43], and (vii) IL-4 gene [44].

In addition, activated effector NK cells and exhausted memory Tregs were reported to be increased in the blood of patients with AIH and decreased in association with steroid therapy, suggesting a role of inadequate regulation of NK cells in the pathogenesis of AIH [45]. In this regard, it has been suggested that the recruitment of cytotoxic NK cells into the liver and not liver resident NK cells expansion may contribute to the progression of AIH [46].

Dysfunction of Kupffer cells and a reduction in the capacity to phagocytize *E. coli* were documented in patients with AIH; how this finding relates to the disease's pathogenesis is unknown [47].

## Epigenetics

"An epigenetic trait is a stably heritable phenotype resulting from changes in a chromosome without alterations in the DNA sequence" [48]. MicroRNAs (miRNAs) are short RNA molecules that can be regulated by genetics and epigenetic mechanisms [49] and that bind to specific mRNAs leading to translational repression and gene silencing; deficiencies or excess in certain microRNAs have been reported in association with disease [50].

Circulating serum levels of miR-21 were reported as significantly higher in patients with AIH than in disease and normal control subjects. Serum levels of miR-21 and miR-122 correlated with serum activity of alanine aminotransferase (ALT) and were significantly reduced in patients with cirrhosis from AIH, in whom they correlated inversely with the degree of fibrosis, with miR-21 correlating with the degree of inflammation. These results have suggested that the circulation of these two microRNAs may reflect an important role of these two microRNAs in the pathogenesis of the disease [51].

## Clinical Manifestations

The key to an expeditious diagnosis of AIH is to recognize that this disease can have variable presentations. More women than men have AIH. Two peaks in the presentation of this disease, in early adolescence and in the fourth to six decades, have been recognized. However, it has been suggested that referral patterns may contribute to this impression [52]. Patients can be asymptomatic, referred to a physician because of incidental identification of an abnormal liver profile or they can present with fatigue, joint pains, and some signs of liver disease in association with an abnormal liver profile suggestive of hepatocellular injury. A history of intermittently abnormal liver profile can be identified sometimes. Hypergammaglobulinemia is a characteristic laboratory finding in AIH. In approximately a third of patients, AIH can present as fulminant hepatitis and laboratory findings not suggestive of that disease, including normal IgG and total serum gammaglobulin concentrations and negative or low titers of ANA. In these patients, liver histology is useful; however, expertise in obtaining a liver biopsy, usually transjugularly, is necessary to get liver tissue in this type of patient. Liver histology tends to show centrilobular massive and submassive necrosis [53].

As hepatitis, including AIH, can be triggered by some medications, information on drug intake or herbal preparations must be sought, and the suspected triggering agent stopped. Drug-induced hepatitis can have features of AIH; a diagnosis of AIH has to be considered in all cases, and also, the suspected agent has to be stopped immediately. In general, drug-induced hepatitis tends to resolve in association with the discontinuation of the medication; however, treatment with corticosteroids is indicated in patients who present with florid features of both diseases as, indeed, AIH may be part of the pathogenetic process in some patients. Histologically, AIH and drug-induced hepatitis have similar features. At presentation, cirrhosis was not found in any of the patients with drug-induced AIH in a retrospective study that included 261 patients, with a prevalence of nine percent [54]. However, it was present in twenty percent of the patients with AIH proper [54]. Minocycline and nitrofurantoin were identified as the most common causes of drug-induced AIH in this study [54]. Only two patients were not treated with corticosteroids, and of those treated, only one patient with drug-induced AIH did not have a complete response to treatment. In patients in whom corticosteroids were discontinued, hepatitis had not recurred during a median follow up of 36 months; however, it did recur in patients with AIH proper [54]. This natural history was interpreted to suggest that the drug-induced AIH was indeed induced by the drug and not by an underlying process of immune-mediated inflammation [54].

## Physical Examination

On physical examination, patients may or may not exhibit signs suggestive of liver disease, including spider angiomata, jaundice, and ascites. Patients with AIH presenting with fulminant liver failure display signs of hepatic encephalopathy.

The common laboratory findings are increased serum activity of transaminases (alanine and aspartate), normal or increased serum concentration of bilirubin, and modestly increased activity of AP and GGTP. The presence of autoantibodies, as discussed below, is characteristic of autoimmune hepatitis. ANA and ASMA are the most prevalent antibodies identified in the serum of patients with this disease.

Hypergammaglobulinemia is also typical of AIH; serum protein electrophoresis displays a peak in the gamma globulin region, consistent with a high serum concentration of immunoglobulin gamma.

## Autoantibodies

AIH is associated with autoantibodies in most cases, although their absence does not exclude the diagnosis in patients with other features characteristics of the disease. AIH type 1 refers to the disease in adults, associated, in general, with antinuclear antibodies (ANA) directed to centromere, ribonucleoproteins, and ribonucleoprotein complexes [55–57] and anti-smooth muscle antibodies (ASMA), directed to actin and other nonactin cellular components [58]. AIH type 2 is characterized by the presence of anti-LKM antibodies, predominantly in children [56]. The occurrence of anti-LKM, together with ANA and anti-SMA, is reported as less than 4% of patients with AIH. Other autoantibodies can be found in the serum of patients with AIH and, when present, help to confirm the diagnosis in atypical cases, including antibodies to soluble liver antigen (anti-SLA) [59] and antibodies to liver cytosol type 1 (anti-LC1) (Table 4.1).

**Table 4.1** Autoantibodies in autoimmune hepatitis

| Type of antibody | Antigen | Indirect immunofluorescence characteristics | Reported clinical relevance | References |
|---|---|---|---|---|
| Antinuclear | Centromere, ribonucleoproteins, and ribonucleoprotein complexes | Homogenous or speckled nuclear staining of hepatocytes | Characterizes AIH 1, long-term prognosis is better than in seronegative, associated with HLA-DR4 | [55] |
| Anti-double stranded DNA | Double stranded-DNA | Stain of kinetoplast Crithidia luciliae, used as substrate | Common in ANA positive AIH 1, associated with HLA DR4, may portend inferior immediate response to steroids | [57] |
| Anti-smooth muscle | Actin and nonactin cellular components including vimentin, skeletin, tubulin, desmin | Smooth muscle fibers within blood vessels and muscularis usually sought on mucosa of murine stomach and kidney | AIH 1 | [58] |

(continued)

**Table 4.1** (continued)

| Type of antibody | Antigen | Indirect immunofluorescence characteristics | Reported clinical relevance | References |
|---|---|---|---|---|
| Anti-LKM 1 Anti-LKM 2 Anti-LKM 3 Anti-LKM | CYP2D6 CYP2C9 UGT CYP1A2 | Cytoplasm of hepatocytes and proximal renal tubules | AIH 2, genetic predisposition to HLA-B14, DR3, and C4A-QO, and AIH in association with APECED | [56] |
| SLA | Sec synthase | N/A | Specific for AIH 1, portends relapse and severe disease, and associated with HLA-DR3 and DR4 | [59] |
| LCI 1 | FTCD | Cytoplasm of hepatocytes sparing those surrounding the central vein | AIH type 2 | [60] |
| ASGPR | Type 2 transmembrane glycoprotein expressed on the hepatocyte membrane | N/A | Correlates with histological severity | [61] |

*ANA* antinuclear antibodies; *Anti-LKM* anti-liver kidney microsomes antibodies; *SLA* soluble liver antigen; *Anti-LC1* anti-liver cytosol antibody; *ASGPR* anti-asialoglycoprotein receptor antibodies; *CYP* cytochrome P 450; *UGT* Uridine diphosphate glucuronosyltransferase, family of enzymes that catalyze the covalent addition of glucuronic acid to several lipophilic chemicals; their function concerns the detoxification of numerous exogenous and endogenous substances by increasing their polarity, improving their suitability to be excreted in bile or urine [62]; *FTCD* formiminotransferase cyclodeaminase enzyme that catalyzes the conversion of histidine to glutamic acid [63]; *Anti-SLA* anti-soluble liver antigen antibodies, identified as being the same as anti-liver pancreas antibodies; *Sec synthase* a pyridoxal phosphate (PLP)-dependent protein that converts the serine attached to tRNA [Ser] Sec to Sec to an aminoacrylyl intermediate that serves as the acceptor for activated selenium; when selenium is donated, selenocysteyl-tRNA[Ser]Sec is formed [64]. Selenocysteyl-tRNA[Ser]Sec is a carrier molecule upon which selenocysteine is biosynthesized and also, donates selenocysteine, the 21st naturally occurring amino acid of protein, to the forming polypeptide chain in response to specific UGA codons [64]; *AIH 1 and 2* Autoimmune hepatitis type 1 and type 2; *APECED* autoimmune polyendocrinopathy-candidiasis-ectodermal dystrophy

# Histology

The histological hallmark of AIH is interface hepatitis (Fig. 4.1) associated with confluent hepatic necrosis and bridging fibrosis [65]. The inflammatory infiltrate of autoimmune hepatitis is comprised of lymphocytes (Fig. 4.2) and plasma cells

**Fig. 4.2** Lymphocytes (arrow) infiltrating between surviving hepatocytes within the inflammatory infiltrate in a case of autoimmune hepatitis. Hematoxylin and Eosin, original magnification 40X

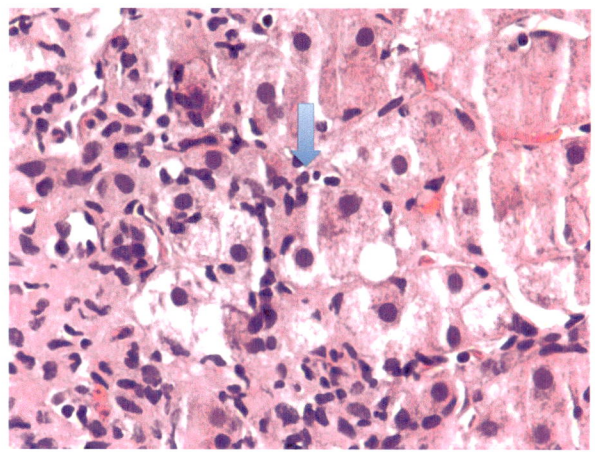

**Fig. 4.3** Plasma cells (arrows) within inflammatory infiltrate in a case of autoimmune hepatitis. Hematoxylin and Eosin, original magnification 40X

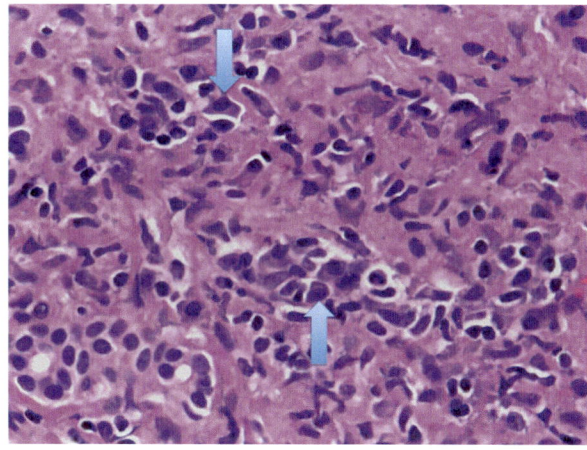

(Fig. 4.3) of the CD8 population [65]. Lobular inflammatory infiltrates may be identified, as well as rosette formation, and even in acute presentation, nodular formation can be present [52, 65]. The predictive value of periportal plasma cells for relapse in patients with autoimmune hepatitis is important. Liver histology from patients who had achieved remission and had been taken off steroids, and subsequently had relapsed had, characteristically, plasma cell infiltration in the portal tracts, in contrast to patients who had not relapsed. These results tend to suggest that liver histology should be reviewed prior to drug discontinuation in patients with AIH. In addition, a pathogenetic mechanism mediated by plasma cells in patients who relapsed is suggested [66]. One of the possible mechanisms of disease perpetuation by plasma cells may be their relationship with activated stellate cells, which are pivotal in the generation of fibrosis, and with which they colocalized in an immunohistochemical study [67]; the number of plasma cells was reported to correlate with stellate cells and fibrosis scores. After treatment, patients in remission had a decreased number of plasma cells, hepatic stellate cells, and degree of fibrosis [66]. Indeed, an immunohistological study of paired biopsies before and after clinical remission from children with AIH was reported to reveal a decrease in hepatic stellate cells activation, as evidenced by attenuation of anti-alpha smooth muscle immunoreactivity, in association with a reduction in inflammation score, although no changes in fibrosis were documented [68]; these results suggest that a decrease in hepatic stellate deactivation, in association with treatment, may be associated with the halting of fibrogenic mechanisms.

Emperipolesis is the penetration of a cell by another of a different lineage that remains intact [65]. It was reported in 65.3% of patients with AIH, from a group of 101, a finding significantly higher than in disease control liver biopsies, and associated with higher serum activity of aminotransferases, inflammatory activity, and degree of fibrosis than in disease control biopsies. CD8 T cells were the majority of lymphocytes identified in emperipolesis, which was associated with induction of cleaved caspase-3 expression, and notable in areas of apoptosis, which has suggested that emperipolesis may induce apoptosis, which then may contribute to the liver injury in AIH [69].

Drug-induced hepatitis and AIH have similar histological features, hence the importance of a detailed history of medications and over the counter preparations taken in relationship with the onset of hepatitis. Prominent intra-acinar lymphocyte infiltrate or canalicular cholestasis without portal inflammation, rosette formation, rich portal plasma infiltrates, and intra-acinar eosinophils has been identified as common features in AIH, whereas a combination of prominent intra-acinar lymphocyte infiltrates, canalicular cholestasis, and fewer than two of the features that were highly exhibited by the livers affected by AIH support a diagnosis of drug-induced hepatitis. Interestingly, eosinophils were more prevalent in AIH than in drug-induced hepatitis [70].

## Diagnostic Scores for AIH

Diagnostic criteria for autoimmune hepatitis have been published and presented as scoring systems to diagnose this disease [52, 71, 72]. The revised scoring system most frequently used during the decade that followed its publication [52] is adapted in Tables 4.2, 4.3, 4.4, 4.5, 4.6, 4.7, and 4.8 and presented from the perspective of approaching a patient in whom AIH is suspected. A simplified score system, the variables of which are titers of autoantibodies, the serum concentration of IgG, liver histological features, and exclusion of viral hepatitis, has been published [71] and summarized in Tables 4.9, 4.10, and 4.11.

Comparative analyses of the two scoring systems have been reported. In a study that comprised 153 patients in whom a diagnosis of definitive AIH had been made

**Table 4.2** Systematic application of the revised scoring system for the diagnosis of autoimmune hepatitis in the evaluation of a patient with suspected disease and scores associated with presence or absence of the factor [52]—History

|  | Yes (score) | No (score) |
|---|---|---|
| Use of potential hepatotoxins (e.g., medications, herbal substances) temporally related to the hepatitis | −4 | +1 |
| History of autoimmune diseases in patient or first-degree relatives | +2 | No score |
| Alcohol intake |  |  |
| <25 g/day | +2 | No score |
| >60 g/day | −2 | No score |

**Table 4.3** Systematic application of the revised scoring system for the diagnosis of autoimmune hepatitis in the evaluation of a patient with suspected disease and scores associated with presence or absence of the factor—Physical exam

|  | Score |
|---|---|
| Female gender | +2 |

**Table 4.4** Systematic application of the revised scoring system for the diagnosis of autoimmune hepatitis in the evaluation of a patient with suspected disease and scores associated with presence or absence of the factor—Laboratory findings

|  | Ratio | Score |
|---|---|---|
| [a]ALP:AST (or ALT) ratio | <1.5 | +2 |
|  | 1.5–3.0 | 0 |
|  | >3.0 | −2 |
|  | >2.0 | +3 |
|  | 1.5–2.0 | +2 |
|  | 1.0–1.5 | +1 |
|  | <1.0 | 0 |
|  | **Titer** |  |
| ANA, SMA, or LKM-1 | >1:80 | +3 |
|  | 1:80 | +2 |
|  | 1:40 | +1 |
|  | <1:40 | 0 |
| AMA | Positive | −4 |
| Hepatitis serology | Positive | Negative |
|  | −3 | +3 |

*AP* alkaline phosphatase; *AST* aspartate aminotransferase; *ALT* alanine aminotransferase
Hepatitis serology: IgM anti-HAV, HBsAg, IgM anti-HBc, anti-HCV, and HCV-RNA. If a viral etiology is considered in spite of negative viral hepatitis serology as listed here, serology for cytomegalovirus, Epstein Barr virus and hepatitis E must be obtained as these viral infections may be the cause of the hepatitis
[a]Ratio calculated as units above the upper limit of normal (ULN) (i.e., (AP IU/L ÷ (ULN) AP ÷ (IU/L AST÷ ULN AST)

**Table 4.5** Systematic application of the revised scoring system for the diagnosis of autoimmune hepatitis in the evaluation of a patient with suspected disease and scores associated with presence or absence of the factor—Histology

|  | Score |
|---|---|
| Interface hepatitis | +3 |
| Predominance of lymphocytes and plasma cells in inflammatory infiltrate | +1 |
| Rosettes formation of hepatocytes | +1 |
| Absence of the three findings cited above | −5 |
| Biliary epithelial cell changes suggestive of PBC (e.g., ductopenia, granulomata, bile ductular proliferation, concentric fibrosis of bile ducts) or PSC (e.g., concentric fibrosis of bile ducts) | −3 |
| Findings suggestive of other etiologies | −3 |

**Table 4.6** Systematic application of the revised scoring system for the diagnosis of autoimmune hepatitis in the evaluation of a patient with suspected disease and scores associated with presence or absence of the factor—Items characterized as optional

|  | Score |
|---|---|
| Presence of autoantibodies identified in AIH including pANCA, anti-LC1, anti-SLA, and anti-ASGPR in the absence of typical autoantibodies (see above) | +2 |
| HLA DR3 or DR4 in Caucasian and Japanese subjects | +1 |
| Any other HLA class II antigen | +1 |

**Table 4.7** Systematic application of the revised scoring system for the diagnosis of autoimmune hepatitis in the evaluation of a patient with suspected disease and scores associated with presence or absence of the factor—Follow-up period under therapy with immunosuppressants

|  | Definition 1 and score | Definition 2 and score |
|---|---|---|
| Complete response as described under definitions 1 or 2 | Notable improvement of symptoms and normalization of serum liver associated enzyme activity, serum bilirubin and IgG concentrations within 1 year and sustained followed by a 6 month period on maintenance therapy or liver histology at any point during the period described above displaying not more than minimal inflammatory activity, or definition 2 | Substantial improvement of symptoms in association with a decrease by 50% of the serum abnormalities of the liver tests from baseline, during the first month of treatment, followed by a continuous decrease in the activity of AST and ALT to less than twice the ULN within 6 months during any reduction toward maintenance therapy, or liver histology within 1 year displaying minimal inflammatory activity |
|  | +2 | +2 |
| Relapse as described under definitions 1 or 2 | Increased activity of AST and ALT activities to higher than twice the ULN, or findings on liver histology consistent with active disease, either in association or not with symptoms, after a complete remission, as defined above, or definition 2 | Return of symptoms requiring administration of therapy, or increase of dose, if the patient is on medications for AIH, after a complete response as defined above |
|  | +3 | +3 |

**Table 4.8** Systematic application of the revised scoring system for the diagnosis of autoimmune hepatitis in the evaluation of a patient with suspected disease and scores associated with presence or absence of the factor—Interpretation of scores

|  | Definite AIH | Probable AIH |
|---|---|---|
| Pre treatment | >15 | 10–15 |
| Post treatment | >17 | 12–17 |

**Table 4.9** Simplified autoimmune hepatitis scoring system [71]—Laboratory variables

|  |  | Titer | Score |
|---|---|---|---|
| Autoantibodies |  |  |  |
|  | ANA or ASMA or | ≥1:40 | 1 |
|  | ANA or ASMA | ≥1:80 |  |
|  | Anti-LKM or | ≥1:40 | 2 |
|  | Anti-SLA | Positive |  |
|  |  | Change |  |
| Serum concentration of IgG |  | >ULN limit | 1 |
|  |  | >1.10 times upper | 2 |
|  |  | Within normal limits |  |
| Absence of viral hepatitis |  |  | 2 |

**Table 4.10** Simplified autoimmune hepatitis scoring system—Histology

| Features | Score |
|---|---|
| Typical of AIH: interface hepatitis, lymphocytic or lymphoplasmacytic infiltration of portal tracts and lobules, emperipolesis, and hepatic rosette formation | 2 |
| Compatible with AIH: lymphocytic infiltration of portal tracts and lobular activity without all the features considered typical | 1 |
| Atypical: findings of other diseases |  |

**Table 4.11** Simplified autoimmune hepatitis scoring system—Interpretation of the summation of scores

| Total score |  |
|---|---|
| ≥6 | Probable AIH |
| ≥7 | Definite AIH |

based on the revised original scoring system [52], 11 (7.1%) were classified as probable AIH by the use of the simplified scoring system [71], and two (1.3%) were identified as not having AIH. With the use of the simplified scoring system [71], five patients were classified as having definitive and five as not having AIH, of the 13 who had been classified as probable AIH. Discordance in the diagnosis between the two scoring systems was 15%, comprising 23 patients, whereas concordance was exhibited in 127 patients (97.7%) for definite and for probable diagnosis in 3

(2.4%) [72]. Remission with treatment in patients diagnosed as having definite or probable AIH by the use of the revised original scoring criteria was 68% and 75%, respectively, and the failure of therapy was 16 and 0%, respectively. Seventy and 50 percent of patients classified by the simplified scoring criteria as having definite and probable AIH, respectively, achieved remission in association with therapy, and 15 and 25% of patients, respectively, failed treatment. These responses were not different in relation to the score used. In this study, five patients had non diagnostic scores as per the simplified scoring criteria, four of whom responded to treatment with remission, and one was still on therapy at the time of the study completion [72]. Neither of the two scoring systems compared classified patients with chronic liver disease from alcohol, viral hepatitis, or primary biliary cholangitis (PBC) with those who had definite AIH; two patients with primary sclerosing cholangitis (PSC) were classified as AIH by both systems [72]. The comparison of sensitivity, specificity, and positive predictability and negative predictability of the original scoring system with the simplified scoring system was 100 and 95%, 73 and 90%, 82 and 92%, 67 and 83%, and 100 and 97%, respectively [72], in this study from a center in the United States. The simplified scoring system has been considered to be simpler in its application than the revised system, of being able to exclude more frequently other liver diseases, and of carrying a higher specificity than that of the latter, with the revised scoring system being reported as 95% specific and 90% sensitive, but a sensitivity of 65% and a specificity of 100% for the simplified scoring system [73]. A study that included patients with overlap syndrome, AIH, and other liver diseases in association with AIH, documented that the simplified and the revised scoring systems were specific at 97.9 and 97%, respectively [74]. However, it was noted that the ability to identify AIH in patients with other liver diseases was significantly lower with the use of the simplified scoring system than with the use of the revised scoring system, liver histology being the only factor able to reveal that information [74]. In this regard, from in a series that included 25 patients from Asia, Europe, and the United States, 20 of whom had chronic hepatitis C and five chronic hepatitis B, it was reported that, according to the revised scoring system, 72% met the criteria for the diagnosis of probable AIH, and 48% met these criteria as per the simplified scoring system [75]; however, none of the patients were diagnosed with definite AIH by either score [73]. These findings underscore the importance of the differential diagnosis in evaluating patients with liver disease. Specifically, the existence of a viral disease, i.e., hepatitis, does not exclude the presence of another liver disease, including metabolic and autoimmune disease. Accordingly, a full liver disease workup is required in the approach to a patient with suspected liver disease. This study [75] tends to support those of the prior report that documented that liver biopsy was necessary to confirm the coexistence of additional liver pathology [73]. It is also emphasized that the use of the scoring systems is complementary to clinical judgment. Autoimmune markers by ELISA methodology have not been used to validate the scoring system [72]; this is necessary as clinical laboratories have moved to this type of assay as the methodology for these tests.

## Overlap Syndromes

There are clinical, histological, and biochemical features of AIH, PBC, and PSC [76] that coexist in a minority of patients with any of these diseases. These entities have been named overlap syndromes, mostly comprising AIH and PBC cases, and have been the subject of some controversy regarding their existence as separate entities, as part of the same disease, as one disease changing to another, or some characteristics of each. The diagnostic criteria for the overlap syndrome of AIH with PBC have been named the Paris criteria [77] and include at least two of the three accepted criteria for the diagnosis of each of those individual diseases, and has a sensitivity and specificity of 92% and 97%, respectively. For PBC, the diagnostic criteria are: (1) serum AP activity at least two times the upper limit of normal or serum GGTP five times the upper limit of normal, (2) positive antimitochondrial antibody (AMA), and (3) liver biopsy exhibiting the lesion of chronic nonsuppurative destructive cholangitis (i.e., florid bile duct lesion). For AIH, the diagnostic criteria are: (1) serum activity of ALT at least five times the upper limit of normal, (2) serum IgG concentrations at least twice the upper limit of normal or positive ASMA, and (3) interface hepatitis on liver histology [77]. The diagnosis of AIH overlapping PSC is the absence of AMA and typical cholangiogram (e.g., strictures) by MRI or ERCP [78, 79].

AIH with overlap to PBC has been reported to occur in approximately 7–10% of patients and AIH with PSC 8–17%. AMA negative PBC, small duct PSC, autoimmune PSC, and immunoglobulin G4-associated cholangitis are considered variants of the overlap syndromes [76]. The difficulty in diagnosing overlap syndromes with a high level of certainty seems to have encouraged scoring systems to classify patients with an overlap of AIH on PBC and PSC. Features of AIH overlap were identified in 137 cases of histologically diagnosed PBC by the use of the revised scoring system, with 2% being found to meet criteria for definite AIH and 62% for probable AIH; no cases of definite AIH overlap were identified, with 19% meeting criteria for probable AIH overlap [80]. The main contribution to identifying overlap AIH in PBC was the presence of ANA, associated autoimmune disorders, and histological findings [80]. In this regard, the serological profile of patients with PBC with an overlap to AIH has been documented to consist of a predominance of anti-dsDNA antibodies, found in 60% of patients with overlap syndrome of AIH and PBC, in contrast to a 4% prevalence in patients with PBC, and 26% of patients with AIH. The dual presence of anti-dsDNA antibodies and AMA was only reported in 2% of patients with PBC or AIH, in contrast to 47% of samples from patients with overlap syndrome, a finding that could help identify this not so distinct entity [81]. Analyses of data from patients with PSC have documented a prevalence of AIH overlap of 6 and 11%, in contrast to what ranged from 30 to 50% by the use of the original scoring system [82]. However, others have documented a prevalence of 19% of overlap of AIH in PSC with the use of the revised system [83]. With the advent of the simplified scoring system, several published retrospective studies have reported the ability of the revised and the simplified scoring system for the diagnosis of AIH to detect an overlap of such on PBC [84] and PSC [83]. By the use of the revised [52] and the simplified [71] scoring systems, 368 patients who had a diagnosis of PBC were examined; 12% were classified as probable overlap PBC-AIH with the revised scoring system, and 6% with the simplified system. Patients with characteristics of overlap syndrome had more complications of portal hypertension, significantly more liver related deaths and liver transplantation surgeries than those with PBC [84], suggesting that the AIH component worsened or accelerated the disease [84]. These selected reports must be interpreted with caution, as has been the recommendation of the International Autoimmune Hepatitis Group, which was responsible for the derivation of the revised scoring system, and which underscores the lack of evidence for the use of the scoring systems for the diagnosis of overlap syndromes. Exhortation to identify patients with overlap syndrome and its variants is documented in the literature [76].

AIH can be associated with other autoimmune diseases, including thyroiditis, the most common co-occurrence, reported in 10% of a study group that included 278 patients, and vitiligo, rheumatoid arthritis, Sjogren's syndrome, inflammatory bowel disease, systemic lupus erythematosus, and celiac disease reported in a few patients [85].

## Treatment of Autoimmune Hepatitis

The goal of treatment of patients with AIH is to control the liver inflammatory response, which is associated with symptoms, can result in liver failure, and is expressed biochemically by increased serum activity of liver associated enzymes and concentration of bilirubin. The practice guidelines supported by the American Association for the Study of Liver Disease (AASLD) divide the indications for treatment of AIH into absolute, relative, and none [86]. The absolute indications are a serum activity of aspartate aminotransferase (AST) ten times the upper limit of normal, AST five times the upper limit of normal and serum concentration of gamma globulin at least twice the upper limit of normal, liver histology revealing bridging necrosis or multiacinar necrosis, and incapacitating symptoms, including fatigue and arthralgias. The relative indications are fatigue, arthralgias, jaundice, a sign included under symptoms in the practice guidelines, and a liver histology exhibiting interface hepatitis. Inactive cirrhosis or mild portal inflammation, absence of symptoms, and normal or close to normal serum activity of AST and serum concentration of gamma globulin are not considered indications for treatment. In this regard, however, almost half of asymptomatic patients with AIH have as much inflammation and fibrosis as patients with symptoms, and, although some patients with mild disease can improve spontaneously, they cannot be distinguished from those who, in the category of mild disease, do progress to liver failure and who may benefit from therapy [87]; thus, it is difficult to withhold treatment in patients with mild disease, in the absence of prognostic factors that correlate with clinical outcomes. Transient elastography was reported to provide improved diagnostic information regarding fibrosis with a documented sensitivity and specificity of 93.6 and 44.4%, respectively, for significant fibrosis, as compared to APRI and FIB-4 scores [88]; the increasing availability of this technology may allow for its incorporation in the investigational approach of patients with AIH and perhaps, to support treatment of patients with fibrosis when there is uncertainty regarding this decision. All patients with AIH attended by the author have been treated.

A study that included 128 patients with AIH reported that 29% had cirrhosis at entry, and 40% of those who did not have cirrhosis developed it during $39 \pm 32$ months [89]. The response to therapy, relapse after discontinuation of treatment, and failure to respond to treatment were similar between patients with and without cirrhosis at entry [89]. In this study, the overall 10 year survival was 93%, comparable to the 94% of an age-and sex-matched group from the general population [89]. Treatment with corticosteroids over 5 years was reported to be associated with decreased fibrosis scores, in association with decreased inflammatory activity, from a study in which 325 liver samples from 87 patients were reviewed [90]. The frequency of cirrhosis, which was 16% at baseline, decreased to 11% [90]. Accordingly, timely diagnosis and treatment of patients with AIH are necessary, a statement that highlights the importance of expeditious workup of an abnormal liver profile.

The treatment goal is to stop the inflammatory process; this outcome is associated with normalization of serum liver profile and markers of autoimmune activity, i.e., serum IgG concentrations, which can be used as indirect indices of disease activity. In this regard, the normalization of AST and ALT activities and normalization of serum concentration of bilirubin predict remission; in one study, this outcome was reported to correlate with a decrease in the proportion of patients who relapsed post treatment from 86% to 60% [91]. Reports from a study that comprised 132 patients with definite type 1 AIH and who met clinical, laboratory, and histological criteria for remission, indicate that the degree of change in laboratory exams at the time of completion of treatment correlates with the probability of relapse. Patients who did not relapse had a mean serum activity of AST of 7 U/L, a mean serum IgG of 337 g/dl, and a mean serum gamma globulin of 0.2 g/dl lower than those who relapsed after treatment discontinuation; the proportion of patients who relapsed after treatment discontinuation, 40, 36, and 25%, had not normalized the AST activity or had a decrease in the serum concentrations of IgG at the time the treatment was stopped, in contrast to 13, 3, and 4 percent, respectively, that did not relapse [91]. These results support the idea of treating patients with AIH until there is complete normalization of these indices of disease. The histological findings were reported to be similar in the groups that relapsed and the group that did not relapse.

Galectins are carbohydrate binding proteins that play a role in inflammation and immune-mediated responses, among other activities [92]. Serum galectin-9 was reported to correlate with disease activity in AIH and was suggested as a potential marker of disease activity [93], which could be used in tandem with serum AST to assess disease activity. In the context of serum markers of liver disease, the angiotensin converting enzyme (ACE) system has been reported to contribute to the mediation of fibrogenesis [94]. In this regard, serum levels of angiotensin converting enzyme (ACE) were reported to correlate with the degree of fibrosis in patients with AIH with a median serum level of 45 U/l identifying patients with fibrosis stage I, and 68 U/L as cut off level in cirrhosis, with 100% sensitivity and 84.4% specificity, with the area under the curve of 0.95 [95]. The use of these serum markers has not been incorporated in clinical use.

The standard treatment of autoimmune hepatitis is comprised of corticosteroids alone or in combination with azathioprine, which is associated with normalization of serum liver profile and degree of fibrosis in most patients [96]. In patients with cytopenias, thiopurine methyltransferase deficiency, pregnancy, malignancy, and anticipated short course (difficult to define), treatment with prednisone alone is favored. In addition, azathioprine can be associated with liver toxicity and with pancreatitis; thus, the use of prednisone or prednisolone alone at the beginning of therapy eliminates the confounding factor of azathioprine side effects and allows for the follow up of a pure response to corticosteroid therapy. Guidelines recommend the initial dose for prednisone to be 60 mg/day [86], or 0.5–1 mg/kg of body weight [97, 86], or, by body weight, azathioprine 1–2 mg/kg [86, 98]. Prednisone is decreased from 60 to 40 mg at the end of week one, and to 30 mg at the end of week 2, and kept at this dose for 2 weeks; after 4 weeks of therapy, the dose of prednisone is decreased to 20 mg/day and gradually decreased by 5–10 mg/week, and subsequently, by 2.5 mg/week to reach the lowest possible dose of prednisone (e.g., 2.5 mg/day) that will maintain normal AST and ALT activities (Table 4.12) [86]. Initiation of combination therapy is done with azathioprine 50 mg (or 1–2 mg/kg) in association with prednisone 30 mg during the first week of treatment; while keeping azathioprine at the same dose, the dose of prednisone is decreased to 20 mg/day for the second week of treatment, to 15 mg/day for the third and fourth weeks of treatment, and 10 mg/day starting at the fifth week of treatment until the goal is achieved (Table 4.13) [86, 98]. Histological resolution of inflammation lags behind the normalization of serum liver profile by 3–8 months; accordingly, therapy is continued beyond the time point of disappearance of peripheral indices of disease, e.g., 12 to 24 months, the latter being more realistic than the former. Liver histology is recommended for assessing response to therapy prior to discontinuation of such [86], although the latest guidelines tend to be liberal regarding this prerequisite. The advantage of having liver histology prior to discontinuation of treatment is that the finding of interface hepatitis in patients on treatment whose AST activity has normalized itself supports the continuation of therapy as its discontinuation is associated with the disease's relapse. If peripheral indices of disease and liver histology

**Table 4.12** Regimen for treatment of autoimmune hepatitis with prednisone

| Days 1–7 | Days 8–14 | Days 15–21st | Days 22th–28th | Taper initiation on Day 29th until treatment goal is reached |
|---|---|---|---|---|
| 60 mg | 40 mg | 30 mg | 20 mg | 10 mg per day ([a]) |

[a]The rate of taper of prednisone from 10 to 2.5 mg is guided by maintenance of a normal serum liver profile. The author tapers at a rate of 5 mg every 4 weeks, until the lowest dose (i.e. 2.5 mg/day) of prednisone associated with persistently normal activity of transaminases is reached. The use of prednisone alone is rare in our practice

**Table 4.13** Regimen for the treatment of autoimmune hepatitis with prednisone (P) and azathioprine (A)

| Days 1–7 | Days 8–14 | Days 15–21st | Days 22th–28th | Taper initiation of P on Day 29th until treatment goal is reached | After P has been tapered and discontinued |
|---|---|---|---|---|---|
| P 60 mg | P 40 mg | P 30 mg plus A 50 mg | P 20 mg plus A 50 mg | 10 mg per day [a] plus continuation of A at 50 mg | A 50 mg per day, which can be increased to twice a day or as per body weight 1–2 mg, in two doses depending on the activity of AST and ALT |

[a]The rate of taper of prednisone from 10 to 2.5 mg is guided by maintenance of normal activity of liver profile. The author tapers slowly at a rate of 5 mg every 4 weeks, until the lowest dose (i.e., 2.5 mg/day) of prednisone associated with persistently normal activity of transaminases is reached. At present, we treat patients for a total of 3 years, two of those consecutively, after normalization of the serum liver panel. We customarily do a liver biopsy prior to discontinuation of therapy; liver biopsy is not done in patients who decline the procedure ($n = 1$ in our practice) and who are followed vigilantly to identify any suggestion of relapse and need to retreat

suggest remission, treatment can be gradually tapered to discontinuation over 6 weeks, checking laboratory tests reflective of liver inflammation every 3 weeks during drug withdrawal and for the 3 months that follow. Adrenal suppression must be considered in patients on long-term steroid therapy; thus, prednisone must be tapered and adrenal function tested as recommended by guidelines [99]. After treatment has been stopped, clinical and laboratory evaluation are recommended every 3 weeks for the first 3 months, then 3 months later, every 6 months for a year, and annually after [86] to confirm ongoing remission. The relapse of AIH is defined as the recurrence of disease after normal histology has been attained during a prior treatment course. In case of relapse, which can occur in 20–28% of patients, therapy is reinstituted [91, 100]. The approach of patients who relapse consists of exclusion of other causes of acute hepatitis and reinstitution of treatment with prednisone, which can be at a dose of 10 mg/day in combination with azathioprine 2 mg/kg/day [101], which may be indefinitely; the long duration of therapy in patients who have a relapse of their hepatitis underscores the relevance of the liver biopsy prior to discontinuation of treatment to document histological remission [102].

Treatment of AIH should be individualized within the published guidelines as a reference. The most recent guidelines from the European Association for the Study of Liver Disease propose a treatment regime that starts with prednisolone 60 (or 1 mg/kg), decreased to 50 mg at the end of week one, and a decrease to 40 mg at the end of week two with the addition of azathioprine at a dose of 50 mg/day and subsequent taper of prednisone by 10 mg at the end of weeks three and four, and reduction by 5 mg (i.e., 25 mg) at the end of week four with a concomitant increase of azathioprine to 100 mg/day (the author prescribes it in two divided doses of 50 mg each), or 1–2 mg/kg of body weight. The dose of azathioprine is maintained as prednisone is decreased by 5 mg over weeks six to eight and by 2.5 mg over weeks eight and nine. From week ten, the dose of prednisone should be 10 mg/day in conjunction with azathioprine 100 mg, which remains unchanged after week five [97].

Response to corticosteroids therapy within 2 weeks of initiation correlates with improved survival [103]. From a retrospective review that comprised 149 patients with AIH, it was documented that patients at least 60 years of age responded to therapy faster, i.e., within 6 months of initiation of treatment, than those aged younger than 40, with a proportion of 18% versus 2%, respectively, and with 94% having responded within 24 months versus 64%, respectively, with all comparisons being statistically significant. The development of cirrhosis was more common in the slow than in the rapid responders, 54% versus 18%, and liver transplantation was also more common in the slow than in the rapid responders, 15% versus 2%, respectively, both comparisons significantly different; however, the proportion of patients who sustained response, and who relapsed was similar between both groups, 10% versus 19% ($p = 0.6$) [104]. These results may guide the clinician when treating patients from different age groups in discussions about prognosis, and relative end of treatment, and also, emphasize that, although the faster response to therapy may limit the amount of immunosuppression required for remission, in the end, relapse was important in both types of responders; however, the advantage of a decrease in the proportion of patients who develop cirrhosis or that need liver transplantation, was noted in the rapid responders, who are of increased age.

The goal of therapy is the normalization of serum transaminase activity, concentrations of serum bilirubin and gamma globulin, and liver histology; however, this is reached in approximately 40% of patients only [91]; patients who achieve this goal on therapy have a decreased probability of relapse, as compared to those who do not when treatment is stopped [91]. In a study where patients who did not respond to corticosteroids were compared to those who did, it was found that acute presentation, age ($33 \pm 3$ years), and serum bilirubin of $4.1 \pm 0.9$ mg/dL at onset were features associated with failure of therapy. The Model of End-Stage Liver Disease (MELD) score of greater than 12 at presentation tended to correlate with failure to respond to corticosteroid therapy [105].

Maintenance therapy with azathioprine alone beyond the first few weeks of treatment has been proposed to spare steroids' side effects [106]; this regimen is effective and associated with the disappearance of steroid-induced side effects, e.g., Cushingnoid facies and increase in body weight [106]. Data from a study that was comprised of 72 patients with AIH have supported the use of this drug for long-term maintenance therapy [106]. The patients had been in remission, which was defined as the absence of symptoms, normal activity of AST, and normal serum concentration of immunoglobulin, and with or without liver histology showing minimal or no disease activity, for at least 1 year on prednisolone 5–15 mg and azathioprine 1 mg/kg of body weight, and had the dose of azathioprine increased to 2 mg/kg/day as the dose of steroids was decreased gradually. On azathioprine alone, 83% of patients remained in remission for over 5 years (67 months, range 12–128); liver histology examined in 42 patients ($n = 48$ biopsies) showed no or minimal inflammation, and three showed moderate disease, at 2 and 8 years of therapy [106]. The shortest time to spontaneous relapse after the initiation of azathioprine alone in the 12 patients who did relapse was 7 months, and the longest was 59; three patients relapsed in association with precipitating factors of infection, pregnancy, and discontinuation of therapy, in this patient at 2 years. In this study, the discontinuation of prednisolone was associated with arthralgias of various duration managed with analgesic or anti-inflammatory drugs and self-limited fatigue, nausea, rash, tendonitis, and pruritus. On the 2 mg/kg dose of azathioprine, four patients developed cytopenias, which was managed with dose reduction to 1 mg/kg; this change was associated with relapse of hepatitis in two patients, who were managed with reinstitution of prednisone therapy. The remission rate of 83% reported in this study has supported the use of azathioprine at a dose of 2 mg/kg of body weight per day for maintenance therapy in AIH after remission had been obtained with combination therapy for at least 1 year [106].

Azathioprine is the pro-drug of 6 mercaptopurine (6-MP); it can be associated with bone marrow suppression and aplastic anemia. The metabolism of these drugs depends on the activity of thiopurine methyltransferase (TPMT), hypoxanthine phosphoribosyl transferase, and xanthine oxidase [107]. Deficiency of TPMT is associated with azathioprine and 6-MP toxicity [108, 109]; thus, phenotype testing for TPMT prior to initiating treatment with these drugs is a prevalent practice to decide whether or not to prescribe these drugs to patients with AIH [110]. Bone marrow suppression can occur independently from the phenotype of TPMT; accordingly, monitoring of the complete blood count is part of the follow up of patients treated with these drugs. In patients with AIH treated with prednisone alone, or in combination with azathioprine, 50 mg/day, the probability of developing malignancy was 1.4 higher (95% CI, 0.6–2.9) than that of a gender and age matched cohort of subjects [111]. The complications of immunosuppression therapy with steroids alone or in combination with azathioprine, or with azathioprine alone, and the relatively long-term treatment required in AIH highlight the importance of individualizing the choice of therapeutic regimens, consistent with the preferences of an informed patient, to improve treatment adherence and to minimize side effects.

Patients who fail treatment, defined as having worsening of histological findings and peripheral indices of disease activity, in spite of adherence to therapy, are managed with prednisone at doses of 60 mg/day, in combination with azathioprine, 150 mg/day for at least 4 weeks, gradually decreasing the doses in response to a decrease in the serum AST activity, as done at the initiation of therapy.

Patients who do not achieve complete remission but exhibit improvement of clinical, histological, and laboratory features of AIH are considered to have had an incomplete response to therapy and are reported to represent thirteen percent of the population treated for 3 years [86]. These patients continue to be managed with prednisone, at the lowest dose associated with a stable and lowest possible serum AST activity, or with azathioprine, 2 mg/kg of body weight, to spare them from steroids' side effects [86].

After 2 years of remission, it was reported from a study of 311 patients from the Netherlands that 47% of patients relapsed, defined as increased activity of ALT to three times the upper limits of normal, and that 42% had lost remission, defined as upward trend of serum ALT activity while in withdrawal phase of therapy. After 3 years of treatment discontinuation, 81% of the patients required treatment, 73% after 2 years, and 59% after 1 year. After one relapse, attempts to discontinue therapy were not successful in half of the patients [112], which has suggested that AIH is a chronic disease for which long-term treatment is required [113]. By applying defined criteria, 28 of 288 patients with AIH who had been in remission for at least

2 years on one immunosuppressant had their immunosuppression stopped. Fifteen (54%) patients remained in remission for a median of 28 months of follow up, with a range of 17–57, but 13 (46%) had to be restarted on treatment; a serum concentration of IgG up to 12 g/L and serum activity of ALT half the upper limit of normal on therapy, and prior to its discontinuation characterized the patients who remain in remission [114]. This report seems useful in the selection of patients considered for discontinuation of therapy. However, disease relapse has been documented to occur as late as 22 years after discontinuation of treatment; accordingly, the recommendation is for long-term follow up in patients who have exhibited a prolonged remission is warranted [115].

There is discordance between biochemical and histological remission in AIH. In patients who had normalized their hepatic panel in association with treatment, a liver biopsy done 6 months a posteriori from the normalization of serum ALT activity and gamma globulin exhibited inflammatory activity in 46% of the subjects who had serum activity of AST and ALT within normal limits (i.e., 27 IU/L and ALT 24 IU/L, respectively) but, still higher than those from whom histology was consistent with remission, i.e., AST 23 IU/L, and ALT 18 IU/L; the degree of regression of fibrosis was also less in the group with higher AST and ALT activities than in the comparison group (32% vs. 60%), and significant excess mortality, i.e., standardized mortality ratio of 1.4 vs. 0.7, due to liver disease. It was documented that continued histological activity was independently associated with all-cause mortality or liver transplantation. On multivariate analysis, persisting histological activity was independently associated with all-cause death and transplantation with a reported hazard ratio of 3.1, 95% confidence interval (CI), 1.2–8.1, $p = 0.02$. These results confirm the importance of histological remission in the natural history of AIH and serve as guidance to consider liver biopsy prior to discontinuation of therapy [116].

The proportion of patients that worsens on therapy for AIH has been reported as seven percent [105, 117]. In these cases, it is the practice to reinitiate treatment with doses recommended as initial therapy for at least 4 weeks, followed by a taper of prednisone (Tables 4.12 and 4.13). This approach has been reported in association with clinical remission and normalization of serum indices of liver disease in 70% of the cases and with histological remission in 20–41% of patients after 2 years of treatment [118].

Budesonide, a steroid drug with 90% first pass through the liver, has been used to treat AIH and studied in a controlled clinical trial of 6 months duration. In this study, first-line therapy with budesonide, at a dose of 3 mg three times a day, in combination with azathioprine, 1–2 mg/kg/day, was associated with normalization of serum activity of transaminases in 47% of the patients, as compared to 18% of the patients treated with prednisone, 40 mg tapered to 10 mg/day, and azathioprine, 1–2 mg/kg/day [119]. Documentation of histological resolution was not reported in this trial, however. Also, the response to standard therapy in the patients included in this study, 18%, is lower than what has been documented by other clinical experiences. The sparing of steroid-induced side effects makes budesonide an acceptable alternative, especially in patients with comorbidities that increase their vulnerability to these types of complications, including hypertension and diabetes. In this regard, from a retrospective study that included two groups of 25 patients each who had been treated with prednisolone and AZA versus budesonide and AZA for a period of 3 years (2015–2018), it was reported that a lower number of side effects was associated with the latter than with the former, with the need to discontinue treatment in 2 (8%) of patients in the prednisolone group versus none in the budesonide group; however, no differences in the biochemical response between the two groups was documented; thus, it was concluded that patients with comorbidities that may worsen in association with prednisolone might be treated with the alternative steroid option with the expectation of a similar beneficial effect [120].

Budesonide does not prevent steroid-induced side effects in patients with cirrhosis because of decreased first pass liver clearance hence increased systemic availability; thus, it is not recommended for this type of patient [121].

Therapy with the standard drug regime of prednisone and azathioprine for over 3 years without evidence of remission is associated with disease progression in approximately half of the patients [104]. In this type of patient, the introduction of alternative immunosuppressants is an option. The calcineurin inhibitors, cyclosporin [122] and tacrolimus [123, 124], and the reversible inhibitor of inosine monophosphate dehydrogenase in purine synthesis, mycophenolate mofetil [125–129], have been used as an alternative therapy for autoimmune hepatitis, usually in patients who have not tolerated conventional treatment with prednisone (or prednisolone) and azathioprine, as first line, and in recalcitrant disease.

Calcineurin inhibitors have not been adopted as an alternative treatment for patients with AIH because of side effects, including nephrotoxicity [130]; however, the use of tacrolimus in patients with AIH refractory to steroids or intolerant to this type of drug was reported from a review of published experiences on the subject, and documented that tacrolimus, dosed between 1 and 8 mg/day, with targeted trough levels between 0.5 and 10.7 ng/mL, and a treatment duration of 1 to 136 months was associated with biochemical response in 121 patients (74.7%), with documented histological remission in 25 of the 83 patients who had had a baseline liver biopsy, with 17.3% of patients from the whole group having had the drug discontinued because of side effects, but with reported stability of renal function. The nature of this publication, i.e., a combined review, and the anticipated heterogeneity of the subjects do not provide strong evidence to use this drug without concerns; however, in cases of recalcitrant disease, the results suggested that the use of tacrolimus may be an option [131], especially when administered by clinicians with expertise in the use of the drug.

From a retrospective review that comprised 128 patients, 29 were identified as having been treated with mycophenolate mofetil [126]. It was reported that mycophenolate mofetil was not well tolerated by almost a third of patients with intolerance to standard therapy or used as first line in combination with prednisone; however, in those who tolerated the drug well, mycophenolate mofetil was associated with response in 84% of patients [126]. As first line, mycophenolate mofetil at doses of 1.5–2 g/day in combination with prednisolone at doses of 0.5–1 mg/kg daily was prescribed to 59 patients with AIH in an open-label study. The treatment was associated with response in 88% of the patients within the first 3 months of therapy; the rest had a partial response, as defined by the Revised Autoimmune Hepatitis Score [129]. Fifty-nine percent of patients exhibited a complete response in association with treatment; 37% of the group reached this goal off prednisolone, which had been discontinued in 58% of the patients by 8 months of treatment. Of the group that experienced a complete response, 29% relapsed. Two patients experienced side effects leading to discontinuation of therapy. Three of the six patients in whom mycophenolate mofetil was discontinued relapsed [129]. A retrospective study reported the experience of a group of 22 patients with AIH who were treated with mycophenolic mofetil; 14 had experienced side effects on therapy with prednisolone and azathioprine (i.e., standard treatment), five had not experienced remission, and three had both reasons not to continue on standard therapy. The group was treated with mycophenolic mofetil, at a dose of 20 mg/kg/day to a maximum of 3 g/day, with variable follow up for 2 years in ten patients; three normalized the serum activity of AST and ALT, and seven exhibited stabilization after three to 30 weeks, with 12 patients having the drug discontinued because of side effects, three changed to cyclosporine, and one had a liver transplant. Ten patients continued mycophenolic mofetil for a period of 20 to 124 months, with one being able to have prednisolone discontinued, five had the dose decreased to less than 5 mg, and four continued on 5–10 mg/day. Based on these results, it was concluded that mycophenolic mofetil might be safely prescribed, and that is associated with control of the disease [132]. However, mycophenolate mofetil has not been studied in controlled clinical trials; thus, recommendations on its use as first-line therapy, including duration of treatment, have not been formulated.

Azathioprine use in pregnancy is not recommended because of its teratogenic potential, falling in the D classification; thus, pregnant women with autoimmune hepatitis are managed with prednisone alone. Flares of autoimmune hepatitis can occur after delivery [126]; thus, follow up over the post-partum period is necessary, and the provision of standard therapy is recommended.

Standard therapy with corticosteroids alone or with azathioprine in combination with UDCA 13–15 mg/kg of body weight is the treatment that has been implemented for patients who exhibit features of AIH overlapping with PBC [133, 134] or PSC [135, 136] with salutary effects [137].

Forty (26%) of 154 patients who presented with fulminant liver failure to several transplant centers were identified as having AIH as the cause in a retrospective review. It was documented that the period from jaundice to encephalopathy was significantly longer in AIH than in the rest, i.e., 26 versus 16 days, and that the Model of End-Stage Liver Disease (MELD) score was significantly lower than in those with other causes of liver failure, i.e., 29 versus 33, with 25 (62%) undergoing liver transplantation, eight (20%) surviving the insult without liver transplantation, and seven (18%) dying. A high MELD score and grade 3 encephalopathy were associated with steroid failure, which was used in 17 patients, seven (41%) of whom survived. Given the high number of patients who required liver transplantation, these data emphasize the importance of suspecting AIH in cases of liver failure, not infrequently with absent autoantibodies, in whom referral to a liver transplant center, as encephalopathy ensues (i.e., grade 2 at the most) is fundamental for appropriate management that may include liver transplantation; in addition, cortico-steroids may benefit a group of patients, which, as per this publication, concerned patients with a MELD lower than 27 [138].

The use of anti-tumor necrosis factor-alpha rituximab and the mammalian target of rapamycin (mTOR) inhibitor sirolimus [139] and the anti-CD20 rituximab [140] as alternative therapies has been published in preliminary studies with encouraging results with regard to short-term response assessed by serum activity of transami-nases. Clinicaltrials.gov provides information regarding clinical trials that are planned or being conducted.

The practice guidelines supported by the AASLD [86] and the British Society of Gastroenterology [98] for the management of autoimmune hepatitis have been char-acterized by a recognized author in the field as being "fraught with uncertainties" [110]. The guidelines offer standards to follow in the management of patients with this complex disease; however, considering their limitations, the need to stay abreast of the progress in the subject of AIH is emphasized, and the recommendation for referral to experienced hepatologists strongly supported.

## Hepatocellular Carcinoma

The percentage of cirrhosis in AIH patients varied from 18.7% to 83.3% in studies from Japan, and from 12% to 50.2% in the other regions, with a mean follow up of the patients with AIH of 10 years [141]. Cirrhosis from AIH is a risk factor for hepa-tocellular carcinoma (HCC). One to nine percent of patients with AIH and cirrhosis develop HCC, with a reported annual incidence of 1.1–1.9%. From Sweden, the reported incidence of HCC was 0.3%, with long-term follow up of 634 well charac-terized patients, who developed this complication only when cirrhosis had been established [142]. An analysis of the published world data from 1989 to 2016 that included 8460 patients with AIH documented a diagnosis of HCC in 0–12.3% of the patients. In patients with AIH and cirrhosis, the proportion of patients with HCC varied between 0.2% and 12.3%, and the estimated proportion of patients without cirrhosis with HCC was 1.03% [143].

Surveillance of hepatocellular carcinoma every 6 months with a liver sonogram, and alpha fetoprotein is recommended [86, 98].

## Autoimmune Hepatitis in Children

Autoimmune hepatitis is particularly aggressive in children, predominantly affect-ing girls. Type 1 AIH can occur in children, whereas type 2 tends to occur mostly in children. In this regard, PSC with characteristics of AIH, including interface hepatitis in association with ANA and ASMA, usually seen in type 1, tends to affect boys and girls. Diagnostic characteristics of PSC are revealed by imaging studies, i.e. magnetic resonance cholangiography. The treatment is comprised of immunosuppression, which is associated with a good response in the hepatocellular injury component of the disease. In contrast, the injurious process of the bile duct is not halted by this type of therapy in approximately half of the affected patients. The need for liver transplantation in this type of liver disease is increased in the PSE AIH variant, as is the disease's recurrence in the liver graft post transplantation [144].

The treatment for AIH in children is prednisone (or prednisolone) in combination with azathioprine; as in adults, treatment should be individualized. A proposed treatment for AIH consists of prednisolone per body weight, orally, daily of 2 to a maximum dose of 60 mg during the first week of treatment, with subsequent decreases by 0.25 mg/kg/day until completion of the seventh week of treatment, to 0.25 during the eighth and ninth weeks, and to 0.1–0.2 during the tenth and eleventh weeks. Evaluation with hepatic panel is recommended weekly prior to decreasing the dose of steroids; if the decrease in AST and ATL activity stops, it is recommended to add AZA at a dose of 0.5 mg/day with increases to 2–2.5 mg/kg/day, until the goal is achieved. The dose of steroids should be decreased to 2–2.5 mg/kg/day over 2 weeks and then discontinued if serious side effects arise during their use [145]. The use of AZA as first-line treatment is not recommended because of potential toxicity, especially in patients with hyperbilirubinemia; however, most patients have been reported to require the addition of this drug to achieve remission. Testing for TPMT is also applied in children, as is the monitoring of AZA metabolites, 6-thioguanine, and 6-methylmercaptopurine, to identify the optimal therapeutic level of AZA, as reported in a prospective study that included 20 children with AIH [146], and as done in the treatment of inflammatory bowel disease. The optimal levels of these metabolites in relation to AZA's salutary effect have not been clearly established [147]. A recent report documented that a majority of children on AZA therapy maintained biochemical remissions at 6-TGN levels ranging from 50 to 250 pmol/$8 \times 10^8$ RBC, in association with the lowest doses of the drug, suggesting that AZA can be used as a steroid sparing agent in children with AIH [148], as it is done in adult subjects. This information can be used as doses are adjusted [106].

The goal of treatment is remission, defined as: (i) no symptoms, (ii) normal serum activity of AST and ALT, and (iii) normal serum concentrations of IgG. In addition, low or absent titers for ANA and ASMA, and anti-LKM are included in the criteria for remission [149].

In general, the duration of standard therapy is 24 months in patients aged 60 or beyond and 36 months in patients up to 40 years of age. Remission of AIH has been defined as normal AST activity in two consecutive months and absence of symptoms. Discontinuation of immunosuppression therapy can be considered after documented normal AST and ALT serum activity every 3 months for at least 1 year and the absence of necroinflammatory activity on liver histology. Serum AST activity was reported to correlate with serum concentrations of IgG in types 1 and 2 AIH and with titers of ASMA in type 1, suggesting that these markers can be included as measures of response to treatment [150].

From a retrospective study that included 20 years of experience in the treatment of children with AIH, it was reported that discontinuation of therapy was possible in 19% of ANA and ASMA positive patients after treatment for a median of 3 years; however, in this series, none of the patients who had anti-LKM antibodies were able to have therapy discontinued [151]. Close monitoring of patients and their laboratory exams are required to identify and treat relapse of disease, defined as an increase in AST activity by two fold from baseline. Relapses of AIH are treated with prednisolone (or prednisone) at 1–2 mg/kg/day, a dose that can be increased to 2–2.5 mg/kg/day until the therapeutic goal is achieved (see above).

Penicillamine, cyclosporin A, and mycophenolic mofetil have been used in children who do not respond to standard therapy [152]; however, alternate treatments have not been tested in randomized clinical trials. The reader is referred to clinicaltrials.gov for information on available clinical studies.

## Liver Transplantation

Liver transplantation is the alternative to the treatment of AIH not responsive to immunosuppressant therapy. Prospectively studied, it was documented that from a group of 1429 patients, 55 (3.8%) were transplanted for AIH, the majority of whom were women, and tended to exhibit episodes of rejection within the first 3, 6, and 12 months; however, the patient and graft survivals were similar to those transplanted for other indications [153]. The survival rate of patients with AIH who undergo liver transplantation is reported as 87% at 1 year and from 80% to 90% at five, and the survival rates of liver grafts are 84% at 1 year and 74–76% at five [154, 155].

AIH recurs in the liver graft. A large prospective study reported that 20% of patients sustained a recurrence of disease, most within the first year after transplantation. However, none of these patients required retransplantation because of disease recurrence [153]. The literature reports the clinical presentation of AIH recurrence from 1 month to 5 years post transplant [155]; recurrences after 15 years have been documented [156] and also, with histological findings in the graft at least 5 years before a clinical presentation suggestive of recurrence in 24% of patients in a published series [156]. A retrospective review did not report any recurrence, though, in the six out of 32 patients who were transplanted for acute liver failure at presentation [157]. The criteria that define recurrent AIH can be summarized as follows: (1) indication of AIH for transplant, (2) autoantibodies at high titers, (3) persistently increase in the activity of ALT over twice the upper limit of normal, (4) high serum immunoglobulin concentration, (5) liver histology compatible for AIH, (6) dependency on corticosteroid to maintain normal liver profile or need to increase steroid dose, and (7) exclusion of other causes of post transplant hepatitis or graft-dysfunction [155, 158].

Post transplant de novo AIH occurs in patients who have received a liver transplant for diseases other than AIH [159]. It was initially reported in children, with

4% of patients from 180 developing the disease over 5 years [160]. Histologically this condition is characterized by interface hepatitis, and an inflammatory infiltrate highly comprised of plasma cells. The factors that have been identified as predisposing to de novo AIH are HLA-DR3 or HLA-DR4 recipient or donor, previous episodes of acute cellular rejection, steroid dependence, female donor, aged donor, and tacrolimus-based immunosuppression [159]. The treatment of post transplant de novo AIH is the standard therapy for AIH, emphasizing the importance of making the diagnosis of de novo post transplant AIH promptly not to deviate treatment efforts to a presumed diagnosis of rejection, to preserve the life of the graft [161]. The importance of treatment with steroids was documented in a case series in which five non-treated patients lost the graft a few months after diagnosis of de novo AIH in contrast to the seven who were treated, none of whom lost their graft after a follow-up period of a mean of 4 years; also, the tapering of steroids was associated with relapse [162]. A long-term study has found that de novo AIH does respond to treatment, but relapse and progression to cirrhosis were documented [163].

**Acknowledgments** The author acknowledges Dr. Cesar del Rosario for having contributed Figures 4.1, 4.2, and 4.3.

# References

1. Hori S, Nomura T, Sakaguchi S. Control of regulatory T cell development by the transcription factor Foxp3. Science. 2003 Feb 14;299(5609):1057–61.
2. Longhi MS, Ma Y, Bogdanos DP, Cheeseman P, Mieli-Vergani G, Vergani D. Impairment of CD4(+)CD25(+) regulatory T-cells in autoimmune liver disease. J Hepatol. 2004 July;41(1):31–7.
3. Longhi MS, Ma Y, Mitry RR, Bogdanos DP, Heneghan M, Cheeseman P, et al. Effect of CD4+ CD25+ regulatory T-cells on CD8 T-cell function in patients with autoimmune hepatitis. J Autoimmun. 2005 Aug;25(1):63–71.
4. Liang M, Liwen Z, Yun Z, Yanbo D, Jianping C. Serum levels of IL-33 and correlation with IL-4, IL-17A, and hypergammaglobulinemia in patients with autoimmune hepatitis. Mediat Inflamm. 2018;2018:7964654.
5. Gutkowski K, Gutkowska D, Kiszka J, Partyka M, Kacperek-Hartleb T, Kajor M, et al. Serum interleukin17 levels predict inflammatory activity in patients with autoimmune hepatitis. Pol Arch Intern Med. 2018 Mar 29;128(3):150–6.
6. Migita K, Horai Y, Kozuru H, Koga T, Abiru S, Yamasaki K, et al. Serum cytokine profiles and Mac-2 binding protein glycosylation isomer (M2BPGi) level in patients with autoimmune hepatitis. Medicine. 2018 Dec;97(50):e13450.
7. Longhi MS, Hussain MJ, Mitry RR, Arora SK, Mieli-Vergani G, Vergani D, et al. Functional study of CD4+CD25+ regulatory T cells in health and autoimmune hepatitis. J Immunol. 2006 Apr 1;176(7):4484–91.
8. Ferri S, Longhi MS, De Molo C, Lalanne C, Muratori P, Granito A, et al. A multifaceted imbalance of T cells with regulatory function characterizes type 1 autoimmune hepatitis. Hepatology. 2010 Sep;52(3):999–1007.
9. Peiseler M, Sebode M, Franke B, Wortmann F, Schwinge D, Quaas A, et al. FOXP3+ regulatory T cells in autoimmune hepatitis are fully functional and not reduced in frequency. J Hepatol. 2012 Jul;57(1):125–32.

10. Zhu C, Anderson AC, Schubart A, Xiong H, Imitola J, Khoury SJ, et al. The Tim-3 ligand galectin-9 negatively regulates T helper type 1 immunity. Nat Immunol. 2005 Dec;6(12): 1245–52.
11. Liberal R, Grant CR, Holder BS, Ma Y, Mieli-Vergani G, Vergani D, et al. The impaired immune regulation of autoimmune hepatitis is linked to a defective galectin-9/tim-3 pathway. Hepatology. 2012 Aug;56(2):677–86.
12. Albert LJ, Inman RD. Molecular mimicry and autoimmunity. N Engl J Med. 1999 Dec 30;341(27):2068–74.
13. Manns MP, Johnson EF, Griffin KJ, Tan EM, Sullivan KF. Major antigen of liver kidney microsomal autoantibodies in idiopathic autoimmune hepatitis is cytochrome P450db1. J Clin Invest. 1989 Mar;83(3):1066–72.
14. Kerkar N, Choudhuri K, Ma Y, Mahmoud A, Bogdanos DP, Muratori L, et al. Cytochrome P4502D6(193–212): a new immunodominant epitope and target of virus/self cross-reactivity in liver kidney microsomal autoantibody type 1-positive liver disease. J Immunol. 2003 Feb 1;170(3):1481–9.
15. Vento S, Cainelli F, Renzini C, Concia E. Autoimmune hepatitis type 2 induced by HCV and persisting after viral clearance. Lancet. 1997 Nov 1;350(9087):1298–9.
16. Zingaretti C, Arigo M, Cardaci A, Moro M, Crosti M, Sinisi A, et al. Identification of new autoantigens by protein array indicates a role for IL4 neutralization in autoimmune hepatitis. MCP. 2012 Dec;11(12):1885–97.
17. Ngu JH, Gearry RB, Frampton CM, Stedman CA. Autoimmune hepatitis: the role of environmental risk factors: a population-based study. Hepatol Int. 2013 Jul;7(3):869–75.
18. Hawrelak JA, Myers SP. The causes of intestinal dysbiosis: a review. Altern Med Rev. 2004 Jun;9(2):180–97.
19. Lin R, Zhou L, Zhang J, Wang B. Abnormal intestinal permeability and microbiota in patients with autoimmune hepatitis. Int J Clin Exp Pathol. 2015;8(5):5153–60.
20. Czaja AJ. Review article: chemokines as orchestrators of autoimmune hepatitis and potential therapeutic targets. Aliment Pharmacol Ther. 2014;40(3):261–79.
21. Kimura N, Yamagiwa S, Sugano T, Horigome R, Setsu T, Tominaga K, et al. Usefulness of chemokine C-C receptor 7(-)\/programmed cell death-1(+) follicular helper T cell subset frequencies in the diagnosis of autoimmune hepatitis. Hepatol Res. 2019 Sep;49(9): 1026–33.
22. Pando M, Larriba J, Fernandez GC, Fainboim H, Ciocca M, Ramonet M, et al. Pediatric and adult forms of type I autoimmune hepatitis in Argentina: evidence for differential genetic predisposition. Hepatology. 1999 Dec;30(6):1374–80.
23. Czaja AJ, Souto EO, Bittencourt PL, Cancado EL, Porta G, Goldberg AC, et al. Clinical distinctions and pathogenic implications of type 1 autoimmune hepatitis in Brazil and the United States. J Hepatol. 2002 Sep;37(3):302–8.
24. Muratori P, Czaja AJ, Muratori L, Pappas G, Maccariello S, Cassani F, et al. Genetic distinctions between autoimmune hepatitis in Italy and North America. World J Gastroenterol. 2005;11(12):1862–6.
25. Strettell MD, Donaldson PT, Thomson LJ, Santrach PJ, Moore SB, Czaja AJ, et al. Allelic basis for HLA-encoded susceptibility to type 1 autoimmune hepatitis. Gastroenterology. 1997;112(6):2028–35.
26. de Boer YS, van Gerven NM, Zwiers A, Verwer BJ, van Hoek B, van Erpecum KJ, et al. Genome-wide association study identifies variants associated with autoimmune hepatitis type 1. Gastroenterology. 2014 Aug;147(2):443–52.
27. Inazawa J, Itoh N, Abe T, Nagata S. Assignment of the human Fas antigen gene (Fas) to 10q24.1. Genomics. 1992 Nov;14(3):821–2.
28. Hiraide A, Imazeki F, Yokosuka O, Kanda T, Kojima H, Fukai K, et al. Fas polymorphisms influence susceptibility to autoimmune hepatitis. Am J Gastroenterol. 2005 June;100(6):1322–9.
29. Ashkenazi A, Dixit VM. Death receptors: signaling and modulation. Science. 1998 Aug 28;281(5381):1305–8.

30. Cookson S, Constantini PK, Clare M, Underhill JA, Bernal W, Czaja AJ, et al. Frequency and nature of cytokine gene polymorphisms in type 1 autoimmune hepatitis. Hepatology. 1999 Oct;30(4):851–6.
31. Old LJ. Tumor necrosis factor (TNF). Science. 1985 Nov 8;230(4726):630–2.
32. Locksley RM, Killeen N, Lenardo MJ. The TNF and TNF receptor superfamilies: integrating mammalian biology. Cell. 2001 Feb 23;104(4):487–501.
33. Paladino N, Flores AC, Fainboim H, Schroder T, Cuarterolo M, Lezama C, et al. The most severe forms of type I autoimmune hepatitis are associated with genetically determined levels of TGF-beta1. Clin Immunol. 2010 Mar;134(3):305–12.
34. Wahl SM, Wen J, Moutsopoulos N. TGF-beta: a mobile purveyor of immune privilege. Immunol Rev. 2006 Oct;213:213–27.
35. Chen S, Zhao W, Tan W, Luo X, Dan Y, You Z, et al. Association of TBX21 promoter polymorphisms with type 1 autoimmune hepatitis in a Chinese population. Hum Immunol. 2011 Jan;72(1):69–73.
36. Szabo SJ, Kim ST, Costa GL, Zhang X, Fathman CG, Glimcher LH. A novel transcription factor, T-bet, directs Th1 lineage commitment. Cell. 2000 Mar 17;100(6):655–69.
37. Vogel A, Strassburg CP, Manns MP. Genetic association of vitamin D receptor polymorphisms with primary biliary cirrhosis and autoimmune hepatitis. Hepatology. 2002 Jan;35(1):126–31.
38. Kamen DL, Tangpricha V. Vitamin D and molecular actions on the immune system: modulation of innate and autoimmunity. J Mol Med. 2010 May;88(5):441–50.
39. Agarwal K, Czaja AJ, Jones DE, Donaldson PT. Cytotoxic T lymphocyte antigen-4 (CTLA-4) gene polymorphisms and susceptibility to type 1 autoimmune hepatitis. Hepatology. 2000 Jan;31(1):49–53.
40. van Gerven NM, de Boer YS, Zwiers A, van Hoek B, van Erpecum KJ, Beuers U, et al. Cytotoxic T Lymphocyte Antigen-4 +49A/G polymorphism does not affect susceptibility to autoimmune hepatitis. Liver Int. 2013 Mar;33:1039–43.
41. Dariavach P, Mattei MG, Golstein P, Lefranc MP. Human Ig superfamily CTLA-4 gene: chromosomal localization and identity of protein sequence between murine and human CTLA-4 cytoplasmic domains. Eur J Immunol. 1988 Dec;18(12):1901–5.
42. Schneider H, Downey J, Smith A, Zinselmeyer BH, Rush C, Brewer JM, et al. Reversal of the TCR stop signal by CTLA-4. Science. 2006 Sep 29;313(5795):1972–5.
43. Chaouali M, Fernandes V, Ghazouani E, Pereira L, Kochkar R. Association of STAT4, TGFbeta1, SH2B3 and PTPN22 polymorphisms with autoimmune hepatitis. Exp Mol Pathol. 2018 Dec;105(3):279–84.
44. Yousefi A, Mahmoudi E, Zare Bidoki A, Najmi Varzaneh F, Baradaran Noveiry B, Sadr M, et al. IL4 gene polymorphisms in Iranian patients with autoimmune hepatitis. Expert Rev Gastroenterol Hepatol. 2016;10(5):659–63.
45. Jeffery HC, Braitch MK, Bagnall C, Hodson J, Jeffery LE, Wawman RE, et al. Changes in natural killer cells and exhausted memory regulatory T Cells with corticosteroid therapy in acute autoimmune hepatitis. Hepatol Commun. 2018 Apr;2(4):421–36.
46. Xiao F, Ai G, Yan W, Wan X, Luo X, Ning Q. Intrahepatic recruitment of cytotoxic NK cells contributes to autoimmune hepatitis progression. Cell Immunol. 2018 May;327:13–20.
47. Lin R, Zhang J, Zhou L, Wang B. Altered function of monocytes/macrophages in patients with autoimmune hepatitis. Mol Med Rep. 2016 May;13(5):3874–80.
48. Berger SL, Kouzarides T, Shiekhattar R, Shilatifard A. An operational definition of epigenetics. Genes Dev. 2009 Apr 1;23(7):781–3.
49. Saito Y, Liang G, Egger G, Friedman JM, Chuang JC, Coetzee GA, et al. Specific activation of microRNA-127 with downregulation of the proto-oncogene BCL6 by chromatin-modifying drugs in human cancer cells. Cancer Cell. 2006 June;9(6):435–43.
50. Ardekani AM, Naeini MM. The role of MicroRNAs in human diseases. Avicenna J Med Biotechnol. 2010 Oct;2(4):161–79.

51. Migita K, Komori A, Kozuru H, Jiuchi Y, Nakamura M, Yasunami M, et al. Circulating microRNA profiles in patients with type-1 autoimmune hepatitis. PLoS One. 2015;10(11):e0136908.
52. Alvarez F, Berg PA, Bianchi FB, Bianchi L, Burroughs AK, Cancado EL, et al. International autoimmune hepatitis group report: review of criteria for diagnosis of autoimmune hepatitis. J Hepatol. 1999 Nov;31(5):929–38.
53. Yasui S, Fujiwara K, Yonemitsu Y, Oda S, Nakano M, Yokosuka O. Clinicopathological features of severe and fulminant forms of autoimmune hepatitis. J Gastroenterol. 2011 Mar;46(3):378–90.
54. Bjornsson E, Talwalkar J, Treeprasertsuk S, Kamath PS, Takahashi N, Sanderson S, et al. Drug-induced autoimmune hepatitis: clinical characteristics and prognosis. Hepatology. 2010 Jun;51(6):2040–8.
55. Czaja AJ, Nishioka M, Morshed SA, Hachiya T. Patterns of nuclear immunofluorescence and reactivities to recombinant nuclear antigens in autoimmune hepatitis. Gastroenterology. 1994 July;107(1):200–7.
56. Czaja AJ, Manns MP. The validity and importance of subtypes in autoimmune hepatitis: a point of view. Am J Gastroenterol. 1995 Aug;90(8):1206–11.
57. Czaja AJ, Morshed SA, Parveen S, Nishioka M. Antibodies to single-stranded and double-stranded DNA in antinuclear antibody-positive type 1-autoimmune hepatitis. Hepatology. 1997;26(3):567–72.
58. Lidman K. Clinical diagnosis in patients with smooth muscle antibodies. A study of a one-year material. Acta Med Scand. 1976;200(5):403–7.
59. Wies I, Brunner S, Henninger J, Herkel J, Kanzler S, Meyer zum Buschenfelde KH, et al. Identification of target antigen for SLA/LP autoantibodies in autoimmune hepatitis. Lancet. 2000;355(9214):1510–5.
60. Martini E, Abuaf N, Cavalli F, Durand V, Johanet C, Homberg JC. Antibody to liver cytosol (anti-LC1) in patients with autoimmune chronic active hepatitis type 2. Hepatology. 1988;8(6):1662–6.
61. McFarlane IG, Hegarty JE, McSorley CG, McFarlane BM, Williams R. Antibodies to liver-specific protein predict outcome of treatment withdrawal in autoimmune chronic active hepatitis. Lancet. 1984;2(8409):954–6.
62. Meech R, Mackenzie PI. Structure and function of uridine diphosphate glucuronosyltransferases. Clin Exp Pharmacol Physiol. 1997;24(12):907–15.
63. Lapierre P, Hajoui O, Homberg JC, Alvarez F. Formiminotransferase cyclodeaminase is an organ-specific autoantigen recognized by sera of patients with autoimmune hepatitis. Gastroenterology. 1999;116(3):643–9.
64. Xu XM, Carlson BA, Mix H, Zhang Y, Saira K, Glass RS, et al. Biosynthesis of selenocysteine on its tRNA in eukaryotes. PLoS biology. 2007;5(1):e4.
65. Bianchi L, Gudat, F. Chronic hepatitis. In: MacSween RNM, Anthony PP, Scheuer PJ, Burt AD, Portman BC, editors. Pathology of the Liver. 1. Third ed. Edinburgh: Churchill Livingstone; 1994. p. 349–95.
66. Czaja AJ, Carpenter HA. Histological features associated with relapse after corticosteroid withdrawal in type 1 autoimmune hepatitis. Liver Int. 2003 Apr;23(2):116–23.
67. Brandao DF, Ramalho FS, Martinelli AL, Zucoloto S, Ramalho LN. Relationship between plasma cells and hepatic stellate cells in autoimmune hepatitis. Pathol Res Pract. 2010;206(12):800–4.
68. Maia JM, Maranhao Hde S, Sena LV, Rocha LR, Medeiros IA, Ramos AM. Hepatic stellate cell activation and hepatic fibrosis in children with type 1 autoimmune hepatitis: an immunohistochemical study of paired liver biopsies before treatment and after clinical remission. Eur J Gastroenterol Hepatol. 2010;22(3):264–9.
69. Miao Q, Bian Z, Tang R, Zhang H, Wang Q, Huang S, et al. Emperipolesis mediated by CD8 T cells is a characteristic histopathologic feature of autoimmune hepatitis. Clin Rev Allergy Immunol. 2015 June;48(2–3):226–35.

70. Suzuki A, Brunt EM, Kleiner DE, Miquel R, Smyrk TC, Andrade RJ, et al. The use of liver biopsy evaluation in discrimination of idiopathic autoimmune hepatitis versus drug-induced liver injury. Hepatology. 2011 Sep;54(3):931–9.

71. Hennes EM, Zeniya M, Czaja AJ, Pares A, Dalekos GN, Krawitt EL, et al. Simplified criteria for the diagnosis of autoimmune hepatitis. Hepatology. 2008 July;48(1):169–76.

72. Czaja AJ. Performance parameters of the diagnostic scoring systems for autoimmune hepatitis. Hepatology. 2008;48(5):1540–8.

73. Munoz-Espinosa L, Alarcon G, Mercado-Moreira A, Cordero P, Caballero E, Avalos V, et al. Performance of the international classifications criteria for autoimmune hepatitis diagnosis in Mexican patients. Autoimmunity. 2011;44(7):543–8.

74. Gatselis NK, Zachou K, Papamichalis P, Koukoulis GK, Gabeta S, Dalekos GN, et al. Comparison of simplified score with the revised original score for the diagnosis of autoimmune hepatitis: a new or a complementary diagnostic score? Digestive and liver disease: official journal of the Italian Society of Gastroenterology and the Italian Association for the Study of the Liver. 2010;42(11):807–12.

75. Efe C, Wahlin S, Ozaslan E, Purnak T, Muratori L, Quarneti C, et al. Diagnostic difficulties, therapeutic strategies, and performance of scoring systems in patients with autoimmune hepatitis and concurrent hepatitis B/C. Scand J Gastroenterol. 2013 Apr;48(4):504–8.

76. Czaja AJ. The overlap syndromes of autoimmune hepatitis. Dig Dis Sci. 2013 Feb;58(2):326–43.

77. Chazouilleres O, Wendum D, Serfaty L, Montembault S, Rosmorduc O, Poupon R. Primary biliary cirrhosis-autoimmune hepatitis overlap syndrome: clinical features and response to therapy. Hepatology. 1998 Aug;28(2):296–301.

78. Gohlke F, Lohse AW, Dienes HP, Lohr H, Marker-Hermann E, Gerken G, et al. Evidence for an overlap syndrome of autoimmune hepatitis and primary sclerosing cholangitis. J Hepatol. 1996;24(6):699–705.

79. van Buuren HR, van Hoogstraten HJE, Terkivatan T, Schalm SW, Vleggaar FP. High prevalence of autoimmune hepatitis among patients with primary sclerosing cholangitis. J Hepatol. 2000 Oct;33(4):543–8.

80. Talwalkar JA, Keach JC, Angulo P, Lindor KD. Overlap of autoimmune hepatitis and primary biliary cirrhosis: an evaluation of a modified scoring system. Am J Gastroenterol. 2002 May;97(5):1191–7.

81. Muratori P, Granito A, Pappas G, Pendino GM, Quarneti C, Cicola R, et al. The serological profile of the autoimmune hepatitis/primary biliary cirrhosis overlap syndrome. Am J Gastroenterol. 2009 June;104(6):1420–5.

82. Boberg KM, Fausa O, Haaland T, Holter E, Mellbye OJ, Spurkland A, et al. Features of autoimmune hepatitis in primary sclerosing cholangitis: an evaluation of 114 primary sclerosing cholangitis patients according to a scoring system for the diagnosis of autoimmune hepatitis. Hepatology. 1996 June;23(6):1369–76.

83. Kaya M, Angulo P, Lindor KD. Overlap of autoimmune hepatitis and primary sclerosing cholangitis: an evaluation of a modified scoring system. J Hepatol. 2000 Oct;33(4):537–42.

84. Neuhauser M, Bjornsson E, Treeprasertsuk S, Enders F, Silveira M, Talwalkar J, et al. Autoimmune hepatitis-PBC overlap syndrome: a simplified scoring system may assist in the diagnosis. Am J Gastroenterol. 2010 Feb;105(2):345–53.

85. Teufel A, Weinmann A, Kahaly GJ, Centner C, Piendl A, Worns M, et al. Concurrent autoimmune diseases in patients with autoimmune hepatitis. J Clin Gastroenterol. 2010 Mar;44(3):208–13.

86. Manns MP, Czaja AJ, Gorham JD, Krawitt EL, Mieli-Vergani G, Vergani D, et al. Diagnosis and management of autoimmune hepatitis. Hepatology. 2010 June;51(6):2193–213.

87. Czaja AJ. Features and consequences of untreated type 1 autoimmune hepatitis. Liver Int. 2009 July;29(6):816–23.

88. Park DW, Lee YJ, Chang W, Park JH, Lee KH, Kim YH, et al. Diagnostic performance of a point shear wave elastography (pSWE) for hepatic fibrosis in patients with autoimmune liver disease. PLoS One. 2019;14(3):e0212771.

89. Roberts SK, Therneau TM, Czaja AJ. Prognosis of histological cirrhosis in type 1 autoimmune hepatitis. Gastroenterology. 1996 Mar;110(3):848–57.
90. Czaja AJ, Carpenter HA. Decreased fibrosis during corticosteroid therapy of autoimmune hepatitis. J Hepatol. 2004 Apr;40(4):646–52.
91. Montano-Loza AJ, Carpenter HA, Czaja AJ. Improving the end point of corticosteroid therapy in type 1 autoimmune hepatitis to reduce the frequency of relapse. Am J Gastroenterol. 2007 May;102(5):1005–12.
92. Johannes L, Jacob R, Leffler H. Galectins at a glance. J Cell Sci. 2018 May;131(9): jcs208884.
93. Matsuoka N, Kozuru H, Koga T, Abiru S, Yamasaki K, Komori A, et al. Galectin-9 in autoimmune hepatitis: correlation between serum levels of galectin-9 and M2BPGi in patients with autoimmune hepatitis. Medicine. 2019 Aug;98(35):e16924.
94. Shim KY, Eom YW, Kim MY, Kang SH, Baik SK. Role of the renin-angiotensin system in hepatic fibrosis and portal hypertension. Korean J Intern Med. 2018 May;33(3): 453–61.
95. Efe C, Cengiz M, Kahramanoglu-Aksoy E, Yilmaz B, Ozseker B, Beyazt Y, et al. Angiotensin-converting enzyme for noninvasive assessment of liver fibrosis in autoimmune hepatitis. Eur J Gastroenterol Hepatol. 2015 June;27(6):649–54.
96. Cook GC, Mulligan R, Sherlock S. Controlled prospective trial of corticosteroid therapy in active chronic hepatitis. Q J Med. 1971 Apr;40(158):159–85.
97. European Association for the Study of the Liver. EASL clinical practice guidelines: autoimmune hepatitis. J Hepatol. 2015 Oct;63(4):971–1004.
98. Gleeson D, Heneghan MA, British Society of Gastroenterology. British Society of Gastroenterology (BSG) guidelines for management of autoimmune hepatitis. Gut. 2011 Dec;60(12):1611–29.
99. Richter B, Neises G, Clar C. Glucocorticoid withdrawal schemes in chronic medical disorders. A systematic review. Endocrinol Metab Clin N Am. 2002 Sep;31(3):751–78.
100. Czaja AJ, Davis GL, Ludwig J, Taswell HF. Complete resolution of inflammatory activity following corticosteroid treatment of HBsAg-negative chronic active hepatitis. Hepatology. 1984 July–Aug;4(4):622–7.
101. Czaja AJ. Low-dose corticosteroid therapy after multiple relapses of severe HBsAg-negative chronic active hepatitis. Hepatology. 1990 June;11(6):1044–9.
102. Mack CL, Adams D, Assis DN, Kerkar N, Manns MP, Mayo MJ, et al. Diagnosis and management of autoimmune hepatitis in adults and children: 2019 practice guidance and guidelines from the american association for the study of liver diseases. Hepatology. 2020;72(2):671–722.
103. Czaja AJ, Rakela J, Ludwig J. Features reflective of early prognosis in corticosteroid-treated severe autoimmune chronic active hepatitis. Gastroenterology. 1988 Aug;95(2): 448–53.
104. Czaja AJ. Rapidity of treatment response and outcome in type 1 autoimmune hepatitis. J Hepatol. 2009 July;51(1):161–7.
105. Montano-Loza AJ, Carpenter HA, Czaja AJ. Features associated with treatment failure in type 1 autoimmune hepatitis and predictive value of the model of end-stage liver disease. Hepatology. 2007 Oct;46(4):1138–45.
106. Johnson PJ, McFarlane IG, Williams R. Azathioprine for long-term maintenance of remission in autoimmune hepatitis. N Engl J Med. 1995 Oct 12;333(15):958–63.
107. Karran P, Attard N. Thiopurines in current medical practice: molecular mechanisms and contributions to therapy-related cancer. Nat Rev Cancer. 2008 Jan;8(1):24–36.
108. Evans WE. Pharmacogenetics of thiopurine S-methyltransferase and thiopurine therapy. Ther Drug Monit. 2004 Apr;26(2):186–91.
109. Fujita K, Sasaki Y. Pharmacogenomics in drug-metabolizing enzymes catalyzing anticancer drugs for personalized cancer chemotherapy. Curr Drug Metab. 2007 Aug;8(6):554–62.
110. Czaja AJ. Review article: the management of autoimmune hepatitis beyond consensus guidelines. Aliment Pharmacol Ther. 2013 Aug;38(4):343–64.

111. Wang KK, Czaja AJ, Beaver SJ, Go VL. Extrahepatic malignancy following long-term immunosuppressive therapy of severe hepatitis B surface antigen-negative chronic active hepatitis. Hepatology. 1989 July;10(1):39–43.

112. van Gerven NM, Verwer BJ, Witte BI, van Hoek B, Coenraad MJ, van Erpecum KJ, et al. Relapse is almost universal after withdrawal of immunosuppressive medication in patients with autoimmune hepatitis in remission. J Hepatol. 2013 Jan;58(1):141–7.

113. Weiler-Normann C, Lohse AW. Autoimmune hepatitis: a life-long disease. J Hepatol. 2013 Jan;58(1):5–7.

114. Hartl J, Ehlken H, Weiler-Normann C, Sebode M, Kreuels B, Pannicke N, et al. Patient selection based on treatment duration and liver biochemistry increases success rates after treatment withdrawal in autoimmune hepatitis. J Hepatol. 2015 Mar;62(3):642–6.

115. Czaja AJ. Late relapse of type 1 autoimmune hepatitis after corticosteroid withdrawal. Dig Dis Sci. 2010 June;55(6):1761–9.

116. Dhaliwal HK, Hoeroldt BS, Dube AK, McFarlane E, Underwood JC, Karajeh MA, et al. Long-term prognostic significance of persisting histological activity despite biochemical remission in autoimmune hepatitis. Am J Gastroenterol. 2015 July;110(7):993–9.

117. Yeoman AD, Westbrook RH, Zen Y, Maninchedda P, Portmann BC, Devlin J, et al. Early predictors of corticosteroid treatment failure in icteric presentations of autoimmune hepatitis. Hepatology. 2011 Mar;53(3):926–34.

118. Selvarajah V, Montano-Loza AJ, Czaja AJ. Systematic review: managing suboptimal treatment responses in autoimmune hepatitis with conventional and nonstandard drugs. Aliment Pharmacol Ther. 2012 Oct;36(8):691–707.

119. Manns MP, Woynarowski M, Kreisel W, Lurie Y, Rust C, Zuckerman E, et al. Budesonide induces remission more effectively than prednisone in a controlled trial of patients with autoimmune hepatitis. Gastroenterology. 2010 Oct;139(4):1198–206.

120. Binicier OB, Gunay S. The efficacy and adverse effects of budesonide in remission induction treatment of autoimmune hepatitis: a retrospective study. Croat Med J. 2019 Aug 31;60(4):345–51.

121. Efe C, Ozaslan E, Kav T, Purnak T, Shorbagi A, Ozkayar O, et al. Liver fibrosis may reduce the efficacy of budesonide in the treatment of autoimmune hepatitis and overlap syndrome. Autoimmun Rev. 2012 Mar;11(5):330–4.

122. Malekzadeh R, Nasseri-Moghaddam S, Kaviani MJ, Taheri H, Kamalian N, Sotoudeh M. Cyclosporin A is a promising alternative to corticosteroids in autoimmune hepatitis. Dig Dis Sci. 2001 June;46(6):1321–7.

123. Van Thiel DH, Wright H, Carroll P, Abu-Elmagd K, Rodriguez-Rilo H, McMichael J, et al. Tacrolimus: a potential new treatment for autoimmune chronic active hepatitis: results of an open-label preliminary trial. Am J Gastroenterol. 1995 May;90(5):771–6.

124. Larsen FS, Vainer B, Eefsen M, Bjerring PN, Adel HB. Low-dose tacrolimus ameliorates liver inflammation and fibrosis in steroid refractory autoimmune hepatitis. World J Gastroenterol: WJG. 2007 June 21;13(23):3232–6.

125. Czaja AJ, Carpenter HA. Empiric therapy of autoimmune hepatitis with mycophenolate mofetil: comparison with conventional treatment for refractory disease. J Clin Gastroenterol. 2005 Oct;39(9):819–25.

126. Hlivko JT, Shiffman ML, Stravitz RT, Luketic VA, Sanyal AJ, Fuchs M, et al. A single center review of the use of mycophenolate mofetil in the treatment of autoimmune hepatitis. Clin Gastroenterol Hepatol. 2008 Sep;6(9):1036–40.

127. Wolf DC, Bojito L, Facciuto M, Lebovics E. Mycophenolate mofetil for autoimmune hepatitis: a single practice experience. Dig Dis Sci. 2009 Nov;54(11):2519–22.

128. Sharzehi K, Huang MA, Schreibman IR, Brown KA. Mycophenolate mofetil for the treatment of autoimmune hepatitis in patients refractory or intolerant to conventional therapy. Can J Gastroenterol. 2010 Oct;24(10):588–92.

129. Zachou K, Gatselis N, Papadamou G, Rigopoulou EI, Dalekos GN. Mycophenolate for the treatment of autoimmune hepatitis: prospective assessment of its efficacy and safety for induction and maintenance of remission in a large cohort of treatment-naive patients. J Hepatol. 2011 Sep;55(3):636–46.

130. Naesens M, Kuypers DR, Sarwal M. Calcineurin inhibitor nephrotoxicity. Clin J Am Soc Nephrol CJASN. 2009 Feb;4(2):481–508.

131. Hanouneh M, Ritchie MM, Ascha M, Ascha MS, Chedid A, Sanguankeo A, et al. A review of the utility of tacrolimus in the management of adults with autoimmune hepatitis. Scand J Gastroenterol. 2019 Jan;54(1):76–80.

132. Giannakopoulos G, Verbaan H, Friis-Liby IL, Sangfelt P, Nyhlin N, Almer S, et al. Mycophenolate mofetil treatment in patients with autoimmune hepatitis failing standard therapy with prednisolone and azathioprine. Dig Liver Dis. 2019 Feb;51(2):253–7.

133. Lohse AW, zum Buschenfelde KH, Franz B, Kanzler S, Gerken G, Dienes HP. Characterization of the overlap syndrome of primary biliary cirrhosis (PBC) and autoimmune hepatitis: evidence for it being a hepatitic form of PBC in genetically susceptible individuals. Hepatology. 1999 Apr;29(4):1078–84.

134. Renou C, Bourliere M, Martini F, Ouzan D, Penaranda G, Larroque O, et al. Primary biliary cirrhosis-autoimmune hepatitis overlap syndrome: complete biochemical and histological response to therapy with ursodesoxycholic acid. J Gastroenterol Hepatol. 2006 Apr;21(4):781–2.

135. McNair AN, Moloney M, Portmann BC, Williams R, McFarlane IG. Autoimmune hepatitis overlapping with primary sclerosing cholangitis in five cases. Am J Gastroenterol. 1998 May;93(5):777–84.

136. Floreani A, Rizzotto ER, Ferrara F, Carderi I, Caroli D, Blasone L, et al. Clinical course and outcome of autoimmune hepatitis/primary sclerosing cholangitis overlap syndrome. Am J Gastroenterol. 2005 July;100(7):1516–22.

137. Czaja AJ. Difficult treatment decisions in autoimmune hepatitis. World J Gastroenterol WJG. 2010 Feb 28;16(8):934–47.

138. Mendizabal M, Marciano S, Videla MG, Anders M, Zerega A, Balderramo DC, et al. Fulminant presentation of autoimmune hepatitis: clinical features and early predictors of corticosteroid treatment failure. Eur J Gastroenterol Hepatol. 2015 June;27(6):644–8.

139. Rubin JN, Te HS. Refractory Autoimmune Hepatitis: Beyond Standard Therapy. Dig Dis Sci. 2016 June;61(6):1757–62.

140. Burak KW, Swain MG, Santodomingo-Garzon T, Lee SS, Urbanski SJ, Aspinall AI, et al. Rituximab for the treatment of patients with autoimmune hepatitis who are refractory or intolerant to standard therapy. Can J Gastroenterol. 2013;27(5):273–80.

141. Valean S, Acalovschi M, Dumitrascu DL, Ciobanu L, Nagy G, Chira R. Hepatocellular carcinoma in patients with autoimmune hepatitis - a systematic review of the literature published between 1989-2016. Med Pharmacy Rep. 2019 Apr;92(2):99–105.

142. Danielsson Borssen A, Almer S, Prytz H, Wallerstedt S, Friis-Liby IL, Bergquist A, et al. Hepatocellular and extrahepatic cancer in patients with autoimmune hepatitis: a long-term follow-up study in 634 Swedish patients. Scand J Gastroenterol. 2015 Feb;50(2):217–23.

143. Valean S, Acalovschi M, Dumitrascu DL, Ciobanu L, Nagy G, Chira R. Hepatocellular carcinoma in patients with autoimmune hepatitis - a systematic review of the literature published between 1989–2016. Med Pharm Rep. 2019;92(2):99–105.

144. Floreani A, Liberal R, Vergani D, Mieli-Vergani G. Autoimmune hepatitis: contrasts and comparisons in children and adults - a comprehensive review. J Autoimmun. 2013 Oct; 46:7–16.

145. Terziroli Beretta-Piccoli B, Mieli-Vergani G, Vergani D. Autoimmune hepatitis: standard treatment and systematic review of alternative treatments. World J Gastroenterol WJG. 2017 Sep 7;23(33):6030–48.

146. Rumbo C, Emerick KM, Emre S, Shneider BL. Azathioprine metabolite measurements in the treatment of autoimmune hepatitis in pediatric patients: a preliminary report. J Pediatr Gastroenterol Nutr. 2002 Sep;35(3):391–8.

147. Czaja AJ. Current and prospective pharmacotherapy for autoimmune hepatitis. Expert Opin Pharmacother. 2014 Aug;15(12):1715–36.

148. Sheiko MA, Sundaram SS, Capocelli KE, Pan Z, McCoy AM, Mack CL. Outcomes in pediatric autoimmune hepatitis and significance of azathioprine metabolites. J Pediatr Gastroenterol Nutr. 2017 July;65(1):80–5.

149. Vergani D, Mackay IR, Mieli-Vergani G. Hepatitis. In: Noel R, Rose IRM, editors. The auto-immune diseases. 5th ed. New York: Elsevier. p. 889–907.
150. Gregorio GV, McFarlane B, Bracken P, Vergani D, Mieli-Vergani G. Organ and non-organ specific autoantibody titres and IgG levels as markers of disease activity: a longitudinal study in childhood autoimmune liver disease. Autoimmunity. 2002 Dec;35(8):515–9.
151. Gregorio GV, Portmann B, Reid F, Donaldson PT, Doherty DG, McCartney M, et al. Autoimmune hepatitis in childhood: a 20-year experience. Hepatology. 1997 Mar;25(3):541–7.
152. Mieli-Vergani G, Vergani D. Autoimmune paediatric liver disease. World J Gastroenterol. 2008 June 7;14(21):3360–7.
153. Molmenti EP, Netto GJ, Murray NG, Smith DM, Molmenti H, Crippin JS, et al. Incidence and recurrence of autoimmune/alloimmune hepatitis in liver transplant recipients. Liver Transp. 2002 June;8(6):519–26.
154. Futagawa Y, Terasaki PI. An analysis of the OPTN/UNOS liver transplant registry. Clin Transpl. 2004;2004:315–29.
155. Mottershead M, Neuberger J. Transplantation in autoimmune liver diseases. World J Gastroenterol WJG. 2008 June 7;14(21):3388–95.
156. Duclos-Vallee JC, Sebagh M, Rifai K, Johanet C, Ballot E, Guettier C, et al. A 10 year follow up study of patients transplanted for autoimmune hepatitis: histological recurrence precedes clinical and biochemical recurrence. Gut. 2003 June;52(6):893–7.
157. Reich DJ, Fiel I, Guarrera JV, Emre S, Guy SR, Schwartz ME, et al. Liver transplantation for autoimmune hepatitis. Hepatology. 2000 Oct;32(4 Pt 1):693–700.
158. Banff Working G, Demetris AJ, Adeyi O, Bellamy CO, Clouston A, Charlotte F, et al. Liver biopsy interpretation for causes of late liver allograft dysfunction. Hepatology. 2006 Aug;44(2):489–501.
159. Liberal R, Zen Y, Mieli-Vergani G, Vergani D. Liver transplantation and autoimmune liver diseases. Liver Transp. 2013 Oct;19(10):1065–77.
160. Kerkar N, Hadzic N, Davies ET, Portmann B, Donaldson PT, Rela M, et al. De-novo autoimmune hepatitis after liver transplantation. Lancet. 1998 Feb 7;351(9100):409–13.
161. Vukotic R, Vitale G, D'Errico-Grigioni A, Muratori L, Andreone P. De novo autoimmune hepatitis in liver transplant: State-of-the-art review. World J Gastroenterol. 2016 Mar 14;22(10):2906–14.
162. Salcedo M, Vaquero J, Banares R, Rodriguez-Mahou M, Alvarez E, Vicario JL, et al. Response to steroids in de novo autoimmune hepatitis after liver transplantation. Hepatology. 2002 Feb;35(2):349–56.
163. Kwon JH, Hanouneh IA, Allende D, Yerian L, Diago T, Eghtesad B, et al. De novo autoimmune hepatitis following liver transplantation. Transplant Proc. 2018 June;50(5):1451–6.

# Chapter 5
# Primary Sclerosing Cholangitis

Nora V. Bergasa

A 51-year-old woman presented to the hospital because of abdominal pain and fever. Her vital signs were notable for a high temperature; she had scleral icterus, abdominal tenderness on the right upper quadrant without rebound, and legs with prominent varicose veins. The relevant laboratory tests were leukocytosis, with a predominance of neutrophils but no bandemia, normal electrolytes, normal coagulation profile, and a serum alkaline phosphatase (AP) of 440 IU/L, serum bilirubin of 3 mg/dL, and a mild increase of AST and ALT activities to less than 100 IU/L. A right upper quadrant sonogram was normal, but a magnetic resonance cholangiopancreatography (MRCP) revealed changes suggestive of primary sclerosing cholangitis (PSC) with intrahepatic biliary strictures and sacculations; she did not have gallstones. Urine and blood cultures were negative for bacterial growth. She was started on empirical antibiotic therapy for cholangitis in the face of suspected PSC. She subsequently provided a colonoscopy report from a few years prior to this presentation, documenting inactive colitis on biopsy. The hepatology service was consulted and subsequently followed the patient in the clinic with relatively good liver function but intermittent increases in serum bilirubin. She did not have pruritus. The patient developed episodes of fever and leukocytosis associated with right upper quadrant discomfort. On one occasion, her blood cultures grew *Klebsiella pneumoniae*. She was referred for liver transplant evaluation because of recurrent cholangitis. After 9 years of follow up, she underwent liver transplantation from a hepatitis B anticore + donor, for which she is on an antiviral. At present, she is doing relatively well; however, she has an anastomotic stricture. She has had normal surveillance colonoscopies over the years. She regularly goes on vacation, has a good

N. V. Bergasa (✉)
Department of Medicine, H+H/Metropolitan, New York, NY, USA

New York Medical College, Valhalla, NY, USA

Hepatology, H+H/Woodhull, Brooklyn, NY, USA

© The Author(s), under exclusive license to Springer-Verlag London Ltd., part of Springer Nature 2022
N. V. Bergasa (ed.), *Clinical Cases in Hepatology*,
https://doi.org/10.1007/978-1-4471-4715-2_5

appetite and energy level, and continues to follow up at our hepatology clinic with scheduled visits to the transplant center where MRCPs and adjustments of her immunosuppression are made and where she was started on ursodeoxycholic acid (UDCA). Her AP activity post-transplantation has been normal, her bilirubin has been around 3 mg/dL, her albumin has been low, without proteinuria, suggestive of synthetic dysfunction. There are no features of PSC on liver histology and no inflammatory activity, but she has cirrhosis, classified as cryptogenic.

## Sclerosing Cholangitis

The patient described in this chapter presented with a picture of cholangitis, associated with cholestasis, and a magnetic resonance cholangiopancreatography that revealed intrahepatic biliary strictures [1]. In the absence of prior biliary tract surgery, the findings are consistent with primary sclerosing cholangitis (PSC). A colonoscopy performed 4 years prior to her initial presentation had revealed inactive colitis. The patient had not had symptoms of inflammatory bowel disease, which is associated with PSC in approximately 70% of the time.

Sclerosing cholangitis is a condition associated with the disappearance of intrahepatic and extrahepatic bile ducts secondary to a fibrosing process that leads to biliary cirrhosis and liver failure. PSC is the term used when no precipitating factor is identified; it may or may not be associated with inflammatory bowel disease. Secondary sclerosing cholangitis is the term used when the precipitating factor(s) of the condition is (are) identified or inferred.

The etiology of PSC is unknown [2, 3]. It has been suggested that this liver disease may have an autoimmune basis. PSC has been diagnosed in association with retroperitoneal fibrosis and mediastinal fibrosis. The syndrome of sclerosing cholangitis has been described in patients with histiocytosis X. In contrast to PSC, some processes lead to secondary sclerosing cholangitis, including hepatic artery infusions of chemotherapeutic agents (e.g., fluorodeoxyuridine (FUDR) [4] for treatment of malignancies, the associated coagulative phenomena due to lupus anticoagulant, infusions of scolicidal solution (formaldehyde, 20% sodium chloride) directly into hydatid cysts, neoplasms of the biliary tract, bacterial or parasitic infections of the biliary tree, opportunistic infections in immunocompromised patients, complications of cholecystectomy, and abdominal trauma [5]. The mechanisms by which these events lead to sclerosing cholangitis are unknown; it has been speculated that invasion of the biliary tract by pathogens and the effects of inflammation lead to cholangitis in the last two conditions. In patients with AIDS, polymicrobial cholangitis (e.g., from cryptosporidium, *Candida albicans, Klebsiella pneumoniae*, and cytomegalovirus) have been reported. Ischemia has been proposed in the pathogenesis of sclerosing cholangitis secondary to intraarterial infusions of FUDR [6]. The instillation of scolicidal solution into intrahepatic Ecchinococcal cysts communicating with the biliary tree is associated with the rapid development of sclerosing cholangitis from caustic injury [7]. As PSC is associated with inflammatory bowel disease (IBD) in 70 to 80 percent of patients, cholestasis in this patient population suggests the diagnosis of this liver disease [3]; in this regard, colon neoplasia in patients with IBD in association with PSC tended to be more frequent than in patients without PSC in one report [8]; in addition, it was documented that patients with PSC and IBD had more rectal sparing and more involvement of the terminal ileum than patients with PSC. The combination of diseases was associated with a decreased survival at 5 years from the time of presentation [9]. Indeed, PSC associated with IBD has been proposed to differ from that not associated with IBD, although reports do not seem consistent. In a study from Sweden, patients with PSC associated with IBD had active inflammation documented histologically but not apparent on inspection. The inflammation was reported to be prominent or exclusively on the right side of the colon, with rectal sparing and backwash ileitis. From this study, it has been suggested that the apparent quiescent state of the colon in patients with IBD may mask active inflammatory activity, hence promoting the development of malignancy [10]. In contrast, in a study from the Netherlands of patients with PSC in association with IBD, the majority had pancolitis, the rectum was infrequently spared, and there were few patients with backwash ileitis, in association with ulcerative colitis; in patients with Crohn's disease, the predominant finding was colitis [11]. PSC presents alone in a substantial number of patients; accordingly, it has to be considered in the differential diagnosis of patients who present with cholestasis regardless of any gastrointestinal comorbidities. It is significantly more common in men than in women. It is most commonly diagnosed around the age of 30 years.

## Etiology

An autoimmune component in the etiology of PSC has been proposed because of its association with autoantibodies. Antinuclear antibodies of the homogenous type, with an approximate prevalence of 35% [12], were reported in PSC. In addition, anticardiolipin, antithyroperoxidase antibodies, and rheumatoid factor have been reported in PSC [13]. Antineutrophil nuclear antibody (ANNA), initially reported as antibodies against a component of the portal tract and subsequently characterized as ANNA, was reported in the serum of 84% of patients with PSC at a relatively high titer, and in 86% of patients with IBD [14]. It was demonstrated by an enzyme-linked immunosorbent assay for immunoglobulin G (IgG) neutrophil antibodies that neutrophil binding in sera from patients with PSC was significantly greater than of patients with other liver diseases, including primary biliary cholangitis (PBC) [15]. Perinuclear immunofluorescence was shown by most serum samples from patients with ulcerative colitis, PSC, and PSC without ulcerative colitis [15]; in one study, circulating antineutrophil antibodies (ANCA) of the perinuclear type (p-ANCA) were reported to occur in 87% of patients with PSC with or without ulcerative colitis, and in 68% of those with ulcerative colitis only [13]. Antineutrophil cytoplasmic antibodies (ANCA) of the IgA class were found in 20% of sera from 35 patients with PSC and in 50% of 40 patients with autoimmune hepatitis in a small study. The staining pattern in patients with PSC showed both an atypical perinuclear staining in PSC and the classical pattern in neutrophils from patients with autoimmune hepatitis. The staining pattern for the IgA class of antibody against ANCA was "classical" and "atypical" in PSC compared to the findings in autoimmune hepatitis in which the staining was the classic perinuclear expression. These findings were interpreted to suggest that there are different target antigens of IgA class ANCA with distinct subcellular localization [16]. Atypical p-ANCA observed in patients with PSC, ulcerative colitis, and autoimmune hepatitis was reported to react with an antigen present in the nuclear lamina of granulocytes [17] that was identified subsequently as a 50-kilodalton myeloid-specific nuclear envelope protein [18]. The 50-kDa ANCA autoantigen has been reported to be β-tubulin isotype 5 (TBB-5). In experiments that included sera from patients with autoimmune hepatitis, and with PSC alone or in association with IBD, p-ANCA recognized human β-tubulin isotype 5 (TBB5) and cross-reacted with filamenting temperature-sensitive mutant Z (FtsZ), its evolutionary bacterial precursor protein. FtsZ is a tubulin homolog and the major cytoskeletal protein in bacterial cell division, during which it is the first protein to move to the division site from where it recruits other proteins that produce a new cell wall between the dividing cells [19]. These results have suggested that the reaction of p-ANCAs against human TBB-5 and their cross reactivity with FtsZ reflects an abnormal immune response to intestinal microorganisms in individuals vulnerable to develop these types of diseases, including PSC [20]. The association of some autoimmune diseases with PSC has been interpreted to suggest an autoimmune component in the pathogenesis of the latter [21].

The high frequency of autoantibodies that bind biliary epithelial cells (BEC) was documented in patients with PSC compared to control and disease control sera. Anti biliary epithelial cell antibodies were reported to induce IL-6 production by BEC from patients with PSC (and PBC); however, IgM and IgG immunoglobulin fractions only from PSC sera significantly induced the expression of CD44, an adhesion molecule [22], which suggested a potential function of biliary epithelial cell antibodies in BEC injury in PSC (and PBC).

## Genetics

Associations with the human leukocyte antigen (HLA) complex located in chromosome 6p21 have been consistently documented in patients with PSC from distinct geographical areas [23–25]. The occurrence of PSC in members of the same family also has suggested its genetic predisposition. The frequency of HLA-DR2 and the haplotype A1 B8 DR3 was increased in patients with the disease, whereas a decrease was documented in the B44 and DR4 haplotype in a study of 81 patients [26]. Another study documented that HLA DR3, DR52a, DR2, and Dw2 were significantly more frequent in the disease group than in the control group [27]. It was also documented that HLA DR4 was associated with rapid disease progression [27], in contrast with a prior study in which no associations with disease progression and HLA alleles were found [26]. In Northern Italy, the frequency of HLA-C2 killer-immunoglobulin receptor (KIR) ligand was significantly decreased in patients with PSC compared to the control group; homozygosity of HLA-C1 was documented in association with an increased risk for PSC. In contrast to the population of Northern Europe in which DRB1*03, *04, or *1301 alleles have been identified as prevalent, no such finding was confirmed in a study from Northern Italy; the association with DRB1*15 and DRB1*07, however, was also detected [25]. By the use of genome-wide association studies (GWAS) in a study of patients from Norway, strong associations were identified in chromosome 6p21 near HLA-B and in chromosomes 13q31 and 2q35 and 3p21, both of which have been identified as susceptibility loci for ulcerative colitis [24]. Other associations outside the HLA complex have been found by the use of GWAS in PSC for a total of 16 risk loci for PSC specifically. Although the association with IBD was found in 72% of the patients studied, 6 of the 12 loci had a stronger association with PSC alone than with IBD, which suggested that although there is overlap in the risk for both, there are genetic distinctions between the two conditions. Association statistics from seven diseases that occur in patients with PSC, i.e., Crohn's disease, celiac disease, psoriasis, rheumatoid arthritis, sarcoidosis, type 1 diabetes, and ulcerative colitis, documented 33 additional pleiotropic risk loci [28].

Most killer immunoglobulin-like receptors (KIRs) are inhibitory [29]. The decrease in natural killer (NK) cells inhibition by a combination of killer immunoglobulin-like receptors (KIRs) and HLA class I ligands have been reported as a risk for the development of autoimmune disease [30]. In a study from Scandinavia, the gene frequency of KIR was not different in patients with PSC than from the control group; however, it was reported that the frequency of HLA-Bw4 and –C2, ligands at the inhibitory KIRs3DL1 and 2DL1, respectively, was significantly reduced in PSC patients as compared with controls. The 5.1 variant of the major HLA class I chain-related A (MICA), which has been documented to influence the predisposition to develop PSC, was prevalent in the patients. In contrast, the DRB1*0301 or DRB1*1501 alleles were absent. These findings have suggested that variants of ligands for NK cell receptors encoded by different genes in the HLA complex may contribute to the genetic predisposition to develop PSC [31].

In a study from Norway, strong associations were identified in chromosome 6p21 near HLA-B and in chromosomes 12q31 and 2q35 and 3p21 by the use of GWAS in patients with PSC. These chromosomes have been identified as susceptibility loci for ulcerative colitis [24]. A relatively large study from Sweden reported that the risk of PSC was significantly higher in first-degree relatives of patients with PSC than in the first-degree relatives of a control group subjects. The hazard ratio and 95% confidence interval (CI) for offsprings were reported as 11.5 (1.6–84.4), for siblings 11.1 (CI = 3.3–37.8), and for parents 2.3 (CI = 0.9–6.1) [32]. Through GWAS, several susceptibility loci carrying SNP in genes, the product of which may reveal their relevance in the pathogenesis of PSC. In a study from Norway, strong associations were identified in chromosome 6p21 near HLA-B and in chromosomes 12q31, and 2q35 and 3p21, identified as susceptibility loci for ulcerative colitis [24].

HLA-B8 was reported in association with PSC in patients identified as European Americans, African Americans, and Hispanic from the United States Organ Sharing database listed for liver transplantation. In contrast, HLA-DR3, which is in linkage disequilibrium with HLA-B8, was found only in European Americans and Hispanic subjects; however, this association was absent from the African American patients, which has suggested an area of further study as a difference among the groups was revealed [33].

SNP rs 9524260 in chromosome 13q31, where glypican 6 is encoded, was also significantly more prevalent in samples from patients with PSC than in those in the control group. Downregulation and upregulation of hundreds of genes were documented in association with silencing of glypican 6 in *in vitro* studies in a cell line of BEC; among the genes that were upregulated were: (i) LIPOCALIN-2, which encodes lipocalin-2, a protein involved in iron delivery to the cell [34] and relevant in the immune response to bacterial infections [35] and in cell growth [36], (ii) NR1H4, which encodes the farsenoid receptor X, a nuclear receptor that induces the expression of the small heterodimer partner (SHP), which inhibits the transcription of the *CYP7A1* gene encoding CYP7A1, the rate-limiting enzyme in the synthesis of bile acids from cholesterol, (iii) the *CXCL3* and *CXCL5*, encoding chemokine ligand 3 (CXCL3), and CXCL5, respectively, involved in cell adhesion processes [37, 38], (iv) MCPT8, which encodes mast cell protease 8 which, as other products of mast cells, participates in inflammatory processes and regulation of immunity [39, 40], and (v) TIMP3, encoding tissue inhibitor of matrix metalloproteinase 3, which inhibits, as other members of this group of proteins, matrix metalloproteinases, a group of peptidases that participate in the degradation of extracellular matrix [41]. These findings have suggested that genes that participate in the regulation of bile acid production and the inflammatory response contribute to the genetic susceptibility to develop PSC [24]. Additional GWAS have identified other loci in association with PSC, including: (i) IL-2RA located in chromosome 10p15 encoding interleukin-2 receptor A [42], an inducible growth factor that mediates immune function through its effects on the development and activity of T and B lymphocytes, natural killer cells, and lymphokine-activated killer cells, and that is located on the surface of activated T lymphocytes [43], (ii) MST1 located in chromosome 3p21, encoding macrophage stimulating 1 (MST1) [42, 44]. The deduced amino acid sequence of MST1 is homologous to hepatocyte growth factor [45, 46]; it is proteolytically activated by caspases during apoptosis, and its biological processes include positive regulation of apoptosis and negative regulation of cell proliferation [47], (iii) IL-2/IL-21 loci in chromosome 4q27 [42]; Il-21 has a role in proliferation and maturation of natural killer cells and proliferation of some stimulated B and T cells [48]; IL-2 is pivotal in the pathway that leads T cells to become effector cells [49], (iv) MMEL1 and TNFRSF14 in chromosome 1p36 [50]; membrane metalloendopeptidase-like 1 (MMEL1) is a metalloprotease that participates in early embryonic development and sperm function, and that degrades a broad variety of small peptides [51], and tumor necrosis factor receptor superfamily member 14 (TNFRSF14), the receptor for B- and T-lymphocyte attenuator and for tumor necrosis factor ligand superfamily member 14. TNFRSF14 is involved in lymphocyte activation [52], (v) *BCL2L11* in 2q13, encoding Bcl2-interacting protein [44], which enhances the antiapoptotic effects of BCL-2. Bcl-2 (B-cell lymphoma 2) is the first member of the Bcl-2 family of apoptosis regulator proteins [53], (vi) 2q37.3 GPR35 [54] encoding G protein-coupled receptor 35, the expression of which is detected in immune cells, in the gastrointestinal tract [55], and gastric cancer [56], in the crypts of Lieberkühn in rats [57], and expressed in gastric cancer cells and normal intestinal mucosa [56], and (vii) 18q21.2 TCF4 encoding transcription factor 4 or immunoglobulin transcription factor 2, which binds to the immunoglobulin enhancer Mu-E5/KE5-motif, and is involved in neuronal differentiation [58]. It recognizes an Ephrussi-box ("E-box") binding site ("CANNTG") that was first identified in immunoglobulin enhancers [59] and is considered important in the development of the nervous system [60], and (viii) CARD9 [50], in chromosome 9q35, encoding caspase recruitment domain-containing protein 9 (CARD9), a member of the caspase recruitment domain-containing family, which participates in the regulation of apoptosis [61].

One of the GWAS reported above [50], which included 715 patients with PSC, 332 from Scandinavia, and 382 from Germany, and a large group of control subjects from both countries also documented a SNP in the fucosyltransferase 2 gene (*FUT2*) in chromosome 19q13, which has suggested some relevance to the susceptibility to PSC because, although their presence was not sufficiently strong for analysis there is a reported association between FUT2 genotypes and infectious diseases [50]. In this regard, nonsense SNP rs601338 (W(TGC) to * (TAG) encodes a nonfunctional FUT2 protein, defining a nonsecretor phenotype [62]. The expression of FTU2 in the bile duct epithelium of patients with PSC was sought by the immunostaining of alpha (1,2) fucose-specific lectin *Ulex europaeus* agglutinin-1; it was documented that samples from the subjects with the secretor phenotype expressed alpha (1,2) fucosylated glycans in bile duct epithelia, in contrast to those with the nonsecretor phenotype, which did not express the immunostain. Bile samples from several patients with PSC and that from other species were used for sequencing human FTU2; from these experiments, differences were documented in the composition of bile samples from patients with the nonsecretor phenotype, which contained a significant increase in the Firmicutes and a decrease in Proteobacteria versus the secretor phenotype [50]. A nonfunctional FUT2 prevents the synthesis of ABH antigens in intestinal mucosa and their presence in secretions [63]; the phenotype of FTU2 contributes to the susceptibility of infections [64]. The phenotype of FUT2 was also associated with the community composition of intestinal microbiota [63]. These findings suggest a role of FTU2 genotype on how microbiota may contribute to the pathogenesis of PSC. Interestingly, rs601338 was significantly more prevalent in patients with ulcerative colitis than in control subjects, in two minority groups of China. However, this finding was not reported in a study from the United States, which documented an association between the nonsecretor phenotype and Crohn's disease, but not with ulcerative colitis [65].

SNPs in the matrix metalloproteinase 3 (MMP3) characterized by homozygosity were identified in patients with PSC and correlated with the risk of progression [66]. The 5A allele in the promoter region of MMT3 is associated with increased transcription of the gene product, and it has been found to correlate with disease risk and possibly disease progression [67]. In this context, patients with PSC and ulcerative colitis also had an increase in the frequency of MMP-3 allele 5A as opposed to patients with PSC without ulcerative colitis. In addition, all patients with cholangiocarcinoma, to which patients with PSC are predisposed, had the allele 1 G in MMP-1 compared to patients without cholangiocarcinoma in whom 72% carried that allele [68].

## Clinical Manifestations

The most common clinical manifestations are fatigue, jaundice, pruritus, weight loss, and right upper quadrant pain; jaundice may manifest itself alone or in combination with episodic cholangitis, which can be associated with fever and shaking chills. The symptoms of secondary sclerosing cholangitis are similar to those of PSC. PSC has been found in association with other diseases, including celiac disease, Hodgkin's lymphoma, retroperitoneal, and mediastinal fibrosis. Accordingly, the primary clinical manifestations may be those of the associated disease.

As in other diseases characterized by cholestasis, the pruritus of sclerosing cholangitis can be mild or severe, with sleep deprivation. Pruritus in patients with PSC may be secondary to cholangitis, which requires antibiotic therapy, and which can be associated with relief of the pruritus.

Fatigue is a complex symptom experienced by patients with liver disease and particularly notable in PBC. PSC can also present with fatigue [69]. Depression and decrease in general health, as measured by a quality of life tool, predicted the presence of this symptom, which did not correlate with the severity of disease [70]. This finding is not supported by another study, in which depression was not a prevalent symptom in patients with PSC [71]. Health-related quality of life was reported to be impaired in a group of 182 unselected patients with PSC that resided in England or Sweden. Pruritus was associated with decreased quality of life; however, fatigue was not found to be more common in patients with PSC than in the control group [72].

## Differential Diagnosis

The differential diagnosis of sclerosing cholangitis includes all cholestatic syndromes. PSC can present alone or, in a substantial number of patients in association with IBD, primarily ulcerative colitis, and less commonly, Crohn's disease. PSC has been associated with other diseases, including thyroid dysfunction [73, 74], celiac disease [75, 76], Hodgkin's [77] and non-Hodgkin's lymphoma, pulmonary fibrosis [78], and systemic sclerosis [79]; accordingly, the dominating clinical presentation may be those of the associated disease. PSC can also be asymptomatic [5].

## Physical Examination

Physical examination may be normal or suggestive of cirrhosis. Dermatological manifestations include those suggestive of cirrhosis and portal hypertension, including palmar erythema, spider angiomata, and hyperpigmentation. In patients with ulcerative colitis, erythema gangrenosum and erythema nodosum may be found. Patients who suffer from pruritus may have cutaneous excoriations and prurigo nodularis. Also, in patients who have undergone proctocolectomy for ulcerative colitis, stomal varices secondary to portal hypertension may be appreciated. New strictures and episodic cholangitis can be associated with jaundice. Hepatomegaly, not infrequently at the expense of the left lobe of the liver, splenomegaly, and ascites may be found, as in other liver diseases.

## Laboratory Findings

Cholestasis is the dominating serum biochemical feature; thus, increased activity of AP and gamma-glutamyl transpeptidase (GGTP) are the characteristic laboratory abnormalities; the serum activity of 5'nucleotidase, an index of cholestasis, can also be high. Modest elevations of the serum activity of transaminases (alanine aminotransferase and aspartate aminotransferase) are common. Hyperbilirubinemia may be present from advanced disease, episodic cholangitis, a benign dominant stricture, or cholangiocarcinoma. Hypoalbuminemia and prolonged prothrombin time suggestive of impaired liver function can be found; because PSC is often associated with IBD and has been reported in association with celiac disease, these two abnormalities can be observed in the context of good liver function but secondary to severe colitis, and malabsorption. Thrombocytopenia secondary to hypersplenism from portal hypertension may be found in the hemogram. Normocytic normochromic anemia secondary to cirrhosis may be observed; however, hypochromic microcytic anemia is not uncommon in patients with PSC and IBD because of chronic fecal blood loss. Eosinophilia has been reported.

## Diagnosis

Magnetic resonance cholangiography (MRC) has supplanted the use of endoscopic retrograde cholangiography (ERC) as the diagnostic test for sclerosing cholangitis, as the former can reveal the classical radiographic picture suggestive of the disease (Fig. 5.1), and it avoids the manipulation of the biliary tract necessary in endoscopic procedures. Four histological stages have been described in PSC; stage I is characterized by an inflammatory infiltrate composed of polymorphonuclear leukocytes and lymphocytes around the ducts, with vacuolation of the epithelium; however, the

**Fig. 5.1** Magnetic resonance cholangiogram in a 59-year-old woman with primary sclerosing cholangitis revealing intrahepatic biliary strictures (straight arrow) and dilatations (curved arrow)

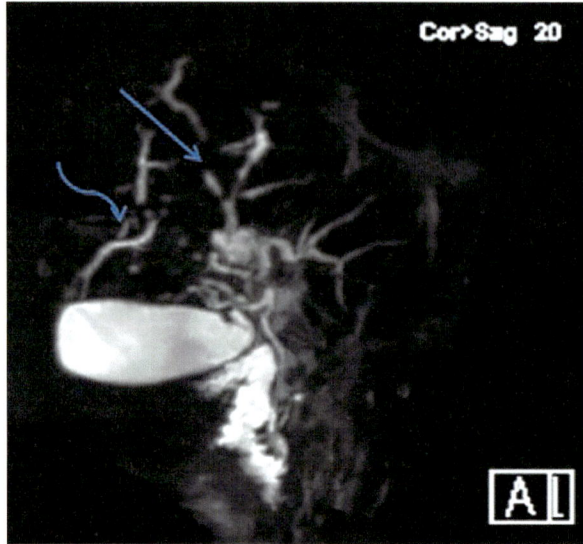

**Fig. 5.2** Liver histology in a patient with primary sclerosing cholangitis exhibiting periportal fibrosis and absence of bile duct, replaced by fibrous tissue (arrow head). Another portal tract exhibits fibrotic changes around a bile duct the lumen of which has been compromised (arrow)

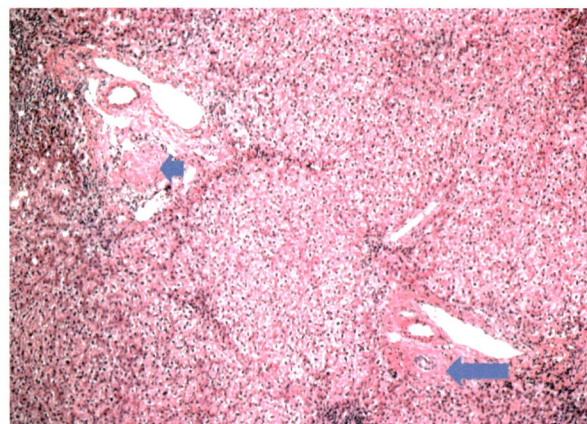

inflammatory infiltrate is less intense than that found in the lesion of nonsuppurative destructive cholangitis of PBC. Concentric layers of fibrotic tissue surrounding the bile duct characterize the onionskin lesion classic of PSC; bile ductular proliferation is also included in this stage. Stage II is characterized by an inflammatory infiltrate and fibrotic changes outside the portal tracts; biliary piecemeal is a feature of this stage, and ductopenia can also be identified (Fig. 5.2). Stage III is characterized by portal-to-portal fibrosis. Stage IV is characterized by biliary cirrhosis. Pseudoxanthomatous changes suggestive of cholestasis are usually found in the last three stages. PSC can be limited to the smallest branches of the intrahepatic bile ducts not appreciated in cholangiograms. In these cases, the appearance of the biliary tree on cholangiogram may be normal; thus, only liver histology may be consistent with the diagnosis. The lesion that affects the smallest branches of the intrahepatic bile ducts has been termed small duct PSC; this lesion may represent the pericholangitis characteristically found in patients with ulcerative colitis and abnormalities in the serum activity of liver associated enzymes. Abnormalities of the pancreatic duct consistent with chronic pancreatitis can also be observed in the pancreatogram.

## Immunology

The mechanisms that mediate the biliary inflammation and fibrosis in PSC are unknown. In this context, cells of the immune system circulate in the blood to tissues and back into the bloodstream [80]. This characteristic movement allows activated neutrophils and monocytes to migrate to sites of infection where there is inflammation, naïve T and B lymphocytes into secondary lymphoid tissues, and effector and memory T cells to sites of infection and tissue injury where they mediate cell-mediated immunity. Recruitment is the process that attracts leukocytes to tissues from the circulation. It requires the adhesion of leukocytes to the endothelium of postcapillary venules and traversal of the endothelium and basement membrane into extravascular tissue. Adhesion molecules and chemokines are fundamental components of recruitment [80]. Intercellular adhesion molecule 1, a ligand for the leukocyte adhesion receptor lymphocyte function-associated antigen 1, was reported to be expressed by interlobular and proliferating bile ducts in PSC and PBC affected livers, suggesting a mechanism for the attraction of lymphocytes to the target tissue [81].

A significant decrease in the number of circulating T cells was reported in patients with PSC. B cells, in contrast with another study, were significantly increased, and a correlation between this change and histologic stage of the disease, serum gamma globulin, and IgG concentrations, and bilirubin was reported, findings interpreted to suggest immunological alterations as relevant in the pathogenesis of PSC [82]. An immune-mediated pathogenetic component has been indicated by immunohistochemical studies on explanted livers from patients with PSC that revealed CD44 positive BEC, which were more preponderant in biliary as opposed to hepatocellular diseases. The proportion of CD44+ ducts was much higher in biliary disease than in chronic hepatitis. By contrast, the expression of HLA-DR was detected in a relatively small percentage of bile ducts. CD4+ activated T lymphocytes were also reported to be increased in the liver parenchyma; CD8+ T cells were found in the inflammatory infiltrate of the biliary epithelium [83]. A small histological study from patients with PSC documented CD3+CD45RO+ cells in liver samples; few cells expressed activation or proliferation markers in the samples that also included tissues from PBC, another liver disease characterized by inflammatory destruction of BEC. In the PSC material, significantly more of the infiltrative lymphocytes were positive for the gut-homing integrin alpha4beta7. There was a variable HLA-DR expression of the biliary epithelium in PSC liver tissues compared to the control and disease control livers (i.e., PBC); however, the adhesion molecule ICAM1 or B7.2 were not detected, suggesting that BEC do not act as antigen-presenting cells [84].

A cDNA library from normal human common bile duct cells was constructed and was screened with sera from patients with PSC. From these experiments, the immunoreactivity against PDZ domain containing 1 (PDZK1), identified as a candidate antigen in patients' sera but not in control sera, was detected in cytoplasmatic granules and apical cell membranes of BEC in a small group of patients with PSC (9% of 35 patients). However, it was not unique to PSC, as it was found in 18% of patients with Grave's disease and a small percentage of patients with IBD and autoimmune hepatitis [85]. The integrin alpha4beta7 and mucosal addressin cell adhesion molecule-1 (MAdCAM-1) participate in the trafficking of lymphocytes between blood and tissues. MAdCAM-1 is expressed in the liver of patients with portal inflammation; its expression correlated with the degree of inflammation in chronic hepatitis C; however, it was not detected in fetal or normal adult liver. These findings have suggested that MAdCAM-1 may contribute to the recruitment of inflammatory cells to the liver [86], an idea that is further supported by the strong expression of MAdCAM-1 in the endothelium of the inflamed portal vein and sinusoids from patients with autoimmune-mediated liver diseases, shown to support the adhesion of gut-derived alpha4beta7+ T lymphocytes from patients with IBD and PSC in an experimental assay [87]. The mechanism by which PSC develops in association with IBD in the absence of active colon inflammation was proposed to relate to the presence of memory T cells stimulated in the gut. These memory T cells reach the liver by the enterohepatic circulation, where, in a permissive environment, lymphocyte recruitment mediates the inflammatory process of PSC [88]. C-C chemokine receptor type 9 (CCR9) or cluster of differentiation w199 (CDw199) is the receptor for CCl25 [89]. CCR9 is expressed by a subset of circulatory memory $\alpha4\beta7$high CD4+ and CD8+ lymphocytes [90]; the $\alpha4\beta7$ integrin is expressed on gut trafficking T lymphocytes, which has suggested that this subset of cells is relevant in immune-mediated processes in the intestines [90, 91]. Mucosal vascular addressin cell adhesion molecule 1 (MAdCAM-1), found in the endothelium of venules, interacts preferentially with $\alpha4\beta7$. Chemokine (C-C motif) ligand 25 (CCL25) is a cytokine that is chemotactic for thymocytes, macrophages, and dendritic cells; CCl25 is also found in the small intestine where it is produced by intestinal epithelium and where it mediates homing of effector CD8+ T cells [92]. The expression of the chemokine CCL25 was reported in the liver sinusoids of patients with PSC, in association with interface hepatitis, and macrophages and dendritic cells in portal tracts; this finding is in contrast to the absence of CCL25 expression in the liver of patients with other liver diseases including PBC. Quantification of mRNA confirmed a marked increase in CCL25 in the liver tissues from patients with PSC compared to livers from disease controls and control tissue. Liver infiltrating lymphocytes had a substantial increase in adhesion of MAdCAM-1 in association with CCL25, as compared to control lymphocytes, an effect that was blocked by anti-$\alpha4\beta7$ antibodies. These results have suggested that the aberrant expression of CCL25 provides the environment necessary for effective recruitment of gut-stimulated lymphocytes, which contribute to PSC development in dormant IBD, or after colectomy [93].

Indeed, it has been suggested that the inflammatory process that triggers or perpetuates IBD or both are also involved in the pathogenesis of the associated liver disease. In this regard, the expression of MAdCAM-1 in the mucosal endothelium of the gut may be a factor in the pathogenesis of IBD. MAdCAM-1 is also detected on the liver vessels of patients with IBD and liver disease, which is suggested to recruit effector cells from the gut, where they were initially activated, to the liver.

In this regards to the etiology of IBD and PSC, it was reported that the deamination of methylamine (MA) by vascular adhesion protein-1 (VAP-1) in the presence of tumor necrosis factor (TNF)-alpha results in the expression of MAdCAM-1 in hepatic endothelial cells, which is associated with increased adhesion of lymphocytes from patients with PSC to hepatic vessels. In laboratory animals, feeding methylamine, which is found in food and cigarette smoke, and in the portal blood, was associated with VAP-1/SSAO-dependent MAdCAM-1 expression in mucosal vessels in vivo. These findings have identified a potential mechanism in the pathogenesis of liver diseases, including PSC, in patients with IBD, and perhaps, potential environmental factors that may be involved in the triggering of this type of liver disease [94].

Altered regulation of toll-like receptors (TLR), which are present in BEC, in response to the stimulation of intracellular signaling by cytokines and pathogen-associated molecular patterns (PAMPs) may be relevant in the pathogenesis of biliary diseases [95]. BEC isolated from PSC liver explants revealed a reversible increase in TLR and nucleotide binding oligomerization domain (NOD) protein expression and activation of the myeloid differentiation primary response gene (MYD88)/interleukin (IL)-1 receptor-associated kinase 1 (IRAK1) pathway [96]. This pathway is associated with a stimulated interleukin-1 receptor and induction of nuclear factor-kappaB (NF kappa B), a rapid-acting transcription factor that participates in cellular responses to numerous stimuli, including regulating genes that play a role in innate and adaptive immune response [97]. In an *in vitro* study, the immune response to endotoxin was altered, and tolerance was not developed after repeated exposure to it [96]. This finding was interpreted to result from the stimulatory effect of interferon-gamma and TNF-alpha, which were strongly expressed in the liver of patients with PSC, and which might have led to an increase in the incorporation of endotoxin from the stimulation of TLR-4-mediated signaling in BEC, and to an impaired inactivation of the TLR-4 signaling cascade [96]. This hyper-responsiveness and lack of tolerance to intestinal endotoxin were interpreted as potential perpetuators of the cholangitis of PSC [96].

## Cellular Pathogenesis

Cellular senescence is a cell state implicated in various physiological processes and a broad spectrum of age-related diseases [98]. It is characterized by a cycle arrest of formerly replicating competent cells induced by stress, which usually is triggered by persistent DNA damage response (DDR) or stress signaling, and executed by constitutive activation of the $p16^{INK4a}$-RB or p53 pathways, or both [99]. Senescent cells exhibit increased expression of the products of the CDKN2a locus, p16INK4a, and ARF, tend to express an increased lysosomal β-galactosidase activity, and to secrete cytokines, composite that has been labeled as senescence-associated secretory phenotype (SASP) [100]. Although senescent cells are in a low hyporeplicative state, they are metabolically active and often can perform functions typical of the cells from which they originate [101]. A pathogenic effect of senescent cells is the formation of lesions that can lead to impaired physiology, e.g., atherosclerotic plaque in blood flow, the grouping of these cells that obstruct tissue homeostasis, and the production of paracrine and endocrine proinflammatory products that promote tissue dysfunction at all levels of the economy.

Transepithelial/transendothelial electrical resistance (TEER) is a quantitative technique to measure the integrity of tight junction dynamics in cell culture models of endothelial and epithelial monolayers [102]. Characterization of cultured biliary BEC isolated from livers of patients with PSC documented a significantly lower proliferation rate and TEER versus those of control BEC; in addition, the amount and expression of IL-6 and IL-8 mRNAs and their translated proteins, and senescence-associated β-galactosidase were significantly higher in PSC-BEC than in the control cells [103]. PSE-BEC in vivo and experimentally induced senescence of BEC was associated with activation of N-Ras, a known inducer of senescence, which was inhibited by the inactivation of Ras, suggesting a mechanistic involvement of the gene in the senescence process. Studies documented an increase in the expression of the senescence-related p16(INK4a) and γH2A.x compared to normal and disease control cells and exhibited the proinflammatory senescence-associated secretory phenotype (SASP) that includes the expression of IL-6, IL-8, CCL2, and PAI-1. The investigators suggested that the use of drugs that inhibit N-RAS activation may provide a pathway to the treatment of PSC [104]. Further involvement of N-Ras was suggested in an *in vitro* experiment that documented an increase of BEC proliferation by LPS, which was inhibited by the inactivation of the gene; in addition, the blocking of IL-6 by a specific antibody prevented the proliferation of BEC induced by stimulation of TLRs. These findings were interpreted to suggest that LPS, which is produced by commensal intestinal bacteria, may contribute to the inflammatory response caused by microbes on the BECs [105].

# Dysbiosis

Dysbiosis is defined as an imbalance in the composition and function of intestinal microbes [106]. Characterization of gut microbiota from stool samples from patients with PSC revealed markedly decreased bacterial diversity as compared to that from the healthy control group, and a different composition from that of patients with ulcerative colitis, and from the healthy control pool. The microbiota from patients with PSC with or without associated IBD were similar. Eleven genera were reduced from the twelve that separated PSC samples from healthy controls, with the *Veillonella* genus being significantly increased in the PSC samples versus those from the healthy control and ulcerative colitis groups, a finding that allowed for the separation of PSC from the healthy control group, with an area under the curve of 0.64, and 0.78 when all the genera from the PSC samples were combined [107]. Anaerobic species, including *Veillonella*, were isolated from sputum samples from patients with cystic fibrosis [108], which indeed has a fibrosis component including biliary strictures [109, 110]; however, the connection between this finding and the gut microbiota is unknown [111]. Altered biodiversity was confirmed in another study that explored the characteristics of the microbiota in PSC and which expanded the findings to include documentation of fungal dysbiosis that had an increase in the representation of *Exophiala* and a decrease in *Saccharomyces cerevisiae* as compared to samples from healthy controls and patients with IBD [112]; the idea of altered interkingdom cross talk in patients with PSC was proposed based on the disruption in bacteria–fungi correlation network [112]. A case of systemic infection in an immunocompetent subject with *Exophiala dermatitidis* has been reported in association with hepatobiliary findings that mimicked PSC [113], and a fatal case of a child with systemic disease complicated by cholestasis and intrahepatic biliary dilatation has also been reported [114]. The pathogenesis of PSC in the context of perturbation of intestinal dysbiosis is a subject of research interest.

## Histology

The lesion of intrahepatic bile ducts of PSC is characterized by concentric fibrosis; finger-like projections or fine undulations of the basal free surfaces with duplicated basal lamina have been documented. The lamina is surrounded by elongated fibroblasts and thickened bundles of collagen fibers outwards. Severe periductal fibrosis was associated with the disappearance of bile ducts, interpreted to suggest that the communication between bile ducts and peribiliary plexus through which the ducts are nourished was interrupted. Lymphocytes infiltrating BEC were observed [115]. Inflammatory lymphoplasmacytic infiltration and fibrosis were reported in peribiliary glands, suggesting that these structures are also affected by the PSC's disease process [116]. *In vitro*, the activation of hepatic stellate cells, which express stem cell factor, attracted mast cells, an effect that was inhibited, in part, by antibodies to that cytokine [117]. Mast cells that expressed c-kit, fibroblast growth factor, tumor necrosis factor-alpha, or both were identified in the periductal and ductal fibrotic changes around the intrahepatic large bile ducts and around proliferative peribiliary glands. Stem cell factor, which binds to c-kit, was also expressed on the BEC epithelium of dilated and stenotic bile ducts that showed periductal fibrosis and inflammation, and by proliferating bile ducts and peribiliary glands in PSC and hepatolithiasis but not in spared bile ducts. These findings were interpreted to suggest that stem cell factor may contribute to the pathogenesis of PSC by stimulating mast cells by the c-kit receptor and inducing the expression of fibrogenic factors [118].

A study examined the status of canalicular transporters in PSC. ATP-binding cassette (ABC) transporters are located in the hepatocyte's canalicular side and transport compounds from the hepatocyte into the bile, including organic anions, bile acids, and phospholipids; they play a pivotal role in bile formation and detoxification. Malfunction of the transporters can lead to cholestasis [119]. A study explored the expression of ABCB11, the bile salt efflux pump of hepatocytes that coordinates cellular excretion of conjugated bile acids into the bile canaliculi, and of ABCB4, and ATP-dependent flippase that translocates phosphatidylcholine from the inner to the outer leaflet of the bile canalicular membrane. In the liver of patients with PSC, the expression of ABCB11 and ABCB4 mRNAs and proteins were significantly increased, exhibiting a correlation with disease stage. These findings tend to suggest that the upregulation of these canalicular transporters is a cellular effort to protect the liver from the toxic effects of substances, including bile acids, that accumulate in the organ as a result of cholestasis [120].

Three conditions that affect the biliary tree have been described in the last decade, IgG-4-related sclerosing cholangitis, follicular cholangitis, and sclerosing cholangitis with granulocytic epithelial lesion. The diagnosis of these conditions requires histology, in contrast to PSC, for which MRCP is the preferred diagnostic test [1], as this modality does not require manipulation of the biliary tree. IgG4+ related cholangitis is characterized by a transmural inflammatory infiltrate composed of lymphocytes and plasma cells. In general, IgG4 cholangiopathy is associated with autoimmune pancreatitis type I, whereas the others present as isolated cholangitis [121]. An aggressive phenotype, however, has been reported in association with IgG4 and classic cholangitis; in a study from the United States that examined stored materials from 98 patients with PSC [122], 23% of liver samples had periductal infiltration with IgG4+ plasma cells, and 22% had elevated serum IgG4 levels, including eight without tissue IgG4 positivity. Dense periductal fibrosis was reported in all cases. There was a strong correlation between IgG4 positivity in the liver and moderate-to-marked periductal lymphoplasmacytic inflammation. The expression of IgG in the liver correlated with shorter disease duration prior to liver transplant and recurrence of disease in the graft compared to serum IgG4. A substantial number of liver samples from patients with PSC had increased IgG4+ periductal plasma cell infiltrates and high IgG4 serum concentration [122]. These findings seem to suggest some relevance of IgG4 in the pathogenesis of classic PSC. In a study from the United Kingdom, however, 95% of 41 explants from patients with PSC had minimal infiltration of IgG4+ plasma cells, and only two cases had a high number of this type of cells, which were present in areas of xanthogranulomatous tissue within large bile ducts; there were no significant findings in common with IgG4+ sclerosing cholangitis identified [123].

## Epidemiology

A literature review on PSC reported an incidence rate of 1.3 per 100,000 subjects per year and a prevalence rate of 0–16.2 per 100,000 [124], and both are likely to vary among different geographical areas. From a pooled analysis of eight studies, the incidence rate ratio for men compared to women was 1.70 (1.34–2.07) [125].

An increase in the incidence of PSC in Scandinavia has been reported. From 1986 to 1995, from a hospital in Oslo, Norway, 70 patients with PSC were registered, with a calculated point prevalence of 8.5 [126]. In a study from southern Sweden, 199 patients with PSC were identified in a retrospective review from 1992 to 2005; the point prevalence of PSC on the last day of 2005 was 16.2 per 100,000 inhabitants, with that for men being 23.7 per 100,000 persons, and for women, 8.9. The annual incidence was calculated as 1.22 per 100,000 inhabitants; for men, it was 1.78 per 100,000 and for women 0.69. The overall incidence rate of PSC increased significantly over the years that comprised the study, with an average annual percent change of 3.06 (95% CI 0.01–6.20). The incidence of inflammatory bowel disease associated with PSC increased at an average annual rate of 7.01 (95% CI 0.24–14.24). The average annual percent change for classic PSC in women was 6.32 (95% CI 0.03–13.02), and for PSC without IBD, the average annual rate was 9.69 (95% CI 0.82–19.33), and for small duct PSC, it was 17.88 (95% CI 0.95–40.25) in men [127].

From a large database of ethnically diverse subjects from Northern California in the United States, 169 patients, 59.7% of whom were male, were identified as having PSC from 2000 to 2006. The age-adjusted point prevalence was 4.15 per 100,000 in 2005. The age-adjusted incidence per 100,000 person-years was 0.45 (95% CI 0.33–0.61) in men and 0.37 (95% CI 0.26–0.51) in women. PSC was associated with IBD in 64.5% of the subjects; 73.3% of men had both conditions, in contrast to women, in whom both conditions existed in 51.5%. The cumulative average mortality rate per year was 1.9% [128].

In a study from Switzerland composed of 950 patients with inflammatory disease, PSC was found in 1% of those with Crohn's disease and 4% of those with ulcerative colitis [129].

## Natural History

The natural history of PSC is variable. It seems to differ depending on the country where the patients reside [130]. However, it is a rare disease, and robust information on its natural history is lacking. The reported period to death or liver transplantation has ranged between 4 and 18 years [124, 131, 132]. In patients from Europe, a median survival rate of approximately 12 years from the time of diagnosis was reported in a group of 305 patients from Sweden [131]; in a group of 28 patients from Italy, the estimated survival rate was 65% at 10 years [133]; in The Netherlands, the estimated median survival in a group of 174 patients diagnosed and followed for almost three decades starting in 1970 was 18 years from the time of diagnosis to death from liver disease or to liver transplantation [132]; from France, survival without liver transplantation was reported to be 4 years in 79% of 150 patients over a period that ranged from 0.1 to 7.2 years [134]; from the United States, the survival rate from a group of 174 was reported to be 11.9 years [135]. Patients without symptoms from PSC were reported to have significantly higher survival than those with symptoms [131]. The Kaplan-Meier curve in adults shows a 65% rate of survival at 10 years. A serum bilirubin concentration four times the upper limit of normal was reflective of advanced disease in one study [130]. Hepatomegaly and a serum bilirubin concentration greater than 1.5 mg/dL at the time of diagnosis were associated with poor prognosis [136]. The importance of bilirubin has been confirmed by a report indicating that a persistent increase in serum bilirubin concentration for longer than 3 months from the time of diagnosis correlated with poor prognosis [137]. The outcome for secondary sclerosing cholangitis has been reported to be worse than that of PSC [138].

## Liver Transplantation

PSC recurs after liver transplantation in 20% to 25% of subjects [139]. Referral for liver transplant evaluation is recommended when the Model for End-Stage Liver Disease (MELD) score is 15 or when complications specific to PSC such as recurrent cholangitis arise. A study that included 150 patients transplanted at one institution with the provision of 174 liver grafts and who were followed for a mean of 55 months reported the actuarial patient survival at 1, 2, 5, and 10 years of 93.7%, 92.2%, 86.4%, and 69.8%, respectively, and graft survival as 83.4%, 83.4%, 79.0%, and 60.5%, respectively. The main indication for retransplantation was hepatic artery thrombosis and the most common cause of death severe infection. The proportion of patients developing acute cellular and chronic ductopenic rejection was higher in patients with PSC than in those with other liver diseases. Frequent complications of biliary strictures, anastomotic, and nonanastomotic were reported in 16.2 and 27.2% of patients, respectively, with disease recurring in 20%; however, these complications were not reported to decrease survival. Four percent of the patients transplanted had cholangiocarcinoma, which was associated with mortality in a patient in whom cancer recurred. Seventy-eight percent of patients had associated IBD, with ulcerative colitis being the most common type, and which did not influence the outcome of transplantation. Colectomy post-transplant was required in some patients because of IBD-related complications [140].

A study explored the outcomes of 5080 adult patients who had had liver transplantation, had been relisted, and had been retransplanted for PSC from 1987 and 2015 with the United Network for Organ Sharing/Organ Procurement and Transplantation Network database as source [141]. It was reported that 1803 experienced graft failure; 762 were relisted, and 636 were retransplanted. The most common types of patients relisted were the young and those with graft failure from vascular thrombosis and biliary complications, with a significant decrease in graft and patient survival at 5 years after retransplantation compared to patients transplanted once. However, the 5-year survival for graft and patients after retransplantation for disease recurrence was similar to that of the primary transplantation and superior to other indications for retransplantation. Features reflective of a postoperative stormy course, including mechanical ventilation and impaired renal function, were associated with inferior outcomes after retransplantation. It was concluded that although retransplantation was associated with a reduced survival versus one transplantation, retransplantation was a good option for patients with recurrent disease, as outcomes post retransplantation at 5 years were similar to those from the primary transplantation [141]. These results are encouraging considering the gravity of PSC and the risk for recurrence after a life-changing procedure.

# Cholangiocarcinoma

Cholangiocarcinoma usually presents with a relatively sudden increase in serum bilirubin concentration, which may be associated with a new biliary stricture or subtle changes in the appearance of the biliary tree on imaging studies, e.g., MRCP. It must be suspected in patients with PSC whose liver function deteriorates itself. The predicted time to develop cholangiocarcinoma was estimated to be 9% at year 10 after the diagnosis of PSC in a group of 211 patients from The Netherlands [142]. The annual incidence of cholangiocarcinoma was reported as 1.2% in a study composed of 230 patients, 23 of whom developed cholangiocarcinoma [143]. Men and patients with large duct PSC and ulcerative colitis seem to be at a higher risk of developing cholangiocarcinoma than women and children, and in patients with small duct PSC or those with associated Crohn's disease [144]. Antibodies to glycoprotein 2, a specific target of pancreatic autoantibodies [PAbs] detected in Crohn's disease and involved in gut innate immunity processes, were reported in association with PSC, correlating with a decrease in transplant-free survival [145]. Antibodies to glycoprotein 2 (GP2) were documented to exhibit a strong association with biliary tract cancer in a group of patients from Norway, found in over 50% of the patients in the study [146]; thus, it has been suggested that they may be a useful marker to detect malignancy in association with PSC.

Cholangiocarcinoma is difficult to differentiate from benign strictures; diagnostic means include cytological analysis of biliary material obtained by brushing suspicious areas during endoscopic examination of the biliary tree by ERC, and by cholangioscopy, and by the measurements of serum markers of biliary tract malignancy. In this regard, the serum concentration of carbohydrate 19-9 (CA 19-9) can be normal or increased in patients with cholangiocarcinoma. The results of some of the studies examining CA 19-9 in patients with cholangiocarcinoma have included the following findings: (i) a serum concentration of CA19-9 > 180 U/mL had a sensitivity of 66.7% (95% CI [34.9, 87.7]) and specificity of 97.7% (95% CI [88.2, 99.9]) in a group of 55 patients [147], (ii) serum concentration of CA 19-9 > 100 U/mL had 75% sensitivity and 80% specificity in identifying patients with PSC and cholangiocarcinoma [148], (iii) in fourteen patients, a serum concentration greater than 129 U/mL was associated with a sensitivity of 78.6% and a specificity of 98.5% for the diagnosis, and an adjusted positive predictive value of 56.6% and a negative predictive value of 99.4%; in addition, it was reported that in the patients with cholangiocarcinoma there was a significant median change over time of 664 U/mL in cholangiocarcinoma as compared to 6.7 U/mL in patients with PSC not complicated by this malignancy. A change of 63.2 U/mL in the median concentration of CA 19-9 gave a sensitivity of 90%, a specificity of 98%, and a positive predictive value of 42% for the presence of cholangiocarcinoma; however, in this study, only patients with advanced disease were identified by CA 19-9 [149], and (iv) in a prospective study that followed 230 patients, 23 of whom developed cholangiocarcinoma, a concentration of serum CA 19-9 of 20 U/mL, was associated with a sensitivity of 78%, a specificity of 67%, a positive predictive value of 23%, and a negative predictive value of 96% [143]. For a diagnosis of cholangiocarcinoma in patients with PSC, the combination of serum CA 19-9 with ultrasonography findings provided a sensitivity of 91%, and a specificity of 62%, a positive predictive value of 23%, and a negative predictive value of 98%, with computed tomography the values were 100% for sensitivity, 38% for specificity, and 22 and 100% for positive and negative predictive values, respectively, and with magnetic resonance imaging (MRI), the sensitivity was 96%, the specificity of 37%, and the positive and negative predictive values were 24 and 98%, respectively.

The use of molecular cytogenetics in clinical testing has increased the diagnostic options for cholangiocarcinoma [150]. Karyotypic characteristics were identified in four cholangiocarcinoma cell lines [151]. In this regard, the application of fluorescence in situ hybridization (FISH) [152] in the diagnostic process of cholangiocarcinoma has revealed cellular features in association with this tumor [153]. Material obtained by brushing and from biliary aspirates from bile ducts of patients with biliary strictures was analyzed by the use of FISH through which chromosomal abnormalities were identified and considered positive for malignancy if five or more cells displayed polysomy; in this study, the sensitivity for malignancy by cytology was 15%, and that of FISH 34%, the sensitivity of FISH for malignancy in bile aspirates and biliary aspirates combined was 35%, and for aspirates alone, it was 23% [154]. From a retrospective study, it was reported that 69% of patients from a total of 13 with PSC and who developed cholangiocarcinoma had had more than one finding of serial polysomy fluorescence in situ hybridization documented 1–2.7 years prior, in contrast to patients who did not have serial FISH polysomy [155].

Cytokeratins are a subfamily of intermediate filament proteins that participate in the cells' cytoskeletal organization and influence the cytoplasm's structural appearance [156]. Cytokeratins are markers of epithelial differentiation; epithelial cells do not lose the characteristic expression of cytokeratins during malignant transformation [156, 157]; thus, characterization of the intermediate filaments can identify tumorous cells, which is particularly helpful in tumors difficult to diagnose. Carcinomas express cytokeratins. Cytokeratin 19 belongs to the acidic cytokeratins; it is the smallest of the cytokeratins and is found in several simple and usually in some non-keratinizing stratified squamous epithelia [157]. Serum fragment of cytokeratin subunit 19 (CYFRA 21-1) can be measured in the serum, its concentration being high in various cancers, including lung [158] and breast [159]. High serum concentrations of CYFRA 21-1 were specific for the diagnosis of cholangiocarcinoma [160]; however, it was less sensitive than CA 19-9 and associated with poor prognosis [160]. From a prospective study that included patients with PSC with and without cholangiocarcinoma, sporadic biliary tract carcinoma, and non-malignant biliary tract disease, it was reported that a serum concentration of CYFRA 21-1 $\geq$ 1.5 ng/mL had a sensitivity of 56% and a specificity of 88% for cholangiocarcinoma, in contrast to serum levels of CA 19-9 ($\geq$37 U/mL), which had a sensitivity and a specificity of 79% and 78%, respectively. A serum concentration of 3 ng/mL of CYFRA 21-1 had a sensitivity of 30% and specificity of 97% and predicted median survival of 2 months. Combining CYFRA 21-1 ($\geq$1.5 ng/mL) and CA 19-9 ($\geq$37 U/mL) increased the sensitivity and the specificity to 45% and 96%, respectively.

Intraductal confocal microscopy is an evolving technique that allows for examining the common bile duct; characteristic findings in cholangiocarcinoma included irregular vessels with a lack of contrast in the common bile duct wall [161].

Determination of bile proteomics by the use of capillary electrophoresis mass spectrometry revealed specific peptide patterns that differentiated cholangiocarcinoma from PSC and choledocholithiasis [162]. In a study of urine proteomics, a cholangiocarcinoma-specific peptide model was designed based on the distribution of several peptides in patients with cholangiocarcinoma, PSC, and benign biliary tract disorders; the model accurately classified the majority of samples from patients with cholangiocarcinoma, as well as patients with PSC, not complicated by this malignancy, and patients with biliary tract disorders. The noninvasive nature of this approach is appealing, considering the preliminary findings reported [163].

Transpapillary cholangioscopy is being advanced as an advantageous technique for diagnosing cholangiocarcinoma that allows for tissue sampling from common bile duct strictures. Cholangioscopy was found to be significantly better at diagnosing malignancy in common bile ducts, documented by histology or cytology, with a sensitivity of 92% and a specificity of 93%, compared to 66 and 51% for ERC in a study composed of 53 patients with dominant common bile duct strictures 12 of whom had malignancy [164].

## Treatment

The treatment of PSC encompasses vigilant follow-up to identify and treat complications, including cholangitis, cholangiocarcinoma, and complications of liver disease. There are no treatments specifically approved for this disease.

The use of UDCA for the treatment of PSC at high, 25–30 mg/kg/day, or low dose, 13 to 15 mg/kg/day, has not been consistently associated with beneficial effects. A meta-analysis that included eight clinical trials of high and low doses of UDCA for PSC and that included 567 patients documented lack of effect on mortality with a calculated odds ratio of 0.6 (95% CI, 0.4–1.4) and on the incidence of cholangiocarcinoma with calculated odds of 1.7 (95% CI, 0.6–5.1); UDCA had no effect on pruritus or fatigue [165]. At doses between 28 and 30 mg/kg/day, studied in a randomized, placebo-controlled trial, UDCA was reported to be harmful, associated with death or liver transplantation, and adverse events in individuals with advanced disease [166] as evidenced by worsening in liver function, in contrast to the effect of placebo in the control group. Subsequently, however, a review of data from a randomized placebo-controlled study of UDCA at doses of 17–23 mg/kg/day for 6 years, and then monitored for another four was published [167]. In that study, a response was defined as normalization or as a decrease in the activity of AP by 40%. More patients met the definition of response in the UDCA group than in the placebo group. In the patients given active drug, those who met response criteria survived for 10 years, in contrast to those who did not meet the criteria. However, patients in whom the activity of AP decreased, and who comprised 27.7% of the participants, survived longer than those without a decrease in the activity of this enzyme, regardless of whether they had been randomized to UDCA or placebo [167]. These results have sparked renewed interest in UDCA for the treatment of PSC. These findings may also highlight two phenomena: (i) the spontaneous changes in enzyme activity, interpreted as a reflection of changes in liver inflammation, and which may be related to the predisposition of some patients to do better than others with the same disease, and (ii) the placebo effect on liver disease. The use of UDCA on PSC remains controversial [2].

Antibiotics are being studied for the treatment of PSC. A case report documented reproducible improvement of serum activity of liver associated enzymes and symptoms of cholestasis in association with azithromycin, used for treatment for severe asthma in a patient with PSC and Crohn's disease, the beneficial effect interpreted to be secondary to the anti-inflammatory effect of the macrolide [168]. The combination of UDCA and metronidazole was reported to be associated with a decrease in serum activity of liver associated enzymes, in comparison to UDCA and placebo in a 3-year study of patients with PSC; there was a decrease in disease stage, and no changes in cholangiography features, as evaluated by endoscopic retrograde cholangiopancreatography (ERCP) [169].

Vancomycin was reported to improve serum markers of liver disease in children with PSC, especially those without cirrhosis [170]; an immunomodulating effect of the drug was postulated [171]. In a comparative study that included 35 patients, metronidazole and vancomycin were tested at two doses, each associated with side effects, which led to discontinuation of the drugs in 17% of the subjects. Both drugs were associated with some efficacy at week 12, the study duration; vancomycin was associated with a significant decrease in the serum activity of AP, metronidazole with a decrease in serum bilirubin concentration, and both drugs with a reduction in the Mayo score, a model to estimate patient survival in PSC. Pruritus was reported to be decreased in association with metronidazole only [172]. At present, there is no consensus on the use of vancomycin for the treatment of PSC [173].

Several clinical studies for the treatment of PSC have been conducted by using a decrease in serum activity of AP as a surrogate marker of disease activity, as it is now being suggested [174]. The reader is referred to clinicaltrials.gov to check the status of follow up studies being conducted in PSC.

24-norursodeoxycholic acid (norUDCA), a side chain-shortened $C_{23}$ homologue of UDCA, was studied in a randomized multicenter controlled trial of 12 weeks duration in 166 patients with PSC, with a reported relative decrease in the serum activity of AP by minus 12.3%, 17.3%, and 26%, with respect to 500, 1000, and 1500 mg/day doses of the medication versus placebo, which was associated with a small increase. As AP is considered a surrogate marker for the disease, these results suggested that *nor*UDCA could be an effective treatment for PSC [175].

Cilofexor, a nonsteroidal farnesoid X receptor agonist (FXR), is a side chain-shortened $C_{23}$ homologue of UDCA studied in a randomized placebo-controlled trial of 12-week duration in 52 patients with PSC, 46% of whom were on UDCA, with 60% of the total having IBD. The drug was reported to be associated with a relative decrease in the serum activity of AP by minus 12.3, 17.3, and 26%, as well as other markers of liver disease, with respect to the medication at daily doses of 500, 1000, and 1500 mg versus placebo, regardless of the coadministration of UDCA; pruritus was a notable symptom in association with the drug and with the placebo [176].

Obeticholic acid (OCA), another FXR agonist, was studied in a randomized dose finding, multicenter controlled trial of 24 weeks duration in 76 patients with PSC, 47% of whom were on UDCA, with 58% of the total having IBD. OCA at doses from 1.5 to 10 mg/day, titrated by protocol, was reported to be associated with significant decreases in serum activity of AP relative to baseline from $-105\%$ to $-110\%$ versus placebo, which was associated with a decrease of minus 37%; the effect of OCA was irrespective of the use of UDCA [177]. Pruritus was a significant side effect of OCA, as already documented in PBC studies [178, 179]. These results suggested that OCA should be studied in properly controlled studies, as AP is considered a surrogate marker of disease [177].

NGM282 is a nontumorigenic FGF19 analogue that regulates CYP7A1-mediated bile acid homeostasis. This drug was studied in a double blind, placebo-controlled phase II trial of 12 weeks duration in 62 patients with PSC with a reported associated significant decrease in liver stiffness at doses of 1 and 3 mg of the drug, bile acid levels, and fibrosis biomarkers, considered predictors of transplant-free survival, in contrast to the placebo associated effects, however, no changes in serum activity of AP [180]; thus, not meeting the endpoint by design, i.e., not effective, or negative study. However, the authors discuss potential reasons for serum AP being unaffected in spite of the potential benefits of the drug. The publication of this study was accompanied by an editorial that raised the matter of AP as a surrogate marker of disease [181]. This is an obvious question that requires discussion as opportunities to study drugs in clinical trials in cholestatic diseases arise.

All-trans retinoic acid (ATRA) reduces the bile acid pool via activation of the FXR/nuclear receptor subfamily 1, group H, member 4 (NR1H4) pathway. In a pilot study, the drug was tested in combination with UDCA in patients with PSC who had not responded optimally to the former. Fifteen patients completed 15 weeks of therapy at which time serum activity of AP had not significantly decreased, as compared to baseline, thus, failing to meet the primary endpoint by design; however, median serum activity of ALT and the bile acid intermediate 7α-hydroxy-4-cholesten-3-one (C4) as a marker of bile acid synthesis, had significantly decreased, returning to baseline after the drug was discontinued [182]. An Efficacy Trial of Low Dose All-trans Retinoic Acid (ATRA) in Patients With Primary Sclerosing Cholangitis is being conducted (clinicaltrials.gov).

The combination of UDCA with fibrates (i.e., bezafibrate and benafibrate) was examined in a retrospective review that included six patients from Barcelona, Spain, and 14 from Paris, France. It was reported that that the combination treatment was associated with a mean reduction of serum activity of AP of 46% and a reduction in pruritus, assessed subjectively; however, liver stiffness increased [183]. The authors suggested that prospective studies with an increase in the number of participants should be conducted to establish the efficacy and safety of fibrates in PSC [183].

Cenicriviroc is an antagonist of the C–C motif chemokine receptor (CCR) types 2 and 5 [184]; based on studies in an animal model of cholestasis, a study in patients with PSC was completed; however, final results have not been published (ClinicalTrials.gov Identifier: NCT02653625).

Vidofludimus is a compound that blocks the replication of activated T and B cells [185]; it was reported to improve findings in a model of colitis in mice [186]. A study that aims at the inflammatory aspect of PSC is being conducted (Clinicaltrials.gov).

BTT1023 (Timolumab) is an antibody against vascular adhesion protein-1 (VAP-1), which propagates inflammation, and which was reported to halt fibrosis in an animal model of IBD. The liver enzymatic activity of VAP-1 was significantly higher in PSC than in disease control tissues. The serum concentration of soluble VAP-1 was reported to be increased and to predict a worse transplant-free survival and the presence of cirrhosis in patients with PSC [187]. A clinical trial with an open-label design to explore this drug's effect on PSC is being conducted (Clinicaltrials.gov) [188].

Modulation of the gut microbiome is an approach that may develop as information regarding intestinal dysbiosis in PSC continues to emerge. In an open-label pilot study that included ten patients with PSC and ulcerative colitis and one with Crohn's disease, fecal microbiota transplantation was associated with a 50% decrease in AP activity in three of the ten patients. An increase in the diversity in the gut microbiota, with an "abundance of engrafter operational taxonomic units …." in patients post fecal transplantation, correlated with the decrease in the AP activity [189]. Additional data regarding this intervention will likely follow (Clinicaltrials.com).

## Therapy of Complications Unique to PSC

Bacterial cholangitis is one of the most common complications of sclerosing cholangitis. Indeed, recurrent cholangitis grants patients exemption points toward liver transplantation; however, the need for such has been recently challenged based on a retrospective study that documented that a history of bacterial cholangitis was not associated with an increased risk of waitlist removal for death or clinical deterioration in multivariate competing-risk models [190]. The use of prophylactic antibiotics to prevent cholangitis can be considered in some cases. Bacterial cholangitis likely results from stagnant bile in association with strictures and sacculations that characterize the biliary tree in this syndrome. It presents with jaundice, pruritus, fever, and chills, and levels of associated liver enzymes and serum bilirubin higher than baseline. Antibiotic treatment should be initiated promptly after appropriate blood cultures are taken.

Cholelithiasis and choledocholithiasis occur in approximately a third of patients with PSC because of cholestasis and cirrhosis.

Dominant biliary strictures are defined as stenosis of the common bile duct with a diameter of ≤1.5 mm, stenosis of the hepatic duct with a diameter of ≤1.0 mm, or both [191]. The treatment of dominant biliary strictures is challenging because of the risk of harboring malignancy; once this is excluded, endoscopic, preferably, and percutaneous dilatations may be associated with patency of the bile duct in 80% of patients at 1 year, and 60% of patients at three [191]. A follow-up study composed of 96 patients with PSC documented an estimated survival time free of liver transplantation after the first dilatation of a dominant stricture of 81% after 5 years and 52% after ten [192]. From a group of 106 patients with PSC, only five required temporary stents and repeat balloon dilatations over 5 years [193]. The limited available literature tends to support the use of balloon dilatation with or without stenting for the treatment of benign strictures for this type of patient [194, 195]. The presence of dominant strictures, all of which were treated endoscopically, in patients with PSC on treatment with UDCA without IBD was not associated with the development of cholangiocarcinoma in a relatively large group of patients followed prospectively for 20 years. Patients with dominant strictures in the absence of IBD did not develop cancer; however, for those with IBD, bile duct cancers were found in six patients, gallbladder cancers in two, and six of the seven patients in whom colorectal cancers were diagnosed also had inflammatory bowel disease. The estimated survival time free of liver transplantation in patients with dominant strictures without IBD at the 18-year point was 77.8%, and that of patients with dominant strictures and IBD was 23% [196].

Experience in the use of covered stents for the management of benign strictures in patients with PSC is not sufficient to generate recommendations [197]. However, it is emphasized that the expertise of the operator and the center where the procedures are performed weigh heavily in the management of this complication of PSC.

PSC is associated with an increased incidence of gallbladder cancer; the presence of a gallbladder mass sized at least 0.8 cm was highly sensitive 100% (95%, CI 77–100%) and specific 70% (95% CI, 35–93%) for a malignant nature in a retrospective study [198]. This study documented substantial complications after cholecystectomy to treat gallbladder masses in patients with PSC; thus, observation rather than surgery was recommended for gallbladder masses smaller than 0.8 cm [198].

Published guidelines have recommended surgical resection of cholangiocarcinoma in the absence of cirrhosis and referral for liver transplantation after neoadjuvant therapy [199]. Liver transplantation is considered an option for patients with cholangiocarcinoma after adequate selection [200]. In this context, it was reported from a series of patients with PSC complicated by cholangiocarcinoma that hepatectomy with Whipple en block, to ensure complete removal of biliary epithelium, followed by liver transplantation was associated with disease-free survival at 10 years in 5 patients; one death was not related to liver disease [201]. It was documented from a series of patients from Scandinavia who had a liver transplant between 1984 and 2005 that subjects with PSC and cholangiocarcinoma classified as TNM less or equal to 2, a CA 19–9 serum concentration lower or equal than 100 ng/mL, and who were transplanted after 1995, had a five-year survival of 58% [202]. The survival rate of patients with a high disease stage was low [202]. These findings have further suggested that the election of patients for transplant is crucial in anticipation of improved survival [202]. Adjuvant therapies, including chemoradiation, chemosensitization, and intraluminal brachytherapy, are options proposed for the treatment of cholangiocarcinoma prior to liver transplantation; the literature on the use of these modalities in cases of cholangiocarcinoma associated with PSC is limited [203].

In patients with advanced cholangiocarcinoma and anticipated life expectancy greater than 4 months, the insertion of metal stents to open the strictures is the recommended approach [204]. Chemotherapy for cholangiocarcinoma is limited and includes the use of gemcitabine or platinum analogues [205]; interest in exploring the potential for molecular therapy is growing [206].

## Liver Transplantation

Liver transplantation is a therapeutic alternative for patients with decompensated liver disease from PSC with an approximate five-year graft survival rate between 80 and 85% [207, 208]. PSC was reported to be associated with acute cellular rejection in 11% of patients and chronic cellular rejection in 32.6% [209]. Early rejection and vascular thrombosis were identified as predictors for retransplantation [207]. The incidence of late acute rejection occurring between 90 and 2922 days from transplant was reported to be 11% from a retrospective study that included almost one thousand. Patients transplantated for PSC had a higher rate of retransplantation than those transplated for other diseases [190]. The disease has been reported to recur in 20% to 25% of patients from 5 to 10 years after transplant [210, 211]. Acute cellular rejection and cytomegalovirus mismatch [212] and live donor liver transplantation [213] were reported to be associated with disease recurrence; however, it was not reported to recur in patients who did not have IBD before or after transplantation [212]. The management of patients with disease recurrence is expectantly and may include retransplantation [214]; the successful use of vancomycin in recurrence of PSC has been reported [215].

As PSC is associated with IBD in a substantial proportion of patients, there is much interest in the impact of liver transplantation on the course of the intestinal disease. Optimization of IBD prior to liver transplantation has been recommended as active IBD in patients with PSC was associated with graft failure [216]; in addition, active smoking at the time of transplantation and cessation of such after the operation was associated with reactivation of IBD [216]. A substantial but not statistically significant number of patients who had IBD prior to liver transplantation experienced an exacerbation of IBD, as documented from a study composed of 59 patients, 79% of whom had IBD diagnosed prior to transplant [212]; however, it was reported from a study composed of 439 patients 80% of whom had IBD at the time of liver transplantation, that 25% developed colon cancer after liver transplantation, and 3% developed de novo IBD [217]; these findings suggested an increase in the risk of colorectal cancer in patients with PSC post transplant. In addition, there was an association between the use of aminosalicylates and ursodeoxycholic acid with the development of colorectal neoplasia [217]. These results highlight the importance of surveillance to detect colon malignancy in patients with PSC post transplant.

A meta-analysis that included studies related to recurrence of PSC after liver transplantation and that included 2159 patients, 17.7% of whom developed recurrent disease identified recurrence with the presence of cholangiocarcinoma prior to transplantation, IBD, and acute cellular rejection among the factors associated with recurrence, and colectomy prior to transplantation, as protective from recurrence [218].

## PSC in Children

In children, PSC is more common in girls than in boys, it tends to respond to immunosuppressant therapy, and it is reported to have a better prognosis than that of adult subjects [219]. A study that included nine children and 28 adult subjects with PSC documented that children had significantly higher serum AST activity, higher serum concentrations of IgG than in adults; also, half of the study group had interface hepatitis. During a follow-up period of 5 years, none of the children died; however, four adult patients underwent liver transplantation (i.e., liver death) [133]. A retrospective study documented that PSC in children was associated with IBD in the majority of cases, 32 of 36 patients (89%); most patients had ulcerative colitis with Crohn's disease being diagnosed in 11% of the subjects [220]. Eleven percent of the children with IBD did not have any symptoms of such. The colitis was documented as universal in the majority of subjects; however, 27% of the reports documented rectal sparing. The patients with Crohn's disease did not develop fistulae, perianal involvement, or strictures. Dysplasia was the indication for colectomy in half of the six patients who had the operation. Four of the five patients in whom an ileal pouch anal anastomosis was performed developed pouchitis. These data have suggested that surveillance for colon malignancy in children with PSC is indicated [220]. The 1 and 5 year survival rates after liver transplant in children with PSC have been reported to be 98.7 and 86.6%, respectively, similar to that of children who had undergone liver transplantation for other indications [221]. PSC was documented to recur in 9.8% of the patients between 1 and 2 years after the transplant. Both the risk of recurrent PSC and the risk of death were increased by the presence of IBD [221]. Treatment with vancomycin has been reported to halt the progression of PSC in children [170].

From a retrospective review that included 781 children, with a median age of 12 years with comorbidities of autoimmune hepatitis in a third, small duct PSC in a small group, and with inflammatory bowel disease in the majority, it was documented that complications from portal hypertension and biliary disease developed in 38 and 25%, respectively, after 10 years of having been diagnosed with PSC, which portended a poor survival, i.e., 3 to 4 years, without liver transplantation, with cholangiocarcinoma developing in 1%; UDCA, which had been prescribed to the majority of patients, did not prevent these complications. Event-free survival was 70% at 5 years and 53% at 10 years. High bilirubin, GGTP, and aspartate aminotransferase-to-platelet ratio index at diagnosis was associated with the worst outcomes. Small duct PSC and PSC associated with IBD were identified as the most favorable phenotype; age, gender, and autoimmune hepatitis overlap did not have an impact on long-term outcome [222].

**Acknowledgments** The author acknowledges Dr. Anatole Sladen for having contributed Figure 5.1.

# References

1. Dave M, Elmunzer BJ, Dwamena BA, Higgins PD. Primary sclerosing cholangitis: meta-analysis of diagnostic performance of MR cholangiopancreatography. Radiology. 2010 Aug;256(2):387–96.
2. Karlsen TH, Schrumpf E, Boberg KM. Update on primary sclerosing cholangitis. Digest Liver Dis. 2010 June;42(6):390–400.
3. Karlsen TH, Folseraas T, Thorburn D, Vesterhus M. Primary sclerosing cholangitis - a comprehensive review. J Hepatol. 2017 Dec;67(6):1298–323.
4. Kemeny MM, Battifora H, Blayney DW, Cecchi G, Goldberg DA, Leong LA, et al. Sclerosing cholangitis after continuous hepatic artery infusion of FUDR. Ann Surg. 1985 Aug;202(2):176–81.
5. Ruemmele P, Hofstaedter F, Gelbmann CM. Secondary sclerosing cholangitis. Nat Rev Gastroenterol Hepatol. 2009 May;6(5):287–95.
6. Loftus EV, Jr., Sandborn WJ, Tremaine WJ, Mahoney DW, Zinsmeister AR, Offord KP, et al. Risk of colorectal neoplasia in patients with primary sclerosing cholangitis. Gastroenterology. 1996;110(2):432–40.
7. Castellano G, Moreno-Sanchez D, Gutierrez J, Moreno-Gonzalez E, Colina F, Solis-Herruzo JA. Caustic sclerosing cholangitis. Report of four cases and a cumulative review of the literature. Hepato-Gastroenterology. 1994 Oct;41(5):458–70.
8. Loftus EV Jr, Sandborn WJ, Tremaine WJ, Mahoney DW, Zinsmeister AR, Offord KP, et al. Primary sclerosing cholangitis is associated with nonsmoking: a case-control study. Gastroenterology. 1996 May;110(5):1496–502.
9. Loftus EV Jr, Harewood GC, Loftus CG, Tremaine WJ, Harmsen WS, Zinsmeister AR, et al. PSC-IBD: a unique form of inflammatory bowel disease associated with primary sclerosing cholangitis. Gut. 2005 Jan;54(1):91–6.
10. Jorgensen KK, Grzyb K, Lundin KE, Clausen OP, Aamodt G, Schrumpf E, et al. Inflammatory bowel disease in patients with primary sclerosing cholangitis: clinical characterization in liver transplanted and nontransplanted patients. Inflamm Bowel Dis. 2012 Mar;18(3):536–45.

11. Boonstra K, van Erpecum KJ, van Nieuwkerk KM, Drenth JP, Poen AC, Witteman BJ, et al. Primary sclerosing cholangitis is associated with a distinct phenotype of inflammatory bowel disease. Inflamm Bowel Dis. 2012 Dec;18(12):2270–6.
12. Zauli D, Schrumpf E, Crespi C, Cassani F, Fausa O, Aadland E. An autoantibody profile in primary sclerosing cholangitis. J Hepatol. 1987 Aug;5(1):14–8.
13. Bansi DS, Fleming KA, Chapman RW. Importance of antineutrophil cytoplasmic antibodies in primary sclerosing cholangitis and ulcerative colitis: prevalence, titre, and IgG subclass. Gut. 1996 Mar;38(3):384–9.
14. Snook JA, Chapman RW, Fleming K, Jewell DP. Anti-neutrophil nuclear antibody in ulcerative colitis, Crohn's disease and primary sclerosing cholangitis. Clin Exp Immunol. 1989 Apr;76(1):30–3.
15. Duerr RH, Targan SR, Landers CJ, LaRusso NF, Lindsay KL, Wiesner RH, et al. Neutrophil cytoplasmic antibodies: a link between primary sclerosing cholangitis and ulcerative colitis. Gastroenterology. 1991 May;100(5 Pt 1):1385–91.
16. Schwarze C, Terjung B, Lilienweiss P, Beuers U, Herzog V, Sauerbruch T, et al. IgA class antineutrophil cytoplasmic antibodies in primary sclerosing cholangitis and autoimmune hepatitis. Clin Exp Immunol. 2003 Aug;133(2):283–9.
17. Terjung B, Herzog V, Worman HJ, Gestmann I, Bauer C, Sauerbruch T, et al. Atypical antineutrophil cytoplasmic antibodies with perinuclear fluorescence in chronic inflammatory bowel diseases and hepatobiliary disorders colocalize with nuclear lamina proteins. Hepatology. 1998 Aug;28(2):332–40.
18. Terjung B, Spengler U, Sauerbruch T, Worman HJ. "Atypical p-ANCA" in IBD and hepatobiliary disorders react with a 50-kilodalton nuclear envelope protein of neutrophils and myeloid cell lines. Gastroenterology. 2000 Aug;119(2):310–22.
19. Osawa M, Anderson DE, Erickson HP. Reconstitution of contractile FtsZ rings in liposomes. Science. 2008 May 9;320(5877):792–4.
20. Terjung B, Sohne J, Lechtenberg B, Gottwein J, Muennich M, Herzog V, et al. P-ANCAs in autoimmune liver disorders recognise human beta-tubulin isotype 5 and cross-react with microbial protein FtsZ. Gut. 2010 June;59(6):808–16.
21. Saarinen S, Olerup O, Broome U. Increased frequency of autoimmune diseases in patients with primary sclerosing cholangitis. Am J Gastroenterol. 2000 Nov;95(11):3195–9.
22. Xu B, Broome U, Ericzon BG, Sumitran-Holgersson S. High frequency of autoantibodies in patients with primary sclerosing cholangitis that bind biliary epithelial cells and induce expression of CD44 and production of interleukin 6. Gut. 2002 July;51(1):120–7.
23. Chapman RW, Varghese Z, Gaul R, Patel G, Kokinon N, Sherlock S. Association of primary sclerosing cholangitis with HLA-B8. Gut. 1983 Jan;24(1):38–41.
24. Karlsen TH, Franke A, Melum E, Kaser A, Hov JR, Balschun T, et al. Genome-wide association analysis in primary sclerosing cholangitis. Gastroenterology. 2010 Mar;138(3):1102–11.
25. Hov JR, Lleo A, Selmi C, Woldseth B, Fabris L, Strazzabosco M, et al. Genetic associations in Italian primary sclerosing cholangitis: heterogeneity across Europe defines a critical role for HLA-C. J Hepatol. 2010 May;52(5):712–7.
26. Donaldson PT, Farrant JM, Wilkinson ML, Hayllar K, Portmann BC, Williams R. Dual association of HLA DR2 and DR3 with primary sclerosing cholangitis. Hepatology. 1991 Jan;13(1):129–33.
27. Mehal WZ, Lo YM, Wordsworth BP, Neuberger JM, Hubscher SC, Fleming KA, et al. HLA DR4 is a marker for rapid disease progression in primary sclerosing cholangitis. Gastroenterology. 1994 Jan;106(1):160–7.
28. Liu JZ, Hov JR, Folseraas T, Ellinghaus E, Rushbrook SM, Doncheva NT, et al. Dense genotyping of immune-related disease regions identifies nine new risk loci for primary sclerosing cholangitis. Nat Genet. 2013 June;45(6):670–5.
29. Vilches C, Parham P. KIR: diverse, rapidly evolving receptors of innate and adaptive immunity. Annu Rev Immunol. 2002;20:217–51.

30. Kusnierczyk P. Killer cell immunoglobulin-like receptor gene associations with autoimmune and allergic diseases, recurrent spontaneous abortion, and neoplasms. Front Immunol. 2013;4:8.

31. Karlsen TH, Boberg KM, Olsson M, Sun JY, Senitzer D, Bergquist A, et al. Particular genetic variants of ligands for natural killer cell receptors may contribute to the HLA associated risk of primary sclerosing cholangitis. J Hepatol. 2007 May;46(5):899–906.

32. Bergquist A, Montgomery SM, Bahmanyar S, Olsson R, Danielsson A, Lindgren S, et al. Increased risk of primary sclerosing cholangitis and ulcerative colitis in first-degree relatives of patients with primary sclerosing cholangitis. Clin Gastroenterol Hepatol. 2008 Aug;6(8):939–43.

33. Bowlus CL, Li CS, Karlsen TH, Lie BA, Selmi C. Primary sclerosing cholangitis in genetically diverse populations listed for liver transplantation: unique clinical and human leukocyte antigen associations. Liver Transpl. 2010 Nov;16(11):1324–30.

34. Yang J, Goetz D, Li JY, Wang W, Mori K, Setlik D, et al. An iron delivery pathway mediated by a lipocalin. Mol Cell. 2002 Nov;10(5):1045–56.

35. Flo TH, Smith KD, Sato S, Rodriguez DJ, Holmes MA, Strong RK, et al. Lipocalin 2 mediates an innate immune response to bacterial infection by sequestrating iron. Nature. 2004 Dec 16;432(7019):917–21.

36. Schmidt-Ott KM, Mori K, Li JY, Kalandadze A, Cohen DJ, Devarajan P, et al. Dual action of neutrophil gelatinase-associated lipocalin. J Am Soc Nephrol. 2007 Feb;18(2):407–13.

37. Smith DF, Galkina E, Ley K, Huo Y. GRO family chemokines are specialized for monocyte arrest from flow. Am J Physiol Heart Circ Physiol. 2005 Nov;289(5):H1976–84.

38. Zlotnik A, Yoshie O. The chemokine superfamily revisited. Immunity. 2012 May 25;36(5):705–16.

39. Galli SJ, Grimbaldeston M, Tsai M. Immunomodulatory mast cells: negative, as well as positive, regulators of immunity. Nat Rev Immunol. 2008 Jun;8(6):478–86.

40. Pejler G, Ronnberg E, Waern I, Wernersson S. Mast cell proteases: multifaceted regulators of inflammatory disease. Blood. 2010 Jun 17;115(24):4981–90.

41. Matrisian LM. Metalloproteinases and their inhibitors in matrix remodeling. Trends Genet. 1990 Apr;6(4):121–5.

42. Srivastava B, Mells GF, Cordell HJ, Muriithi A, Brown M, Ellinghaus E, et al. Fine mapping and replication of genetic risk loci in primary sclerosing cholangitis. Scand J Gastroenterol. 2012 Jul;47(7):820–6.

43. Kuziel WA, Greene WC. Interleukin-2 and the IL-2 receptor: new insights into structure and function. J Invest Dermatol. 1990 June;94(6 Suppl):27S–32S.

44. Melum E, Franke A, Schramm C, Weismuller TJ, Gotthardt DN, Offner FA, et al. Genome-wide association analysis in primary sclerosing cholangitis identifies two non-HLA susceptibility loci. Nat Genet. 2011 Jan;43(1):17–9.

45. Han S, Stuart LA, Degen SJ. Characterization of the DNF15S2 locus on human chromosome 3: identification of a gene coding for four kringle domains with homology to hepatocyte growth factor. Biochemistry. 1991 Oct 8;30(40):9768–80.

46. Yoshimura T, Yuhki N, Wang MH, Skeel A, Leonard EJ. Cloning, sequencing, and expression of human macrophage stimulating protein (MSP, MST1) confirms MSP as a member of the family of kringle proteins and locates the MSP gene on chromosome 3. J Biol Chem. 1993 July 25;268(21):15461–8.

47. Hornbeck PV, Kornhauser JM, Tkachev S, Zhang B, Skrzypek E, Murray B, et al. PhosphoSitePlus: a comprehensive resource for investigating the structure and function of experimentally determined post-translational modifications in man and mouse. Nucleic Acids Res. 2012 Jan;40(Database issue):D261–70.

48. Parrish-Novak J, Dillon SR, Nelson A, Hammond A, Sprecher C, Gross JA, et al. Interleukin 21 and its receptor are involved in NK cell expansion and regulation of lymphocyte function. Nature. 2000 Nov 2;408(6808):57–63.

49. Cantrell DA, Smith KA. The interleukin-2 T-cell system: a new cell growth model. Science. 1984 Jun 22;224(4655):1312–6.

50. Folseraas T, Melum E, Rausch P, Juran BD, Ellinghaus E, Shiryaev A, et al. Extended analysis of a genome-wide association study in primary sclerosing cholangitis detects multiple novel risk loci. J Hepatol. 2012 Aug;57(2):366–75.

51. Bond J, Beynon R. The astacin family od metalloendopeptidases. Protein Sci. 1995;4(7):1247–61.

52. Marsters SA, Ayres TM, Skubatch M, Gray CL, Rothe M, Ashkenazi A. Herpesvirus entry mediator, a member of the tumor necrosis factor receptor (TNFR) family, interacts with members of the TNFR-associated factor family and activates the transcription factors NF-kappaB and AP-1. J Biol Chem. 1997 May 30;272(22):14029–32.

53. Cleary ML, Smith SD, Sklar J. Cloning and structural analysis of cDNAs for bcl-2 and a hybrid bcl-2/immunoglobulin transcript resulting from the t(14;18) translocation. Cell. 1986 Oct 10;47(1):19–28.

54. Ellinghaus D, Folseraas T, Holm K, Ellinghaus E, Melum E, Balschun T, et al. Genome-wide association analysis in primary sclerosing cholangitis and ulcerative colitis identifies risk loci at GPR35 and TCF4. Hepatology. 2013 Sep;58:1074–83.

55. Wang J, Simonavicius N, Wu X, Swaminath G, Reagan J, Tian H, et al. Kynurenic acid as a ligand for orphan G protein-coupled receptor GPR35. J Biol Chem. 2006 Aug 4;281(31):22021–8.

56. Okumura S, Baba H, Kumada T, Nanmoku K, Nakajima H, Nakane Y, et al. Cloning of a G-protein-coupled receptor that shows an activity to transform NIH3T3 cells and is expressed in gastric cancer cells. Cancer Sci. 2004 Feb;95(2):131–5.

57. O'Dowd BF, Nguyen T, Marchese A, Cheng R, Lynch KR, Heng HH, et al. Discovery of three novel G-protein-coupled receptor genes. Genomics. 1998 Jan 15;47(2):310–3.

58. D'Rozario M, Zhang T, Waddell EA, Zhang Y, Sahin C, Sharoni M, et al. Type I bHLH Proteins Daughterless and Tcf4 Restrict Neurite Branching and Synapse Formation by Repressing Neurexin in Postmitotic Neurons. Cell Rep. 2016;15(2):386–97.

59. Bain G, Murre C. The role of E-proteins in B- and T-lymphocyte development. Semin Immunol. 1998 Apr;10(2):143–53.

60. Henthorn P, McCarrick-Walmsley R, Kadesch T. Sequence of the cDNA encoding ITF-2, a positive-acting transcription factor. Nucleic Acids Res. 1990 Feb 11;18(3):678.

61. Bertin J, Guo Y, Wang L, Srinivasula SM, Jacobson MD, Poyet JL, et al. CARD9 is a novel caspase recruitment domain-containing protein that interacts with BCL10/CLAP and activates NF-kappa B. J Biol Chem. 2000 Dec 29;275(52):41082–6.

62. Kelly RJ, Rouquier S, Giorgi D, Lennon GG, Lowe JB. Sequence and expression of a candidate for the human secretor blood group alpha(1,2)fucosyltransferase gene (FUT2). Homozygosity for an enzyme-inactivating nonsense mutation commonly correlates with the non-secretor phenotype. J Biol Chem. 1995 Mar 3;270(9):4640–9.

63. Wacklin P, Makivuokko H, Alakulppi N, Nikkila J, Tenkanen H, Rabina J, et al. Secretor genotype (FUT2 gene) is strongly associated with the composition of Bifidobacteria in the human intestine. PLoS One. 2010;6(5):e20113.

64. Silva LM, Carvalho AS, Guillon P, Seixas S, Azevedo M, Almeida R, et al. Infection-associated FUT2 (Fucosyltransferase 2) genetic variation and impact on functionality assessed by in vivo studies. Glycoconj J. 2010 Jan;27(1):61–8.

65. McGovern DP, Jones MR, Taylor KD, Marciante K, Yan X, Dubinsky M, et al. Fucosyltransferase 2 (FUT2) non-secretor status is associated with Crohn's disease. Hum Mol Genet. 2010 Sep 1;19(17):3468–76.

66. Juran BD, Atkinson EJ, Schlicht EM, Larson JJ, Ellinghaus D, Franke A, et al. Genetic polymorphisms of matrix metalloproteinase 3 in primary sclerosing cholangitis. Liver Int. 2011 Jul;31(6):785–91.

67. Satsangi J, Chapman RW, Haldar N, Donaldson P, Mitchell S, Simmons J, et al. A functional polymorphism of the stromelysin gene (MMP-3) influences susceptibility to primary sclerosing cholangitis. Gastroenterology. 2001 July;121(1):124–30.

68. Wiencke K, Louka AS, Spurkland A, Vatn M, Schrumpf E, Boberg KM. Association of matrix metalloproteinase-1 and -3 promoter polymorphisms with clinical subsets of Norwegian primary sclerosing cholangitis patients. J Hepatol. 2004 Aug;41(2):209–14.

69. Wiesner RH, LaRusso NF, Ludwig J, Dickson ER. Comparison of the clinicopathologic features of primary sclerosing cholangitis and primary biliary cirrhosis. Gastroenterology. 1985 Jan;88(1 Pt 1):108–14.

70. Bjornsson E, Simren M, Olsson R, Chapman RW. Fatigue in patients with primary sclerosing cholangitis. Scand J Gastroenterol. 2004 Oct;39(10):961–8.

71. van Os E, van den Broek WW, Mulder PG, ter Borg PC, Bruijn JA, van Buuren HR. Depression in patients with primary biliary cirrhosis and primary sclerosing cholangitis. J Hepatol. 2007 June;46(6):1099–103.

72. Benito de Valle M, Rahman M, Lindkvist B, Bjornsson E, Chapman R, Kalaitzakis E. Factors that reduce health-related quality of life in patients with primary sclerosing cholangitis. Clin Gastroenterol Hepatol. 2012 July;10(7):769–75.

73. Silveira MG, Mendes FD, Diehl NN, Enders FT, Lindor KD. Thyroid dysfunction in primary biliary cirrhosis, primary sclerosing cholangitis and non-alcoholic fatty liver disease. Liver Int. 2009 Aug;29(7):1094–100.

74. Lamberts LE, Janse M, Haagsma EB, van den Berg AP, Weersma RK. Immune-mediated diseases in primary sclerosing cholangitis. Dig Liver Dis. 2011 Oct;43(10):802–6.

75. Venturini I, Cosenza R, Miglioli L, Borghi A, Bagni A, Gandolfo M, et al. Adult celiac disease and primary sclerosing cholangitis: two case reports. Hepato-Gastroenterology. 1998 Nov–Dec;45(24):2344–7.

76. Fracassetti O, Delvecchio G, Tambini R, Lorenzi N, Gavazzeni G. Primary sclerosing cholangitis with celiac sprue: two cases. J Clin Gastroenterol. 1996 Jan;22(1):71–2.

77. Man KM, Drejet A, Keeffe EB, Garcia-Kennedy R, Imperial JC, Esquivel CO. Primary sclerosing cholangitis and Hodgkin's disease. Hepatology. 1993 Nov;18(5):1127–31.

78. Jonard P, Geubel A, Wallon J, Rahier J, Dive C, Meunier H. Primary sclerosing cholangitis and idiopathic pulmonary fibrosis: a case report. Acta Clin Belg. 1989;44(1):24–30.

79. Fraile G, Rodriguez-Garcia JL, Moreno A. Primary sclerosing cholangitis associated with systemic sclerosis. Postgrad Med J. 1991 Feb;67(784):189–92.

80. Abbas A, Lichtman A, Pillai S. Leukocytes migration into tissues. In: Abbas A, Lichtman A, Pillai S, editors. Cellular and molecular immunology. Philadelphia: Elsevier; 2012.

81. Adams DH, Hubscher SG, Shaw J, Johnson GD, Babbs C, Rothlein R, et al. Increased expression of intercellular adhesion molecule 1 on bile ducts in primary biliary cirrhosis and primary sclerosing cholangitis. Hepatology. 1991 Sep;14(3):426–31.

82. Lindor KD, Wiesner RH, Katzmann JA, LaRusso NF, Beaver SJ. Lymphocyte subsets in primary sclerosing cholangitis. Dig Dis Sci. 1987 Jul;32(7):720–5.

83. Cruickshank SM, Southgate J, Wyatt JI, Selby PJ, Trejdosiewicz LK. Expression of CD44 on bile ducts in primary sclerosing cholangitis and primary biliary cirrhosis. J Clin Pathol. 1999 Oct;52(10):730–4.

84. Ponsioen CY, Kuiper H, Ten Kate FJ, van Milligen de Wit M, van Deventer SJ, Tytgat GN. Immunohistochemical analysis of inflammation in primary sclerosing cholangitis. Eur J Gastroenterol Hepatol. 1999 Jul;11(7):769–74.

85. Ardesjo B, Portela-Gomes GM, Rorsman F, Grimelius L, Ekwall O. Identification of a novel staining pattern of bile duct epithelial cells in primary sclerosing cholangitis. Inflamm Bowel Dis. 2010 Feb;16(2):305–11.

86. Hillan KJ, Hagler KE, MacSween RN, Ryan AM, Renz ME, Chiu HH, et al. Expression of the mucosal vascular addressin, MAdCAM-1, in inflammatory liver disease. Liver. 1999 Dec;19(6):509–18.

87. Grant AJ, Lalor PF, Hubscher SG, Briskin M, Adams DH. MAdCAM-1 expressed in chronic inflammatory liver disease supports mucosal lymphocyte adhesion to hepatic endothelium (MAdCAM-1 in chronic inflammatory liver disease). Hepatology. 2001 May;33(5):1065–72.

88. Grant AJ, Lalor PF, Salmi M, Jalkanen S, Adams DH. Homing of mucosal lymphocytes to the liver in the pathogenesis of hepatic complications of inflammatory bowel disease. Lancet. 2002 Jan 12;359(9301):150–7.

89. Zaballos A, Gutierrez J, Varona R, Ardavin C, Marquez G. Cutting edge: identification of the orphan chemokine receptor GPR-9-6 as CCR9, the receptor for the chemokine TECK. J Immunol. 1999 May 15;162(10):5671–5.
90. Zabel BA, Agace WW, Campbell JJ, Heath HM, Parent D, Roberts AI, et al. Human G protein-coupled receptor GPR-9-6/CC chemokine receptor 9 is selectively expressed on intestinal homing T lymphocytes, mucosal lymphocytes, and thymocytes and is required for thymus-expressed chemokine-mediated chemotaxis. J Exp Med. 1999 Nov 1;190(9):1241–56.
91. Kunkel EJ, Campbell JJ, Haraldsen G, Pan J, Boisvert J, Roberts AI, et al. Lymphocyte CC chemokine receptor 9 and epithelial thymus-expressed chemokine (TECK) expression distinguish the small intestinal immune compartment: epithelial expression of tissue-specific chemokines as an organizing principle in regional immunity. J Exp Med. 2000 Sep 4;192(5):761–8.
92. Kunkel EJ, Butcher EC. Chemokines and the tissue-specific migration of lymphocytes. Immunity. 2002 Jan;16(1):1–4.
93. Eksteen B, Grant AJ, Miles A, Curbishley SM, Lalor PF, Hubscher SG, et al. Hepatic endothelial CCL25 mediates the recruitment of CCR9+ gut-homing lymphocytes to the liver in primary sclerosing cholangitis. J Exp Med. 2004 Dec 6;200(11):1511–7.
94. Liaskou E, Karikoski M, Reynolds GM, Lalor PF, Weston CJ, Pullen N, et al. Regulation of mucosal addressin cell adhesion molecule 1 expression in human and mice by vascular adhesion protein 1 amine oxidase activity. Hepatology. 2011 Feb;53(2):661–72.
95. Harada K, Isse K, Nakanuma Y. Interferon gamma accelerates NF-kappaB activation of biliary epithelial cells induced by toll-like receptor and ligand interaction. J Clin Pathol. 2006 Feb;59(2):184–90.
96. Mueller T, Beutler C, Pico AH, Shibolet O, Pratt DS, Pascher A, et al. Enhanced innate immune responsiveness and intolerance to intestinal endotoxins in human biliary epithelial cells contributes to chronic cholangitis. Liver Int. 2011 Nov;31(10):1574–88.
97. Gilmore TD. Introduction to NF-kappaB: players, pathways, perspectives. Oncogene. 2006 Oct 30;25(51):6680–4.
98. Gorgoulis VG, Pratsinis H, Zacharatos P, Demoliou C, Sigala F, Asimacopoulos PJ, et al. p53-dependent ICAM-1 overexpression in senescent human cells identified in atherosclerotic lesions. Lab Invest. 2005 Apr;85(4):502–11.
99. He L, Chen Y, Feng J, Sun W, Li S, Ou M, et al. Cellular senescence regulated by SWI/SNF complex subunits through p53/p21 and p16/pRB pathway. Int J Biochem Cell Biol. 2017 Sep;90:29–37.
100. Coppe JP, Patil CK, Rodier F, Sun Y, Munoz DP, Goldstein J, et al. Senescence-associated secretory phenotypes reveal cell-nonautonomous functions of oncogenic RAS and the p53 tumor suppressor. PLoS Biol. 2008 Dec 2;6(12):2853–68.
101. Dorr JR, Yu Y, Milanovic M, Beuster G, Zasada C, Dabritz JH, et al. Synthetic lethal metabolic targeting of cellular senescence in cancer therapy. Nature. 2013 Sep 19;501(7467):421–5.
102. Srinivasan B, Kolli AR, Esch MB, Abaci HE, Shuler ML, Hickman JJ. TEER measurement techniques for in vitro barrier model systems. J Lab Autom. 2015 Apr;20(2):107–26.
103. Tabibian JH, Trussoni CE, O'Hara SP, Splinter PL, Heimbach JK, LaRusso NF. Characterization of cultured cholangiocytes isolated from livers of patients with primary sclerosing cholangitis. Lab Invest. 2014 Oct;94(10):1126–33.
104. Tabibian JH, O'Hara SP, Splinter PL, Trussoni CE, LaRusso NF. Cholangiocyte senescence by way of N-ras activation is a characteristic of primary sclerosing cholangitis. Hepatology. 2014 June;59(6):2263–75.
105. O'Hara SP, Splinter PL, Trussoni CE, Gajdos GB, Lineswala PN, LaRusso NF. Cholangiocyte N-Ras protein mediates lipopolysaccharide-induced interleukin 6 secretion and proliferation. J Biol Chem. 2011 Sep 2;286(35):30352–60.
106. Iebba V, Totino V, Gagliardi A, Santangelo F, Cacciotti F, Trancassini M, et al. Eubiosis and dysbiosis: the two sides of the microbiota. New Microbiol. 2016 Jan;39(1):1–12.

107. Rogosa M, Bishop FS. The genus Veillonella. 3. Hydrogen sulfide production by growing cultures. J Bacteriol. 1964 July;88:37–41.
108. Tunney MM, Field TR, Moriarty TF, Patrick S, Doering G, Muhlebach MS, et al. Detection of anaerobic bacteria in high numbers in sputum from patients with cystic fibrosis. Am J Respir Crit Care Med. 2008 May 1;177(9):995–1001.
109. Nagel RA, Westaby D, Javaid A, Kavani J, Meire HB, Lombard MG, et al. Liver disease and bile duct abnormalities in adults with cystic fibrosis. Lancet. 1989 Dec 16;2(8677):1422–5.
110. Elborn JS. Cystic fibrosis. Lancet. 2016 Nov 19;388(10059):2519–31.
111. Tunney MM, Einarsson GG, Wei L, Drain M, Klem ER, Cardwell C, et al. Lung microbiota and bacterial abundance in patients with bronchiectasis when clinically stable and during exacerbation. Am J Respir Crit Care Med. 2013 May 15;187(10):1118–26.
112. Lemoinne S, Kemgang A, Ben Belkacem K, Straube M, Jegou S, Corpechot C, et al. Fungi participate in the dysbiosis of gut microbiota in patients with primary sclerosing cholangitis. Gut. 2020 Jan;69(1):92–102.
113. Oztas E, Odemis B, Kekilli M, Kurt M, Dinc BM, Parlak E, et al. Systemic phaeohyphomycosis resembling primary sclerosing cholangitis caused by Exophiala dermatitidis. J Med Microbiol. 2009 Sep;58(Pt 9):1243–6.
114. Hong KH, Kim JW, Jang SJ, Yu E, Kim EC. Liver cirrhosis caused by Exophiala dermatitidis. J Med Microbiol. 2009 May;58(Pt 5):674–7.
115. Nakanuma Y, Hirai N, Kono N, Ohta G. Histological and ultrastructural examination of the intrahepatic biliary tree in primary sclerosing cholangitis. Liver. 1986 Dec;6(6):317–25.
116. Terasaki S, Nakanuma Y, Unoura M, Kaneko S, Kobayashi K. Involvement of peribiliary glands in primary sclerosing cholangitis: a histopathologic study. Intern Med. 1997 Nov;36(11):766–70.
117. Gaca MD, Pickering JA, Arthur MJ, Benyon RC. Human and rat hepatic stellate cells produce stem cell factor: a possible mechanism for mast cell recruitment in liver fibrosis. J Hepatol. 1999 May;30(5):850–8.
118. Tsuneyama K, Kono N, Yamashiro M, Kouda W, Sabit A, Sasaki M, et al. Aberrant expression of stem cell factor on biliary epithelial cells and peribiliary infiltration of c-kit-expressing mast cells in hepatolithiasis and primary sclerosing cholangitis: a possible contribution to bile duct fibrosis. J Pathol. 1999 Dec;189(4):609–14.
119. Kipp H, Arias IM. Trafficking of canalicular ABC transporters in hepatocytes. Annu Rev Physiol. 2002;64:595–608.
120. Thoeni C, Waldherr R, Scheuerer J, Schmitteckert S, Roeth R, Niesler B, et al. Expression analysis of ATP-binding cassette transporters ABCB11 and ABCB4 in primary Sclerosing cholangitis and variety of pediatric and adult Cholestatic and Noncholestatic liver diseases. Can J Gastroenterol Hepatol. 2019;2019:1085717.
121. Zen Y, Nakanuma Y, Portmann B. Immunoglobulin G4-related sclerosing cholangitis: pathologic features and histologic mimics. Semin Diagn Pathol. 2012 Nov;29(4):205–11.
122. Zhang L, Lewis JT, Abraham SC, Smyrk TC, Leung S, Chari ST, et al. IgG4+ plasma cell infiltrates in liver explants with primary sclerosing cholangitis. Am J Surg Pathol. 2010 Jan;34(1):88–94.
123. Zen Y, Quaglia A, Portmann B. Immunoglobulin G4-positive plasma cell infiltration in explanted livers for primary sclerosing cholangitis. Histopathology. 2011 Feb;58(3):414–22.
124. Boonstra K, Beuers U, Ponsioen CY. Epidemiology of primary sclerosing cholangitis and primary biliary cirrhosis: a systematic review. J Hepatol. 2012 May;56(5):1181–8.
125. Molodecky NA, Kareemi H, Parab R, Barkema HW, Quan H, Myers RP, et al. Incidence of primary sclerosing cholangitis: a systematic review and meta-analysis. Hepatology. 2011 May;53(5):1590–9.
126. Boberg KM, Aadland E, Jahnsen J, Raknerud N, Stiris M, Bell H. Incidence and prevalence of primary biliary cirrhosis, primary sclerosing cholangitis, and autoimmune hepatitis in a Norwegian population. Scand J Gastroenterol. 1998 Jan;33(1):99–103.

127. Lindkvist B, Benito de Valle M, Gullberg B, Bjornsson E. Incidence and prevalence of primary sclerosing cholangitis in a defined adult population in Sweden. Hepatology. 2010 Aug;52(2):571–7.
128. Toy E, Balasubramanian S, Selmi C, Li CS, Bowlus CL. The prevalence, incidence and natural history of primary sclerosing cholangitis in an ethnically diverse population. BMC Gastroenterol. 2011;11:83.
129. Vavricka SR, Brun L, Ballabeni P, Pittet V, Prinz Vavricka BM, Zeitz J, et al. Frequency and risk factors for extraintestinal manifestations in the Swiss inflammatory bowel disease cohort. Am J Gastroenterol. 2011 Jan;106(1):110–9.
130. Lebovics E, Palmer M, Woo J, Schaffner F. Outcome of primary sclerosing cholangitis. Analysis of long-term observation of 38 patients. Arch Intern Med. 1987 Apr;147(4):729–31.
131. Broome U, Olsson R, Loof L, Bodemar G, Hultcrantz R, Danielsson A, et al. Natural history and prognostic factors in 305 Swedish patients with primary sclerosing cholangitis. Gut. 1996;38(4):610–5.
132. Ponsioen CY, Vrouenraets SM, Prawirodirdjo W, Rajaram R, Rauws EA, Mulder CJ, et al. Natural history of primary sclerosing cholangitis and prognostic value of cholangiography in a Dutch population. Gut. 2002 Oct;51(4):562–6.
133. Floreani A, Zancan L, Melis A, Baragiotta A, Chiaramonte M. Primary sclerosing cholangitis (PSC): clinical, laboratory and survival analysis in children and adults. Liver. 1999 June;19(3):228–33.
134. Garioud A, Seksik P, Chretien Y, Corphechot C, Poupon R, Poupon RE, et al. Characteristics and clinical course of primary sclerosing cholangitis in France: a prospective cohort study. Eur J Gastroenterol Hepatol. 2010 Jul;22(7):842–7.
135. Wiesner RH, Grambsch PM, Dickson ER, Ludwig J, MacCarty RL, Hunter EB, et al. Primary sclerosing cholangitis: natural history, prognostic factors and survival analysis. Hepatology. 1989 Oct;10(4):430–6.
136. Helzberg JH, Petersen JM, Boyer JL. Improved survival with primary sclerosing cholangitis. A review of clinicopathologic features and comparison of symptomatic and asymptomatic patients. Gastroenterology. 1987 June;92(6):1869–75.
137. Tischendorf JJ, Hecker H, Kruger M, Manns MP, Meier PN. Characterization, outcome, and prognosis in 273 patients with primary sclerosing cholangitis: a single center study. Am J Gastroenterol. 2007 Jan;102(1):107–14.
138. Gossard AA, Angulo P, Lindor KD. Secondary sclerosing cholangitis: a comparison to primary sclerosing cholangitis. Am J Gastroenterol. 2005 June;100(6):1330–3.
139. Dyson JK, Beuers U, Jones DEJ, Lohse AW, Hudson M. Primary sclerosing cholangitis. Lancet. 2018 June 23;391(10139):2547–59.
140. Graziadei IW, Wiesner RH, Batts KP, Marotta PJ, LaRusso NF, Porayko MK, et al. Recurrence of primary sclerosing cholangitis following liver transplantation. Hepatology. 1999 Apr;29(4):1050–6.
141. Henson JB, Patel YA, Wilder JM, Zheng J, Chow SC, King LY, et al. Differences in phenotypes and liver transplantation outcomes by age group in patients with primary Sclerosing cholangitis. Dig Dis Sci. 2017 Nov;62(11):3200–9.
142. Claessen MM, Vleggaar FP, Tytgat KM, Siersema PD, van Buuren HR. High lifetime risk of cancer in primary sclerosing cholangitis. J Hepatol. 2009 Jan;50(1):158–64.
143. Charatcharoenwitthaya P, Enders FB, Halling KC, Lindor KD. Utility of serum tumor markers, imaging, and biliary cytology for detecting cholangiocarcinoma in primary sclerosing cholangitis. Hepatology. 2008 Oct;48(4):1106–17.
144. Song J, Li Y, Bowlus CL, Yang G, Leung PSC, Gershwin ME. Cholangiocarcinoma in patients with primary Sclerosing cholangitis (PSC): a comprehensive review. Clin Rev Allergy Immunol. 2019 Aug;28:159–65.
145. Tornai T, Tornai D, Sipeki N, Tornai I, Alsulaimani R, Fechner K, et al. Loss of tolerance to gut immunity protein, glycoprotein 2 (GP2) is associated with progressive disease course in primary sclerosing cholangitis. Sci Rep. 2018 Jan 10;8(1):399.

146. Jendrek ST, Gotthardt D, Nitzsche T, Widmann L, Korf T, Michaels MA, et al. Anti-GP2 IgA autoantibodies are associated with poor survival and cholangiocarcinoma in primary sclerosing cholangitis. Gut. 2017 Jan;66(1):137–44.

147. Siqueira E, Schoen RE, Silverman W, Martin J, Rabinovitz M, Weissfeld JL, et al. Detecting cholangiocarcinoma in patients with primary sclerosing cholangitis. Gastrointest Endosc. 2002 July;56(1):40–7.

148. Chalasani N, Baluyut A, Ismail A, Zaman A, Sood G, Ghalib R, et al. Cholangiocarcinoma in patients with primary sclerosing cholangitis: a multicenter case-control study. Hepatology. 2000 Jan;31(1):7–11.

149. Levy C, Lymp J, Angulo P, Gores GJ, Larusso N, Lindor KD. The value of serum CA 19-9 in predicting cholangiocarcinomas in patients with primary sclerosing cholangitis. Dig Dis Sci. 2005 Sep;50(9):1734–40.

150. Kipp BR, Barr Fritcher EG, Pettengill JE, Halling KC, Clayton AC. Improving the accuracy of pancreatobiliary tract cytology with fluorescence in situ hybridization: a molecular test with proven clinical success. Cancer Cytopathol. 2013 Nov;121:610–9.

151. Kim DG, Park SY, You KR, Lee GB, Kim H, Moon WS, et al. Establishment and characterization of chromosomal aberrations in human cholangiocarcinoma cell lines by cross-species color banding. Genes Chromosomes Cancer. 2001 Jan;30(1):48–56.

152. Langer-Safer PR, Levine M, Ward DC. Immunological method for mapping genes on Drosophila polytene chromosomes. Proc Natl Acad Sci U S A. 1982 July;79(14):4381–5.

153. Barr Fritcher EG, Caudill JL, Blue JE, Djuric K, Feipel L, Maritim BK, et al. Identification of malignant cytologic criteria in pancreatobiliary brushings with corresponding positive fluorescence in situ hybridization results. Am J Clin Pathol. 2011 Sep;136(3):442–9.

154. Kipp BR, Stadheim LM, Halling SA, Pochron NL, Harmsen S, Nagorney DM, et al. A comparison of routine cytology and fluorescence in situ hybridization for the detection of malignant bile duct strictures. Am J Gastroenterol. 2004 Sep;99(9):1675–81.

155. Barr Fritcher EG, Kipp BR, Voss JS, Clayton AC, Lindor KD, Halling KC, et al. Primary sclerosing cholangitis patients with serial polysomy fluorescence in situ hybridization results are at increased risk of cholangiocarcinoma. Am J Gastroenterol. 2011 Nov;106(11):2023–8.

156. Osborn M, Weber K. Tumor diagnosis by intermediate filament typing: a novel tool for surgical pathology. Lab Invest. 1983 Apr;48(4):372–94.

157. Moll R, Franke WW, Schiller DL, Geiger B, Krepler R. The catalog of human cytokeratins: patterns of expression in normal epithelia, tumors and cultured cells. Cell. 1982 Nov;31(1):11–24.

158. Pujol JL, Grenier J, Parrat E, Lehmann M, Lafontaine T, Quantin X, et al. Cytokeratins as serum markers in lung cancer: a comparison of CYFRA 21-1 and TPS. Am J Respir Crit Care Med. 1996 Sep;154(3 Pt 1):725–33.

159. Nakata B, Takashima T, Ogawa Y, Ishikawa T, Hirakawa K. Serum CYFRA 21-1 (cytokeratin-19 fragments) is a useful tumour marker for detecting disease relapse and assessing treatment efficacy in breast cancer. Br J Cancer. 2004 Aug 31;91(5):873–8.

160. Chapman MH, Sandanayake NS, Andreola F, Dhar DK, Webster GJ, Dooley JS, et al. Circulating CYFRA 21-1 is a specific diagnostic and prognostic biomarker in biliary tract Cancer. J Clin Exp Hepatol. 2011 Jun;1(1):6–12.

161. Giovannini M, Bories E, Monges G, Pesenti C, Caillol F, Delpero JR. Results of a phase I-II study on intraductal confocal microscopy (IDCM) in patients with common bile duct (CBD) stenosis. Surg Endosc. 2011 July;25(7):2247–53.

162. Lankisch TO, Metzger J, Negm AA, Vosskuhl K, Schiffer E, Siwy J, et al. Bile proteomic profiles differentiate cholangiocarcinoma from primary sclerosing cholangitis and choledocholithiasis. Hepatology. 2011 Mar;53(3):875–84.

163. Metzger J, Negm AA, Plentz RR, Weismuller TJ, Wedemeyer J, Karlsen TH, et al. Urine proteomic analysis differentiates cholangiocarcinoma from primary sclerosing cholangitis and other benign biliary disorders. Gut. 2013 Jan;62(1):122–30.

164. Tischendorf JJ, Kruger M, Trautwein C, Duckstein N, Schneider A, Manns MP, et al. Cholangioscopic characterization of dominant bile duct stenoses in patients with primary sclerosing cholangitis. Endoscopy. 2006 July;38(7):665–9.

165. Triantos CK, Koukias NM, Nikolopoulou VN, Burroughs AK. Meta-analysis: ursodeoxycholic acid for primary sclerosing cholangitis. Aliment Pharmacol Ther. 2011 Oct;34(8):901–10.
166. Lindor KD, Kowdley KV, Luketic VA, Harrison ME, McCashland T, Befeler AS, et al. High-dose ursodeoxycholic acid for the treatment of primary sclerosing cholangitis. Hepatology. 2009 Sep;50(3):808–14.
167. Lindstrom L, Hultcrantz R, Boberg KM, Friis-Liby I, Bergquist A. Association between reduced levels of alkaline phosphatase and survival times of patients with primary Sclerosing cholangitis. Clin Gastroenterol Hepatol. 2013 July;11:841–6.
168. Boner AL, Peroni D, Bodini A, Delaini G, Piacentini G. Azithromycin may reduce cholestasis in primary sclerosing cholangitis: a case report and serendipitous observation. Int J Immunopathol Pharmacol. 2007 Oct–Dec;20(4):847–9.
169. Farkkila M, Karvonen AL, Nurmi H, Nuutinen H, Taavitsainen M, Pikkarainen P, et al. Metronidazole and ursodeoxycholic acid for primary sclerosing cholangitis: a randomized placebo-controlled trial. Hepatology. 2004 Dec;40(6):1379–86.
170. Davies YK, Cox KM, Abdullah BA, Safta A, Terry AB, Cox KL. Long-term treatment of primary sclerosing cholangitis in children with oral vancomycin: an immunomodulating antibiotic. J Pediatr Gastroenterol Nutr. 2008 July;47(1):61–7.
171. Abarbanel DN, Seki SM, Davies Y, Marlen N, Benavides JA, Cox K, et al. Immunomodulatory effect of vancomycin on Treg in pediatric inflammatory bowel disease and primary sclerosing cholangitis. J Clin Immunol. 2013 Feb;33(2):397–406.
172. Tabibian JH, Weeding E, Jorgensen RA, Petz JL, Keach JC, Talwalkar JA, et al. Randomised clinical trial: vancomycin or metronidazole in patients with primary sclerosing cholangitis - a pilot study. Aliment Pharmacol Ther. 2013 Mar;37(6):604–12.
173. Damman JL, Rodriguez EA, Ali AH, Buness CW, Cox KL, Carey EJ, et al. Review article: the evidence that vancomycin is a therapeutic option for primary sclerosing cholangitis. Aliment Pharmacol Ther. 2018 Apr;47(7):886–95.
174. Lammers WJ, van Buuren HR, Hirschfield GM, Janssen HL, Invernizzi P, Mason AL, et al. Levels of alkaline phosphatase and bilirubin are surrogate end points of outcomes of patients with primary biliary cirrhosis: an international follow-up study. Gastroenterology. 2014 Dec;147(6):1338–49.e5.
175. Fickert P, Hirschfield GM, Denk G, Marschall HU, Altorjay I, Farkkila M, et al. norUrsodeoxycholic acid improves cholestasis in primary sclerosing cholangitis. J Hepatol. 2017 Sep;67(3):549–58.
176. Trauner M, Gulamhusein A, Hameed B, Caldwell S, Shiffman ML, Landis C, et al. The nonsteroidal Farnesoid X receptor agonist Cilofexor (GS-9674) improves markers of cholestasis and liver injury in patients with primary Sclerosing cholangitis. Hepatology. 2019 Sep;70(3):788–801.
177. Larusso NF, Levy C, Vuppalanchi R, Floreani A, Andreone P, Srestha R, Trotter J, Goldgerg D, Rushbrook S, Hirschfield GM, Van Biene C, Penceck R, Macconell DS. The AESOP trial: a randomized, double-blind, placebo-controlled, phase 2 study of obeticholic acid in patients with primary sclerosing cholangitis. Dig Liver Dis. 2018;50(2):e67.
178. Nevens F, Andreone P, Mazzella G, Strasser SI, Bowlus C, Invernizzi P, et al. A placebo-controlled trial of Obeticholic acid in primary biliary cholangitis. N Engl J Med. 2016 Aug 18;375(7):631–43.
179. Kowdley KV, Luketic V, Chapman R, Hirschfield GM, Poupon R, Schramm C, et al. A randomized trial of obeticholic acid monotherapy in patients with primary biliary cholangitis. Hepatology. 2018 May;67(5):1890–902.
180. Hirschfield GM, Chazouilleres O, Drenth JP, Thorburn D, Harrison SA, Landis CS, et al. Effect of NGM282, an FGF19 analogue, in primary sclerosing cholangitis: a multicenter, randomized, double-blind, placebo-controlled phase II trial. J Hepatol. 2019 Mar;70(3):483–93.
181. Tabibian JH, Lindor KD. Ursodeoxycholic acid in primary sclerosing cholangitis: if withdrawal is bad, then administration is good (right?). Hepatology. 2014 Sep;60(3):785–8.
182. Assis DN, Abdelghany O, Cai SY, Gossard AA, Eaton JE, Keach JC, et al. Combination therapy of all-trans retinoic acid with Ursodeoxycholic acid in patients with primary Sclerosing cholangitis: a human pilot study. J Clin Gastroenterol. 2017 Feb;51(2):e11–e6.

183. Lemoinne S, Pares A, Reig A, Ben Belkacem K, Kemgang Fankem AD, Gaouar F, et al. Primary sclerosing cholangitis response to the combination of fibrates with ursodeoxycholic acid: French-Spanish experience. Clin Res Hepatol Gastroenterol. 2018 Dec;42(6):521–8.

184. Yu D, Cai SY, Mennone A, Vig P, Boyer JL. Cenicriviroc, a cytokine receptor antagonist, potentiates all-trans retinoic acid in reducing liver injury in cholestatic rodents. Liver Int. 2018 June;38(6):1128–38.

185. Leban J, Kralik M, Mies J, Baumgartner R, Gassen M, Tasler S. Biphenyl-4-ylcarbamoyl thiophene carboxylic acids as potent DHODH inhibitors. Bioorg Med Chem Lett. 2006 Jan 15;16(2):267–70.

186. Fitzpatrick LR, Deml L, Hofmann C, Small JS, Groeppel M, Hamm S, et al. 4SC-101, a novel immunosuppressive drug, inhibits IL-17 and attenuates colitis in two murine models of inflammatory bowel disease. Inflamm Bowel Dis. 2010 Oct;16(10):1763–77.

187. Trivedi PJ, Tickle J, Vesterhus MN, Eddowes PJ, Bruns T, Vainio J, et al. Vascular adhesion protein-1 is elevated in primary sclerosing cholangitis, is predictive of clinical outcome and facilitates recruitment of gut-tropic lymphocytes to liver in a substrate-dependent manner. Gut. 2018 June;67(6):1135–45.

188. Arndtz K, Corrigan M, Rowe A, Kirkham A, Barton D, Fox RP, et al. Investigating the safety and activity of the use of BTT1023 (Timolumab), in the treatment of patients with primary sclerosing cholangitis (BUTEO): a single-arm, two-stage, open-label, multi-Centre, phase II clinical trial protocol. BMJ Open. 2017 July 3;7(6):e015081.

189. Allegretti JR, Kassam Z, Carrellas M, Mullish BH, Marchesi JR, Pechlivanis A, et al. Fecal microbiota transplantation in patients with primary Sclerosing cholangitis: a pilot clinical trial. Am J Gastroenterol. 2019 July;114(7):1071–9.

190. Goldberg DS, Camp A, Martinez-Camacho A, Forman L, Fortune B, Reddy KR. Risk of waitlist mortality in patients with primary sclerosing cholangitis and bacterial cholangitis. Liver Transpl. 2013;19(3):250–8.

191. Aljiffry M, Renfrew PD, Walsh MJ, Laryea M, Molinari M. Analytical review of diagnosis and treatment strategies for dominant bile duct strictures in patients with primary sclerosing cholangitis. HPB. 2011 Feb;13(2):79–90.

192. Gotthardt DN, Rudolph G, Kloters-Plachky P, Kulaksiz H, Stiehl A. Endoscopic dilation of dominant stenoses in primary sclerosing cholangitis: outcome after long-term treatment. Gastrointest Endosc. 2010 Mar;71(3):527–34.

193. Stiehl A, Rudolph G, Kloters-Plachky P, Sauer P, Walker S. Development of dominant bile duct stenoses in patients with primary sclerosing cholangitis treated with ursodeoxycholic acid: outcome after endoscopic treatment. J Hepatol. 2002 Feb;36(2):151–6.

194. Kaya M, de Groen PC, Angulo P, Nagorney DM, Gunderson LL, Gores GJ, et al. Treatment of cholangiocarcinoma complicating primary sclerosing cholangitis: the Mayo Clinic experience. Am J Gastroenterol. 2001 Apr;96(4):1164–9.

195. Baluyut AR, Sherman S, Lehman GA, Hoen H, Chalasani N. Impact of endoscopic therapy on the survival of patients with primary sclerosing cholangitis. Gastrointest Endosc. 2001 Mar;53(3):308–12.

196. Rudolph G, Gotthardt D, Kloeters-Plachky P, Rost D, Kulaksiz H, Stiehl A. In PSC with dominant bile duct stenosis, IBD is associated with an increase of carcinomas and reduced survival. J Hepatol. 2010 Aug;53(2):313–7.

197. Pausawasadi N, Soontornmanokul T, Rerknimitr R. Role of fully covered self-expandable metal stent for treatment of benign biliary strictures and bile leaks. Korean J Radiol. 2012 Jan–Feb;13(Suppl 1):S67–73.

198. Eaton JE, Thackeray EW, Lindor KD. Likelihood of malignancy in gallbladder polyps and outcomes following cholecystectomy in primary sclerosing cholangitis. Am J Gastroenterol. 2012 Mar;107(3):431–9.

199. Chapman R, Fevery J, Kalloo A, Nagorney DM, Boberg KM, Shneider B, et al. Diagnosis and management of primary sclerosing cholangitis. Hepatology. 2010 Feb;51(2):660–78.

200. Grossman EJ, Millis JM. Liver transplantation for non-hepatocellular carcinoma malignancy: indications, limitations, and analysis of the current literature. Liver Transpl. 2010 Aug;16(8):930–42.

201. Wu Y, Johlin FC, Rayhill SC, Jensen CS, Xie J, Cohen MB, et al. Long-term, tumor-free survival after radiotherapy combining hepatectomy-Whipple en bloc and orthotopic liver transplantation for early-stage hilar cholangiocarcinoma. Liver Transpl. 2008 Mar;14(3):279–86.

202. Friman S, Foss A, Isoniemi H, Olausson M, Hockerstedt K, Yamamoto S, et al. Liver transplantation for cholangiocarcinoma: selection is essential for acceptable results. Scand J Gastroenterol. 2011 Mar;46(3):370–5.

203. Gringeri E, Bassi D, D'Amico FE, Boetto R, Polacco M, Lodo E, et al. Neoadjuvant therapy protocol and liver transplantation in combination with pancreatoduodenectomy for the treatment of hilar cholangiocarcinoma occurring in a case of primary sclerosing cholangitis: case report with a more than 8-year disease-free survival. Transplant Proc. 2011 May;43(4):1187–9.

204. Alvaro D, Cannizzaro R, Labianca R, Valvo F, Farinati F. Italian Society of G, et al. cholangiocarcinoma: a position paper by the Italian Society of Gastroenterology (SIGE), the Italian Association of Hospital Gastroenterology (AIGO), the Italian Association of Medical Oncology (AIOM) and the Italian Association of Oncological Radiotherapy (AIRO). Dig Liver Dis. 2010 Dec;42(12):831–8.

205. Dasanu CA, Majumder S, Trikudanathan G. Emerging pharmacotherapeutic strategies for cholangiocarcinoma. Expert Opin Pharmacother. 2011 Aug;12(12):1865–74.

206. Sia D, Tovar V, Moeini A, Llovet JM. Intrahepatic cholangiocarcinoma: pathogenesis and rationale for molecular therapies. Oncogene. 2013 Jan;32:4861.

207. Brandsaeter B, Friman S, Broome U, Isoniemi H, Olausson M, Backman L, et al. Outcome following liver transplantation for primary sclerosing cholangitis in the Nordic countries. Scand J Gastroenterol. 2003 Nov;38(11):1176–83.

208. Singal AK, Guturu P, Hmoud B, Kuo YF, Salameh H, Wiesner RH. Evolving frequency and outcomes of liver transplantation based on etiology of liver disease. Transplantation. 2013 Mar 15;95(5):755–60.

209. Florman S, Schiano T, Kim L, Maman D, Levay A, Gondolesi G, et al. The incidence and significance of late acute cellular rejection (>1000 days) after liver transplantation. Clin Transpl. 2004 Apr;18(2):152–5.

210. Graziadei IW. Recurrence of primary sclerosing cholangitis after liver transplantation. Liver Transpl. 2002 July;8(7):575–81.

211. Graziadei IW, Wiesner RH, Marotta PJ, Porayko MK, Hay JE, Charlton MR, et al. Long-term results of patients undergoing liver transplantation for primary sclerosing cholangitis. Hepatology. 1999 Nov;30(5):1121–7.

212. Moncrief KJ, Savu A, Ma MM, Bain VG, Wong WW, Tandon P. The natural history of inflammatory bowel disease and primary sclerosing cholangitis after liver transplantation: a single-Centre experience. Can J Gastroenterol. 2010 Jan;24(1):40–6.

213. Graziadei IW. Live donor liver transplantation for primary sclerosing cholangitis: is disease recurrence increased? Curr Opin Gastroenterol. 2011 May;27(3):301–5.

214. Fosby B, Karlsen TH, Melum E. Recurrence and rejection in liver transplantation for primary sclerosing cholangitis. World J Gastroenterol WJG. 2012 Jan 7;18(1):1–15.

215. Davies YK, Tsay CJ, Caccamo DV, Cox KM, Castillo RO, Cox KL. Successful treatment of recurrent primary sclerosing cholangitis after orthotopic liver transplantation with oral vancomycin. Case Rep Transpl. 2013;2013:314292.

216. Joshi D, Bjarnason I, Belgaumkar A, O'Grady J, Suddle A, Heneghan MA, et al. The impact of inflammatory bowel disease post-liver transplantation for primary sclerosing cholangitis. Liver Int. 2013 Jan;33(1):53–61.

217. Jorgensen KK, Lindstrom L, Cvancarova M, Castedal M, Friman S, Schrumpf E, et al. Colorectal neoplasia in patients with primary sclerosing cholangitis undergoing liver transplantation: a Nordic multicenter study. Scand J Gastroenterol. 2012 Sep;47(8–9):1021–9.

218. Steenstraten IC, Sebib Korkmaz K, Trivedi PJ, Inderson A, van Hoek B, Rodriguez Girondo MDM, et al. Systematic review with meta-analysis: risk factors for recurrent primary sclerosing cholangitis after liver transplantation. Aliment Pharmacol Ther. 2019 Mar;49(6):636–43.

219. Mieli-Vergani G, Vergani D. Unique features of primary sclerosing cholangitis in children. Curr Opin Gastroenterol. 2010 May;26(3):265–8.

220. Faubion WA Jr, Loftus EV, Sandborn WJ, Freese DK, Perrault J. Pediatric "PSC-IBD": a descriptive report of associated inflammatory bowel disease among pediatric patients with PSC. J Pediatr Gastroenterol Nutr. 2001 Sep;33(3):296–300.
221. Miloh T, Anand R, Yin W, Vos M, Kerkar N, Alonso E, et al. Pediatric liver transplantation for primary sclerosing cholangitis. Liver Transpl. 2011 Aug;17(8):925–33.
222. Deneau MR, El-Matary W, Valentino PL, Abdou R, Alqoaer K, Amin M, et al. The natural history of primary sclerosing cholangitis in 781 children: a multicenter, international collaboration. Hepatology. 2017 Aug;66(2):518–27.

# Chapter 6
# Chronic Hepatitis C

Nora V. Bergasa

A 50-year-old man was referred to the Hepatology clinic for evaluation of chronic hepatitis C diagnosed 10 year prior to the referral. His risk factors included intravenous drug use and multiple tattoos done in prison. He felt well. His exam was notable for absent cutaneous stigmata of chronic liver disease, and several tattoos (Fig. 6.1). His hemogram and liver function were normal, the serum alanine (ALT ) and aspartate (AST) transaminase activities were twice the upper limit of normal consistently, with normal bilirubin and coagulation profile. He was infected with genotype 1a, and his viral load was 1 million IU/L. He was immune to hepatitis A and B. His liver ultrasound was normal. Liver disease workup done at the time of the first clinic visit excluded other causes of liver disease. This patient's risk for viral hepatitis included tattoos done in prison; of interest, he placed tattoos on both antecubital fossae to cover needle tracts from his intravenous injection of drugs. He continued to use heroin intranasally. He reported that the environment in which he lived was not supportive of his wish to stop using illicit drugs and, thus, had decided to move to another state where he would seek treatment for chronic HCV.

N. V. Bergasa (✉)
Department of Medicine, H+H/Metropolitan, New York, NY, USA

New York Medical College, Valhalla, NY, USA

Hepatology, H+H/Woodhull, Brooklyn, NY, USA

N. V. Bergasa (ed.), *Clinical Cases in Hepatology*,
https://doi.org/10.1007/978-1-4471-4715-2_6

**Fig. 6.1** Tattoo on needle tracts on the left antecubital fossa of a patient who had used intravenous drugs. The dragon alludes to the phrase "chasing the dragon", which refers to inhaling the vapor from a heated solution of drugs including heroin

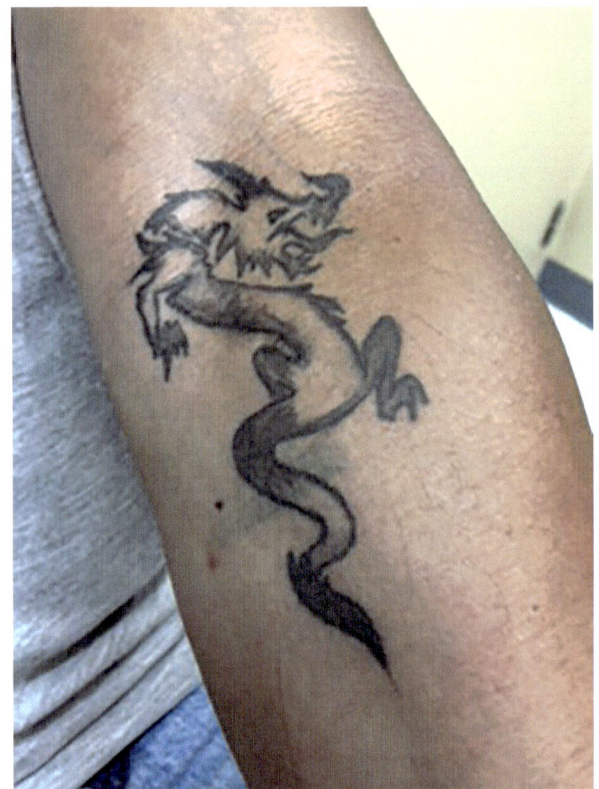

## Etiology

The hepatitis C virus (HCV) belongs to the genus Hepacivirus of the Flaviviridae family [1]. It is an RNA virus of 60 nm in dimension, surrounded by a protein shell that is further encased by a lipid envelope, in which two glycoproteins are anchored [2]. The virus has a positive sense single-stranded RNA genome that consists of a single open reading frame 9600 nucleotide bases long that produces one protein [1], which is processed by proteases to generate ten polypeptides [3]. The structural region is comprised of the core, E (envelope) 1, and E2, and the nonstructural region of p7, NS2, NS3, NS4A, NS4B, NS5A, and NS5B. NS2 and NS4A function as proteases, NS3 as a helicase protease, and NS5B as an RNA polymerase [4]. An HCV antigen is considered to be encoded, at least in part, by an alternate reading frame (ARF) overlapping the core-encoding region [5, 6]. The variabilities in the NS5B region of the virus has led to the identification of several genotypes, 1 through 7, comprised of subtypes [7]. The HCV circulates in the form of quasispecies [8], which are closely related genomes that result from mutations in the nucleotide sequence [9, 10]; this characteristic allows the virus to survive different replication environments including the appearance of neutralizing antibodies and cytotoxic T cells, contributing to the chronic state of the infection [11], and resistance to antiviral drugs [12]. The virus replicates within the hepatocyte; the entry sites include the CD81, highly sulfated heparan sulfate, the low-density lipoprotein receptor, and scavenger receptor class B type I and claudin-1 [13, 14]. Hepatocyte specific factors that facilitate the entrance of the virus and that have not been identified seem necessary to explain the predilection for the hepatocyte as a site for replication [14]; however, there are experimental findings to suggest that this virus also replicates in cells outside the liver, including the peripheral mononuclear cells compartment [15], central nervous system [16], and epithelial cells [17], including the small intestine [18].

## Genetics

Eighty to eighty-five percent of subjects who acquire HCV infection develop chronic disease. Factors associated with spontaneous HCV clearance included acute clinical hepatitis and female gender [19], as concluded from an analysis of the course of viral hepatitis from a group of studies that comprised 675 subjects, with a rate of spontaneous resolution calculated to be 26% [19]. The genetic characteristics of the host are relevant in the evolution of an HCV infection as distinct MHC class I and II alleles have been reported in association with clearance of the virus in human beings [20]. From a study of a group of patients infected from a single source, the majority of subjects that cleared the infection exhibited A*03, B*27, and Cw*01 more frequently than those who did not. The haplotypes associated with the resolution of the infection were A*03-B*07-DRB1*15-DQB1*0602 and A*02-B*27-Cw*01-DRB1*0101-DQB1*0501. The alleles A*03, DRB1*0101, *0401, *15, and B*27 were reported to be associated with viral clearance, with the latter exhibiting the strongest association. The haplotype A*01-B*08-Cw*07-DRB1*03011-DQB1*0201 was reported in association with chronicity [20]. HLA-B 57 and HLA DRB1* have been associated with resolution in contrast to HLA-B 08, which was reported in association with chronicity [21]. A group of patients typed as HLA-B57 that had not been protected from developing chronic hepatitis C was stated to have sequence variations in HLA-B 57-restricted T-cell epitopes, which seem to have prevented HLA-B 57-mediated immune pressure [21]. Along the same line, another study from this well-characterized group of patients also revealed HLA-B27 in association with chronicity and HCV clearance. An HLA-B27 restricted hepatitis C virus (HCV)-specific CD8+ T cell epitope was recognized in the majority of HLA-B27 positive women who had resolved the acute HCV infection. In patients who had developed chronic hepatitis C, the viral sequence was strongly associated with sequence variations within this epitope and expression of HLA-B27, which was interpreted to suggest an allele-specific selection pressure at the population level. It was further documented that the new viral epitopes are escape mutations. These results identified HLA-B27 as having a fundamental role in HCV infection resolution, and evolution of the HCV in relationship to a dominant CD8+ T cell epitope [22].

The genetic characteristics of the host also influence the progression of chronic hepatitis C to cirrhosis. In this regard, the polymorphism rs738409 GG genotype of the patatin-like phospholipase domain-containing 3 (PNPLA3) encoding for the I148M protein variant has been reported in significant association with the stage of fibrosis and presence of cirrhosis [23, 24].

Viral behavior is fundamental in determining the course of infection, including the slow evolution of the heterogeneous viral population, defined as quasispecies, correlating with the resolution, and viral escape mutations in epitopes targeted by cytotoxic T lymphocytes associated with chronicity [24].

Changes in the sequence have been demonstrated to occur mainly within the hypervariable region 1 of the E2 gene, confirmed to be temporarily related to antibody seroconversion, which has suggested that it is a behavior to escape immunological pressure from the immune system [11]. Acute infection associated with the size of the inoculum, low and high, has both been associated with spontaneous resolution. A single nucleotide polymorphism (rs12979860) in chromosome 19q13, 3 kilobases upstream of the IL28B gene, which encodes the type III interferon IFN-3, and a high viral load in the acute infection (i.e., 7 log(10) IU/ml) were associated with spontaneous viral clearance, as compared to subjects with the IL28B-T allele in whom chronic infection prevailed [25]; this allele is also associated with sustained virological response in association with treatment with interferon [26]. Other genetic polymorphisms have been identified in association with clearance of the hepatitis C virus infection, including genotype −509C in the gene that codes for transforming growth factor (TGF)-β1 [27], and which suppresses the proliferation and cytotoxicity of cells [28]. Genes encoding KIR2DL3, a receptor on the NK cell, and its human leukocyte antigen C group 1 (HLA-C1) ligand also contribute to the resolution of acute hepatitis C [29]. Over 50% of patients with genotype CC in the gene that codes for IL 28B cleared an acute hepatitis C viral infection, in contrast to those with genotypes CT, and TT, the least favorable genotype in association with clearance [30].

What determines the outcome of the infection also relates to the manner in which the host immune system handles the virus. Natural killer (NK) cells are fundamental in response to viral infections. In hepatitis C, there is an activation of natural killer cells during acute infection regardless of its outcome [31]. In the realm of NK cells, the population of peripheral CD56(neg) NK cells was expanded in acute, resolved, and chronic HCV infection. Increased frequency of HLA-C-binding KIR(+) NK cells was documented in patients who had resolved the acute infection. There was a reported increase in NKG2A(+) and CD94(+) NK cells in acute and chronic HCV infection, but this was not documented in patients who had resolved the infection. In addition, a decrease in the frequency of NKp30(+), NKp46(+), CD161(+), and NKG2D(+) cells was reported in patients who in follow up, resolved the infection [32]. Patients who did not develop hepatitis after documented exposure to the hepatitis C virus exhibited signs of natural killer (NK) T cell activation, increased serum concentrations of chemokines, and NK cell responses with increased expression of

CD122, NKp44, NKp46, and NKG2A, TRAIL and CD107a, and production of gamma interferon. The NK response manifested itself earlier in the subjects who did not develop hepatitis than in the one individual who did. The production of interferon gamma by NK cells differed from what is documented to happen in patients with chronic hepatitis C, whose NK cells fail to produce interferon gamma appropriately. The degree of NKT cell activation and cytotoxicity was reported to correlate with the specific HCV-T cell response expressed subsequently. There was evidence of active replication in the absence of systemic viremia, as indicated by the response of T cells targeting nonstructural proteins of the hepatitis C genome, which require translation of viral RNA and hence, suggested replication. These findings tend to support the idea that a vigorous response by NKT cells is associated with a subsequent effective T cell response and potential immunity against the hepatitis C virus [33]. Also, in chronic infection, continued expansion in the NK population of cells has been documented, with an increased presence of this type of cell in the liver versus peripheral blood. The NK cells in the chronic stage of the infection were reported to express tumor necrosis factor-related apoptosis-inducing ligand (TRAIL), NKp44, NKG2C, and CD122 in contrast to a control group of non-infected subjects. There was an increased frequency of CD107a expression indicative of degranulation (i.e., cytotoxicity); however, no increase in interferon gamma production of CD56(dim) NK cells was noted. The use of interferon alpha to stimulate in vitro NK cells from infected and non-infected individuals was documented to be associated with the NK phenotype of patients. These results were interpreted to suggest that the exposure of NK cells to alpha interferon may contribute to the liver injury associated with HCV infection via TRAIL and cytotoxicity, with the low expression of gamma interferon contributing to chronicity [34]. In patients with chronic hepatitis C, NKp46(High) NK cells displayed a greater cytolytic activity and production of interferon gamma than NKp46(Dim) NK cells, and in vitro, NKp46(High) NK cells blocked the production of HCV in the replicon system. An increase in the density of NKp46(High) NK cells correlated inversely with hepatitis C RNA load, suggesting an in situ and in vivo antiviral effect and with hepatic fibrosis, suggesting an antifibrotic function of this type of NK cells [35]. The chemokine CXCR3 receptor and its ligands have been reported as increased in chronic hepatitis C. In further support of a role of NK cells in liver fibrosis in chronic hepatitis C is the increase in the density of CXCR3(+)CD56Bright NK cells, which were documented to display impaired degranulation and impaired production of interferon gamma in association with exposure to hepatic stellate cells [36]. Thus, emerging data support the activation of innate immune responses after acute infection with the hepatitis C virus and NK's role in the evolution of hepatitis C virus infection and potential mediation of liver fibrosis.

Spontaneous resolution of acute HCV infection is associated with the production of neutralizing antibodies and the development of CD4+ and CD8+ T cells specific to the virus [37]. In vitro studies by the use of an infectious retroviral HCV pseudoparticle model system with sera from subjects who had experienced acute HCV after the receipt of contaminated immunoglobulin D [38] revealed that resolution of infection was associated with high titers of neutralizing antibodies in the early phase, defined as the first 6 months after it, in contrast to what was reported from patients who had developed chronic infection in whom low titers or absence of this type of antibodies was documented [39]. Neutralizing antibodies, which were recorded to cross-react with genotypes different from the one that caused the index infection, decreased or disappeared after the resolution of the acute infection, consistent with prior reports [40]; this peculiarity may be related to the absence of protection from new HCV infections [41].

CD4+ T cells are considered essential in the clearance of the HCV in acute infection and prolonged protection against recurrent infections, as supported from studies of reinfection with HCV in chimpanzees in which CD4+ T cells had been antibody-depleted. Persistence and immune evasion on a repeat exposure to the HCV were reported in this model of the human disease in spite of functional CD8+ T cells [42]. In the initial stages of the infection, HCV-specific CD8+ T cells exhibit a deficiency in the production of interferon gamma [43]. In the subsequent stage, interferon gamma is produced by HCV-specific CD8+ T cells [44]; this event coincides with the appearance of HCV-specific CD4+ T cells, a decrease in viral load, and an increase in serum activity of transaminases [44]. Ex vivo studies with cells from patients with chronic hepatitis C and from those who recovered from the infection have been reported to reveal a significantly greater response of HCV-specific type-1 T-cell in patients who had recovered from the infection than in those who had not. Chronicity of the infection was associated with a reversible CD4-mediated suppression of HCV-specific CD8 T cells and with an increase in the number of CD4(+) CD25(+) regulatory T cells in the material from patients with chronic infection able to suppress HCV-specific type-1 CD8 T cells [45].

In contrast to the disappearance of antibodies, helper and cytotoxic T cell responses characterized by interferon gamma production have been documented to remain for years after the infection [40]. However, the characteristic features of T cells have also been reported in patients who clear or fail to clear the virus on the index infection. Clearance of the virus was stated to be associated with a production of Th1 cytokines upon stimulation of CD4+ T cells by NS3 and NS4, nonstructural proteins of the virus in vitro, as compared to cells from patients who developed chronic disease, which did not produce any Th1 cytokines [46]. In the liver, CD4+ FOXP3+ cells were abundant in the inflammatory infiltrate of samples from patients with chronic hepatitis C virus infection [47].

T cell-mediated cytotoxic mechanisms also contribute to the response to an HCV infection. Peripheral blood mononuclear cells from patients with resolved hepatitis C viral infection were reported to exhibit a specific response to recombinant nonstructural viral protein 3 characterized by the production of interferon gamma. A response was observed by peripheral mononuclear cells from some patients with progression to chronic hepatitis C infection found from only a minority of samples from patients with chronic infection [48]. A strong proliferative response to the recombinant viral proteins core, E1, E2, NS3, NS4, and NS5 by peripheral T cells was characteristic of cells derived from subjects who exhibited normalization of serum activity of transaminases, a reflection of hepatic inflammation, in response to an acute HCV infection, and viral clearance, than from cells derived from subjects who developed the chronic disease. T cells' response to the viral proteins was detected early in the course of the infection, suggesting that its magnitude determines the natural history of the infection, i.e., resolution or chronicity [49]. The loss of specific CD4+ T cell proliferation in response to the virus has been associated with recurrence of the disease, suggesting that for the infection to be permanently controlled, the CD4+ cells must remain responsive to the viral proteins [49].

An important role of CD8+ T cells in the mediation of chronic hepatitis C has also been identified and considered fundamental in the evolution of the acute HCV infection. In this regard, it was demonstrated that in early HCV infection, a robust T helper and cytotoxic response was characteristic; however, the cytotoxic activated lymphocytes were deficient in the production of interferon gamma, which gradually increased as the viral load decreased. Hepatitis C responses from cytotoxic lymphocytes were more common in patients who cleared the virus than in those with chronic disease [43].

The events that characterized the course of acute hepatitis C were: (i) the appearance of hepatitis C virus specific T cells 1 month after infection, (ii) a CD38+ IFN-gamma—CD8+ T cell response, in association with a decrease in viral load, (iii) a robust CD4+ T cell response, and (iv) the appearance of CD 38-CD8+ T cells that produced interferon gamma, which coincided with a marked decrease in viral load, not associated with an apparent increase in disease activity. In patients in whom the viral infection became chronic, there was no substantial T cell response or a response that was, although strong, transient [44]. A central role of CD8+ T cells has been further suggested by the reported association between protective HLA alleles, including HLA-B27, HLA-B57, and HLA-A3 and resolution of HCV infection in relationship with dominant CD8+ T cell epitopes [37, 50, 51].

The mechanism by which CD8+ T cells eliminate virus infected hepatocytes is mostly non-cytolytic and mainly mediated by interferon gamma [52]. A fundamental role of CD8+ T cells has also been supported by an in vitro study in which depletion of CD4(+)CD25(+) T regulatory (T(reg)) cells from patients with chronic hepatitis C was associated with increased HCV (and EBV) peptide driven expansion and in the number of CD8(+) T cells expressing IFN-gamma; also, the suppressive effect of CD4(+)CD25(+) regulatory T cells on CD8(+) T-cell proliferation was not prevented by the addition of antibodies to IL-10 and to transforming growth factor beta to block the expressed receptors by the CD8+T cells. These experiments have supported the idea of a marked CD4(+)CD25(+) regulatory T-cell activity in patients with chronic hepatitis C, associated with a suboptimal response to the HCV by CD8+ T cells [53], consistent with the proper function of memory CD8+ T as a prerequisite for protection from chronic hepatitis C [54].

It was also demonstrated that in early HCV infection a robust T helper and cytotoxic response was characteristic; however, the cytotoxic activated lymphocytes were deficient in the production of interferon gamma, which gradually increased as the viral load decreased. Hepatitis C responses from cytotoxic lymphocytes were more common in patients who cleared the virus, as compared to those with chronic disease [43].

Also, in patients who develop chronic hepatitis C, an abnormal function of CD8+ T cells, including their inability to produce IL-2, interferon gamma and other cytokines, and to proliferate, has been documented [55, 56]. In this respect, studies on the role of the immunoinhibitory receptor programmed death-1 (PD-1), which is upregulated in dysfunctional virus specific CD8+ T cells, revealed that in the liver of patients with chronic hepatitis C, HCV-specific CD8 T cells from chronically HCV-infected patients expressed PD-1 intensely, exhibited dysfunctional behavior, and were not responsive to the reparatory effect of PD-1/PD-L blockade. However, in the periphery, CD8+ T cells expression was lower than that of the intrahepatic cells and did exhibit a response to PD-1/PD-L blockade [57]. The expression of PD-1 in CD8+ T cells during the acute phase of the HCV infection was high, regardless of the course of the disease, i.e., resolution vs. chronicity, and subsequently decreased, in association with differentiation of CD8+ T cells to a memory CD127+ phenotype and resolution of infection [58]. The degree of PD-1 expression in the acute phase of the infection has also been reported to be significantly higher on T cells specifically responsive to the HCV in patients who develop chronic hepatitis than in those who resolve the infection [59].

IL-10, a cytokine that prevents inflammation but that also has been reported to facilitate viral prevalence, has been reported to contribute to the development of chronic hepatitis C. In this context, intrahepatic CD8+ T cells responsive to the hepatitis C virus produce IL-10 and not gamma interferon, and, although their presence was reported to prevent liver injury, these cells are not effective in eliminating the virus [60]. In addition, CD8+ T cells that produce IL-10 were documented to be present in the early stages of the acute infection and to prevail in chronic disease; these findings were reported to correlate with poor CD4+ effector function, and with high viral load in acute infection. Although interleukin secretion in response to the hepatitis C virus was high in patients without cirrhosis, the blockade of IL-10 was associated with an increased antiviral effect mediated by IFN-gamma, suggesting that a proviral environment is facilitated by IL-10 [60].

An important role of CD8+ T cells has also been supported by an in vitro study in which depletion of CD4(+)CD25(+) T regulatory cells in samples from patients with chronic viral hepatitis C was associated with increased HCV (and EBV) peptide driven expansion and in the number of CD8(+) T cells expressing IFN-gamma; also, the suppressive effect of CD4(+)CD25(+) regulatory T cells on CD8(+) T-cell proliferation was not prevented by the addition of antibodies to IL-10 and to transforming growth factor beta to block the expressed receptors by the CD8+ T cells. These experiments have supported the idea of a marked CD4(+)CD25(+) regulatory T-cell activity in patients with chronic hepatitis C, associated with a suboptimal response to the HCV by CD8+ T cells [53], consistent with the proper function of memory CD8+ T as a prerequisite for protection from chronic HCV infection [54]. Escaping CD8+ T cells by rapid mutations is another mechanism by which the HCV survives in the body of the host. The lack of T cell receptor diversity does not allow recognition of the mutant variant against which cellular activation and effector functions would have been expected to occur, thus providing a way for the virus to escape the immune system.

## Epidemiology

The World Health Organization (WHO) reports that every year 3–4 million people contract hepatitis C virus infection [61]. Numbers as high as one hundred and fifty (150) million chronically infected individuals worldwide are quoted [61]. However, there is uncertainty about the prevalence and incidence of this infection because epidemiological studies come from certain parts of the globe only. Most importantly, statistics from vulnerable populations, including homeless and incarcerated people, are not available. Yearly, the WHO reports that 350,000 people die from chronic hepatitis C related complications [61]. In the United States, between 1999 and 2007, deaths from HCV increased significantly to 15,106 in a study that used death certificates as sources of information [62]. In this regard, the generation of baby boomers, comprised of individuals born from 1945 to 1965, is considered as having been at risk for exposure, which, according to a Canadian group of investigators, concerns health care practices [63], and not the societal events that included drug use and that affected that generation [64, 65]; this concern has led to the recommendation of the Centers for Disease Control and the United States Preventive Task Force to screen persons from that generation and which now has been extended to include subjects aged at least 18 years [66].

The hepatitis C virus is transmitted by contaminated blood products, body fluids, and supplies used in procedures including injections; thus, the factors for hepatitis C virus infection include: (i) blood transfusions given before 1992, and blood products, including factors, before 1987, (ii) organ transplantation before 1992, (iii) injections with contaminated needles including those used for illicit drugs, or those used by lay injectors, e.g., unsafe therapeutic injections, (iv) use of contaminated needles such as injection of illicit drugs, (v) drug snorting, e.g., cocaine and heroin, (vi) body piercing and tattoos done with contaminated needles or contaminated ink, (vii) sex between men, multiple sexual partners, or sexual intercourse with an infected partner 6 months prior to clinical expression of the infection [67], (viii) children born to HCV-positive mothers [68].

The prevention of hepatitis C virus infection concerns avoidance of high risk behavior and practices, including unsafe injection practices, sharing sharp objects of personal use, e.g., razors, sharing of drug paraphernalia, unprotected sex with people with chronic hepatitis C, body piercing, acupuncture and tattoos with potentially contaminated equipment.

## Natural History

The clinical manifestation of acute hepatitis C is preceded by an incubation period between 2 weeks and 6 months after inoculation with the virus.

Studies of populations at risk or analysis of stored samples from patients subsequently identified as having chronic hepatitis C have provided information on the natural history of acute HCV infection [69, 70]. In one such study, it was docu-mented that 85% of patients presented with clinical findings of acute hepatitis, and of those, 52% exhibited spontaneous clearance of the virus, measured by reverse transcriptase (RT) polymerase chain reaction (PCR) [71], the concentration of which fluctuates during the acute phase of the infection, varying from hundreds to millions of international units per ml [72], within 12 weeks of the determined time of infection, in contrast to the patients who developed chronic hepatitis C, who had stable serum RNA concentrations [72], and who did not have any clinical manifes-tations [70], further supporting the idea of a host-specific response in the determina-tion of the course of the infection [20]. The development of anti-HCV antibodies measured by documented antibody seroconversion by enzyme immunoassay (EIA) and recombinant immunoblot assay occurs in the majority of patients after acute HCV [69]. In transfusion associated acute hepatitis C, it was documented that anti-bodies appeared 22 weeks after infection, or 15 weeks after the onset of clinical hepatitis [69], and persist over many years. In patients in whom the infection resolves itself, the antibody has been documented to disappear after 4 years [69].

Most patients who resolve the acute hepatitis C infection clear the virus within 6 months [72, 73]. Thus, chronic hepatitis C has been defined as the presence of the hepatitis C RNA in serum 6 months after infection. However, the spontaneous clear-ance of the virus has been documented up to 2 years after the time of infection [74]. The resolution of acute hepatitis C virus infection has been reported in association with race, being less common in individuals of the black race, versus non-black subjects [74]. Approximately 75–85% of patients develop chronic infection, 60 to 70% chronic liver disease, and 5–20% cirrhosis over 20–30 years [68, 72, 75], with up to 4% per year proceeding to decompensated disease and hepatocellular carci-noma (HCC) [76].

The natural history of chronic hepatitis C (and chronic hepatitis B) was studied over 8.4 years in a representative sample from individuals from Northern Italy. It was documented that progression to cirrhosis was 4.5 per 1000 person-year, and the development of hepatocellular carcinoma 2.0 per 1000 person-year; the intake of alcohol was reported as an independent predictor of cirrhosis with a rate ratio of 4.5, with a 95% confidence interval (CI) ranging from 1.02 to 41.2 and a death rate of 8.53 (95% CI 1.40–24.61) for increments by 30 g/day of alcohol intake at base-line [77].

By the use of the METAVIR score system, a study that included 2235 patients with chronic hepatitis C documented that patients with chronic hepatitis C could be categorized as slow fibrosers, defined as patients infected for more than 20 years, and liver histology not exhibiting septa fibrosis (F0 or F1), rapid fibrosers, defined as patients who had developed cirrhosis (F4) before the age of 50 years, and inter-mediate fibrosers (F2 or F3, by inference); this finding suggested that progression was not "universal" or "inevitable" [75]. Age older than 40 years at the time of infection, male gender, and alcohol intake of more than 50 g/day were identified in association with disease progression, the latter being associated with an increase in the progression of fibrosis of 34% [75]. The median expected time to cirrhosis was

30 years, with 33% of patients having an expected time to cirrhosis of fewer than 20 years, and with 31% not progressing to cirrhosis at all, or not progressing for at least 50 years [75].

A study that included 33 patients who were infected from a common source revealed chronic hepatitis in the majority of the liver samples obtained 17 and 19 years after the infection with little progression over the 2 year period; only one patient had developed cirrhosis [78]. From the same group of patients, a non-aggressive course was documented 22 years of after infection [79].

Steatosis is documented to accelerate disease progression in association with chronic hepatitis C genotype 3 [80] and to impede response to antiviral therapy [80]. Steatosis was reported in significant association with fibrosis, infection with genotype 3 hepatitis C virus, high body mass index (BMI), alcohol use, and age [80]. In patients with chronic hepatitis C coinfected with the human immunodeficiency virus and who had a high BMI, diabetes and hepatic steatosis were associated with fibrosis; in addition, persistently increased serum activity of transaminases related to fibrosis progression, which occurred over 2.5 years [81].

In a study published in 1997 that included 2235 patients with chronic hepatitis C, factors identified with disease progression were age older than 40 at the time of infection, alcohol intake of at least 50 g/day, and male gender. The median time to progression to cirrhosis was 30 years from infection, with a range from 28 to 32. In men infected after age 40, cirrhosis could be established after 13 years of the infection. In women, cirrhosis could be established 42 years after the infection in the absence of alcohol use. Thirty-three percent of patients who were not treated had an expected median time to cirrhosis of 20 years, with 31% not expected to progress to cirrhosis for at least 50 years [75]. In regard to cirrhosis, the polymorphism rs738409 GG genotype of the patatin-like phospholipase domain-containing 3 (PNPLA3) encoding for the I148M protein variant was reported in significant association with the stage of fibrosis and presence of cirrhosis [23, 24], supporting a role of genetic predisposition to the progression of the disease.

## Clinical Manifestations

20 to 30% of patients with acute hepatitis C have symptoms, fatigue being the most common. A subgroup of women who acquired hepatitis C virus from a common source [68, 74, 82] was studied at the time of the infection and 22 years afterward [79]. Jaundice was reported at the time of the infection by 20.6% of those who did not have hepatitis C viral RNA by polymerase chain reaction (PCR) at the time of the follow-up study [74], versus 3.4% of those in whom hepatitis C RNA was detected. These findings suggested that jaundice may predict the resolution of acute hepatitis C. Other signs include choluria and acholic stools. Other symptoms include arthralgia, anorexia, abdominal pain, nausea, and vomiting.

# Physical Exam

In general, the physical exam in patients with acute hepatitis C would be notable for jaundice, in cases of hyperbilirubinemia. In patients with chronic hepatitis C, the findings depend on the degree of liver disease; patients may or may not exhibit cutaneous stigmata of liver disease and signs of decompensation, including ascites and edema.

Acute hepatitis C is associated with increased activity of ALT, usually higher than 400 IU/ml, and rarely in the thousands. Hyperbilirubinemia may be present. Patients with chronic hepatitis C can have a normal liver profile, e.g., ALT activity; 66% of patients with chronic hepatitis C 20 years after the infection were reported to have increased serum activity of ALT (>40 IU/l) [79]. The serum activity of ALT can fluctuate throughout the disease; in a prospective study, this pattern was documented in 21% of patients with chronic hepatitis C over several years [79]. A fluctuating pattern has also been reported, emphasizing the importance of screening for hepatitis C virus infection regardless of a normal liver profile [66]. As the disease progresses and cirrhosis ensues, serum AST activity increases over that of the ALT as it happens in most chronic liver diseases [83, 84]. Increased activity of alkaline phosphatase, and gamma glutamyl transpeptidase, in association with increased activity of transaminases, is the profile typical of advanced disease. Hyperbilirubinemia, hypoalbuminemia, and coagulopathy are features of hepatic dysfunction, as in that from other etiologies. Thrombocytopenia is a sign of hypersplenism, from portal hypertension; however, it can be seen in patients with chronic hepatitis C without portal hypertension, considered to be an effect of the virus per se, with normalization of platelet count after successful antiviral therapy. In chronic hepatitis C, there is also suppression of all hematological cell lines, characteristic of liver disease in general.

Several methods have been developed to test antibodies in blood and in saliva. The methodology includes enzyme immunoassay (EIA), enhanced chemiluminescence immunoassay (CIA), microparticle enzyme immunoassay (MEIA), recombinant immunoblot assay (RIBA), and chemiluminescent microparticle immunoassay (CMIA) [85–87]; the presence of hepatitis C RNA can be qualitatively and quantitatively detected by polymerase chain reaction (PCR) methodology [87].

Anti-hepatitis C antibodies (anti-HCV) can be detected in serum 4–10 weeks after infection with the hepatitis C virus, with a 96% detectability 6 months after the infection [69, 88]. Anti-HCV tends to persist. However, a rate of antibody loss has been reported as 0.6 per 100 person-years [88].

Testing for genotype in patients with chronic hepatitis C has been necessary as the duration of treatment has varied according to the genotype [89]. The presence of anti-HCV antibodies should be followed by testing for serum HCV RNA, and when appropriate, e.g., in the face of acute hepatitis, the latter should be repeated over several weeks. The absence of anti-HCV antibodies in the presence of infection, i.e., a false negative result, can occur when the viral titer is low, as in very early stages of infection, or in persons who are immunocompromised. Thus, the presence of risk factors in a subject with absent anti-HCV antibody requires repeat testing, including HCV-RNA [90].

Antinuclear antibodies, anti-smooth muscle antibodies, and anti-liver/kidney microsomal type 1 antibodies can be detected in the serum of patients with chronic hepatitis C with a reported wide prevalence of approximately 20 to 40% in some series [91, 92]. The presence of non-organ specific autoantibodies has not been consistently associated with the stage of liver disease. In some studies, serum auto-antibodies have been associated with a high degree of inflammation and fibrosis, and elevated serum concentrations of gamma globulins [93, 94]. However, in other studies, including an observational study that included 24,306 patients [95], the presence of autoantibodies in chronic hepatitis C has been documented to correlate with histology, decision to start standard antiviral therapy, or response to it [92, 95]. The interpretation of the clinical relevance of autoantibodies has to be individualized [95], especially, if a diagnostic procedure, e.g., liver biopsy, or treatment for another liver disease, e.g. autoimmune hepatitis, is considered based on serum auto-antibody profile.

## Differential Diagnosis

Causes of hepatitis, including viral, autoimmune, metabolic, and toxic (e.g., drug-induced), must be excluded in patients who present with increase serum activity of transaminases, with or without hyperbilirubinemia. Identifying risk factors is fundamental for prompt diagnosis, which is confirmed by laboratory findings, i.e., serum hepatitis C RNA.

## Histology

Some of the features documented from liver histology in acute hepatitis C include confluent liver necrosis, sinusoidal inflammatory infiltrates, steatosis, dense portal lymphoid aggregates, and bile duct injury, i.e., the Poulsen–Christoffersen lesions [96, 97], the latter having been documented to portend evolution to chronic liver disease in one study [96].

The principal histological findings that have been reported in chronic hepatitis C include portal and lobular inflammation, and interface hepatitis, steatosis, lymphoid aggregates, and bile duct injury, apoptotic and Mallory bodies, steatosis, bile duct lesions, and lymphoid cell follicles within portal tracts (Fig. 6.2) [79, 98–100].

The bile duct lesion of hepatitis, most commonly seen in chronic hepatitis C, is characterized by swelling, vacuolization, and irregular nuclei, with a basement membrane that appears ruptured, lymphocytes, some plasma cells, and neutrophils, invading the bile ducts; the lesion is reminiscent of the florid bile duct lesion of primary biliary cholangitis (PBC); however, it is not considered to lead to bile duct

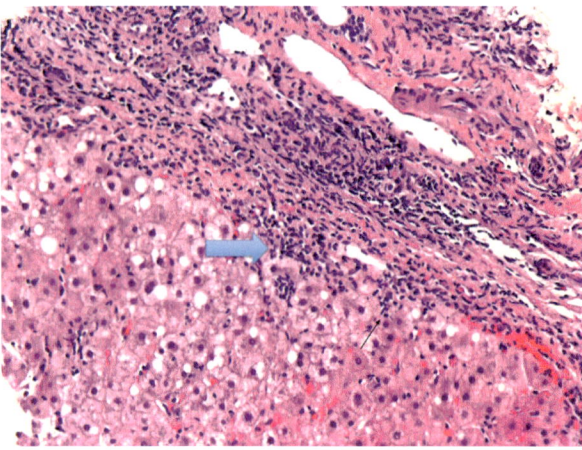

**Fig. 6.2** Liver histology in a patients with chronic hepatitis C displaying interface hepatitis (arrow) (Hematoxylin and Eosin stain)

destruction and ductopenia in most cases, as happens in PBC. This bile duct lesion of hepatitis, and mostly of chronic hepatitis C, i.e., the Poulsen–Christoffersen lesion [101], has been documented to represent diverticular bile duct lesions that may represent Hering ducts and groups of periportal liver cells that have escaped the piecemeal necrosis [102].

Early immunohistochemical studies documented the constitution of the lymphoid aggregates or follicles, characteristic of chronic hepatitis C, as functional lymphoid follicles that contain activated B cells in the midst of a follicular dendritic cell network, and a mantle zone of B cells, surrounded by a T cell zone, consisting of CD4-positive helper T cells and CD8-positive suppressor/cytotoxic T cells [103, 104] some of which expressed CD25 and IL-2 receptor, as well as human leukocyte antigen DR, suggesting an activated state [104]. The necrotic inflammatory infiltrate that comprised the necrosis, piecemeal type (currently known as interface) in the samples studied was composed of CD4 helper T cells, and those identified in the lobule were predominantly CD8 suppressor/cytotoxic T cells [103]. The characteristics of the hepatic lymphoid follicles were reported as similar to those found in autoimmune diseases. They suggested that a component of the liver injury in chronic hepatitis C may be immune mediated [103, 104]. One immunohistochemical study of liver tissue from patients with chronic hepatitis C (and B) documented the cellular inflammatory infiltrate to be comprised of T lymphocytes, 50% of which was CD4CD45RO(+), consistent with activated cells, and 25% CD8CD45RO(+), and of B lymphocytes, 15% of which was CD20(+)CD45RA (+), and 10% of which was a combination of CD20(−)CD45RA(+) and NK cells. Most cells in the portal area expressed HLA class II molecules suggesting a response to antigen presentation, i.e., the HCV [104].

Foxp3 is a member of the forkhead transcription factors group, which regulates the development and function of regulatory T cells, CD4(+)CD25(+)Treg (Tregs) [105]; these cells are a key suppressive component of the immune system [106]. The presence of activated CD4+FoxP3+ Treg, as evidenced by the expression of

CD45RO, CCR7, CTLA-4, and HLA-DR, has been documented in the livers of patients with chronic hepatitis C and limited fibrosis, suggesting that this type of cell may decrease fibrogenesis by suppression of an immunological response to the virus [107]. In this context, intrahepatic FoxP3+CD4+ regulatory T cells were documented to produce IL-8 in patients with chronic hepatitis C [107]. An increase in the number of activated GARP-positive IL-8(+) Tregs was identified close to areas of fibrosis in liver tissue from patients with chronic hepatitis C. In addition, it was reported that Tregs increased the expression of markers of fibrosis including TIMP1, MMP2, TGF-beta1, alpha-SMA, collagen, and CCL2 in primary human hepatic stellate cells (HSC) studied ex vivo, an effect that was blocked by anti-IL-8 antibodies; these findings were interpreted to support the idea that, in addition to mediating immune response to the HCV infection, Foxp3(+)CD4(+) Tregs contribute to the development of fibrosis [108]. Further characterization of intrahepatic mononuclear cells documented the presence of intrahepatic CD4(+)FoxP3(+)T cells within the inflammatory infiltrate in close association with a few CD8(+)FoxP3(+)T cells; this finding has suggested that the inhibition of CD8+ T cell is mediated by cell to cell contact. Advanced fibrosis was associated with a reduction in the FoxP3(+)/CD8(+) cell ratio because of a low number of FoxP3 cells [109]. Activated CD4+FoxP3+ Treg lymphocytes, as evidenced by the expression of CD45RO, CCR7, CTLA-4, and HLA-DR, have been documented in the livers of patients with chronic hepatitis C and limited fibrosis, suggesting that this type of cell may decrease the fibrosis process in association with this viral infection [107].

Fibrosis in chronic hepatitis is exhibited as portal to portal bridges of collagen, and also as central to central and as central to portal, known as passive septa, which is considered to result from bouts of necrosis in zone 3, and repair of episodes of intra-acinar necrosis [110]. The contraction of fibrous septa is associated with nodule formation, changing the liver's architecture, which defines cirrhosis; the association with nodules, incomplete or complete, with necroinflammatory activity, is termed active cirrhosis [110].

Several non-invasive tests and indices have been developed or derived to predict the presence of fibrosis in the liver of patients with chronic hepatitis C, including the platelet count, age-platelet index, aspartate aminotransferase-platelet ratio index (APRI), FibroIndex, FibroTest, Forns index, and for identification of cirrhosis, the platelet count, age-platelet index, and Hepascore [111]. Examination of liver histology by liver biopsy is the gold standard to assess the presence and degree of liver disease, including fibrosis and cirrhosis [112].

## Extrahepatic Manifestations

Extrahepatic manifestations of chronic hepatitis C have been reported in 38–76% of patients, and they include cryoglobulinemia complicated by systemic vasculitis, sicca syndrome, lymphoproliferative diseases, and lichen planus [113]. The association with sarcoidosis has been documented in case reports [114, 115]. An association between cardiomyopathy and chronic hepatitis C was supported by the recovery of cardiac function in a patient with chronic hepatitis C treated with antiviral therapy that was associated with sustained virological response [116]. This association was initially reported in Japan [117–119]. However, it was not confirmed in studies from Italy [120], Brazil [121], nor Brooklyn, New York [122], which has suggested a racial, ethnic, and/or genetic predisposition to this potential complication of chronic hepatitis C.

Cryoglobulinemia is the presence of serum immunoglobulin that precipitates in vitro at temperatures lower than 37 °C, and dissolves itself after rewarming [123]. The cryoglobulins are classified into three types, based on their composition. Type I tends to be composed of monoclonal immunoglobulin IgM or IgG, type II is a mixture of monoclonal IgM with rheumatoid factor activity, which binds to the Fc portion of IgG, and type III, a combination of polyclonal IgM and IgG [123, 124]. The prevalence of HCV in cryoglobulinemia has been reported to be between 30% to nearly 100% [123, 125], with the development of cryoglobulinemic vasculitis in 10–15% of patients [125]. Non-enveloped HCV core protein has been documented in the cryoprecipitate of type II mixed cryoglobulinemia [126]. In patients with chronic hepatitis C, serum cryoglobulins have been documented with an annual incidence of 3%, and most commonly, in patients with advanced disease [113, 123, 127, 128]. The pathogenesis of cryoglobulinemia in chronic hepatitis C seems to concern the tropism of the hepatitis C virus for lymphoid tissue. The E2 protein of the hepatitis C envelope interacts with an extracellular loop of tetraspanin CD81, a protein expressed by hepatocytes and B and T cells [129], which has been proposed to mediate the proliferation and clonal expansion of B lymphocytes.

The manifestations of cryoglobulinemia-associated vasculitis include rash, palpable purpura, and chronic ulcers, fatigue, arthralgia, motor-sensory axonopathy, arterial hypertension, glomerulonephritis, and nephrotic syndrome [129]. As the hepatitis C virus is considered the stimulus of B cells [130], the treatment aims to eradicate the virus.

The association of lymphoma with chronic hepatitis C was also documented from a retrospective cohort study of subjects who attended US Veterans Affairs health care facilities from 1997 to 2004 and that included 146,394 individuals. The hazard risk for non-Hodgkin's lymphoma was 1.21, with a 95% confidence interval (CI) between 1.07 and 1.37, and a hazard ratio of 2.72 (95% CI 2.00–3.72) both significantly higher than in the group of patients without chronic hepatitis C [131]. This report followed a published meta-analysis from which the pooled relative risk (RR) for all NHL among all patients with chronic hepatitis C was 2.5, (95% CI 2.1–3, and a pooled RR of 2.5 (95% CI, 2.1–3.1) and a pooled RR of 2.0 (95% CI, 1.8–2.2) from case control and cohort studies, respectively [132].

There is literature suggesting an association between chronic hepatitis C and diabetes mellitus type 2; however, analysis of population-based data from the U.S. National Health and Nutrition Examination Survey from 1999 to 2010, which included 15,128 subjects, documented a lack of association between hepatitis C antibody in serum and pre-diabetes or diabetes [133].

There is literature reporting an association between chronic hepatitis C infection and porphyria cutanea tarda (PCT) [134–138]. PCT is characterized by skin fragility, erythema, bullae, erosions, hypertrichosis, and milia in sun-exposed areas and by increased concentration of porphyrins in the urine [139]. PCT is classified as type I, comprising 75–80% of the cases, defined as an acquired deficiency limited to the hepatocyte of uroporphyrinogen decarboxylase (UROD), a key enzyme in the synthesis of heme, type II, hereditary, comprising 20–25% of the cases, and characterized by a decreased activity of UROD in all tissues by approximately 50%, and type III, also hereditary, for which the genetic defect has not been described, comprising less than 1% of the cases, and characterized by a decrease in UROD hepatocyte activity [134, 139]. A reduction of activity of UROD in the liver in the absence of decreased protein levels of UROD has suggested that an inhibitor of UROD is made in the hepatocytes; in support of this idea seems to be the finding of normal protein concentration of UROD in association with reduction of enzyme activity. Studies in a mouse model of PCT have lent support to this line of thinking by revealing the inhibitor of recombinant human URO-D (rhURO-D) to be uroporphomethene; however, the identity of the inhibitor has not been consistently confirmed [140]. An inhibitor of rhURO-D was also isolated from the cytosol of hepatocytes obtained from liver samples from patients with PCT. These results have suggested that the clinical expression of PCT is due to the iron dependent oxidation of uroporphyrinogen to uroporphomethene, a competitive inhibitor of URO-D [134, 141], suggesting that iron itself may contribute to the pathophysiology of PCT [134].

A meta-analysis that included 2167 patients from 50 studies documented the prevalence of hepatitis C RNA in serum of 50% [137]. The prevalence of chronic hepatitis C in PCT varied according to the type of porphyria, 57% for the sporadic form (Type I), and 26% for the familial form (Type II) [137]. From another meta-analysis, the prevalence of chronic hepatitis C in PCT was reported as 17% in Northern Europe, 20% in Australia and New Zealand, and 65% in Southern Europe, and 94% (16 of 17 PCT) in a study from one hospital in Indianapolis, Indiana in the United States [142]. These results have suggested that the HCV contributes to the pathogenesis of PCT [137, 142]. Infection with the HCV alone does not seem sufficient to trigger PCT [143]; however, the HCV may alter porphyrin metabolism facilitating the clinical expression of PCT in patients predisposed to it and with this type of viral hepatitis. How the hepatitis C virus mediates the events that result in PCT has been a matter of speculation; in this regard, it has been proposed that iron may be the factor that predisposes PCT in patients with chronic hepatitis C, in which iron has been reported as a factor contributing to liver injury [144] as also reported for PCT. In this context, it has been suggested that high iron content in PCT is secondary to abnormal regulation of hepcidin, a protein made in the hepatocyte, which regulates iron absorption in human beings. Infection with the HCV was reported to be associated with decreased hepcidin expression [145], which has suggested a mechanism by which there may be a relationship between hepatocellular iron and chronic hepatitis C-mediated liver disease. In this proposed model, the HCV may also contribute to the pathogenesis of PCT as iron mediates the reaction that produces an inhibitor of URO-D, reported to contribute to the pathogenesis of PCT [141].

The prevalence of chronic hepatitis C antibodies in patients with renal disease was 7.9% in contrast to blood donors and pregnant women in whom the prevalence was 1.03% and 0.98%, respectively. Chronic hepatitis C infection has been reported in association with membranoproliferative glomerulonephritis, membranous nephropathy, focal segmental sclerosis, fibrillary glomerulonephritis, immunotac-toid nephropathy, IgA nephropathy, tubulointerstitial nephritis, and thrombotic microangiopathy, usually associated with cryoglobulinemia [146]. The most common renal disease in patients with chronic hepatitis C associated with mixed cryo-globulinemia is type I membranoproliferative glomerulonephritis exhibiting proteinuria and microscopic hematuria, which may be complicated by impaired renal function [131, 147, 148]. Population-based studies have reported an associa-tion between proteinuria and hepatitis C virus infection, interpreted to suggest that the association may be more common than what has been recognized [146].

Histologically, the renal lesion of hepatitis C associated nephropathy includes a cellular infiltrate comprised of monocytes, eosinophils, and intraluminal thrombi. Subendothelial deposits of IgG, IgM, and complement components are prevalent, and vasculitis of small renal arteries has been reported [146, 149]. It has been sug-gested that high binding of immunoglobulin M kappa rheumatoid factor from type II cryoglobulins to cellular fibronectin in the glomerular mesangium contributes to the pathogenesis of glomerulopathies associated with type II cryoglobulinemia and chronic hepatitis C [150].

Xerostomia and xerophthalmia, symptoms typically comprising the sicca syn-drome, have been reported as extrahepatic manifestations of chronic hepatitis C [151–155]. The prevalence of chronic hepatitis C was stated as 19% in patients with sicca syndrome in one study [152], and sicca syndrome was present in 62% of patients with chronic hepatitis C studied prospectively [155]. Antibodies identified with primary Sjogren's syndrome, anti-SS-A/SS-B, were documented as signifi-cantly more prevalent in patients with sicca syndrome without chronic hepatitis C than those with the syndrome without chronic hepatitis C [152, 153, 155] differen-tiating primary from secondary Sjogren's syndrome. Evidence of glandular dys-function in chronic hepatitis C has been documented [153]. An inflammatory infiltrate characterized by activated lymphocytes similar to that found in patients with primary Sjorgren's syndrome has been described in patients with chronic hepa-titis C [156]. The pathogenesis of sicca syndrome with regard to hepatitis C viral infection is not known. In this context, HCV RNA has been detected in saliva and in salivary gland extracts in patients with Sjogren's syndrome and chronic hepatitis C, which has suggested that the virus may localize itself in the salivary glands and trig-ger an inflammatory response resulting in sialoadenitis and sicca symptoms [157]; however, viral particles have not been consistently detected in the affected glands [153].

Lichen planus is histologically characterized by interface dermatitis that mani-fests itself as purple polygonal pruritic papulosquamous lesions that can affect the skin, scalp, nails, and mucous membranes, of unknown etiology, for which an immune-mediated pathogenesis is hypothesized [158]. Lichen planus has been documented in association with chronic hepatitis C [159]. In a cross-sectional study, the prevalence was 5 percent [160]. Two meta-analyses have reported a significantly higher risk for patients with lichen planus to have chronic hepatitis C and patients with chronic hepatitis C to develop lichen planus than those of control groups [161, 162].

The association between adrenal tumors and chronic hepatitis C has been reported [163, 164]. In a series of three patients, two of the tumors were functional, as evidenced by hypokalemia and hypertension. The likely mode of acquiring hepatitis C in the patients preceded the manifestation of hyperaldosteronism by many years; thus, it was inferred that the hepatitis C infection was the first event. The association was confirmed in a retrospective review of patients with adrenal tumors over 10 years, 2001 to 2010 [164]. Of 23 patients with adrenal tumors, 15 (65.2%) had hepatitis C antibody, and 11 (47.8%) had hepatitis C RNA in serum, consistent with chronic hepatitis C, significantly different from the findings in the control group in which only one of 23 (4.3%) patients had hepatitis C antibody in the serum [164]. The mechanism by which chronic hepatitis C may lead to the formation of adrenal tumors may include replication of the hepatitis C virus in the adrenal gland [165], by the systemic effects of IGF, reported as high in patients with chronic viral hepatitis including hepatitis C [166], and by insulin, increased in patients with metabolic syndrome, which has been reported in association with chronic hepatitis C. Both insulin and IGF increased the growth of bovine adrenal fasciculate cells in culture [167]. As chronic hepatitis C and hypertension are prevalent conditions, HCV infection should be excluded in patients with hypertension, even if not necessarily difficult to control, as hyperaldosteronism is more prevalent than previously considered [168], and thus, the exclusion of chronic hepatitis C in patients with adrenal tumors seems warranted.

## Diagnosis

The laboratory findings of hepatitis C virus infection have been described above. The diagnosis of acute HCV infection is made in the presence of hepatitis accompanied by hepatitis C viral RNA in serum, which disappears over the 16 weeks that follow the infection in the patients who clear it, or that remains consistently detected when the infection becomes chronic [88, 169]. Hepatitis C antibody, which can be found from 4 to 15 weeks from infection, remains detected in patients who have been infected, regardless of RNA clearance. The presence of hepatitis C antibody is suggestive of chronic hepatitis C in 80% of the patients. The serum liver profile is usually abnormal with increase serum activity of liver associated transaminases, but periods of normal activity occur.

# Treatment

The treatment of chronic hepatitis C has changed from regimes associated with limited sustained virological response (SVR), defined as no viral RNA detected in serum 24 months after completion of therapy, and considered a cure [170], to regimes associated with SVRs from 90% to 100% in most of the hepatitis C virus genotypes 12 weeks after completion of treatment [170–172]. A negative RNA at 12 weeks post treatment completion was defined as sustained virological response (SVR), i.e., cure in pivotal trials, however, to confirm SVR at 24 and 48 weeks post treatment provides confirmatory evidence of cure [172, 173].

Interferon is a cytokine that participates in the innate immune response to viral infections [174]. Recombinant alpha interferon was approved for the treatment of chronic hepatitis C in 1992 [175]. Alpha interferon therapy was associated with normalization of serum activity of transaminases in patients with chronic hepatitis C but not with (SVR), which was defined as the absence of hepatitis C virus RNA in serum 24 weeks after completion of antiviral therapy [176]. Ribavirin, a nucleoside analogue with antiviral activity against flavivirus, decreased serum activity of aminotransferases and some improvement in liver histology in patients with chronic hepatitis C [177] but, not with a decrease in the serum HCV RNA [177]. In combination with interferon, ribavirin was associated with SVR s of 34% and 38%, when administered for 24 and 48 weeks, respectively [178]. Ribavirin was approved for the treatment of chronic hepatitis C in combination with interferon in 1999. Pegylation of interferon led to its prolonged bioavailability, which allowed for weekly subcutaneous administration. Pegylated interferon and ribavirin for 48 weeks (depending on viral load) was associated with an SVR in 41% to 56% of patients with genotype 1, 74–81% in those with genotypes 2 and 3, and 77% in those with genotype 4 [89]. The proportion of African American patients who achieved SVR with this type of regimen was 28% [179]; this result suggested that racial and genetic factors had a substantial impact on the response to this therapeutic regimen. Subsequently, it was discovered that subjects with a favorable genetic polymorphism in IL28B had an increased probability of reaching SVR in association with treatment with pegylated interferon alpha and ribavirin in contrast to those patients with an unfavorable IL28B genotype. In this regard, a gene coding for IFN-lambda 4 (IFNL4) was documented to be associated with hepatitis C virus clearance in African American patients [180].

Breakthrough findings of the HCV life cycle [181–183], and identification of proteins fundamental in the replication of the HCV [184] have facilitated the development of drugs that act directly on the virus, known as direct-acting antiviral agents (DAA) (Fig. 6.3). The hepatitis C virus undergoes a series of steps to perpetuate infection: (1) entry into the hepatocyte via receptor binding and endocytosis, (2) fusion and uncoating of the virion, (3) translation and polyprotein processing, (4) replication, (5) virion assembly, and (6) transport and release. Telaprevir and boceprevir are inhibitors of the protease NS3-4A, DAAs that were approved in 2011 for the treatment of chronic hepatitis C. The NS3-4A protease breaks the junctions

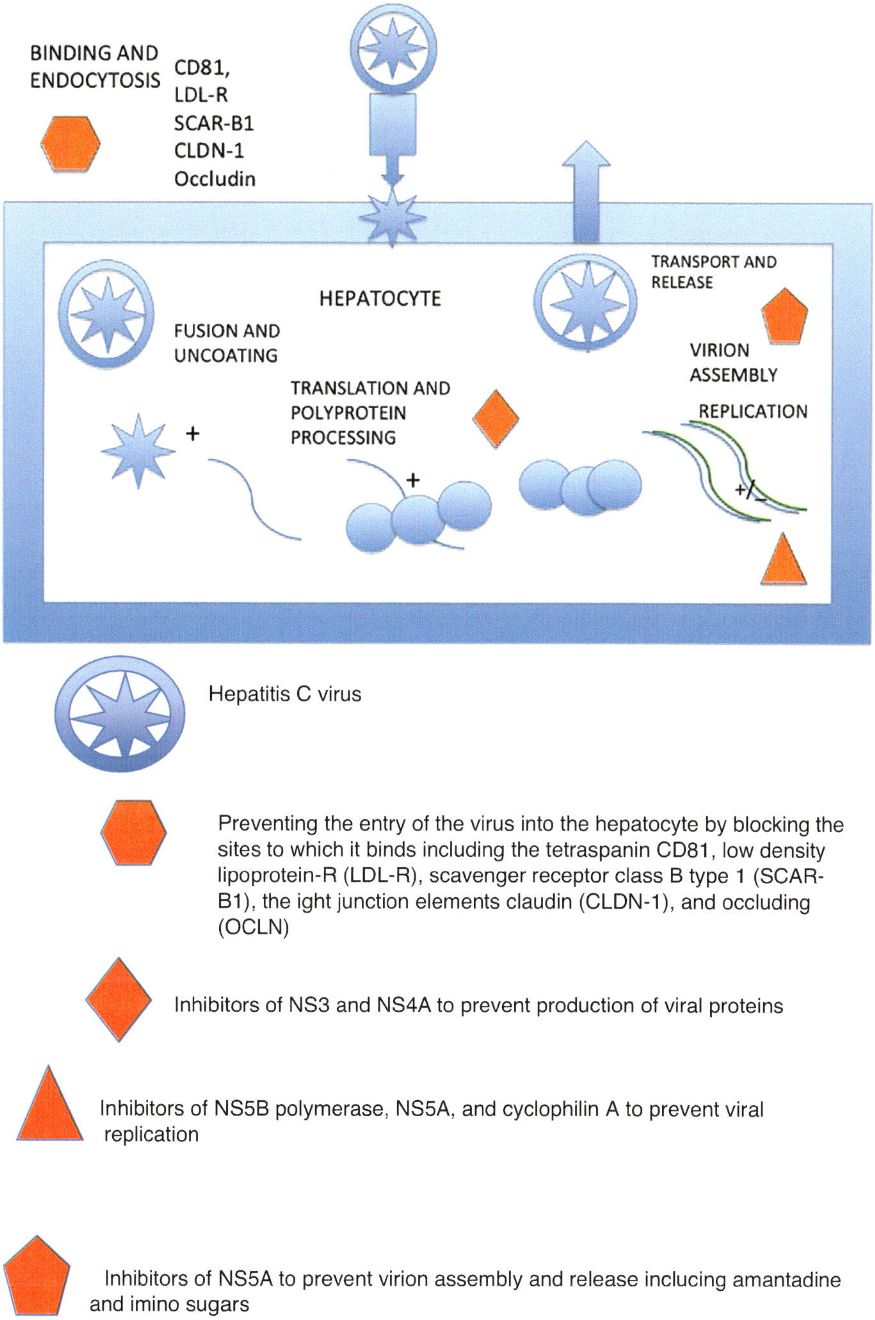

BINDING AND
ENDOCYTOSIS   CD81,
              LDL-R
              SCAR-B1
              CLDN-1
              Occludin

TRANSPORT AND
RELEASE

HEPATOCYTE

FUSION AND
UNCOATING

VIRION
ASSEMBLY

TRANSLATION AND
POLYPROTEIN
PROCESSING

REPLICATION

+

+

+/-

Hepatitis C virus

Preventing the entry of the virus into the hepatocyte by blocking the sites to which it binds including the tetraspanin CD81, low density lipoprotein-R (LDL-R), scavenger receptor class B type 1 (SCAR-B1), the ight junction elements claudin (CLDN-1), and occluding (OCLN)

Inhibitors of NS3 and NS4A to prevent production of viral proteins

Inhibitors of NS5B polymerase, NS5A, and cyclophilin A to prevent viral replication

Inhibitors of NS5A to prevent virion assembly and release inclucing amantadine and imino sugars

**Fig. 6.3** The diagram depicts the hepatitis C virus cycle from entrance into the hepatocyte to the exit of a new virion and therapeutic targets

between NS3/NS4A, NS4A/NS4B, NS4B/NS5A, and NS5A/NS5B [185]. In addition to its role in polyprotein processing, NS3 is necessary for HCV replication and viral assembly and production [186]. Triple therapy with either telaprevir or boceprevir, in combination with pegylated interferon and ribavirin was associated with SVR rates of 75 and 66%, respectively [187, 188], in patients with chronic hepatitis C genotype 1; for boceprevir, the response rate could vary depending on whether patients responded to pegylated interferon and ribavirin with the absence of HCV RNA at week four of treatment, milestone defined as interferon responsivity, which, when achieved, was associated with SVRs of 90%. In patients who had not experienced an SVR in association with standard therapy, the response to triple therapy was lower than in patients who had not been treated [187, 188]. These therapeutic regimes were associated with complications inherent to those of what had been considered standard therapy, i.e., pegylated interferon and ribavirin, such as anemia [187, 188]. The complications added to the regimen from telaprevir included rash, which could be severe, requiring medication discontinuation, in 55% of patients, and anal discomfort in approximately 26%; from boceprevir, dysgeusia was reported by 37% of patients [188]. As both drugs inhibit drug-metabolizing enzymes from the cytochrome P-450 complex, e.g., CYP2C, CYP3A4, and CYP1A, drug interactions were a substantial problem, requiring a change in medication regimen or dose reductions in the medications used to treat comorbidities. Treatment with telaprevir or boceprevir paradigms were also associated with the risk of resistant associated amino acid variants, the prevention of which required absolute adherence to the treatment regimen, and the additional risk of persistence in patients who did not respond to the protease inhibitors paradigm; follow-up studies, however, documented that the prevalence of the resistant mutants decreased over time, with a reversal to a wild-type predominance [189]. The use of telaprevir and boceprevir is not the standard of therapy as new medications with improved efficacy and tolerability have been approved [190].

In 2013, two new medications were approved for the treatment of chronic hepatitis C, including genotypes 1 through 6. Simeprevir is an NS3-4A protease inhibitor that has activity against genotypes 1, 2, and 4, although it is inactive against the resistant associated amino acid variant that carries the Q80K substitution in the NS3 sequence. In combination with standard therapy, simeprevir treatment in patients with chronic hepatitis C genotype 1 for 24 or 48 weeks was associated with an SVR of 74.7–86.1% [191]; in patients who had been treated and who had not responded to therapy, i.e., treatment-experienced patients, simeprevir therapy for 12, 24, and 48 weeks, in combination with pegylated interferon alpha 2 a and ribavirin for 48 weeks, was associated with an SVR of 38% to 89%, depending on the type of failure to prior treatment, e.g., null or partial response, or relapse after response [192]. Sofosbuvir is a uridine nucleotide analogue that inhibits HCV RdRp, which is phosphorylated to its triphosphate form and incorporated into forming RNA chains, resulting in chain termination; it has activity against genotypes 1 through 6, referred to as having pangenotypic activity. In vitro, sofosbuvir does not act against variants that have an S282T in the RdRp sequence; however, these variants did not appear to replicate successfully in vitro or in vivo and had not been associated with a virological breakthrough in patients on treatment, and were only found in those patients who relapsed after treatment had been stopped [193]. The drugs could be administered in combination with standard therapy, i.e., pegylated interferon and ribavirin, or in combination with ribavirin, depending on the infecting genotype, on prior response to standard therapy, and eligibility to receive interferon.

The availability of DDA in interferon-free regimens revolutionized the treatment of chronic hepatitis C, as predicted during the conduct of fundamental clinical trials [170, 171, 194].

Medications including ledipasvir, ombitasvir, daclatasvir, elbasvir, velpatasvir, and pibrentasvir are NS5A inhibitors with coverage against several genotypes, and an intermediate barrier to resistance. NS5A inhibitors inhibit hyperphosphorylation of NS5A phosphoprotein, which is required for HCV RNA replication, and also, cause the transfer of NS5A from the endoplasmic reticulum to lipid droplets in HCV replicon-containing cells leading to a significant reduction of HCV RNA in cell culture [195].

Harvoni® is a combination tablet that contains 90 mg of ledipasvir, an NS5A inhibitor, and 400 mg of sofosbuvir, an NS5B inhibitor that was approved by the FDA in 2014. The NS5B inhibitors act on the catalytic site of NS5B polymerase; after they incorporate themselves into the RNA chain, they cause mRNA termination. Sofosbuvir a nucleotide NS5B polymerase inhibitor and [196]. Results from a meta-analysis showed that the addition of ribavirin did not add benefit to sofosbuvir/ledipasvir for the treatment genotype 1 infection. In a controlled clinical trial, the overall SVR associated with sofosbuvir/ledipasvir in chronic HCV infection genotype 1 was 96%, 98% in the treatment-naïve group versus 95% in the treatment-experienced group, 95% in the 12-week therapy group versus 98% in the 24-week therapy group, 95% without ribavirin vs. 97% with ribavirin [197].

Velpatasvir is a pangenotypic second generation NS5A inhibitor with a higher barrier to resistance than ledipasvir and daclatasvir and which acts as a defective substrate for NS5A to prevent HCV replication. It is used as a fixed dose co-formulation with sofosbuvir under the name of Epclusa®. In a double blind placebo controlled study of 12 weeks, the use of sofosbuvir-velpatasvir in patients with chronic HCV genotypes 1 to 6 was associated with a 99% SVR regardless of prior exposure to treatment, including patients with compensated cirrhosis [198].

Pibrentasvir is a second generation NS5A inhibitor provided in a tablet in combination with glecaprevir under the name of Mavyret®, with a pangenotypic effect, and approved for use in patients with renal failure including patients on hemodialysis.

Sofosbuvir a nucleotide NS5B polymerase inhibitor and [196] ledipasvir, an NS5A inhibitor for the treatment of hepatitis C genotypes 1, 4, 5, and 6 infections is effective. A meta-analysis showed no additional benefit when ribavirin was added to sofosbuvir/ledipasvir for the treatment genotype 1 infection [199].

Dasabuvir is a non-nucleoside NS5B polymerase inhibitor, which binds to the palm domain of NS5B preventing the elongation of HCV RNA, used in combination with paritaprevir/ritonavir-ombitasvir with or without ribavirin for the treatment of hepatitis C genotype 1 infection with or without cirrhosis but, in the compensated state (Child–Pugh A).

The guidelines to treat chronic hepatitis C are updated regularly by the collaboration of the American Association for the Study of Liver Disease (AASLD) and the Infectious Diseases Society of America (IDSA), and they will not be reviewed in this chapter. The reader is referred to the AASLD-IDSA HCV guidance website (www.HCVGuidelines.org), where indication to test for resistance and treatment duration is provided [200]. In general, in preparation for treatment, factors to consider are viral load, genotype, degree of fibrosis, presence or absence of cirrhosis in compensated versus decompensated state, prior treatment, and drug interactions. At present, current illicit drug use is not a contraindication for the treatment of chronic HCV [172]. The SVR rates between patients who use drugs during treatment versus those who do not use tend to be similar. Furthermore, the probability of transmitting HCV from patients being treated for HCV to other individuals, especially if drug paraphernalia is shared, decreases, although patients must be informed of the risk of reinfection by usual transmission modes after successful treatment of chronic HCV.

Hepatitis B reactivation can occur in patients treated with DAA for chronic HCV. A retrospective study that included 62,920 subjects who had been treated for HCV with this type of medications documented that nine had evidence of HBV reactivation during treatment; of these, eight were HBsAg positive, and one was hepatitis B anti-core positive. Seventeen other patients had some increases in serum HBV DNA concentrations not sufficiently high to meet the definition of reactivation as per the study (i.e., HBV >1000 IU/mL or HBsAg detection in a person who was previously negative), and only three of the nine had an increase in ALT twice the upper limit of normal [201]. These results suggested that the probability of major flares is low; however, it is recommended that patients coinfected with HBV be treated to suppression prior to HCV treatment with DAA and that all patients be screened for hepatitis B virus infection prior to initiation of therapy; it is recommended in patients who have hepatitis B anti-core in serum, to check concentrations of HBV DNA. Post treatment follow up is also recommended to determine if flares occur overtime.

Improvement of quality of life measures has been documented in patients who have exhibited an SVR in association with antiviral therapy [202]. Specifically, at baseline (i.e., before antiviral therapy), patients with chronic hepatitis C showed impairment in several functions of the short form (SF)-36 questionnaire including physical function, general health, vitality, and social function, in contrast to a control group of subjects; in association with SVR post treatment, there was documented improvement in health stress, vitality, and social functioning [90], findings generally supported in combined analyses of clinical studies [203]. In addition, antiviral therapy in association with SVR has been reported to decrease cirrhosis progression, deter the development of liver disease complications, and improve survival [204]. Generalized pain and manifestations of sicca syndrome associated with chronic hepatitis C virus infection, measured by the Health-Related Quality of Life (HRQOL), have also been documented to decrease in association with SVR [90].

## Treatment of Conditions Associated with Chronic Hepatitis C

### *Cryoglobulinemia*

There is some reported experience on the effect of direct-acting antiviral (DAA) drugs on cryoglobulinemic vasculitis with encouraging results, i.e., eradication of the virus is associated with a reduction of cryoglobulins and increase in C4 levels, and a substantial decrease in the vasculitis complications [205]. In patients with serious complications of vasculitis, including glomerulonephritis, peripheral neuropathy, and chronic skin ulcers, rituximab may be considered. Rituximab is a chimeric monoclonal antibody against the CD20 antigen expressed on pre-B cells and mature lymphocytes. It is also expressed by the cells expanded and activated in patients with cryoglobulinemic vasculitis. High-dose pulsed glucocorticoid therapy may be useful in severe conditions and can be considered in combination with rituximab; the chronic use of low or medium doses of glucocorticoids has not been supported [206]. Apheresis was recommended for the treatment of complications from severe hyperviscosity syndrome [206]. The addition of cyclophosphamide to apheresis has been proposed, although the experience is minimal [206]. Colchicine was reported as a therapeutic option, but the reported experience is also limited [206].

A prospective 15-year study has offered the opportunity to document the natural history of patients with chronic hepatitis C and cryoglobulinemia. Nine hundred fifty patients with chronic hepatitis C, 246 (25.8%) of whom had mixed cryoglobulinemia, and 184 of these (74%) cryoglobulinemia syndrome were included; 141 patients with cryoglobulinemia syndrome and 601 without mixed cryoglobulinemia completed the study, which was from 1990 to 2010. None of the patients had a spontaneous clearance of cryoglobulins. A switch from type II to type III cryoglobulinemia was documented in 1.6% at a rate of 0.08% per year. The 15-year probability of developing cirrhosis was significantly higher in patients without mixed cryoglobulinemia, 24.9%, than in patients with cryoglobulinemia syndrome, 14.2%, and the risk of developing hepatocellular carcinoma was also significantly different, 20.3% in patients without mixed cryoglobulinemia and 7.5% with cryoglobulinemia syndrome. Renal insufficiency, neuropathies, and B cell non-Hodgkin lymphoma were developed significantly more frequently in patients with cryoglobulinemia syndrome, 32.6, 31.2, and 15%, respectively; in those without mixed cryoglobulinemia, the rate of developing the complications reported was less than 10%. Antiviral therapy with interferon and ribavirin was associated with a sustained virological response, defined as the absence of serum hepatitis C RNA 6 months after treatment and associated with improved prognosis [176], was 44% in patients with cryoglobulinemia syndrome, and 53% in patients without mixed cryoglobulinemia. The 15-year survival rate was 70% for both groups, despite the complications reported to be more common in patients with cryoglobulinemia syndrome [131].

## Porphyria Cutanea Tarda

The treatment of porphyria cutanea tarda (PCT) includes avoiding the sun and other known triggers of expression, including alcohol, cigarette smoking, and estrogen exposure, and removal of iron, and anti-malarial medications that remove tissue porphyrins. The published experience of the treatment of patients with PCT in association with chronic hepatitis C is minimal and inconsistent, with reports documenting response [141, 207, 208] or lack of it [209] to antiviral therapy with interferon and ribavirin. In addition, reports document the development of PCT after this type of antiviral therapy [210, 211]. The literature on treatment with DAA in patients with HCV and PCT is limited; in a series of 12 patients, two patients had PCT and, on therapy with DAA, one experienced a reduction of plasma porphyrins, and the other its disappearance, at the end of treatment [212].

## Nephropathy

The treatment goal of hepatitis C associated glomerulopathies is to eradicate the virus by antiviral therapy; however, there are limited data on the success of this approach. In patients with rapidly progressing renal disease, steroids, immunosuppressors, plasmapheresis, and monoclonal antibody rituximab are recommended [150].

## Xerostomia and Xerophthalmia

Therapy of primary Sjogren's syndrome with interferon has been reported to be associated with improvement in glandular function [213]. A study published in French reported improvement of sicca symptoms in patients with chronic hepatitis C treated and cured with interferon and ribavirin. Specific reports on the effect of DAAs on this complication of chronic hepatitis C were not found.

## Lichen Planus

The therapy of lichen planus has been corticosteroids and other various immunosuppressants orally or topically, depending on the location, and phototherapy [162]. Antiviral therapy with interferon alone or with ribavirin in patients with chronic hepatitis C has been associated with worsening of lichen planus [214, 215]. Improvement of symptoms secondary to oral lichen planus has been associated with treatment with DAAs [216, 217].

## Liver Transplantation

Liver disease from chronic hepatitis C is a common indication for liver transplantation in Europe and the United States (www.unos.org); however, infection of the graft happens in all the patients [218, 219] and which has been calculated to progress to cirrhosis within 5–10 years post transplantation [220]. Graft infection is associated with graft loss and the need for retransplant [219, 220]. Ballooning degeneration and hyperbilirubinemia are histological and clinical features that predict the development of cirrhosis in the transplanted liver in patients with recurrent hepatitis C [221]. Fibrosing cholestatic hepatitis is a particularly aggressive type of liver injury associated with recurrent hepatitis C that leads to graft loss in months after its presentation, which is characterized by marked hyperbilirubinemia [222, 223]. Post transplant immunosuppression is one of the factors contributing to the recurrence of HCV infection in the graft and the rapid progression to fibrosis and cirrhosis [222]. It has been reported that the administration of corticosteroid boluses and anti-lymphocyte antibodies to treat rejection are associated with increased severity of liver disease upon viral recurrence and that relatively low doses of steroids and their slow tapering, and the absence of steroids in pharmacological maintenance regimens are associated with a decrease in disease progression [219, 224]; however, hard conclusions have not been derived.

A retrospective study that included 39 patients who had undergone liver transplantation between 1991 to 1999 and who had cirrhosis post liver transplantation documented that 18 had one episode of decompensation within a median of 7.8 months after the operation with 93% of patients developing ascites [220]. The variables associated with decompensation, retransplantation, or death have been reported to be a Child–Pugh class B or C, serum albumin lower than 3.5 g, presence of cirrhosis within 15.3 (range 3.7–46.1) months from the operation, high serum cyclosporine levels at the time of the diagnosis of cirrhosis, and hepatic venous pressure gradient (HVPG) $\geq 10$ mmHg [220, 225]. The cumulative probability for decompensation, and graft and patient survival at 1 year was 42%, 71%, and 74%, respectively [220], and significantly lower than that of patients who have not undergone liver transplantation [220, 224]. In association with sustained virological response, antiviral therapy has been reported to deter the progression of liver disease in graft viral hepatitis C [226]. SVR rates in the post transplant setting had been relatively low, but, have improved in association with treatment with DAA [227].

A systematic review and meta-analysis from studies published on the subject of treatment of chronic HCV post recurrence in liver transplant patients with genotype 1 and that included 885 patients documented an overall pooled estimate proportion of SVR12 as 93% (95% CI: 0.89, 0.96) with moderate heterogeneity identified ($\tau^2 = 0.01$, $P < 0.01$, I2 = 75%). The highest pooled estimate SVR12 proportion was for sofosbuvir/ledipasvir, followed by paritaprevir/ritonavir/ombitasvir/dasabuvir, daclatasvir/simeprevir ± ribavirin, sofosbuvir/simeprevir ± RBV, and asunaprevir/daclatasvir. The METAVIR is an algorithm for the grading of activity in chronic hepatitis C [75]. The pools of patients with METAVIR stages F0 to F2 tended to show a higher proportion of SVR12, 97% (95% CI: 0.93, 0.99) versus 85% (95% CI: 0.79, 0.90) for stages F3-F4 ($P < 0.01$); the use of ribavirin was not associated with any significant differences in outcome. These data suggested that DAAs are well tolerated and efficacious in treating recurrent HCV post liver transplantation [228]. The use of DAA in the post transplant setting continues to evolve.

Patients with chronic hepatitis C should be evaluated for treatment, and monitored for disease progression, including the development of hepatocellular carcinoma; in cases of fibrosis stages 3 to 4, or documented cirrhosis, surveillance for HCV should continue regardless of HCV cure, as patients remain at risk for HCC. Vaccination against viral hepatitis A and B is recommended.

**Acknowledgments** The author acknowledges Dr. Cesar del Rosario for having contributed Figure 6.2.

# References

1. Kato N. Genome of human hepatitis C virus (HCV): gene organization, sequence diversity, and variation. Microb Comp Genomics. 2000;5(3):129–51.
2. Op De Beeck A, Dubuisson J. Topology of hepatitis C virus envelope glycoproteins. Rev Med Virol. 2003 July–Aug;13(4):233–41.
3. Dubuisson J. Hepatitis C virus proteins. World J Gastroenterol WJG. 2007 May 7;13(17):2406–15.
4. Lindenbach BD, Rice CM. Unravelling hepatitis C virus replication from genome to function. Nature. 2005 Aug 18;436(7053):933–8.
5. Walewski JL, Keller TR, Stump DD, Branch AD. Evidence for a new hepatitis C virus antigen encoded in an overlapping reading frame. RNA. 2001 May;7(5):710–21.
6. Branch AD, Stump DD, Gutierrez JA, Eng F, Walewski JL. The hepatitis C virus alternate reading frame (ARF) and its family of novel products: the alternate reading frame protein/F--protein, the double-frameshift protein, and others. Semin Liver Dis. 2005 Feb;25(1):105–17.
7. Bartenschlager R, Lohmann V. Replication of hepatitis C virus. J Gen Virol. 2000 Jul;81(Pt 7):1631–48.
8. Martell M, Esteban JI, Quer J, Genesca J, Weiner A, Esteban R, et al. Hepatitis C virus (HCV) circulates as a population of different but closely related genomes: quasispecies nature of HCV genome distribution. J Virol. 1992 May;66(5):3225–9.
9. Domingo E, Sabo D, Taniguchi T, Weissmann C. Nucleotide sequence heterogeneity of an RNA phage population. Cell. 1978 Apr;13(4):735–44.
10. Holland JJ, De La Torre JC, Steinhauer DA. RNA virus populations as quasispecies. Curr Top Microbiol Immunol. 1992;176:1–20.
11. Farci P, Shimoda A, Coiana A, Diaz G, Peddis G, Melpolder JC, et al. The outcome of acute hepatitis C predicted by the evolution of the viral quasispecies. Science. 2000 Apr 14;288(5464):339–44.
12. Simmonds P. Genetic diversity and evolution of hepatitis C virus--15 years on. J Gen Virol. 2004 Nov;85(Pt 11):3173–88.
13. Agnello V, Abel G, Elfahal M, Knight GB, Zhang QX. Hepatitis C virus and other flaviviridae viruses enter cells via low density lipoprotein receptor. Proc Natl Acad Sci USA. 1999 Oct 26;96(22):12766–71.
14. Zeisel MB, Barth H, Schuster C, Baumert TF. Hepatitis C virus entry: molecular mechanisms and targets for antiviral therapy. Front Biosci. 2009;14:3274–85.

15. Farci P. New insights into the HCV quasispecies and compartmentalization. Semin Liver Dis. 2011 Nov;31(4):356–74.
16. Forton DM, Karayiannis P, Mahmud N, Taylor-Robinson SD, Thomas HC. Identification of unique hepatitis C virus quasispecies in the central nervous system and comparative analysis of internal translational efficiency of brain, liver, and serum variants. J Virol. 2004 May;78(10):5170–83.
17. Bartenschlager R. Unexpected host range of hepatitis C virus replicons. Hepatology. 2004 Mar;39(3):835–8.
18. Deforges S, Evlashev A, Perret M, Sodoyer M, Pouzol S, Scoazec JY, et al. Expression of hepatitis C virus proteins in epithelial intestinal cells in vivo. J Gen Virol. 2004 Sep;85(Pt 9):2515–23.
19. Micallef JM, Kaldor JM, Dore GJ. Spontaneous viral clearance following acute hepatitis C infection: a systematic review of longitudinal studies. J Viral Hepat. 2006 Jan;13(1):34–41.
20. McKiernan SM, Hagan R, Curry M, McDonald GS, Kelly A, Nolan N, et al. Distinct MHC class I and II alleles are associated with hepatitis C viral clearance, originating from a single source. Hepatology. 2004 Jul;40(1):108–14.
21. Kim AY, Kuntzen T, Timm J, Nolan BE, Baca MA, Reyor LL, et al. Spontaneous control of HCV is associated with expression of HLA-B 57 and preservation of targeted epitopes. Gastroenterology. 2011 Feb;140(2):686–96.
22. Neumann-Haefelin C, McKiernan S, Ward S, Viazov S, Spangenberg HC, Killinger T, et al. Dominant influence of an HLA-B27 restricted CD8+ T cell response in mediating HCV clearance and evolution. Hepatology. 2006 Mar;43(3):563–72.
23. Valenti L, Rumi M, Galmozzi E, Aghemo A, Del Menico B, De Nicola S, et al. Patatin-like phospholipase domain-containing 3 I148M polymorphism, steatosis, and liver damage in chronic hepatitis C. Hepatology. 2011 Mar;53(3):791–9.
24. Trepo E, Pradat P, Potthoff A, Momozawa Y, Quertinmont E, Gustot T, et al. Impact of patatin-like phospholipase-3 (rs738409 C>G) polymorphism on fibrosis progression and steatosis in chronic hepatitis C. Hepatology. 2011 Jul;54(1):60–9.
25. Liu L, Fisher BE, Thomas DL, Cox AL, Ray SC. Spontaneous clearance of primary acute hepatitis C virus infection correlated with high initial viral RNA level and rapid HVR1 evolution. Hepatology. 2012 Jun;55(6):1684–91.
26. Tanaka Y, Nishida N, Sugiyama M, Kurosaki M, Matsuura K, Sakamoto N, et al. Genome-wide association of IL28B with response to pegylated interferon-alpha and ribavirin therapy for chronic hepatitis C. Nat Genet. 2009 Oct;41(10):1105–9.
27. Kimura T, Saito T, Yoshimura M, Yixuan S, Baba M, Ji G, et al. Association of transforming growth factor-beta 1 functional polymorphisms with natural clearance of hepatitis C virus. J Infect Dis. 2006 May 15;193(10):1371–4.
28. Castriconi R, Cantoni C, Della Chiesa M, Vitale M, Marcenaro E, Conte R, et al. Transforming growth factor beta 1 inhibits expression of NKp30 and NKG2D receptors: consequences for the NK-mediated killing of dendritic cells. Proc Natl Acad Sci U S A. 2003 Apr 1;100(7):4120–5.
29. Khakoo SI, Thio CL, Martin MP, Brooks CR, Gao X, Astemborski J, et al. HLA and NK cell inhibitory receptor genes in resolving hepatitis C virus infection. Science. 2004 Aug 6;305(5685):872–4.
30. Thomas DL, Thio CL, Martin MP, Qi Y, Ge D, O'Huigin C, et al. Genetic variation in IL28B and spontaneous clearance of hepatitis C virus. Nature. 2009 Oct 8;461(7265):798–801.
31. Amadei B, Urbani S, Cazaly A, Fisicaro P, Zerbini A, Ahmed P, et al. Activation of natural killer cells during acute infection with hepatitis C virus. Gastroenterology. 2010 Apr;138(4):1536–45.
32. Alter G, Jost S, Rihn S, Reyor LL, Nolan BE, Ghebremichael M, et al. Reduced frequencies of NKp30+NKp46+, CD161+, and NKG2D+ NK cells in acute HCV infection may predict viral clearance. J Hepatol. 2011 Aug;55(2):278–88.

33. Werner JM, Heller T, Gordon AM, Sheets A, Sherker AH, Kessler E, et al. Innate immune responses in hepatitis C virus-exposed healthcare workers who do not develop acute infection. Hepatology. 2013 Nov;58(5):1621–31.
34. Ahlenstiel G, Titerence RH, Koh C, Edlich B, Feld JJ, Rotman Y, et al. Natural killer cells are polarized toward cytotoxicity in chronic hepatitis C in an interferon-alfa-dependent manner. Gastroenterology. 2010 Jan;138(1):325–35.e1-2.
35. Kramer B, Korner C, Kebschull M, Glassner A, Eisenhardt M, Nischalke HD, et al. Natural killer p46High expression defines a natural killer cell subset that is potentially involved in control of hepatitis C virus replication and modulation of liver fibrosis. Hepatology. 2012 Oct;56(4):1201–13.
36. Eisenhardt M, Glassner A, Kramer B, Korner C, Sibbing B, Kokordelis P, et al. The CXCR3(+) CD56Bright phenotype characterizes a distinct NK cell subset with anti-fibrotic potential that shows dys-regulated activity in hepatitis C. PLoS One. 2012;7(7):e38846.
37. Neumann-Haefelin C, Thimme R. Adaptive immune responses in hepatitis C virus infection. Curr Top Microbiol Immunol. 2013;369:243–62.
38. Bartosch B, Dubuisson J, Cosset FL. Infectious hepatitis C virus pseudo-particles containing functional E1-E2 envelope protein complexes. J Exp Med. 2003 Mar 3;197(5):633–42.
39. Pestka JM, Zeisel MB, Blaser E, Schurmann P, Bartosch B, Cosset FL, et al. Rapid induction of virus-neutralizing antibodies and viral clearance in a single-source outbreak of hepatitis C. Proc Natl Acad Sci U S A. 2007 Apr 3;104(14):6025–30.
40. Takaki A, Wiese M, Maertens G, Depla E, Seifert U, Liebetrau A, et al. Cellular immune responses persist and humoral responses decrease two decades after recovery from a single-source outbreak of hepatitis C. Nat Med. 2000 May;6(5):578–82.
41. Lai ME, Mazzoleni AP, Argiolu F, De Virgilis S, Balestrieri A, Purcell RH, et al. Hepatitis C virus in multiple episodes of acute hepatitis in polytransfused thalassaemic children. Lancet. 1994 Feb 12;343(8894):388–90.
42. Grakoui A, Shoukry NH, Woollard DJ, Han JH, Hanson HL, Ghrayeb J, et al. HCV persistence and immune evasion in the absence of memory T cell help. Science. 2003 Oct 24;302(5645):659–62.
43. Lechner F, Wong DK, Dunbar PR, Chapman R, Chung RT, Dohrenwend P, et al. Analysis of successful immune responses in persons infected with hepatitis C virus. J Exp Med. 2000 May 1;191(9):1499–512.
44. Thimme R, Oldach D, Chang KM, Steiger C, Ray SC, Chisari FV. Determinants of viral clearance and persistence during acute hepatitis C virus infection. J Exp Med. 2001 Nov 19;194(10):1395–406.
45. Sugimoto K, Ikeda F, Stadanlick J, Nunes FA, Alter HJ, Chang KM. Suppression of HCV-specific T cells without differential hierarchy demonstrated ex vivo in persistent HCV infection. Hepatology. 2003 Dec;38(6):1437–48.
46. Aberle JH, Formann E, Steindl-Munda P, Weseslindtner L, Gurguta C, Perstinger G, et al. Prospective study of viral clearance and CD4(+) T-cell response in acute hepatitis C primary infection and reinfection. J Clin Virol. 2006 May;36(1):24–31.
47. Ward SM, Fox BC, Brown PJ, Worthington J, Fox SB, Chapman RW, et al. Quantification and localisation of FOXP3+ T lymphocytes and relation to hepatic inflammation during chronic HCV infection. J Hepatol. 2007 Sep;47(3):316–24.
48. Diepolder HM, Zachoval R, Hoffmann RM, Wierenga EA, Santantonio T, Jung MC, et al. Possible mechanism involving T-lymphocyte response to non-structural protein 3 in viral clearance in acute hepatitis C virus infection. Lancet. 1995 Oct 14;346(8981):1006–7.
49. Missale G, Bertoni R, Lamonaca V, Valli A, Massari M, Mori C, et al. Different clinical behaviors of acute hepatitis C virus infection are associated with different vigor of the anti-viral cell-mediated immune response. J Clin Invest. 1996 Aug 1;98(3):706–14.
50. Fitzmaurice K, Petrovic D, Ramamurthy N, Simmons R, Merani S, Gaudieri S, et al. Molecular footprints reveal the impact of the protective HLA-A*03 allele in hepatitis C virus infection. Gut. 2011 Nov;60(11):1563–71.

51. Neumann-Haefelin C, Thimme R. Success and failure of virus-specific T cell responses in hepatitis C virus infection. Dig Dis. 2011;29(4):416–22.
52. Jo J, Aichele U, Kersting N, Klein R, Aichele P, Bisse E, et al. Analysis of CD8+ T-cell-mediated inhibition of hepatitis C virus replication using a novel immunological model. Gastroenterology. 2009 Apr;136(4):1391–401.
53. Rushbrook SM, Ward SM, Unitt E, Vowler SL, Lucas M, Klenerman P, et al. Regulatory T cells suppress in vitro proliferation of virus-specific CD8+ T cells during persistent hepatitis C virus infection. J Virol. 2005 Jun;79(12):7852–9.
54. Shoukry NH, Grakoui A, Houghton M, Chien DY, Ghrayeb J, Reimann KA, et al. Memory CD8+ T cells are required for protection from persistent hepatitis C virus infection. J Exp Med. 2003 Jun 16;197(12):1645–55.
55. Gruener NH, Lechner F, Jung MC, Diepolder H, Gerlach T, Lauer G, et al. Sustained dysfunction of antiviral CD8+ T lymphocytes after infection with hepatitis C virus. J Virol. 2001 Jun;75(12):5550–8.
56. Spangenberg HC, Viazov S, Kersting N, Neumann-Haefelin C, McKinney D, Roggendorf M, et al. Intrahepatic CD8+ T-cell failure during chronic hepatitis C virus infection. Hepatology. 2005 Oct;42(4):828–37.
57. Nakamoto N, Kaplan DE, Coleclough J, Li Y, Valiga ME, Kaminski M, et al. Functional restoration of HCV-specific CD8 T cells by PD-1 blockade is defined by PD-1 expression and compartmentalization. Gastroenterology. 2008 June;134(7):1927–37.e1-2.
58. Urbani S, Amadei B, Tola D, Massari M, Schivazappa S, Missale G, et al. PD-1 expression in acute hepatitis C virus (HCV) infection is associated with HCV-specific CD8 exhaustion. J Virol. 2006 Nov;80(22):11398–403.
59. Rutebemberwa A, Ray SC, Astemborski J, Levine J, Liu L, Dowd KA, et al. High-programmed death-1 levels on hepatitis C virus-specific T cells during acute infection are associated with viral persistence and require preservation of cognate antigen during chronic infection. J Immunol. 2008 Dec 15;181(12):8215–25.
60. Abel M, Sene D, Pol S, Bourliere M, Poynard T, Charlotte F, et al. Intrahepatic virus-specific IL-10-producing CD8 T cells prevent liver damage during chronic hepatitis C virus infection. Hepatology. 2006 Dec;44(6):1607–16.
61. http://www.who.int/mediacentre/factsheets/fs164/en/.
62. Ly KN, Xing J, Klevens RM, Jiles RB, Ward JW, Holmberg SD. The increasing burden of mortality from viral hepatitis in the United States between 1999 and 2007. Ann Intern Med. 2012 Feb 21;156(4):271–8.
63. Joy JB, McCloskey RM, Nguyen T, Liang RH, Khudyakov Y, Olmstead A, et al. The spread of hepatitis C virus genotype 1a in North America: a retrospective phylogenetic study. Lancet Infect Dis. 2016 June;16(6):698–702.
64. Yarnell S, Li L, MacGrory B, Trevisan L, Kirwin P. Substance use disorders in later life: a review and synthesis of the literature of an emerging public health concern. Am J Geriatr Psychiatry. 2020 Feb;28(2):226–36.
65. Geboy AG, Mahajan S, Daly AP, Sewell CF, Fleming IC, Cha HA, et al. High hepatitis C infection rate among baby boomers in an urban primary care clinic: results from the HepTLC initiative. Public Health Rep. 2016 May-Jun;131(Suppl 2):49–56.
66. US Preventive Services Task Force, Owens DK, Davidson KW, Krist AH, Barry MJ, Cabana M, et al. Screening for hepatitis C virus infection in adolescents and adults: US preventive services task Force recommendation statement. JAMA. 2020 Mar;323:970–5.
67. Alter MJ. HCV routes of transmission: what goes around comes around. Semin Liver Dis. 2011 Nov;31(4):340–6.
68. http://www.cdc.gov/hepatitis/hcv/hcvfaq.htm.
69. Alter HJ, Purcell RH, Shih JW, Melpolder JC, Houghton M, Choo QL, et al. Detection of antibody to hepatitis C virus in prospectively followed transfusion recipients with acute and chronic non-A, non-B hepatitis. N Engl J Med. 1989 Nov 30;321(22):1494–500.

70. Gerlach JT, Diepolder HM, Zachoval R, Gruener NH, Jung MC, Ulsenheimer A, et al. Acute hepatitis C: high rate of both spontaneous and treatment-induced viral clearance. Gastroenterology. 2003 July;125(1):80–8.

71. Thomas DL, Astemborski J, Rai RM, Anania FA, Schaeffer M, Galai N, et al. The natural history of hepatitis C virus infection: host, viral, and environmental factors. JAMA. 2000 July 26;284(4):450–6.

72. Villano SA, Vlahov D, Nelson KE, Cohn S, Thomas DL. Persistence of viremia and the importance of long-term follow-up after acute hepatitis C infection. Hepatology. 1999 Mar;29(3):908–14.

73. Hofer H, Watkins-Riedel T, Janata O, Penner E, Holzmann H, Steindl-Munda P, et al. Spontaneous viral clearance in patients with acute hepatitis C can be predicted by repeated measurements of serum viral load. Hepatology. 2003 Jan;37(1):60–4.

74. Larghi A, Zuin M, Crosignani A, Ribero ML, Pipia C, Battezzati PM, et al. Outcome of an outbreak of acute hepatitis C among healthy volunteers participating in pharmacokinetics studies. Hepatology. 2002 Oct;36(4 Pt 1):993–1000.

75. Poynard T, Bedossa P, Opolon P. Natural history of liver fibrosis progression in patients with chronic hepatitis C. the OBSVIRC, METAVIR, CLINIVIR, and DOSVIRC groups. Lancet. 1997 Mar 22;349(9055):825–32.

76. Sangiovanni A, Prati GM, Fasani P, Ronchi G, Romeo R, Manini M, et al. The natural history of compensated cirrhosis due to hepatitis C virus: a 17-year cohort study of 214 patients. Hepatology. 2006 June;43(6):1303–10.

77. Bedogni G, Miglioli L, Masutti F, Ferri S, Castiglione A, Lenzi M, et al. Natural course of chronic HCV and HBV infection and role of alcohol in the general population: the Dionysos study. Am J Gastroenterol. 2008 Sep;103(9):2248–53.

78. Albloushi SS, Murray FE, Callagy G, Courtney MG, O'Keane JC, Kay E. Changes in liver histopathology in women infected with hepatitis C through contaminated anti-D immuno-globulin injections in Ireland. Eur J Gastroenterol Hepatol. 1998 Jan;10(1):69–73.

79. Barrett S, Goh J, Coughlan B, Ryan E, Stewart S, Cockram A, et al. The natural course of hepatitis C virus infection after 22 years in a unique homogenous cohort: spontaneous viral clearance and chronic HCV infection. Gut. 2001 Sep;49(3):423–30.

80. Rubbia-Brandt L, Fabris P, Paganin S, Leandro G, Male PJ, Giostra E, et al. Steatosis affects chronic hepatitis C progression in a genotype specific way. Gut. 2004 Mar;53(3):406–12.

81. Konerman MA, Mehta SH, Sutcliffe CG, Vu T, Higgins Y, Torbenson MS, et al. Fibrosis progression in human immunodeficiency virus/hepatitis C virus coinfected adults: prospective analysis of 435 liver biopsy pairs. Hepatology. 2014 Mar;59(3):767–75.

82. Kenny-Walsh E. Clinical outcomes after hepatitis C infection from contaminated anti-D immune globulin. Irish Hepatology Research Group. N Engl J Med. 1999 Apr 22;340(16):1228–33.

83. Williams AL, Hoofnagle JH. Ratio of serum aspartate to alanine aminotransferase in chronic hepatitis. Relationship to cirrhosis. Gastroenterology. 1988 Sep;95(3):734–9.

84. Nyblom H, Berggren U, Balldin J, Olsson R. High AST/ALT ratio may indicate advanced alcoholic liver disease rather than heavy drinking. Alcohol Alcohol. 2004 Jul-Aug;39(4):336–9.

85. Alter MJ, Kuhnert WL, Finelli L, Centers for Disease Control and Prevention. Guidelines for laboratory testing and result reporting of antibody to hepatitis C virus. Centers for Disease Control and Prevention. MMWR Recommendations and reports : Morbidity and mortality weekly report Recommendations and reports/Centers for Disease Control. 2003 Feb 7;52(RR-3):1–13.

86. Lee SR, Kardos KW, Schiff E, Berne CA, Mounzer K, Banks AT, et al. Evaluation of a new, rapid test for detecting HCV infection, suitable for use with blood or oral fluid. J Virol Methods. 2011 Mar;172(1–2):27–31.

87. http://www.fda.gov.

88. Alter MJ, Margolis HS, Krawczynski K, Judson FN, Mares A, Alexander WJ, et al. The natural history of community-acquired hepatitis C in the United States. The sentinel counties chronic non-A, non-B Hepatitis Study Team. N Engl J Med. 1992 Dec 31;327(27):1899–905.
89. Fried MW, Shiffman ML, Reddy KR, Smith C, Marinos G, Goncales FL Jr, et al. Peginterferon alfa-2a plus ribavirin for chronic hepatitis C virus infection. N Engl J Med. 2002 Sep 26;347(13):975–82.
90. Ware JE Jr, Bayliss MS, Mannocchia M, Davis GL. Health-related quality of life in chronic hepatitis C: impact of disease and treatment response. The Interventional Therapy Group. Hepatology. 1999 Aug;30(2):550–5.
91. Cassani F, Cataleta M, Valentini P, Muratori P, Giostra F, Francesconi R, et al. Serum auto-antibodies in chronic hepatitis C: comparison with autoimmune hepatitis and impact on the disease profile. Hepatology. 1997 Sep;26(3):561–6.
92. Narciso-Schiavon JL, Freire FC, Suarez MM, Ferrari MV, Scanhola GQ, Schiavon Lde L, et al. Antinuclear antibody positivity in patients with chronic hepatitis C: clinically relevant or an epiphenomenon? Eur J Gastroenterol Hepatol. 2009 Apr;21(4):440–6.
93. Chretien P, Chousterman M, Abd Alsamad I, Ozenne V, Rosa I, Barrault C, et al. Non-organ-specific autoantibodies in chronic hepatitis C patients: association with histological activity and fibrosis. J Autoimmun. 2009 May-Jun;32(3–4):201–5.
94. Marconcini ML, Fayad L, Shiozawa MB, Dantas-Correa EB, Lucca Schiavon L, Narciso-Schiavon JL. Autoantibody profile in individuals with chronic hepatitis C. Rev Soc Bras Med Trop. 2013 Mar-Apr;46(2):147–53.
95. Mauss S, Berger F, Schober A, Moog G, Heyne R, John C, et al. Screening for autoantibodies in chronic hepatitis C patients has no effect on treatment initiation or outcome. J Viral Hepat. 2013 Apr;20(4):e72–7.
96. Schmid M, Pirovino M, Altorfer J, Gudat F, Bianchi L. Acute hepatitis non-A, non-B; are there any specific light microscopic features? Liver. 1982 Mar;2(1):61–7.
97. Kryger P, Christoffersen P. Light microscopic morphology of acute hepatitis non-A, non-B. A comparison with hepatitis type A and B. Liver. 1982 Sep;2(3):200–6.
98. Scheuer PJ, Ashrafzadeh P, Sherlock S, Brown D, Dusheiko GM. The pathology of hepatitis C. Hepatology. 1992 Apr;15(4):567–71.
99. Gerber MA, Krawczynski K, Alter MJ, Sampliner RE, Margolis HS. Histopathology of community acquired chronic hepatitis C. the sentinel counties chronic non-A, non-B Hepatitis Study Team. Mod Pathol. 1992 Sep;5(5):483–6.
100. Roberts JM, Searle JW, Cooksley WG. Histological patterns of prolonged hepatitis C infection. Gastroenterol Jpn. 1993 May;28(Suppl 5):37–41.
101. Poulsen H, Christoffersen P. Abnormal bile duct epithelium in liver biopsies with histological signs of viral hepatitis. Acta Pathol Microbiol Scand. 1969;76(3):383–90.
102. Vyberg M. Diverticular bile duct lesion in chronic active hepatitis. Hepatology. 1989 Nov;10(5):774–80.
103. Mosnier JF, Degott C, Marcellin P, Henin D, Erlinger S, Benhamou JP. The intraportal lymphoid nodule and its environment in chronic active hepatitis C: an immunohistochemical study. Hepatology. 1993 Mar;17(3):366–71.
104. Walewska-Zielecka B, Madalinski K, Jablonska J, Godzik P, Cielecka-Kuszyk J, Litwinska B. Composition of inflammatory infiltrate and its correlation with HBV/HCV antigen expression. World J Gastroenterol WJG. 2008 July 7;14(25):4040–6.
105. Zhang L, Zhao Y. The regulation of Foxp3 expression in regulatory CD4(+)CD25(+)T cells: multiple pathways on the road. J Cell Physiol. 2007 Jun;211(3):590–7.
106. de Goer de Herve MG, Jaafoura S, Vallee M, Taoufik Y. FoxP3(+) regulatory CD4 T cells control the generation of functional CD8 memory. Nat Commun. 2012;3:986.
107. Claassen MA, de Knegt RJ, Tilanus HW, Janssen HL, Boonstra A. Abundant numbers of regulatory T cells localize to the liver of chronic hepatitis C infected patients and limit the extent of fibrosis. J Hepatol. 2010 Mar;52(3):315–21.

108. Langhans B, Kramer B, Louis M, Nischalke HD, Huneburg R, Staratschek-Jox A, et al. Intrahepatic IL-8 producing Foxp3(+)CD4(+) regulatory T cells and fibrogenesis in chronic hepatitis C. J Hepatol. 2013 Aug;59(2):229–35.
109. Sturm N, Thelu MA, Camous X, Dimitrov G, Ramzan M, Dufeu-Duchesne T, et al. Characterization and role of intra-hepatic regulatory T cells in chronic hepatitis C pathogenesis. J Hepatol. 2010 Jul;53(1):25–35.
110. Goodman ZD, Ishak KG. Histopathology of hepatitis C virus infection. Semin Liver Dis. 1995 Feb;15(1):70–81.
111. Poynard T, Ngo Y, Perazzo H, Munteanu M, Lebray P, Moussalli J, et al. Prognostic value of liver fibrosis biomarkers: a meta-analysis. Gastroenterol Hepatol. 2011 July;7(7):445–54.
112. Asselah T, Marcellin P, Bedossa P. Improving performance of liver biopsy in fibrosis assessment. J Hepatol. 2014 Aug;61(2):193–5.
113. Cacoub P, Renou C, Rosenthal E, Cohen P, Loury I, Loustaud-Ratti V, et al. Extrahepatic manifestations associated with hepatitis C virus infection. A prospective multicenter study of 321 patients. The GERMIVIC. Groupe d'Etude et de Recherche en Medecine Interne et Maladies Infectieuses sur le Virus de l'Hepatite C. Medicine. 2000 Jan;79(1):47–56.
114. Yamada S, Mine S, Fujisaki T, Ohnari N, Eto S, Tanaka Y. Hepatic sarcoidosis associated with chronic hepatitis C. J Gastroenterol. 2002;37(7):564–70.
115. Bonnet F, Morlat P, Dubuc J, De Witte S, Bonarek M, Bernard N, et al. Sarcoidosis-associated hepatitis C virus infection. Dig Dis Sci. 2002 Apr;47(4):794–6.
116. Sanchez MJ, Bergasa NV. Hepatitis C associated cardiomyopathy: potential pathogenic mechanisms and clinical implications. Med Sci Monitor. 2008 May;14(5):RA55–63.
117. Matsumori A, Matoba Y, Sasayama S. Dilated cardiomyopathy associated with hepatitis C virus infection. Circulation. 1995 Nov 1;92(9):2519–25.
118. Matsumori A, Ohashi N, Nishio R, Kakio T, Hara M, Furukawa Y, et al. Apical hypertrophic cardiomyopathy and hepatitis C virus infection. Jpn Circ J. 1999 Jun;63(6):433–8.
119. Matsumori A. Hepatitis C virus and cardiomyopathy. Herz. 2000 May;25(3):249–54.
120. Prati D, Poli F, Farma E, Picone A, Porta E, De Mattei C, et al. Multicenter study on hepatitis C virus infection in patients with dilated cardiomyopathy. North Italy Transplant Program (NITP). J Med Virol. 1999 Jun;58(2):116–20.
121. Reis FJ, Viana M, Oliveira M, Sousa TA, Parana R. Prevalence of hepatitis C and B virus infection in patients with idiopathic dilated cardiomyopathy in Brazil: a pilot study. Braz J Infect Dis. 2007 Jun;11(3):318–21.
122. Boyella V, Onyebueke I, Farraj N, Graham-Hill S, El Younis C, Bergasa NV. Prevalence of hepatitis C virus infection in patients with cardiomyopathy. Ann Hepatol. 2009 Apr-Jun;8(2):113–5.
123. Ramos-Casals M, Stone JH, Cid MC, Bosch X. The cryoglobulinaemias. Lancet. 2012 Jan 28;379(9813):348–60.
124. Tedeschi A, Barate C, Minola E, Morra E. Cryoglobulinemia. Blood Rev. 2007 Jul;21(4):183–200.
125. Ferri C, Greco F, Longombardo G, Palla P, Moretti A, Marzo E, et al. Association between hepatitis C virus and mixed cryoglobulinemia [see comment]. Clin Exp Rheumatol. 1991 Nov-Dec;9(6):621–4.
126. Sansonno D, Lauletta G, Nisi L, Gatti P, Pesola F, Pansini N, et al. Non-enveloped HCV core protein as constitutive antigen of cold-precipitable immune complexes in type II mixed cryoglobulinaemia. Clin Exp Immunol. 2003 Aug;133(2):275–82.
127. Lunel F, Musset L, Cacoub P, Frangeul L, Cresta P, Perrin M, et al. Cryoglobulinemia in chronic liver diseases: role of hepatitis C virus and liver damage. Gastroenterology. 1994 May;106(5):1291–300.
128. Stefanova-Petrova DV, Tzvetanska AH, Naumova EJ, Mihailova AP, Hadjiev EA, Dikova RP, et al. Chronic hepatitis C virus infection: prevalence of extrahepatic manifestations and association with cryoglobulinemia in Bulgarian patients. World J Gastroenterol WJG. 2007 Dec 28;13(48):6518–28.

129. Pileri P, Uematsu Y, Campagnoli S, Galli G, Falugi F, Petracca R, et al. Binding of hepatitis C virus to CD81. Science. 1998 Oct 30;282(5390):938–41.
130. Franzin F, Efremov DG, Pozzato G, Tulissi P, Batista F, Burrone OR. Clonal B-cell expansions in peripheral blood of HCV-infected patients. Br J Haematol. 1995 Jul;90(3):548–52.
131. Giordano TP, Henderson L, Landgren O, Chiao EY, Kramer JR, El-Serag H, et al. Risk of non-Hodgkin lymphoma and lymphoproliferative precursor diseases in US veterans with hepatitis C virus. JAMA. 2007;297(18):2010–7.
132. Dal Maso L, Franceschi S. Hepatitis C virus and risk of lymphoma and other lymphoid neoplasms: a meta-analysis of epidemiologic studies. Cancer Epidemiol Biomarkers Prevent. 2006 Nov;15(11):2078–85.
133. Ruhl CE, Menke A, Cowie CC, Everhart JE. The relationship of Hepatitis C virus infection with diabetes in the United States population. Hepatology. 2014 Feb 5;60(4):1139–49.
134. Ryan Caballes F, Sendi H, Bonkovsky HL. Hepatitis C, porphyria cutanea tarda and liver iron: an update. Liver Int. 2012 July;32(6):880–93.
135. Hussain I, Hepburn NC, Jones A, O'Rourke K, Hayes PC. The association of hepatitis C viral infection with porphyria cutanea tarda in the Lothian region of Scotland. Clin Exp Dermatol. 1996 Jul;21(4):283–5.
136. Bonkovsky HL, Poh-Fitzpatrick M, Pimstone N, Obando J, Di Bisceglie A, Tattrie C, et al. Porphyria cutanea tarda, hepatitis C, and HFE gene mutations in North America. Hepatology. 1998 Jun;27(6):1661–9.
137. Gisbert JP, Garcia-Buey L, Pajares JM, Moreno-Otero R. Prevalence of hepatitis C virus infection in porphyria cutanea tarda: systematic review and meta-analysis. J Hepatol. 2003 Oct;39(4):620–7.
138. Jalil S, Grady JJ, Lee C, Anderson KE. Associations among behavior-related susceptibility factors in porphyria cutanea tarda. Clin Gastroenterol Hepatol. 2010 Mar;8(3):297–302.
139. Kauppinen R. Porphyrias. Lancet. 2005 Jan;365(9455):241–52.
140. Danton M, Lim CK. Porphomethene inhibitor of uroporphyrinogen decarboxylase: analysis by high-performance liquid chromatography/electrospray ionization tandem mass spectrometry. Biomed Chromatogr BMC. 2007 Jul;21(7):661–3.
141. Phillips JD, Bergonia HA, Reilly CA, Franklin MR, Kushner JP. A porphomethene inhibitor of uroporphyrinogen decarboxylase causes porphyria cutanea tarda. Proc Natl Acad Sci U S A. 2007 Mar 20;104(12):5079–84.
142. Chuang TY, Brashear R, Lewis C. Porphyria cutanea tarda and hepatitis C virus: a case-control study and meta-analysis of the literature. J Am Acad Dermatol. 1999 Jul;41(1):31–6.
143. O'Reilly FM, Darby C, Fogarty J, O'Moore R, Courtney MG, O'Connor J, et al. Porphyrin metabolism in hepatitis C infection. Photodermatol Photoimmunol Photomed. 1996 Feb;12(1):31–3.
144. Haque S, Chandra B, Gerber MA, Lok AS. Iron overload in patients with chronic hepatitis C: a clinicopathologic study. Hum Pathol. 1996 Dec;27(12):1277–81.
145. Fujita N, Sugimoto R, Takeo M, Urawa N, Mifuji R, Tanaka H, et al. Hepcidin expression in the liver: relatively low level in patients with chronic hepatitis C. Mol Med. 2007 Jan–Feb;13(1–2):97–104.
146. Fabrizi F, Plaisier E, Saadoun D, Martin P, Messa P, Cacoub P. Hepatitis C virus infection, mixed cryoglobulinemia, and kidney disease. Am J Kidney Dis. 2013 Apr;61(4):623–37.
147. Garcia-Valdecasas J, Bernal C, Garcia F, Cerezo S, Umana WO, von Albertini B, et al. Epidemiology of hepatitis C virus infection in patients with renal disease. J Am Soc Nephrol JASN. 1994 Aug;5(2):186–92.
148. Fabrizi F, Lunghi G, Messa P, Martin P. Therapy of hepatitis C virus-associated glomerulonephritis: current approaches. J Nephrol. 2008 Nov–Dec;21(6):813–25.
149. Fabrizi F. Hepatitis C virus, cryoglobulinemia, and kidney: novel evidence. Scientifica. 2012;2012:128382.
150. Fornasieri A, Armelloni S, Bernasconi P, Li M, de Septis CP, Sinico RA, et al. High binding of immunoglobulin M kappa rheumatoid factor from type II cryoglobulins to cellular

fibronectin: a mechanism for induction of in situ immune complex glomerulonephritis? Am J Kidney Dis. 1996 Apr;27(4):476–83.

151. Roy K, Bagg J. Hepatitis C virus and oral disease: a critical review. Oral Dis. 1999 Oct;5(4):270–7.

152. Jorgensen C, Legouffe MC, Perney P, Coste J, Tissot B, Segarra C, et al. Sicca syndrome associated with hepatitis C virus infection. Arthritis Rheum. 1996 Jul;39(7):1166–71.

153. Verbaan H, Carlson J, Eriksson S, Larsson A, Liedholm R, Manthorpe R, et al. Extrahepatic manifestations of chronic hepatitis C infection and the interrelationship between primary Sjogren's syndrome and hepatitis C in Swedish patients. J Intern Med. 1999 Feb;245(2):127–32.

154. Ramos-Casals M, Garcia-Carrasco M, Cervera R, Rosas J, Trejo O, de la Red G, et al. Hepatitis C virus infection mimicking primary Sjogren syndrome. A clinical and immunologic description of 35 cases. Medicine. 2001 Jan;80(1):1–8.

155. Loustaud-Ratti V, Riche A, Liozon E, Labrousse F, Soria P, Rogez S, et al. Prevalence and characteristics of Sjogren's syndrome or Sicca syndrome in chronic hepatitis C virus infection: a prospective study. J Rheumatol. 2001 Oct;28(10):2245–51.

156. Coll J, Gambus G, Corominas J, Tomas S, Esteban JI, Guardia J. Immunohistochemistry of minor salivary gland biopsy specimens from patients with Sjogren's syndrome with and without hepatitis C virus infection. Ann Rheum Dis. 1997 Jun;56(6):390–2.

157. Toussirot E, Le Huede G, Mougin C, Balblanc JC, Bettinger D, Wendling D. Presence of hepatitis C virus RNA in the salivary glands of patients with Sjogren's syndrome and hepatitis C virus infection. J Rheumatol. 2002 Nov;29(11):2382–5.

158. Sharma A, Bialynicki-Birula R, Schwartz RA, Janniger CK. Lichen planus: an update and review. Cutis. 2012 Jul;90(1):17–23.

159. Jubert C, Pawlotsky JM, Pouget F, Andre C, DeForges L, Bretagne S, et al. Lichen planus and hepatitis C virus—related chronic active hepatitis. Arch Dermatol. 1994 Jan;130(1):73–6.

160. Pawlotsky JM, Ben Yahia M, Andre C, Voisin MC, Intrator L, Roudot-Thoraval F, et al. Immunological disorders in C virus chronic active hepatitis: a prospective case-control study. Hepatology. 1994 Apr;19(4):841–8.

161. Lodi G, Pellicano R, Carrozzo M. Hepatitis C virus infection and lichen planus: a systematic review with meta-analysis. Oral Dis. 2010 Oct;16(7):601–12.

162. Shengyuan L, Songpo Y, Wen W, Wenjing T, Haitao Z, Binyou W. Hepatitis C virus and lichen planus: a reciprocal association determined by a meta-analysis. Arch Dermatol. 2009 Sep;145(9):1040–7.

163. Bergasa NV, Holguin GE, Martinez M, Chen YL, Baumstein D. Adrenal tumors in patients with chronic hepatitis C. Gastroenterol Hepatol. 2010 Jun;6(6):385–7.

164. Singla M, Sy A, Baumstein D, Kadeishvili K, Matari HM, Bergasa N. Chronic Hepatitis C is associated with adrenal tumors. J Gastroenterol Hepatol Res. 2013;2(7):680–2.

165. Yan FM, Chen AS, Hao F, Zhao XP, Gu CH, Zhao LB, et al. Hepatitis C virus may infect extrahepatic tissues in patients with hepatitis C. World J Gastroenterol WJG. 2000 Dec;6(6):805–11.

166. Okan A, Comlekci A, Akpinar H, Okan I, Yesil S, Tankurt E, et al. Serum concentrations of insulin-like growth factor-I and insulin-like growth factor binding protein-3 in patients with chronic hepatitis. Scand J Gastroenterol. 2000 Nov;35(11):1212–5.

167. Penhoat A, Chatelain PG, Jaillard C, Saez JM. Characterization of insulin-like growth factor I and insulin receptors on cultured bovine adrenal fasciculata cells. Role of these peptides on adrenal cell function. Endocrinology. 1988 Jun;122(6):2518–26.

168. Brown JM, Siddiqui M, Calhoun DA, Carey RM, Hopkins PN, Williams GH, et al. The unrecognized prevalence of primary aldosteronism: a cross-sectional study. Ann Intern Med. 2020 Jul 7;173(1):10–20.

169. Farci P, Alter HJ, Wong D, Miller RH, Shih JW, Jett B, et al. A long-term study of hepatitis C virus replication in non-a, non-B hepatitis. N Engl J Med. 1991 Jul 11;325(2):98–104.

170. Liang TJ, Ghany MG. Therapy of hepatitis C--back to the future. N Engl J Med. 2014 May 22;370(21):2043–7.

171. Chung RT, Baumert TF. Curing chronic hepatitis C—the arc of a medical triumph. N Engl J Med. 2014 Apr 24;370(17):1576–8.

172. Panel A-IHG. Hepatitis C guidance 2018 update: AASLD-IDSA recommendations for testing, managing, and treating hepatitis C virus infection. Clin Infect Dis. 2018 Oct 30;67(10):1477–92.

173. Terrault NA. Care of patients following cure of Hepatitis C virus infection. Gastroenterol Hepatol (N Y). 2018 Nov;14(11):629–34.

174. Feld JJ, Hoofnagle JH. Mechanism of action of interferon and ribavirin in treatment of hepatitis C. Nature. 2005 Aug 18;436(7053):967–72.

175. Hoofnagle JH. A step forward in therapy for hepatitis C. N Engl J Med. 2009 Apr 30;360(18):1899–901.

176. Swain MG, Lai MY, Shiffman ML, Cooksley WG, Zeuzem S, Dieterich DT, et al. A sustained virologic response is durable in patients with chronic hepatitis C treated with peginterferon alfa-2a and ribavirin. Gastroenterology. 2010 Nov;139(5):1593–601.

177. Di Bisceglie AM, Conjeevaram HS, Fried MW, Sallie R, Park Y, Yurdaydin C, et al. Ribavirin as therapy for chronic hepatitis C. a randomized, double-blind, placebo-controlled trial. Ann Intern Med. 1995 Dec 15;123(12):897–903.

178. McHutchison JG, Gordon SC, Schiff ER, Shiffman ML, Lee WM, Rustgi VK, et al. Interferon alfa-2b alone or in combination with ribavirin as initial treatment for chronic hepatitis C. Hepatitis Interventional Therapy Group. N Engl J Med. 1998 Nov 19;339(21):1485–92.

179. Conjeevaram HS, Fried MW, Jeffers LJ, Terrault NA, Wiley-Lucas TE, Afdhal N, et al. Peginterferon and ribavirin treatment in African American and Caucasian American patients with hepatitis C genotype 1. Gastroenterology. 2006 Aug;131(2):470–7.

180. Prokunina-Olsson L, Muchmore B, Tang W, Pfeiffer RM, Park H, Dickensheets H, et al. A variant upstream of IFNL3 (IL28B) creating a new interferon gene IFNL4 is associated with impaired clearance of hepatitis C virus. Nat Genet. 2013 Feb;45(2):164–71.

181. Lindenbach BD, Evans MJ, Syder AJ, Wolk B, Tellinghuisen TL, Liu CC, et al. Complete replication of hepatitis C virus in cell culture. Science. 2005 Jul 22;309(5734):623–6.

182. Lohmann V, Korner F, Koch J, Herian U, Theilmann L, Bartenschlager R. Replication of subgenomic hepatitis C virus RNAs in a hepatoma cell line. Science. 1999 Jul 2;285(5424):110–3.

183. Wakita T, Pietschmann T, Kato T, Date T, Miyamoto M, Zhao Z, et al. Production of infectious hepatitis C virus in tissue culture from a cloned viral genome. Nat Med. 2005 Jul;11(7):791–6.

184. Bartenschlager R, Lohmann V, Penin F. The molecular and structural basis of advanced antiviral therapy for hepatitis C virus infection. Nat Rev Microbiol. 2013 Jul;11(7):482–96.

185. Morikawa K, Lange CM, Gouttenoire J, Meylan E, Brass V, Penin F, et al. Nonstructural protein 3-4A: the Swiss army knife of hepatitis C virus. J Viral Hepat. 2011 May;18(5):305–15.

186. Lindenbach BD, Rice CM. The ins and outs of hepatitis C virus entry and assembly. Nat Rev Microbiol. 2013 Oct;11(10):688–700.

187. Jacobson IM, McHutchison JG, Dusheiko G, Di Bisceglie AM, Reddy KR, Bzowej NH, et al. Telaprevir for previously untreated chronic hepatitis C virus infection. N Engl J Med. 2011 Jun 23;364(25):2405–16.

188. Poordad F, McCone J Jr, Bacon BR, Bruno S, Manns MP, Sulkowski MS, et al. Boceprevir for untreated chronic HCV genotype 1 infection. N Engl J Med. 2011 Mar 31;364(13):1195–206.

189. Halfon P, Sarrazin C. Future treatment of chronic hepatitis C with direct acting antivirals: is resistance important? Liver Int. 2012 Feb;32(Suppl 1):79–87.

190. Goldenberg MM. Pharmaceutical approval update. P T. 2014 Feb;39(2):112–8.

191. Fried MW, Buti M, Dore GJ, Flisiak R, Ferenci P, Jacobson I, et al. Once-daily simeprevir (TMC435) with pegylated interferon and ribavirin in treatment-naive genotype 1 hepatitis C: the randomized PILLAR study. Hepatology. 2013 Dec;58(6):1918–29.

192. Zeuzem S, Berg T, Gane E, Ferenci P, Foster GR, Fried MW, et al. Simeprevir increases rate of sustained virologic response among treatment-experienced patients with HCV genotype-1 infection: a phase IIb trial. Gastroenterology. 2014 Feb;146(2):430–41.

193. Lawitz E, Gane EJ. Sofosbuvir for previously untreated chronic hepatitis C infection. N Engl J Med. 2013 Aug 15;369(7):678–9.

194. Pawlotsky JM. New hepatitis C virus (HCV) drugs and the hope for a cure: concepts in anti-HCV drug development. Semin Liver Dis. 2014 Feb;34(1):22–9.

195. Targett-Adams P, Graham EJ, Middleton J, Palmer A, Shaw SM, Lavender H, et al. Small molecules targeting hepatitis C virus-encoded NS5A cause subcellular redistribution of their target: insights into compound modes of action. J Virol. 2011 Jul;85(13):6353–68.

196. Bhatia HK, Singh H, Grewal N, Natt NK. Sofosbuvir: a novel treatment option for chronic hepatitis C infection. J Pharmacol Pharmacother. 2014 Oct;5(4):278–84.

197. Afdhal N, Zeuzem S, Kwo P, Chojkier M, Gitlin N, Puoti M, et al. Ledipasvir and sofosbuvir for untreated HCV genotype 1 infection. N Engl J Med. 2014 May 15;370(20):1889–98.

198. Feld JJ, Jacobson IM, Hezode C, Asselah T, Ruane PJ, Gruener N, et al. Sofosbuvir and velpatasvir for HCV genotype 1, 2, 4, 5, and 6 infection. N Engl J Med. 2015 Dec 31;373(27):2599–607.

199. Ferreira VL, Assis Jarek NA, Tonin FS, Borba HH, Wiens A, Muzzillo DA, et al. Ledipasvir/sofosbuvir with or without ribavirin for the treatment of chronic hepatitis C genotype 1: a pairwise meta-analysis. J Gastroenterol Hepatol. 2017 Apr;32(4):749–55.

200. Ghany MG, Marks KM, Morgan TR, Wyles DL, Aronsohn AI, Bhattacharya D, et al. Hepatitis C guidance 2019 update: AASLD-IDSA recommendations for testing, managing, and treating hepatitis C virus infection. Hepatology. 2019 Dec 9;71(2):686–721.

201. Belperio PS, Shahoumian TA, Mole LA, Backus LI. Evaluation of hepatitis B reactivation among 62,920 veterans treated with oral hepatitis C antivirals. Hepatology. 2017 Jul;66(1):27–36.

202. Gentzsch J, Brohm C, Steinmann E, Friesland M, Menzel N, Vieyres G, et al. Hepatitis C virus p7 is critical for capsid assembly and envelopment. PLoS Pathogens. 2013;9(5):e1003355.

203. Spiegel BM, Younossi ZM, Hays RD, Revicki D, Robbins S, Kanwal F. Impact of hepatitis C on health related quality of life: a systematic review and quantitative assessment. Hepatology. 2005 Apr;41(4):790–800.

204. Alberti A. Impact of a sustained virological response on the long-term outcome of hepatitis C. Liver Int. 2011 Jan;31(Suppl 1):18–22.

205. Saadoun D, Resche Rigon M, Thibault V, Longuet M, Pol S, Blanc F, et al. Peg-IFNalpha/ribavirin/protease inhibitor combination in hepatitis C virus associated mixed cryoglobulinemia vasculitis: results at week 24. Ann Rheum Dis. 2014 May;73(5):831–7.

206. Pietrogrande M, De Vita S, Zignego AL, Pioltelli P, Sansonno D, Sollima S, et al. Recommendations for the management of mixed cryoglobulinemia syndrome in hepatitis C virus-infected patients. Autoimmun Rev. 2011 Jun;10(8):444–54.

207. Takikawa H, Yamazaki R, Shoji S, Miyake K, Yamanaka M. Normalization of urinary porphyrin level and disappearance of skin lesions after successful interferon therapy in a case of chronic hepatitis C complicated with porphyria cutanea tarda. J Hepatol. 1995 Feb;22(2):249–50.

208. Sheikh MY, Wright RA, Burruss JB. Dramatic resolution of skin lesions associated with porphyria cutanea tarda after interferon-alpha therapy in a case of chronic hepatitis C. Dig Dis Sci. 1998 Mar;43(3):529–33.

209. Furuta M, Kaito M, Gabazza E, Fujita N, Ishida S, Tamaki S, et al. Ineffective interferon treatment of chronic hepatitis C-associated porphyria cutanea tarda, but with a transient decrease in HCV RNA levels. J Gastroenterol. 2000;35(1):60–2.

210. Azim J, McCurdy H, Moseley RH. Porphyria cutanea tarda as a complication of therapy for chronic hepatitis C. World J Gastroenterol WJG. 2008 Oct 14;14(38):5913–5.

211. Jessner W, Der-Petrossian M, Christiansen L, Maier H, Steindl-Munda P, Gangl A, et al. Porphyria cutanea tarda during interferon/ribavirin therapy for chronic hepatitis C. Hepatology. 2002 Nov;36(5):1301–2.

212. Singal AK, Venkata KVR, Jampana S, Islam FU, Anderson KE. Hepatitis C treatment in patients with porphyria cutanea tarda. Am J Med Sci. 2017 Jun;353(6):523–8.
213. Ferraccioli GF, Salaffi F, De Vita S, Casatta L, Avellini C, Carotti M, et al. Interferon alpha-2 (IFN alpha 2) increases lacrimal and salivary function in Sjogren's syndrome patients. Preliminary results of an open pilot trial versus OH-chloroquine. Clin Exp Rheumatol. 1996 Jul-Aug;14(4):367–71.
214. Areias J, Velho GC, Cerqueira R, Barbedo C, Amaral B, Sanches M, et al. Lichen planus and chronic hepatitis C: exacerbation of the lichen under interferon-alpha-2a therapy. Eur J Gastroenterol Hepatol. 1996 Aug;8(8):825–8.
215. Grossmann Sde M, Teixeira R, de Aguiar MC, do Carmo MA. Exacerbation of oral lichen planus lesions during treatment of chronic hepatitis C with pegylated interferon and ribavirin. Eur J Gastroenterol Hepatol. 2008 Jul;20(7):702–6.
216. Misaka K, Kishimoto T, Kawahigashi Y, Sata M, Nagao Y. Use of direct-acting antivirals for the treatment of hepatitis C virus-associated Oral lichen planus: a case report. Case Rep Gastroenterol. 2016 Sep–Dec;10(3):617–22.
217. Nagao Y, Nakasone K, Maeshiro T, Nishida N, Kimura K, Kawahigashi Y, et al. Successful treatment of oral lichen planus with direct-acting antiviral agents after liver transplantation for hepatitis C virus-associated hepatocellular carcinoma. Case Rep Gastroenterol. 2017 Sep-Dec;11(3):701–10.
218. Chopra KB, Demetris AJ, Blakolmer K, Dvorchik I, Laskus T, Wang LF, et al. Progression of liver fibrosis in patients with chronic hepatitis C after orthotopic liver transplantation. Transplantation. 2003 Nov 27;76(10):1487–91.
219. Samonakis DN, Germani G, Burroughs AK. Immunosuppression and HCV recurrence after liver transplantation. J Hepatol. 2012 Apr;56(4):973–83.
220. Berenguer M, Prieto M, Rayon JM, Mora J, Pastor M, Ortiz V, et al. Natural history of clinically compensated hepatitis C virus-related graft cirrhosis after liver transplantation. Hepatology. 2000 Oct;32(4 Pt 1):852–8.
221. Rosen HR, Gretch DR, Oehlke M, Flora KD, Benner KG, Rabkin JM, et al. Timing and severity of initial hepatitis C recurrence as predictors of long-term liver allograft injury. Transplantation. 1998 May 15;65(9):1178–82.
222. Schluger LK, Sheiner PA, Thung SN, Lau JY, Min A, Wolf DC, et al. Severe recurrent cholestatic hepatitis C following orthotopic liver transplantation. Hepatology. 1996 May;23(5):971–6.
223. Lim HL, Lau GK, Davis GL, Dolson DJ, Lau JY. Cholestatic hepatitis leading to hepatic failure in a patient with organ-transmitted hepatitis C virus infection. Gastroenterology. 1994 Jan;106(1):248–51.
224. Samonakis DN, Triantos CK, Thalheimer U, Quaglia A, Leandro G, Teixeira R, et al. Immunosuppression and donor age with respect to severity of HCV recurrence after liver transplantation. Liver Transpl. 2005 Apr;11(4):386–95.
225. Kalambokis G, Manousou P, Samonakis D, Grillo F, Dhillon AP, Patch D, et al. Clinical outcome of HCV-related graft cirrhosis and prognostic value of hepatic venous pressure gradient. Transpl Int. 2009 Feb;22(2):172–81.
226. Vinaixa C, Rubin A, Aguilera V, Berenguer M. Recurrence of hepatitis C after liver transplantation. Ann Gastroenterol. 2013;26(4):304–13.
227. Chen T, Terrault NA. Perspectives on treating hepatitis C infection in the liver transplantation setting. Curr Opin Organ Transplant. 2016 Apr;21(2):111–9.
228. Liu J, Ma B, Cao W, Li M, Bramer WM, Peppelenbosch MP, et al. Direct-acting antiviral agents for liver transplant recipients with recurrent genotype 1 hepatitis C virus infection: systematic review and meta-analysis. Transpl Infect Dis. 2019 Apr;21(2):e13047.

# Chapter 7
# Chronic Hepatitis B

**Nora V. Bergasa**

A 43-year-old woman had been diagnosed with chronic hepatitis B virus infection, e antigen negative, e antibody positive associated with serum hepatitis B viral DNA greater than 20,000 IU/ml, and abnormal serum activity of alanine aminotransferase (ALT) at diagnosis. Serology for delta hepatitis was negative. The patient was born in the Dominican Republic. She did not have any risk factors for viral hepatitis or comorbidities. Her physical examination was notable for the absence of stigmata of chronic liver disease. Her ALT was normal, and HBV DNA was undetected, and her liver sonogram was normal. She had been started on lamivudine, changed to adefovir, and subsequently to tenofovir when approved for the treatment of chronic hepatitis B, all of which had been associated with viral suppression and normal liver panel but not with seroconversion to anti-HBs or loss of surface antigen. After 8 years of treatment, her antiviral medication (i.e., tenofovir) was discontinued, and the patient followed for any signs of hepatitis flares, which she did not exhibit. Four years after discontinuation of therapy, the patient lost surface antigen and developed anti-HBs 6 months later, which she has had for 3 years.

## Etiology of Chronic Hepatitis B: Hepatitis B Virus

The hepatitis B virus is a DNA virus that belongs to the Hepadnaviridae family. The identification of the virus was reported as A "New" Antigen in Leukemia Sera in 1965 [1]. The circulating viral particles of the hepatitis B virus have a common

N. V. Bergasa (✉)
Department of Medicine, H+H/Metropolitan, New York, NY, USA

New York Medical College, Valhalla, NY, USA

Hepatology, H+H/Woodhull, Brooklyn, NY, USA

N. V. Bergasa (ed.), *Clinical Cases in Hepatology*,
https://doi.org/10.1007/978-1-4471-4715-2_7

protein in their surface, the hepatitis B surface antigen (HBsAg), against which neutralizing antibodies are generated. The viral particles circulate in different forms; the largest is the Dane particle, a double shelled structure of 42–47 nm, which is the infectious virion, a 20 nm sphere, the most abundant of the particles by thousands of units, and a 20 nm filament of variable length. Inside the envelope of the Dane particle is the core, mostly comprised of C protein, also known as core antigen; within the core is the viral DNA and a polymerase activity. The other particles are composed of HBsAg only and are not infectious because they lack nucleic acid; however, they stimulate a robust immunological response associated with the development of hepatitis B surface antibody, anti-HBs. This response is not sufficient, nevertheless, to prevent the progression of chronic infection, as it is believed that it allows the virion to escape from the host's antibody, which seems to be adsorbed by the most abundant particles.

The HBV has in its inner icosahedral core its DNA as a relaxed circular (RC) partially double stranded structure of approximately 3200 base pairs and is characterized by asymmetric DNA strands, the negative strand being of unit length, covalently bound to P protein at its 5' end, and the positive strand being of less than unit length, capped at its 5' end; each 5' end maps to an 11 nucleotide long region of direct repeats (DRs) in viral DNA, which is involved in the priming of the synthesis of their RNA, DR1 for the negative and DR2 for the positive strands. The gap left by the less than one unit of the positive strand is filled by a polymerase activity primed by the 3' end of the positive strand to synthesize over the negative strand; the product produced, thus, is entirely of positive polarity [2].

The genome of the hepatitis B virus is comprised of four open reading frames (ORFs): (1) ORF *P* encodes the viral polymerase and the terminal protein of the negative strand, (2) ORF *C* (core) encodes the structural protein of the nucleocapsid and another pre-core sequence that contains a signal peptide that allows for translocation into the endoplasmic reticulum; the initiator codon of the pre C region is in the 5' terminally extended precore RNA and produces a precore precursor protein, the HBeAg, which does not participate in replication, and that is independently secreted, (3) ORF *S/preS* encodes three cocarboxyterminal HBV (HBs) proteins, large (L), or pre-S1, middle (M) or pre-S2 (M) and small (S), and (4) ORF *X*, which encodes for the X protein [2–5]. The surface proteins are surrounded by a lipid membrane rich in cholesterol, derived from the endoplasmic reticulum. The capacity of replication is extended in this virus by the overlaps of its ORF, which are the partial overlap of the polymerase with the precore/core and X-ORF and the complete overlap with the surface proteins.

The HBV enters the hepatocyte after making contact with the sodium taurocholate cotransporting polypeptide (NTCP) receptor [6] for which it has high affinity and with the heparan-sulfate proteoglycans for which it has a low affinity. It was recently reported that epidermal growth factor receptor (EGFR) is a host-entry cofactor to NTCP in the internalization of the HBV [7]. It enters the cytoplasm via endocytosis [8], and it is actively transported via microtubules to the nucleus, which the virus enters via the nuclear pore, where the capsid disintegrates to enter the nucleus as polymers and dimers [8]. The partially double stranded DNA is released into the karyoplasm, where it is converted to covalently closed circular DNA (cccDNA) that accumulates in the hepatocyte in association with histone and non-histone viral and cellular proteins, considered to be a stable minichromosome [8–11]. Several factors, although not all have been identified, have been reported to be involved in the process of cccDNA formation, which is maintained in the nucleus and functions as a template for viral replication [12]. The Pol-linked terminal redundant sequence in the 5'-end of the minus strand DNA and the RNA oligonucleotide attached at the 5' end of the plus strand DNA are removed from the relaxed circular (rc)DNA, and the gaps in both strands are filled and ligated to generate cccDNA. By the use of cccDNA as a template four RNAs of different lengths are transcribed, process regulated by preS1, preS2, core, and X, as promoters, and Enhancer I and Enhancer II, as enhancers, a function mediated by the host RNA polymerase II machinery-dependent transcription [13].

Epigenetic factors, and idiosyncrasies of the virus itself, and not only the host, seem to contribute to the formation of cccDNA, which have been proposed as potentially useful in the development of effective anti-hepatitis B virus medications [11]. The host RNA pol II, a nuclear enzyme, binds to the encapsidation signal epsilon, an RNA structure located near the 5' end of the pregenomic RNA. The binding takes place with the assistance of chaperone proteins and transcribes the cccDNA to all the viral RNAs that are subsequently translated in the endoplasmic reticulum to P, C, pre S/S, and X gene products. Viral pregenomic RNAs and the P product, the viral reverse transcriptase, are encapsidated within core particles in the cytoplasm where viral DNA synthesis is initiated [14]. First, the negative strand is synthesized from the template that is the pregenomic RNA, i.e., a participant in genomic replication [14], and that supports transcription by the co-packaged P protein [14, 15] in parallel with degradation by viral RNase H of the RNAs templates. Subsequently, the positive strand, which keeps the HBV polymerase active center attached to the variable 3' end of the DNA product, is synthesized. The process of HBV replication occurs in the cytoplasm; however, newly formed core particles enter the nucleus from the cytoplasm, allowing for the availability of cccDNA for further replication within the infected cells [14, 15].

After the synthesis of genomic DNA is completed, the newly formed cores bud onto the membranes of the endoplasmic reticulum or Golgi apparatus to acquire the glycoprotein envelope, and in this form, they are secreted by the hepatocyte via cellular transport mechanisms [16, 17]. The budding process of the HBV virion, crucial in the manner in which the virus exits the hepatocyte, has not been completely elucidated; however, it is reported to be mediated by the L-like domain (PPAY) expressed on the HBV core, which may bind to the recruitment of the endosomal-sorting-complex-required-for-transport (ESCRT) system or by the use of cellular proteins including Nedd4 and gamma-adaptin [18].

HBV is a noncytopathic virus that causes liver disease in acute infections as acute hepatitis and fulminant liver failure, and that can proceed to chronic viral hepatitis, cirrhosis, and its complications, including liver failure and hepatocellular carcinoma [19, 20]. Acute hepatitis B is associated with an immune-mediated resolution with the development of antibodies, including hepatitis e antibody (anti-HBe), anti-core antibody, IgM in the acute phase, and IgG reflective of prior infection (anti-HB core). The mode in which the HBV infects the hepatocyte seems to evade the immune system by its cryptic navigation through the cytoplasm and installation in the nucleus, where it remains as cccDNA, a perpetuator of viral replication and chronicity.

## Genetics

The response of the host's immune system and characteristics of the virus contribute to the natural history of this infection, i.e., acute followed by resolution, or acute followed by chronicity. Studies conducted in chimpanzees revealed that early infection with HBV was not associated with the induction of genes and their products from the innate immune system associated with antiviral effects. This tepid response has also been reported in human beings. In contrast to a control group of patients with acute hepatitis A, patients with acute hepatitis B exhibited minimal measurable concentrations of interferon (IFN)-α during the incubation phase [21], peak and decline of viral replication, and activity of ALT, as a marker of liver inflammation, and significantly higher serum concentrations of interleukin-15 (IL-15), an inducer of natural killer (NK) cells effector function [22]. In addition, the concentration of interferon gamma-1 was substantially higher in the group of patients with acute hepatitis A [21]. IFN-λ1 was reported as induced by HVB infection, not higher than in samples from healthy controls, and in fact, suppressed at the peak of viremia; this finding was in contrast to the results found in a group of patients with acute hepatitis A in which the concentration of both types of interferon was significantly increased [21]. Several potential pathways through which the HBV may interfere with interferon production have been suggested from in vitro studies including: (i) the inhibition of virus-triggered interferon-regulatory factor 3 and the induction of IFN-B by HBV protein X [23], (ii) the degradation of mitochondrial antiviral signaling (MAVS) protein through $Lys^{136}$ ubiquitin and also by HBV protein X [24]; MAVS protein is part of the signal pathway stimulated by virus to induce the activation of NF-kappa B and of IFN regulatory factor-3 to induce the production of type I IFN, (iii) the inhibition of TANK-binding kinase 1 (TBK1)/IκB kinase-ε (IKKε) activity, by the HBV polymerase, which was reported to disturb the interaction between IKKε and DDX3 DEAD box RNA helicase, and which increases the activity of the kinases, effector kinases of interferon regulatory factor signaling [25], suggesting a possible pathway for the lack of interferon production in acute HBV infection [21], and (iv) the inhibition of activation of IFN B by the binding of HBV protein X to adaptor protein IPS-1. It was also documented that markers of natural killer (NK) cell activation, CD69 on the CD3 − CD56+ subset, examined ex vivo, revealed that in acute hepatitis B, the highest degree of NK activation was at the peak of ALT activity, as HBV DNA serum concentration was decreasing, and it was significantly lower at all stages of the acute infection, as compared to the healthy control group. Furthermore, stimulation of NK cells from patients with acute HBV infection exhibited a decrease in the production of IFN gamma and alpha, cytokines with antiviral properties, which tended to increase as viremia declined. As it relates to NK cells, their state of activation seems to vary according to the phase of the chronic viral infection, i.e., immune active vs. immune tolerant as it has been reported that activated NK exhibiting a cytolytic profile have been identified in patients with immunologically active disease, although not in association with IFN-gamma production, and higher liver expression of interleukin (IL)-12, IL-15, and IL-18, and lower expression of IL-10, a cytokine that can activate and induce degranulation of NK cells in normal control subjects; also, liver NK cells were documented to exhibit increased cytolytic activity as compared to peripheral NK cells, finding that correlated with liver inflammation and activity of serum ALT. These findings, consistent with cell activation, were not documented in the liver of patients who were in the immune tolerant phase or in healthy control subjects [26], suggesting that NK cells contribute to the inflammatory response of the liver to infection with the HBV in active immunological phase [26]. Furthermore, a correlation between chronic hepatitis B flares with fluctuations of IL-8, IFN-alpha, and NK cell expression of tumor necrosis factor-related apoptosis-inducing ligand (TRAIL) in an ex vivo experiment was documented; in addition, abundant activated TRAIL-expressing NK cells and hepatocytes expressing TRAIL death-inducing receptor in situ were reported, as well as NK activation in response to interferon alpha in vitro. These findings were interpreted to suggest that NK cells activated by cytokines produced during the acute exposure contribute to the liver inflammation in response to HBV infection [27]. Divergent from the cytokines that stimulate innate immunity was the documented behavior of IL-10, a cytokine that suppresses the innate immune response, the concentration of which was reported as highest at the time of maximal viral replication, as defined in this study [21]; in addition, HBV-specific CD4 and CD8 T-cell responses were also ameliorated at the time of high serum HBV DNA and recovered after the resolution of the infection [21]. These findings were supported by a study that examined the serum cytokine profile in the acute phase of HBV infection, which, in contrast to HIV, was not associated with an increase in serum concentrations of cytokines, including IFN alpha and IL-15 [28]. These data were interpreted to suggest that the vigorous response to HIV may result in loss of T cells, state that would contribute to chronicity, in contrast to the acute HBV infection, which, in the majority of adult subjects, is associated with antibody response and resolution. In the context of a limited response of the innate immune system, it was reported that acute HBV infection was associated with a transient and strong production of IL-6 by liver macrophages. IL-6 inhibits the expression of hepatocyte nuclear factor 1 alpha and HNF 4 alpha, which stimulate HBV replication, thus helping to control the infection, in the absence of a strong inflammatory response by the innate immune system that would result in cell death [29].

Constituents of the HBV contribute to its evasion of the immune response, with HBx having been reported to interfere with the activation of type I interferons by HBV ds DNA [30], by inhibiting HBV mediated activation of IFN-regulatory factor-3 (IRF3) [23]. The RNA helicase enzyme retinoic acid-inducible gene I (RIG-I) functions as a pattern recognition receptor for short viri; the interaction of RIG-I with unanchored lysine-63 (K63) polyubiquitin chains activates the mitochondrial protein MAVS [31]. Virus infection is associated with conformational changes in MAVS, which lead to what has been defined as prion-like aggregates that trigger the production of interferon regulatory factor (IRF) 3 and NF-κB to induce type I interferons as an antiviral defense mechanism [31]. It was reported from in-vitro studies that HBV protein X promoted the degradation of MAVS, preventing the induction of IFN-β, a mechanism by which the virus could contribute to a reduced antiviral response in association with HBV infection [24]. HBV polymerase has also been implicated in the evasion of the immune system by the virus. DDX3 DEAD box RNA helicase increases the activity of the IRF effector kinases, TANK-binding kinase 1 (TBK1)/IkappaB kinase-epsilon (IKKepsilon). It was reported that the HVB polymerase inhibited these kinases by interfering with the interaction between IKKepsilon and DDX3 DEAD box RNA helicase [25].

Interference with toll-like receptor-mediated immunity by HBV was also reported from in vitro studies, suggesting another mechanism by which the virus itself may curtail the immune response to this viral infection [32]. In samples from patients with chronic hepatitis B e antigen positive, the expression of TLR2 on hepatocytes, Kupffer cells, and peripheral monocytes was significantly decreased compared to that from control subjects and patients with e antigen negative disease. Also, the production of TNF-alpha and the expression of the phospho-p-38 kinase in the samples from e antigen positive patients were reduced, in contrast to the e antigen negative group, which expressed upregulation of the TLR-2 pathway and increased TNF- alpha production [33].

Studies in the early phases after inoculation with HBV virus have provided information from which how the immune system handles the virus at the first encounter can be inferred [34, 35]. Adaptive immune responses to acute HBV infection and significant decreases in viral replication, as assessed by serum HBV DNA, have been documented to occur during the incubation period before the demonstration of liver injury [34]. Specific responses mediated by CD-4+ and CD-8+ cells have been reported in acute HBV infection [35]. Time ex-vivo studies in acute HBV infection have documented that the maximal activity of NK and NT, a subgroup of T cells that co-express an αβ T cell receptor (TCR) as well as NK cell markers [36], is exhibited at the peak of HBV DNA, and that of CD4 and CD8 when the viral load has decreased, and innate immune responses are down [35]. High proportions of NK cells in peripheral blood have also been documented early in the incubation period, decreasing in number in association with a decrease in serum HBV DNA in a study that included patients whose infection source and date were known [34]. Serum analysis at different time points of the immunological response in two patients with acute HBV infections exhibited evidence of activation, including expression of CD69 and NKG2D, on the surface of CD56⁺CD3⁻ NK and CD56⁺CD3⁺ NT cells, within the first 2 weeks of surface antigen detection. NK cytotoxic activity was documented to peak at the zenith of HBV replication, measured as serum HBV DNA; serum IFN gamma production displayed a picture similar to cytotoxicity.

In contrast to the behavior of markers of the innate response, the production of IFN-gamma by HBV-specific T cells peaked when HBV DNA was not detectable, and it was mostly contributed by CD8[+] T cells. HBV specific CD8+ cells have also been documented in peripheral blood several weeks prior to clinical hepatitis [34]. By intracellular cytokine staining, the maximum expression of IL-2, documented in CD4+ and CD8+ cells, was reported prior to that of IFN-gamma; this was interpreted to suggest that early IL2 production may be fundamental for resolution of HBV infection. The expression of IL-4 and IL-10 by CD4+ was detected from the initial phase to a peak documented at the decline of IL-2, and as anti-HBs was found in serum. It was also reported that the earliest production of IFN gamma was stimulated by HBeAg, and the strongest was by the core protein, at the time of viral load; this observation has suggested an association between specific T cell responses to the core protein and resolution of the viral infection [35, 37].

Activated professional antigen presenting cells that result from the priming of CD4+ T cells induces an appropriate antiviral CD8+ cytotoxic T lymphocyte response that leads to resolution of the acute viral infection. In this regard, it was reported that peripheral mononuclear cells (PMNC) from patients who had self-limited HBV hepatitis infection exhibited a response to the hepatitis B core Ag and HBeAg that was stronger than that from patients who developed chronic infection. In addition, a detectable lymphocyte response to antigen nucleocapsid that was associated with clearance of hepatitis e antigen was stronger in patients who cleared the infection than in those who developed chronic disease, in which it was undetectable or limited. These results have suggested that a robust immunological response is fundamental for the resolution of the acute HBV infection [37].

T regulatory cells, CD4+CD25+ Treg, have also been proposed to contribute to the fate of HBV infection in a host to resolution or chronicity [38]. This type of cell was found in high proportion in peripheral blood, correlating with serum concentration of HBV DNA, and as components of the lymphocytic inflammatory infiltrate, as were FoxP3(+)-cells in patients with chronic hepatitis B as compared to control samples. In addition, peripheral and hepatic CD4+CD25+ regulatory T cells also influence the antiviral immune response and disease progression in patients with hepatitis B. A significant increase in CD4+CD25+ Treg, which correlated with viral load, in both cell pools was documented in what was characterized as severe chronic hepatitis B, with a marked increase in FoxP3(+)-cell and inflammatory infiltrate. Acute hepatitis B infection was characterized by an increase in the proportion of CD4+CD25+ Treg frequency. In addition, depletion of CD4+CD25+ Treg was associated with an increase in IFN-gamma by peripheral blood mononuclear cells (PBMN) cells that had been stimulated by HBV Ag. Also, the CD4+CD25+ Treg suppressed proliferation of autologous PBMC, expected from stimulation by HBs Ag. These findings suggested the generation of HBV-Ag-specific Treg in the periphery and liver tissue of patients with HBV infection [38].

A strong CD4+ response in acute HVB infection and the size of the viral inoculum contribute to the outcome of HBV infection [39]. Clearance was heralded by early CD4+ T-cell priming either before or at the onset of detectable viral spread. It coincided with a sharply synchronized influx of HBV-specific CD8+ T cells into the liver and a corresponding increase in intrahepatic CD8 mRNA, serum ALT activity, and histological evidence of acute viral hepatitis. In a primate model of HBV infection in which the percentage of infected hepatocytes was examined, it was demonstrated that inoculation with different concentrations of HBV DNA was associated with extreme differences in the percentage of cells infected, duration and clearance of infection, and different degrees of liver inflammation. Clearance of the virus was associated with priming of CD4+ and detection of HBV specific CD8+ T cells with histological evidence of hepatitis. The depletion of CD4+ cells prior to inoculation was associated with infection of 100% of hepatocytes, persistent inflammation, and persistent infection [39]. In support of the role of CD8+ in the clearance of HBV infection are the findings from studies in human beings with HBV infection where a high number of intrahepatic HBV-specific CD8 cells were documented in the absence of inflammation; however, virus specific cells, although in a similar number, were dispersed in a rich inflammatory infiltrate. Suppression of viral replication was associated with a circulating pool of CD8(+), not detected in patients with high viremia and inflammation, with the ability to expand upon recognition of the virus. These findings were interpreted to suggest that an effective HBV-specific response can be independent from liver injury. In the absence of a specific CD8 response able to control virus replication, a CD8 mediated recruitment of non-virus specific cells can contribute to the liver pathology [40].

As a robust response of CD4+ T cells is important in the resolution of HBV infection, a role of MHCII, which presents antigens to this type of cells, has been considered important in the course of the hepatitis. In this context, in a group of children and adult black subjects from Gambia, the class II allele HLA-DRB1*1302 was reported significantly more frequently in individuals who resolved the infection than in those who did not [41]. In Caucasian subjects from Europe, the class II allele HLA-DRB1*1301-02 was found in 5.7% of those with chronic hepatitis B, significantly lower than in the control group, and in 33.3% of subjects who cleared the virus, significantly higher than in subjects with chronic infection, suggesting that this allele offers protection against chronicity [42]. In patients from Korea, HLA-DR6 was reported in 28.4% of patients who had resolved an acute HBV infection, which was significantly higher than the 9.6% in subjects with chronic disease. Also, HLA-DR9 was significantly higher in patients with chronic infection than in those who cleared it. In addition, HLA-DR13 was associated with an increase in the HBV resolution of infection [43]. In a group of patients from Qatar, it was reported that HLA-DR7 was relatively common in patients with chronic infection, whereas HLA-DR2 was relatively uncommon [44]. From a study conducted in military personnel in China, it was reported that the frequency of the HLA-DRB1*0301, HLA-DQA1*0501, and HLA-DQB1*0301 alleles was significantly higher in patients with chronic hepatitis B, 35.58%, 25.96%, and 35.58%, respectively, compared to that in a control group of subjects in which it was 18.87%, 13.68%, and 18.87%, which has suggested that those alleles predisposed to chronicity. In contrast, the frequency HLA-DRB1*1101/1104 and HLA-DQA1*0301 was 0.96% and 14.42%, both significantly lower in patients with chronic hepatitis B than that of the control group in which it was 13.33% and 30%, respectively, suggesting that these alleles may offer some protection from chronicity of the viral infection [45]. These series of studies covering different racial and possibly ethnic groups have suggested that the host's MHC II composition has an impact on how it responds to the acute viral infection and identifies a genetic vulnerability for its chronicity.

Genetic polymorphisms in cytokines that contribute to endogenous antiviral mechanisms, including TNF-alpha, have also been identified as contributors to chronicity [46–50]; these reports, however, have been inconsistent in the identification of common characteristics in different ethnic groups, which is not unexpected because of genetic heterogeneity. A meta-analysis that included 12 studies that added up to 2754 patients with chronic HBV infection and 1630 subjects who had cleared the virus documented polymorphisms −863 A and − 308 G in the promoter region of TNF-alpha, which is important for the optimal expression of this cytokine, in individuals with chronic viral infection [51]. In contrast to chronicity, IFN I, IFN-AR2 receptor genes, and IL-10RB gene, localized to chromosome 21q22, were reported in association with HBV infection clearance in patients from Gambia where this infection is prevalent [52].

The use of genome-wide association studies (GWAS) has also identified variants in the HLA-DP locus in patients with chronic HBV infection in Asia. HLA-DPA1(*)0202-DPB1(*)0501, HLA-DPA1(*)0202-DPB1(*)0301, and HLA-DPB1*09:01 were reported as haplotypes in association with chronicity, and HLA-DPA1(*)0103-DPB1(*)0402, HLA-DPA1(*)0103-DPB1(*)0401, DPB1*02:01 as haplotypes protective of chronic infection [52, 53].

Characteristics of the virus itself, including genotype and genomic mutations, have also been identified as determinants of the natural history of the HBV infection [54]. Infection with HBV genotypes A and D has been reported in association with chronicity, in contrast to that with B and C, findings that may relate to the virus's geographic distribution. In Japan, where genotypes A, B, and C are prevalent, acute infection with hepatitis B genotype A, was reported to be associated with chronic infection [55–57], reported as 23% in one study [56] and 1%, for subtype Ae in another study [55]. Spontaneous e antigen seroconversion, i.e., e antigen loss and development of anti e antibodies, has been reported more frequently in patients infected with genotypes A and B, being delayed, when it happens, with C and D genotype infections [58]. Mutations in the B hepatitis genome have also been reported to influence the natural history of the infection. Infections with viri with the mutation G1896A at the precore and A1762T/G1764A at the core-promoter regions were six and three times, respectively, more frequent in patients with fulminant hepatitis than in those with than acute self-limited hepatitis [55]. It was documented among subjects from Eastern India that HBV genotype D2 was the most common subgenotype in acute hepatitis B and genotype C most common in patients with chronic HBV. Mutations in the S, BCP/PC, and X gene were relatively low in acute hepatitis B compared with the case of chronic HBV infection, with A1762T and G1764A being the most common mutation in the BCP and most notable indicators of chronicity [59]. Although these findings may be related or modified by the mode of transmission and temporal period of acquisition, it may reflect the virus's ability to lead to persistence.

It has been reported that men who have sex with men and drug users have a greater risk of developing chronic HBV virus infection than the general population. Possible explanations for this observation include degree of immunological function and genetic vulnerability [60]. In this regard, the HLA-DPA1 and HLA-DPB1 genes have been associated with protection against chronic hepatitis B in an Asian population [52, 53, 61], and in an African population. Coding changes in two genes located in chromosome 21q22, the type I IFN receptor gene, IFN-AR2, and the IL-10RB gene, which encodes a receptor chain for IL-10-related cytokines including the IFN-lambdas, are associated with viral clearance were identified [52]. In contrast, genes associated with chronicity include rs652888 on euchromatic histone-lysine-methyltransferase 2 (EHMT2) and rs1419881 on transcription factor 19 (TCF19) in the HLA of chromosome 6 [62], rs3130542 at 6p21.33 (near *HLA-C*), and rs4821116 at 22q11.21 in *UBE2L3* [63]. In addition, single nucleotide polymorphisms (SNPs) that affect the production of Mannose binding lectin, an important component of the innate immune response, have also been found in association with chronic hepatitis B [64].

# Epidemiology

The Centers for Disease Control (CDC) documented that the reported cases of acute HBV infections ranged from 4713 in 2006 to 3218 in 2016; however, it is estimated that the cases of acute HBV infections are 6.5 times higher than what has been reported with estimated numbers of 18,800 (range 10,800–46,100) in 2011 and 20,900 (range 11,900–51,200) in 2016 with the number of cases of chronic hepatitis B being 850,000–2.2 million. The deaths certified from chronic hepatitis B from 1700 to 1800 from 2006 to 2016, with HBV infection listed as an underlying or contributing factor in 1715 in 2016 [65].

The World Health Organization has reported hepatitis B as the most common cause of death worldwide, with a shocking 4000 deaths per day [66]. However, the number of estimated new infections has decreased from over 18 million/year in 1990 to 4.7 million in 2015 in association with the introduction with vaccination against HBV infection [67]; this is a fundamental preventive intervention that the health care system worldwide must provide to eradicate this viral infection. The global effort to eliminate hepatitis B (and C) viral infection has been divided into four categories: (I) policy and data: (1) plans and strategy, (2) reliable national epidemiological data, (3) estimates of economic burden, and (4) mandatory screening of donated blood, (II) prevention of transmission: (1) harm-reduction programs and (2) free at birth and third dose of vaccination coverage, and (III) screening and treatment: (1) publicly funded screening programs, and (2) hepatitis B treatment and availability in national essential medication lists or government subsidized. In the USA, I (3) and III (1) and (2) are in development; the rest is available [66].

## Clinical Manifestations

Signs of HBV virus infection are exhibited by an incubation period from 45 to 120 days (more extended periods have been described), with an average of 90 days in human beings. Symptoms and signs, when present, include fatigue, decreased appetite, and jaundice and tend to appear 12 weeks after exposure, when evidence for infection and viral replication is fully exhibited by serology and laboratory findings of acute liver injury, e.g., high serum activity of ALT and aspartate aminotransferase (AST), which may persist for 12 weeks [68].

## Extrahepatic Manifestations

Polyarteritis nodosa (PAN) is a type of necrotizing vasculitis that affects middle size arteries. It is reported to be associated with HBV infection in a third of the patients. The pathogenesis of polyarteritis nodosa is considered to be from the deposition of immune-complexes in association with HBsAg in the renal lesions. From a large retrospective study in France that comprised 150 patients, it was documented that seroconversion to e antibody was higher when antiviral therapy, which included interferon and ribavirin, was added to cyclophosphamide and plasmapheresis. It was also associated with complete remission, after which relapses were uncommon after seroconversion. Antineutrophil cytoplasmic antibodies (ANCA) were not detected in any of the patients. Renal disease was always associated with renal vasculitis, and glomerulonephritis was not [69].

Renal disease associated with HBV infection includes membranous nephropathy, membranoproliferative glomerulonephritis (MPGN), and PAN (see above). The pathogenesis of HBV-related kidney disease concerns the deposition of HBsAg-antibody complexes in renal lesions and that of HBeAg in membranous nephropathy. In addition, mesangial proliferative glomerulonephritis, immunoglobulin A (IgA) nephropathy, crescentic glomerulonephritis, focal segmental glomerulosclerosis (FSGS), and minimal change disease have been reported in association with HBV infection [70].

Membranous nephropathy is characterized by the deposition of immune complexes in the subepithelial region of the glomerular basement membrane. Proteinuria and nephrotic syndrome are clinical manifestations, and in adults, microscopic hematuria was common. In children, the condition tends to be self-limited and resolves in association with seroconversion from e antigen to anti e antibody; in adults, spontaneous resolution is not common, and the disease can progress to end stage renal disease [71].

MPGN associated with HBV infection manifests itself with proteinuria, hematuria, renal insufficiency, and hypertension. In this condition, antigen-antibody complexes are deposited in the mesangium and subendothelial space [70]. MPGN can be associated with hepatitis B related mixed cryoglobulinemia [72]. In addition to the clinical presentation of MPGN, patients with cryoglobulinemia present with a purpuric rash and low serum complement and rheumatoid factor in serum. The condition can progress to end stage renal disease in spite of antiviral and immunosuppressive therapy [72].

Extrahepatic manifestations that include Guillain Barre syndrome [73], myopathies [74], and hearing loss [75] have also been reported.

## Characteristics of Chronic Hepatitis B Virus Infection

Certain serological, biochemical, and histological features that characterize chronic hepatitis B have been labeled as phases, immune tolerant (or *low inflammatory phase* based on the findings of specific T cell response to HVB [76]), immune active, and inactive (Table 7.1) [77, 78].

One of the features of chronic hepatitis B is the episodic increases in serum AST and ALT activities sometimes accompanied by hyperbilirubinemia, known as flares, which are described in Table 7.2. The flares have been generally defined as an abrupt increase in serum ALT activity to greater than five times the upper limit of normal [90] and associated with: (i) an increase in immune mediated inflammatory activity that includes an increase in HBcAg/HBeAg-specific precursor T cell frequencies [96], (ii) increased production in interferon gamma [97], increased hepatic expression of IL-2 and IFN-gamma mRNA, mostly in the increased ALT activity phase, with IL-4 mRNA in the decreased activity phase, findings suggestive of augmented liver inflammatory response by Th-1 related cytokines, and decreased inflammatory response by Th-2 related cytokines [98], (iii) a decline in HBcAg-specific T(reg) in association with an increase in HBcAg peptide-specific cytotoxic T lymphocyte frequencies, features interpreted to suggest that the former cells mediate the immune tolerant phase of the infection, and that their decline favors spontaneous flares [99], (iv) an increase in IL-10-producing B cells [99], (v) an increase in TRAIL mediated hepatocyte death by NK cells [27], high serum levels of CXCL-9 and CXCL-10 [100], and circulating and intra-hepatic programmed cell death (PD1) levels and expression of its ligand PD-L1, finding interpreted to suggest that the local hepatic PD-L1 may contribute to the persistence of the viral infection by creating an immunosuppressive environment, thus inhibiting anti-HBV T cell expansion [101] that could result in seroconversion from e antigen to anti e antibody status. The appearance of increasing T cell responses to HBcAg/HBeAg usually occurs in the early phase of acute exacerbations. These findings imply that HBcAg/HBeAg-specific T cells play an important role in exacerbating chronic hepatitis B and HBeAg seroconversion. HBcAg/HBeAg-specific precursor T cell frequencies were serially studied in selected cases by limiting dilution assay. Elevation (two- to fourfold) of HBcAg/HBeAg-specific precursor T cell frequencies contributed to increased HBcAg/HBeAg-specific T cell proliferation during acute exacerbations (Table 7.2).

**Table 7.1** Phases of hepatitis B virus infection [77, 78]

|  | HBV DNA (IU/ml) | ALT (IU/ml) | E antigen in serum | Anti e antibody in serum | Histology | Mode of transmission/natural history [79] |
|---|---|---|---|---|---|---|
| Immune tolerant phase | 200,000 IU/mL or beyond | WNL | Positive | Negative | Minimal or no inflammation or fibrosis | • Usually perinatally acquired<br>• Long duration (years)<br>• May be associated with HCC at long term<br>• May change to immune active phase (usually in genotype C) [80, 81] |
| Immune active phase | >20,000 | Increased | Positive | Negative | Inflammation with or without fibrosis | • HBV DNA may decrease<br>• Spontaneous seroconversion, i.e. loss of e Ag and development of anti e antibody<br>• Seroconversion may be associated with hepatitis flare, decreased rate of decompensation and increased survival [79, 82, 83] |
| Immune active | >2000 | Increased | Negative | Positive | Inflammation with or without fibrosis | • Remains in association with activity<br>• Changes to inactive phase and exhibits episodes of reactivation [79, 83, 84] |
| Inactive phase | <2000 IU/ml | WNL |  | Positive | Minimal or absent inflammation, presence of fibrosis that can decrease over years | • Histological improvement overtime<br>• HBV DNA remains low or not detectable [85–88] |

*HBV DNA* hepatitis B deoxyribonucleic acid; *ALT* alanine aminotransferase; *WNL* within normal limits

**Table 7.2** Characteristics of chronic hepatitis B flares [89]

| | Proposed precipitants/ proportion of patients that experience flares | Population/serology/ clinical manifestations/ serum transaminases activity | Immunology | Serology | Histology | Outcomes |
|---|---|---|---|---|---|---|
| Spontaneous flares | Change in immune recognition of HBV/10–30% per year | Mostly adults and[a]/ MSM, infection with HIV, bacterial infections, surgery/ pregnancy/ asymptomatic or anorexia, fatigue, nausea; liver failure can occur especially in advanced disease/2 to 5 times ULN | Expansion of T cells reactive to HBeAg and HBcAg in early phase with subsequent decrease if seroconversion to anti e Ab occurs | (1) Anti e Ab+ and negative HBV DNA (2) + HBeAg and + HBV DNA, or – HBV DNA if ongoing flare activity has been followed seroconversion to anti e Ab (3) In precore mutant HBV with + HBV DNA but – HBeAg IgM anti-core can reappear during chronic hepatitis B flares | CD8+ CTL reactive to hepatocyte surface associated HBcAg peptides/ hepatocellular necrosis with lobular hepatitis/ flares associated with disease progression | Seroconversion to anti e Ab in 50% of patients with serum ALT >5 times ULN, and >60% at 12–18 months of follow-up post flare [90] |

| Proposed precipitants/ proportion of patients that experience flares | Population/serology/ clinical manifestations/ serum transaminases activity | Immunology | Serology | Histology | Outcomes |
|---|---|---|---|---|---|
| In association with cytotoxic and immunosuppressive therapy | | | | | |
| Increased replication and infection to a large hepatocyte population and enhanced recognition of HBV by immune system | Chemotherapy, biological, and post organ transplantation recipients/14 to 72% of subjects with chronic or prior exposure to HBV infection/HB sAg+ (most common), + anti core Ab alone and + anti HBs/hepatitis with and without hyperbilirubinemia, fulminant hepatitis | | HBsAg+, anti-core Ab+ and anti-HBs, alone or in combination. Titers of all tended to decrease during therapy | Lobular hepatitis, submassive hepatic necrosis, fibrosing cholestatic hepatitis (in post OLT patients) | (1) For review [91] (2) Mortality of 5.2% (vs 0.0% in association with prophylaxis with NA in patients on chemotherapy for lymphoma [92] (3) 50% reactivation during chemotherapy in hematological malignancies, 20% after chemotherapy; no deaths [93] (4) In solid tumors, in comparison with early identification, late identification of chronic HBV infection associated with flares, HR, 4.02[b]; hepatic impairment, HR = 8.48[c]; liver failure = HR, 9.38[d]; death = HR, 3.90[e] [94] (5) Hematological malignancies, death was increased by 7.8 times in patients with late identification of HVB[f] [94] |
| In association with antiviral therapy with interferon | | | | | |
| Increased immune recognition | 25% of subjects on treatment | | | | Decrease and ultimate suppression of serum HBV DNA and seroconversion to anti e Ab |

(continued)

**Table 7.2** (continued)

| Proposed precipitants/proportion of patients that experience flares | Population/serology/clinical manifestations/serum transaminases activity | Immunology | Serology | Histology | Outcomes |
|---|---|---|---|---|---|
| HBsAg+ in association with lamivudine (nucleoside analogue)[g] — (1) Increased immunological recognition of HBV in association with reduction of viral replication (2) Resurgence of wild-type HBV virus | (1) 10% of subjects on treatment/AST and ALT 3 times over baseline (2) Flare in association with discontinuation of treatment | | | | |
| In association with HBV genotypic variations: (1) Pre-core mutants (2) Basal core promoter (BCP) — Absence of e Ag production possibly associated with decreased immune tolerance and increased immunologic response to core Ag on hepatocyte surface | (1) Common at the time mutations appear and decrease in frequency when the majority of the infecting HVB is comprised of the pre-core mutant variant (2) BCP | | (2) Decrease in e antigen production and increase in HBV DNA | (2) Active histology | |

| | Proposed precipitants/proportion of patients that experience flares | Population/serology/clinical manifestations/serum transaminases activity | Immunology | Serology | Histology | Outcomes |
|---|---|---|---|---|---|---|
| In association with infections with hepatitis A, C, and D | Superimposed liver injury; may be severe and fulminant | Patients with chronic hepatitis B | | Decrease in serum HBV DNA and loss of e Ag possibly from interference to viral replication | | |
| In association with HIV | (1) Clearance of serum HBV DNA from immune reconstitution from anti HIV treatment (2) Reactivation of HVB due to decrease in serum HIV RNA with subsequent loss of cytokine control on HBV replication | | | (1) Loss of HBV DNA in association with flare | | |

[a]e anti + children

HR = hazard ratio, 95% confidence interval [CI] [b](1.26–12.86); [c](1.86–38.66; [d](1.50–58.86; [e](1.19–12.83); [f](1.73–35.27)

[g]Fialuridine is a nucleoside analogue that was associated with marked decrease in HBV DNA but also with lactic acidosis and death. It is not in use and it will not be discussed in this chapter [95]

ULN upper limit of normal; CTL cytotoxic T lymphocytes; NA nucleos(t)ide analogues

## Laboratory Findings and Serology

Following the incubation and prodrome, frank hepatitis with serum ALT activity from several hundred to low thousands, mild to modest hyperbilirubinemia, hypoalbuminemia, and sometimes short lasting coagulopathy; there can be leukopenia with a predominance of lymphocytes. The hepatic panel, which most strikingly exhibits high serum activity of ALT, normalizes itself over approximately 12 weeks from the initial documented abnormality. The liver profile of patients with chronic hepatitis B varies in reference to the stage of the disease and it can be normal, or with serum activity of transaminases several times the upper limit of normal.

In the context of viral hepatitis B markers, HBsAg can be detected in the serum of acutely infected persons for a period of 1–9 weeks, with an average of four, and it is the only marker of hepatitis B detected after the initial infection; patients who clear the infection do not have any measurable surface antigen by 15 weeks, in general, after the start of symptoms. HBV DNA at high concentrations, indicative of viral replication, is detected in serum soon after the time of infection until 15 weeks after such, its absence coinciding with the disappearance of HBsAg. In fifty percent of patients who clear the acute infection, HBV DNA and HBsAg cannot be detected in serum by week seven after initial clinical manifestations. HBe antigen, which correlates with high HBV DNA levels and is a reflection of high infectivity, is detected in the serum from the time of infection until approximately 14 weeks after, followed by the rise of anti HBe antibody, which remains present as immunological evidence of infection. Total and IgM anti-core antibodies rise to detectable levels 6 weeks after infection; IgM anti-core antibody peaks at week 16 and decreases gradually to undetectability by week 30 post infection, whereas IgG anti-core peaks at week 20 and remains, usually for life, as evidence of prior infection. The window period is characterized by the absence of HBsAg and anti HBs; at this time, the presence of HBV infection can only be confirmed if anti-core antibodies are measured, highlighting the importance of the development of this assay [102] in medicine and epidemiology [103, 104]. The case definition of chronic hepatitis B by the CDC is the absence of IgM anticore antibodies and positive HBsAg, or HBeAg, or hepatitis B virus DNA, including qualitative, quantitative, and genotype testing, or HBsAg positive or HBV DNA positive, also including qualitative, quantitative, and genotype testing or HBeAg positive in two occasions at least 6 months apart [105]. High HBV DNA in serum and the presence of HBe antigen is characteristic of patients who have entered the chronic phase of viral hepatitis B; the rate of seroconversion, i.e., loss of e antigen and development of anti e antibody is 8–12% per year in patients who develop chronic infection. Patients with chronic hepatitis B with and without cirrhosis can develop hepatocellular carcinoma (HCC), as well as complications of chronic liver disease, including portal hypertension and its consequences, and liver failure.

## Differential Diagnosis

Causes of acute or chronic hepatitis, including viral, autoimmune, metabolic, and toxic (e.g., drug-induced), must be excluded in patients who present with increased serum activity of transaminases, with or without hyperbilirubinemia.

## Liver Histology

The histology of acute HBV infection is similar to that of other forms of acute hepatitis. It is noted that in acute hepatitis B, lymphocytes and macrophages are identified in contact with infected hepatocytes, consistent with the immune mediated mechanism recognized to mediate HBV hepatitis. The mechanisms by which hepatocellular death is mediated include rupture of ballooned hepatocytes and apoptosis, the latter having been defined as the most relevant [106]. The feature that characterizes HBV infected hepatocytes is the ground-glass hepatocyte, which can be identified by its expression of HBsAg by immunohistochemistry, or by the orcein or Victoria blue stains. It is a feature of chronic infection as the identification of HBsAg, as expressed by ground-glass hepatocytes, in acute and fulminant cases is uncommon (Fig. 7.1) [106]. Hepatitis B core antigen is found in the cytoplasm in association with active inflammatory activity [106]; it is also found in the nucleus, where it is believed to represent empty nucleocapsids [107].

The histological diagnostic features of chronic HBV infection include marked hepatocellular polymorphism and what has been described as dysplastic

**Fig. 7.1** Liver histology from a patient with chronic hepatitis B and diffuse surface antigen hepatocyte expression as evidenced by orcein stain (arrow) (40X)

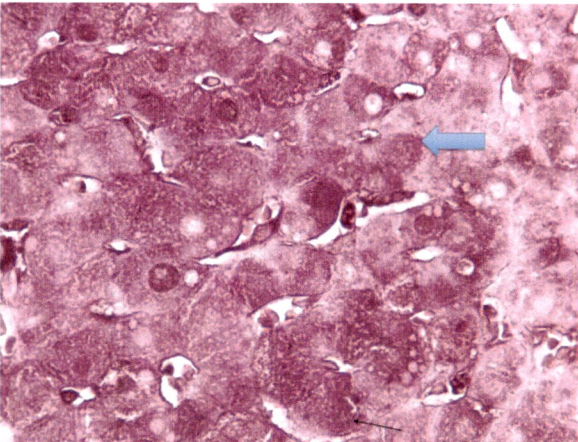

hepatocytes [108], characterized by enlargement of hyperbasophilic nuclei and eosinophilic swelling of the cytoplasm of perivenular hepatocytes [107]. Inflammatory changes in bile ducts and lymphoid follicles are not common; when present, coinfection with HCV or HDV is suggested. Satellitosis, defined as single hepatocytes surrounded by lymphocytes, can also be found. Flares tend to affect zone III, i.e., pericentrally, and characterized by ballooning of hepatocytes.

## Natural History of Chronic Hepatitis B

In patients with chronic hepatitis B, spontaneous losses of hepatitis B surface antigen (HBsAg) occur in 0.2–0.8% per year [109]. This event, which has been termed recovery phase, is associated with a decrease in fibrosis; however, HBV DNA can be detected in serum at a reported frequency of 21% 5 years after antigen loss. A study on the HBsAg seroclearance in 92 Chinese patients with chronic hepatitis B documented HBsAg loss at a mean age of 48.8 years [110]. Seroconversion was reported to be associated with a significant decrease in serum ALT activity. Clearance of HBsAg was documented more frequently in patients infected with genotype B than in those infected with genotype C. Ninety-eight percent of the patients did not have HBV DNA in serum, and 37% had HBV DNA in the liver, mostly in the form of cccDNA. Liver histology was reported as almost normal in association with seroclearance of HBsAg; however, there was no difference in the risk of development of HCC between patients with and without HBsAg seroclearance, although the age at which seroclearance occurred was greater in patients with HCC [110]. These results underscore the importance of screening for HCC in patients who have had chronic hepatitis B. It also highlights the fact that the recovery phase is not always associated with the absence of complications from chronic HBV infection.

In regard to patients with chronic hepatitis B, e antigen negative, anti-e positive serology there is a consensus that supports that a serum concentration of HBV DNA greater than 2000 IU/ml (greater than $10^4$ genomic copies/ml) can be associated with liver injury; thus, it is the level at which a liver biopsy may be considered if information on liver histology is required, e.g., prior to starting therapy in patients with normal ALT and HBV DNA consistently documented as described above [77, 78]. It was documented that liver inflammation and fibrosis were present in 90% of subjects with HBV DNA greater than 20,000 IU/ml and high serum ALT activity, in 10% of those with HBV DNA between 2000 and 20,000 IU/ml, and in 1% of those with serum HBV DNA less than 2000 IU/ml [110]. A series of studies have documented a relationship between gender, age, HBV DNA, and the presence of cirrhosis with the development of HCC in patients with chronic HBV infection [111]. In 28,870 subjects from Taiwan with chronic hepatitis B with a median age of 46 years at study entry, 4155 of whom were HBsAg-positive and 3653 had a baseline HBV DNA available, were followed for 11.4 years. It was documented that subjects who had an HBV DNA greater than 2000 IU/ml at entry and at the end of the follow-up period were at risk for the development of HCC. This information has contributed to the recommendation to screen for HCC in person at least 40 years of age with chronic hepatitis B [111].

Mutations in the BCP region of the HBV to A1762T and G1764A have been reported as independent factors that predict the development of HCC in patients with chronic HBV genotypes A2, B, C, and D [112]; mutations in the pre-core region have been inconsistently reported in association with risk for HCC, although they have been reported in association with active inflammation in patients who are in the HBe-antigen + immune active chronic hepatitis B phase (Table 7.1).

Chronic HBV infection is associated with cirrhosis and its complications and with HCC. From a study that comprised 1536 natives of Alaska with chronic HBV, 41.7% of whom were HBeAg-positive and who were enrolled in a surveillance program for detection of HCC over a follow-up period of 12.3 years, the reported observed probability to clear HBeAg within 10 years of diagnosis was 72.5%, with 7% of subjects losing HBsAg, events associated with increased age and presence of anti-HBe antibodies. The incidence of complications from liver disease was reported as 2.3 per 1000 carrier-years, and that of HCC, which was related to reversion from anti-HBe antibodies to e Ag positivity, as 1.9 per 1000 carrier-years, being documented as more common in men, 2.3, than in women, 1.2 [109].

Seroconversion from e antigen to its loss is an important step in the natural history of chronic HBV virus infection, as it is associated with histological improvement. Seroconversion from e Ag positive to anti-HBe was reported not to be influenced by HBV genotype; however, sustained seroconversion was more common in patients infected with genotype A than in those infected with genotype D. In addition, death from complications of liver disease was significantly higher in patients infected with genotype F than in those infected with genotype D [113]. Infection with HBV genotype C was reported in association with high viral load and with a greater risk for development of HCC in a study comprised of 154 patients from Taiwan who had developed this type of cancer over 14 years of follow-up compared to a control group of subjects [114]. A less aggressive disease was reported in patients with HBV genotype B infection in a study from Japan; however, the long-term complications were not documented to be significantly different between infections from genotypes B and C [114]. However, from another study conducted in Taiwan, HBV infection with genotype B or C was significantly associated with the development of HCC [115]. In the presence of the G1896A variant, HCC was significantly more common than when the infection was associated with G1896 (wild type); for patients infected with a virus that had the BCP A1762T/G1764A double mutation, the risk for HCC was also higher than that in patients infected with a virus that had the BCP A1762/G1764 (wild type). The highest risk to develop HCC was for patients infected with HBV genotype C, wild type precore variant and mutant for the BCP 1762/1764 variant (adjusted hazard ratio = 2.99, 95% CI = 1.57 to 5.70, $p < 0.001$) [115]. In Alaska, genotype F was found in the majority of patients with HCC from a cohort of 47 patients with chronic HBV and HCC, but no association with mutations in the core promoter and precore regions was demonstrated [116].

A retrospective study from the hepatology clinic in a community hospital in Northern Brooklyn attended by the author documented that patients with chronic hepatitis B came from all continents [117]. The most common genotypes in this study were A, D, and E, which are the most prevalent in North America, Southern Europe, the Middle East, and sub-Saharan Africa [54], a reflection of the geographical areas of origin of the population that the hospital serves. The patients with high levels of serum HBV DNA in association with a pre-core mutation and negative anti-HBe antibody were infected with genotype D mostly, consistent with other reports [118].

The impact of HBV treatment on the natural history of the disease was examined in a prospective study in which 103 patients with chronic hepatitis B, with e antigen + disease who had been treated with interferon alpha, were followed for a mean period of 50.0 (±SD) ±19.8 months. Treatment with interferon alpha was associated with the disappearance of HBeAg and HBV DNA in 53 of 103 (51%) patients. Of these, ten lost HBsAg, with estimates of a cumulative clearance at 5 years of 56% for HBeAg loss, and 11.6% for HBsAg, by the Kaplan-Meier analysis. These results were significantly different from those of the control group, which was comprised of 53 patients who had not been treated, and from whom seven lost HBeAg spontaneously at 5 years, and none of whom lost HBsAg. Of the treated patients, six died of liver failure, and two had a liver transplant, all of whom had remained HBeAg+. Eight other patients who had also maintained e Ag+ status developed complications of cirrhosis. Survival and survival without complications were reported to be significantly longer in patients who had lost e Ag in association with therapy than those who had remained e Ag+. HBeAg loss was reported as the strongest predictor of survival in association with treatment. In the control group, 13 of the 53 patients who had remained HBeAg+ developed complications of liver disease, including death and liver transplantation [119].

The probability of survival at 1, 3, and 5 years was reported as 92%, 79%, and 71%, respectively, in a group of 98 patients with cirrhosis in association with chronic HBV infection that was followed for a mean period of 4.3 years, with age, serum bilirubin concentration, and ascites independently related to survival. Decompensated liver disease was associated with a survival of 14% at 5 years, in contrast to that of patients with compensated cirrhosis of 84%. In this study, the presence of hepatitis B e antigen was associated with the probability of survival at 5 years of 72% compared to 97% for patients who were e antigen negative. The importance of e antigen seroconversion was also confirmed, as it was associated with a decrease in the risk of death [120].

Indeed, studies from different geographical areas have documented the morbidity and mortality risk in patients with chronic hepatitis B. From a study conducted in Italy, it was reported that regardless of a specific serology at the time of diagnosis, chronic hepatitis B, with cirrhosis and inflammatory activity as contributing factors, was associated with increased mortality, 5.2 times that of the general population [121]. From Taiwan, it was documented from a study that included 1506 patients with chronic HBV infection that cirrhosis, inferred by clinical and sonographic changes, was a risk factor for HCC, which was identified in a group of patients after 7 years of follow-up, with a multivariate-adjusted relative risk (RR) of 11.8 (95% confidence interval (CI) 3.9–35.8); the presence of e antigen and consistent increase in the serum activity of ALT for 6 months were identified by multivariate analysis as risk factors for cirrhosis [82]. In Japan, 3769 women diagnosed as carrying hepatitis B surface antigen during blood donation were followed from 1977 to 1985; the population attributable risk was estimated to be 6.5% for HCC, significantly higher than that found in the general population of women of the same age [122].

Most of the complications associated with chronic hepatitis B were reported in association with cirrhosis [123], with an estimated 5-year survival of 80% reported from a study that enrolled 76 patients at the time the diagnosis of cirrhosis was made and that were followed for 34.4 months. The annual incidence of acute exacerbations, which tended to occur 2 years after enrollment, which were usually in association with the presence of e antigen, was reported to be 11.9%. Reactivation of HBV infection was the cause of the acute exacerbation in the majority of patients. In 30% of subjects, it was associated with seroconversion from e antigen + to anti-HBe, with the loss of surface antigen being uncommon. The incidence of hepatic decompensation, esophageal variceal bleeding, and HCC was reported as 2.3%, 2.3%, and 2.8%, respectively. Liver failure and variceal bleeding were the cause of death in 9.2% of the patients [123]. Important information was provided by a multicenter European study that examined survival and prognostic factors in 366 patients with compensated cirrhosis in association with chronic hepatitis B. The study followed patients with compensated cirrhosis for a mean period of 72 months (6–202 months). At enrollment, 35% of the patients were HBeAg positive, serum HBV DNA was present in 48% of the patients in whom it was measured, and 20% had antibodies against the delta hepatitis virus. Eighty-four (23%) of the patients died, 45 of complications of liver failure, and 23 of HCC. The cumulative probability of survival was reported as 84 and 68% at 5 and 10 years, respectively. Hepatitis B virus replication, evidenced by the presence of HBV DNA in serum, increased age, portal hypertension, as suggested by splenomegaly and hypersplenism, and synthetic hepatic dysfunction correlated with a decrease in survival. Absence of serum HBV DNA and normal activity of transaminases highly correlated with survival [124].

The incidence of cirrhosis was studied in a histological follow-up study of 105 patients with HBsAg in serum, 59 of whom were reported to have chronic active hepatitis (i.e., presence of interface hepatitis, Fig. 7.2) without cirrhosis, and 46 were reported to have no interface hepatitis at enrollment. Liver histology, reexamined after a mean follow-up of 3.7 years, was reported to show cirrhosis in 21 patients (20%) 1 to 13 years after entry into the study, with a calculated annual incidence of 5.9%. The presence of interface hepatitis (Fig. 7.2) and bridging fibrosis increased the probability of cirrhosis development significantly over findings of limited inflammation. Advanced age, the presence of bridging necrosis on histology, and active replication, as suggested by the detection of HBV DNA in serum, were reported as independent variables that portended poor prognosis [125].

**Fig. 7.2** Liver histology exhibiting interface hepatitis (arrows) in a patients with chronic hepatitis B (40X)

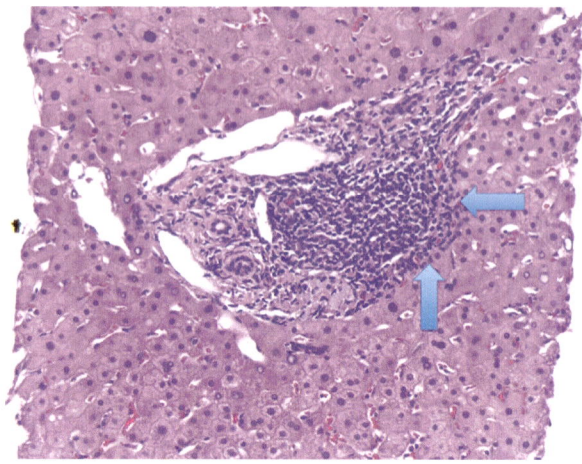

## Impact of Coinfection with HIV, HCV, and Delta Hepatitis Viri on the Natural History of Chronic Hepatitis B

Coinfection with the hepatitis C virus also contributes to the development of HCC in patients with chronic hepatitis B. In a study comprised of 231 black patients with HCC from South Africa, the risk for HCC was increased by 23.3 fold in those patients positive for HBsAg, and 6.6 in those positive for HCV, as compared to those without markers of viral hepatitis infection. The relative risk to develop HCC in patients with markers of hepatitis B and C viral infections was 82.5 [126]. A dominating presence of HBV infection and the contribution of coinfection with HCV was confirmed by a study from Gambia, West Africa, in which 216 incident cases of HCC and 408 control were enrolled and from which it was reported a 61% infection state for HBV in patients with HCC versus 16% of the control subjects, and 19% HCV positive serology in the HCC group versus 3% in the control group. The increased risk for HCC in patients with chronic hepatitis B was calculated as an odds ratio (OR) of 16.7, 95% CI, 9.7–28.7, and for patients with HCV infection, an OR of 16.7; 95% CI, 6.9–40.1, with marked increase by coinfection, with an OR of 35.3; 95% CI, 3.9–323 [127]. Studies from Europe have confirmed the findings of those from Africa. Patients with chronic hepatitis B co-infected with HCV, which tends to be the predominant virus with associated suppression HBV DNA [128], and be associated with loss of HBsAg on long-term follow-up [129], tend to develop advanced disease and are at risk for HCC. A synergism between HBV and HCV infection has been reported towards the risk of development of HCC, with the odds ratio for this type of cancer being reported as 165 (95% CI: 81.2–374), in a meta-analysis of epidemiological studies that examined the combined effect of hepatitis B and C virus infections in causing hepatocellular carcinoma [130]. Also, fulminant liver failure from acute HCV has been documented in patients who are carriers for

HBsAg with a reported incidence of 23.1% (95% CI = 9.9–36.3%), compared to that in patients who did not have HCV infection, in whom the incidence of fulminant liver failure was 2.9% (95% CI = −1.0–6.8%) in a study from Taiwan [131].

## Delta Hepatitis

The delta hepatitis virus is 36 nm in diameter. It is comprised of a single-stranded, circular RNA genome of negative polarity; eight genotypes have been identified, genotype1 being the most prevalent in North America [132] and also the most virulent [133]. HBsAg proteins are embedded in the lipid envelope that surrounds the HDV genome, which encodes a small delta antigen and the large delta antigen, and which uses the HBV envelope proteins for its assembly and propagation of infection; thus, the presence of the HBV is required for HDV replication, which occurs in the nucleus of the hepatocyte, and perpetuation of the infection.

Infection with HDV occurs simultaneously with that of HBV, or as superinfection, in a subject already infected with HBV. In contrast to HBV, HDV does have cytopathic effects on hepatocytes, mostly related to the small deltal antigen SHDAg, via innate and adaptive immunity, which tends to be weak and thus facilitates disease progression. The clinical presentation of coinfection is similar to that of mono infection with HBV, but the inflammatory response is severe, and it can be associated with acute liver failure [134]. Because replication of HDV requires HBV, characteristically, there are two peaks in serum activity of ALT separated by several weeks because the establishment of HBV infection is required [134, 135]. Infection with HDV in patients with chronic hepatitis B, i.e., superinfection, is more severe than coinfection, associated with an increased risk for acute liver failure. In patients with chronic HVB infection, superinfection with delta can be misinterpreted as flares; thus, it is important to rule out HBV superinfection in those cases. HDV RNA can be detected in serum only in the first 2 weeks of infection and transiently after that; IgM antibodies tend to appear within 2 to 3 weeks of infection, usually lasting from 2 to 9 months, occasionally followed by IgG. It is recommended to test HDV RNA when HDV IgG is detected to confirm infection.

The definition of chronic delta hepatitis is anti-HDV antibody positivity. In adults, HDV coinfection becomes chronic in less than 5% of cases. The probability of chronicity is greater than 90% when the infection is acquired in the neonatal period [77, 78]. Progression to cirrhosis can occur in 10–15% of patients within 2 years of infection, and in 80% after 5–10 years of infection [136]. There is a reported two-fold increase in the risk of hepatic decompensation and HCC in HDV than in chronic HBV infection. A report from the European Concerted Action on Viral Hepatitis from a retrospective cohort study of 200 patients from Western Europe with compensated cirrhosis, 20% of whom were infected with the delta hepatitis virus with 6.6 years of follow-up, documented that, as determined by Kaplan-Meier analysis, the 5-year probability of developing HCC was 6, 10, and 9% in patients who had anti-HDV antibodies, e antigen negative, negative for both anti-HDV antibodies and e Ag, and negative for anti-HDV antibody and e Ag positive, respectively; the probability of developing decompensated liver disease was 22, 16, and 19%, respectively, and that for survival was 92, 89, and 83%, respectively. The calculated risk for development of HCC was three times higher for patients with HBV associated cirrhosis co-infected with the delta hepatitis infection, and the probability of death two times greater than those not coinfected [137].

The liver in chronic delta hepatitis exhibits panacinar involvement where there is extensive interface hepatitis; progression to cirrhosis is accelerated. Lymphoid follicles and bile duct lesions can be found in cases of chronic delta hepatitis. The presence of fat was reported in a study that examined autopsy material from Indigenous Venezuelan Indians who exhibited liver failure or rapid progression to cirrhosis in association with HDV infection [107, 138].

Chronic hepatitis B in patients infected with the human immunodeficiency virus (HIV) is associated with a decrease in all the events that lead to seroconversion and resolution of the HBV infection. Patients coinfected with these two viri have increased mortality from liver related complications. From a study comprised of 5293 men who had sex with men, 326 (6%) of whom were HBsAg positive with 213 (65%) of this group being HIV-1 positive and in whom the documented mortality rate was 14.2/1000 as compared to that of subjects who were not coinfected with HBV, in whom it was 1.7/1000, or that of those with chronic HBV, in whom it was 0.8/1000, both significantly different from the coinfected patients [139].

## Treatment of Chronic Hepatitis B

The cure of chronic hepatitis B would be the eradication of cccDNA, the template used for viral replication, from the nucleus of the hepatocyte; however, at present, this has not been accomplished with interferon alpha or nucleos(t)ide reverse transcriptase inhibitors (NRTIs), the therapies available. Loss of surface antigen and the development of anti-HBs are considered a successful response to treatment, but this outcome is infrequent in association with the available medications.

The indications for treatment of chronic hepatitis B include inflammatory activity, indirectly assessed by serum activity of ALT, or documented on liver histology, viral replication, i.e., HBV DNA greater than 2000 IU/ml, and in all cirrhotic patients regardless of serum HBV DNA [140, 141]. In pregnant women, treatment in the third trimester when serum HBV DNA is greater than 200,000 IU//ml with nucleoside analogues, e.g., tenofovir, telbivudine, is indicated to decrease the mother to baby transmission [140, 141].

As it can be appreciated from the natural history of HBV reactivation and flares, inflammatory activity is relevant in the timing to treat patients with chronic hepatitis B. In regard to flares, it is necessary to follow patients with chronic hepatitis B for some time to determine the optimal time to treat because there is a greater than 50% probability of e antigen positive to anti e antibody seroconversion post flares at 18 months of follow-up, and close to 50% at 1 year post flares, a fact that changes the indication for treatment, as reported in a study [90]. In this context, there are notable differences between patients with chronic hepatitis B from the USA and those from Asia; the proportion of subjects that experience seroconversion in association with flares, and which changes the indication for treatment, is higher in the former than in the latter, where not only they tend to recur but do not tend to be associated with seroconversion [89, 90].

Robust flares increase the probabilities of seroconversion; however, flares are also associated with hepatocellular necrosis, fibrosis, and progression to cirrhosis; thus, treatment at the time of flares can be beneficial in terms of HBV DNA suppression, which eventually may lead to seroconversion to anti e and over time, to loss of s Ag and development of anti-HBs. Patients who experience flares associated with serum ALT activity greater than five times the upper limit of normal and hyperbilirubinemia must be closely followed as decompensation may follow [90]. Patients who undergo modest HBV flares with serum activity less than five times the upper limit of normal are unlikely to experience seroconversion, thus, they are the patients in whom treatment is indicated, as documented in the guidelines [90, 141].

Current guidelines recommend that patients with + serum HBV DNA and those with + anti core with or without detected HBV DNA in serum who are going to receive immunosuppressive therapy be treated with antiviral medications, tenofovir being the preferred medication (there are limited data with the use of tenofovir alafenamide for this indication) [90, 142, 143].

Treatment with interferon, which stimulates T and NK cells activity, in all its preparations and doses, can be associated with flares that tend to occur around the eighth week of treatment and after its completion (Table 7.2). Flares can be associated with seroconversion, and thus, it is a good prognostic sign; however, in patients with cirrhosis, flares can lead to liver failure; accordingly, interferon should not be used in this group of patients or used with extreme caution in patients with Child's A classification only. Interferon is contraindicated in patients with decompensated liver disease, i.e., Child's B and C.

Oral antiviral therapy with nucleoside and nucleotide analogues is associated with a marked decrease in HBV DNA and low probability of seroconversion, and with halted disease progression. During treatment with lamivudine, there is an increase in serum ALT activity during the first 4–6 weeks of treatment; however, the proportion of patients who exhibited a flare was not different from those treated with the placebo. Lamivudine therapy, which is not the drug of choice at present, can be associated with flares in association with the development of mutations in the polymerase gene, which are resistant to the drug, leading to the reappearance of HBV DNA [144]. Flares have also been reported in patients co-infected with HIV on treatment with lamivudine for the latter now considered to be from the development of HBV mutants [145].

## Indications for Treatment of Hepatitis B

The goal of treatment of chronic hepatitis B is the prevention of cirrhosis and its complications, including hepatocellular carcinoma. It is recommended that patients with chronic hepatitis B and chronic liver injury, as suggested by the high serum activity of ALT, be treated. Patients with high HBV serum levels and normal ALT activity do not tend to lose e antigen or seroconvert in association with antiviral treatment; thus, it is not recommended that this type of patients be treated; however, follow-up to detect any immune activity resulting in an inflammatory response as indicated by high serum ALT activity is necessary to identify a point in time where treatment may be indicated.

In patients with e antigen + chronic hepatitis B, serum ALT activity twice the upper limit of normal, serum HBV DNA lower than $2.0 \times 10(8)$ IU/mL, and no prior treatment with interferon was associated with sustained virologic response (SVR), defined as serum HBV DNA less than 2000 IU/mL at 6 months after treatment. Patients with genotype A, high serum activity of ALT, and relatively low HBV DNA had a predicted probability of SVR greater than 30% [146]; surface antigen loss in association with IFN treatment has also been associated with this genotype. The strongest predictor of response in patients with genotype B was high serum activity of ALT, and in those with genotype C, it was low HBV DNA; the probability of response to interferon in patients with genotype D was low, regardless of the serum activity of ALT or HBV DNA concentration [146]. There are no predictors of SVR in association with treatment with IFN or nucleoside or nucleotide analogues in patients with e antigen negative chronic HBV infection. A decrease in serum concentration of HBsAg has been identified as a predictor of response in patients with e antigen + chronic hepatitis B, and a predictor of sustained suppression of HBV DNA in serum in patients with e antigen negative chronic hepatitis B. These factors have been used as the basis to discontinue therapy with interferon at 12 or 24 weeks because of predicted futility [147].

Treatment is recommended for patients with cirrhosis, or suggestion of cirrhosis by clinical, laboratory, radiological, and by the technique of Fibroscan to prevent decompensation of liver disease, which will happen in time, or in association of hepatitis flares, which can lead to liver failure, and development of HCC regardless of the degree of viral replication, as measured by serum HBV DNA. Patients who experience worsening of their hepatitis as evidenced by increased serum ALT activity and hyperbilirubinemia and patients with acute liver failure in association with HBV infection should also get treated.

As the risk of developing cirrhosis increases over time in patients who have remained in the immune tolerant phase, patients should be treated at age 30–40 years [140, 141, 148, 149]; this recommendation also applies to patients with a family history of HCC [141, 148].

In pregnant women, a serum HBV DNA > 200,000 IU/ml is an indication for treatment with oral antiviral drugs, e.g., tenofovir, in the third trimester, regardless of the serum activity of ALT for over 8–12 weeks after delivery [141, 150, 151]. In addition, the infant receives hepatitis B immunoglobulin (HBIG) and vaccination against HBV is initiated at birth to prevent HBV transmission to the infant [141, 150, 151].

Patients who are HBsAg + or HBsAg – and anti-core + are at risk for HBV reactivation in association with treatment with immunosuppressants, including anticancer drugs; thus, prophylaxis therapy with oral antiviral medications, e.g., tenofovir, is indicated [141].

Treatment with oral antivirals is recommended in acute infections associated with impaired liver function, i.e., coagulopathy (INR > 1.5) [152, 153] and persistent hyperbilirubinemia, i.e., bilirubin >3 mg/dl for more than 4 weeks after presentation [141]. It is also recommended that patients with extrahepatic manifestations of chronic HBV infections be treated [153].

## Drugs for the Treatment of Chronic Hepatitis B

Interferon alpha is endogenously produced as a host defense against viral infection. Its effects include the induction of interferon-stimulated genes, which have antiviral properties, a decrease in the amount of intracellular HBV nucleocapsids, and the acceleration of the decline of HBV replication-competent nucleocapsids [154]. Interferon is also an immunomodulator. Treatment with interferon alpha was documented to deplete CD8-T cells and to stimulate the production of IL-15, a proproliferation cytokine, and an expansion in the number of CD56(bright) NK cells that exhibited increased activation markers and also, the activation receptor NKp46, in association with an enhanced expression of TRAIL and interferon gamma [155]. This observation coincided with the peak in the decrease in viral replication, supporting the idea that NK cells contribute to interferon's antiviral effect. Another proposed mechanism of action of interferon alpha against HBV replication is the decrease in the transcription of pregenomic RNA (pgRNA) and subgenomic RNA from the HBV covalently closed circular DNA (cccDNA) minichromosome, as documented in cultured cells and mouse livers populated with human hepatocytes infected with this virus [156]. In addition, specific degradation of nuclear viral DNA by the upregulation of APOBEC3A, a DNA cytidine deaminase with antiviral effects, by interferon alpha was reported as another mechanism of action of the drug [157].

The pegylation of interferon facilitated this medication's use by allowing its administration to be once a week for the duration of treatment, determined to be 48 weeks. Peginterferon alfa-2a has a 40 kilodalton branched polyethylene glycol, which significantly increased its serum half-life and plasma concentration [158]; this form of interferon was documented to be more efficacious in the treatment of chronic hepatitis C prior to its approval for use in chronic hepatitis B [159]. The results of one of the pivotal studies on which the approval of pegylated interferon was based are shown in Table 7.3 [160, 161]. A systematic review identified four studies for analysis that documented that pegylated interferon for at least 6 months was superior to lamivudine on viral and biochemical suppression in patients with e antigen + chronic hepatitis B, supporting the use of the former as the first line of therapy [163].

The DNA polymerase of the HBV virus synthesizes DNA via its reverse transcriptase activity [164]. HBV polymerase's priming activity is inhibited by purine analogues, which exert this effect by direct inhibition, through competitive binding with endogenous substrates or through incorporation into the viral DNA to act as chain terminators. The approved oral medications for the treatment of chronic HBV are lamivudine, entecavir, and telbivudine, which are nucleoside analogues, and adefovir dipivoxil and tenofovir disoproxil fumarate (TDF) and its prodrug tenofovir alafenamide (TAF), which are nucleotide analogues [20, 165] (Tables 7.4 and 7.5).

**Table 7.3** Effect of pegylated interferon on chronic hepatitis B

| Study design/drugs/duration | Number of adult patients per drug | Histologic response (%) in inflammation Pegylated interferon/lamivudine | Histologic response (%) in fibrosis Pegylated interferon/lamivudine | HBV DNA Response (%) Pegylated interferon/lamivudine | ALT normalization (%) Pegylated interferon/lamivudine | Serology (HeAg seroconversion (%) Pegylated interferon/lamivudine |
|---|---|---|---|---|---|---|
| HBe Antigen positive | | | | | | |
| Randomized to pegylated interferon or lamivudine/48 weeks duration and 24 weeks of follow-up | 271, pegylated interferon/272, lamivudine | 41/40 | Improved 25/32 Unchanged 25/20 Worsened 26/16 | 32/22 | 41/28 | 32/19 |

| Study design/drugs/duration | Number of adult patients per drug | [a,b]Histologic response (%) in inflammation Pegylated interferon/lamivudine | [c]Histologic response (%) in fibrosis Pegylated interferon/lamivudine | HBV DNA response (%) Pegylated interferon/lamivudine | ALT normalization (%) Pegylated interferon/lamivudine |
|---|---|---|---|---|---|
| HBe Antigen negative | | | | | |
| Randomized to pegylated interferon or lamivudine/48 weeks duration and at 24 weeks of follow-up | 177, pegylated interferon/181, lamivudine | 48/41 | Improved 32/31 Unchanged 30/23 Worsened 19/15 | 43/29 | 59/44 |

HBV DNA response defined as less than 100,000 copies/mL for HBeAg positive and less than 20,000 copies/mL for HBeAg negative

[a]The proportion of unavailable paired liver biopsies in the pegylated interferon group was 31% and in the lamivudine group, 32%

[b]Histological response was defined as greater than or equal to 2-point decrease in Ishak necroinflammatory activity and no worsening of Ishak fibrosis score

[c]Change by one point or more in the Ishak fibrosis score [162]

**Table 7.4** Effect of tenofovir and adefovir on the treatment of chronic hepatitis B [166]

| Study design | Number of patients/HBV serology/age/race/ethnicity | 48 weeks duration/drug (dose (orally))/% complete responders | Histologic[a] response (%) tenofovir/adefovir | HBV DNA response (%) tenofovir/adefovir | ALT normalization (%) tenofovir/adefovir | Serology (HeAg loss/seroconversion tenofovir/adefovir (%) | HBsAg Loss/Seroconversion (%) tenofovir/adefovir |
|---|---|---|---|---|---|---|---|
| Randomized, double blind active-controlled | 375/e Ag negative and + e Ab/mean 44 years/77% men, 25% Asian, 65% Caucasian, 17% previously exposed to interferon/18% previously treated with nucleoside analogues | Tenofovir, 300 mg/71% vs adefovir 10 mg/49% | 72/69 | 93/63 | 76/77 | NA | 0/0 |
| Randomized, double blind active-controlled | 266/e Ag + /and + e Ab/ mean 34 years/69% men, 36% Asian, 52% Caucasian, 16% previously exposed to interferon/, <1% previously treated with nucleoside analogues | Tenofovir, 300 mg/67% vs adefovir 10 mg/12% | 74/68 | 76/13 | 68/54 | 20/16 19/16 | 3/1 0 |

[a]Primary efficacy endpoint was complete response to treatment defined as a 2-point decrease in the Knodell Histologic Activity Index (HAI) at week 48 compared with pretreatment HAI without worsening of fibrosis score, and decrease in HVB DNA to <400 copies/mL (69 IU/mL) [162]. Combination therapy with another nucleoside analogue, adefovir, decreased the proportion of patients in whom mutants were detected; however, combination therapy is not being proposed anymore, as it has not been associated with therapeutic advantages and has been associated with increased nephrotoxicity

**Table 7.5** Effect of TAF on chronic hepatitis B [167]

| Study design | Dose (orally and daily) | Response[a] HBeAg-, N responders/total (%) Baseline HBV DNA <7 log 10 IU/mL Risk difference TAF-TDF (95% CI) | Response[a] HBeAg-, N responders/total (%) Baseline HBV DNA >7 log HBV DNA IU/mL Risk difference TAF-TDF (95% CI) | Response[a] HBeAg+, N responders/total (%) Baseline HBV DNA 7 to <8 log 10 IU/mL Risk difference TAF-TDF (95% CI) | Response[a] HBeAg+, N responders/ total (%) Baseline HBV DNA ≥ 8 log 10 IU/mL Risk difference TAF-TDF (95% CI) |
|---|---|---|---|---|---|
| Randomized-controlled phase III noninferiority[b] TAF to TDF (2:1 randomization) | TAF 25 mg or TEN 300 mg | TAF: 221/230 (96%) vs TDF: 106/116 (92%) +3.8% (−1 to 11%) p = 0.13 | TAF: 47/55 (85%) vs TDF: 23/24 (96%) −10% (23% to +9%) p = 0.23 | TAF: 122/159 (77%) vs TDF: 66/73 (86%) −10% (−20% to +2%), p = 0.009 | TAF: 117/272 (43%) vs TDF: 72/142 (51%) −8% (−18% to +2%), p = 0.14 |

[a]Response was defined as HBV DNA < 29 IU/mL at 48 weeks of treatment
[b]Non-inferiority margin = 10%
*TAF* tenofovir alafenamide; *DF* tenofovir disoproxil fumarate

A randomized controlled phase 3 noninferiority trial, with a margin of 10%, was conducted to compare the effects of TDF 300 mg/day to TAF 25 mg/day, in chronic hepatitis B, e antigen positive and e antigen negative. The randomization was 2:1 for TAF:TDF. Response was defined as serum HBV DNA less than 29 IU/ml at 48 weeks of treatment. In patients with e antigen negative chronic hepatitis B, with serum HBV DNA less than 7 $\log_{10}$ IU/ml the risk difference for TAF-TDF was 96% versus 92% ($p = 0.13$ CI = +3.8 (−1–11%)), and in patients with HBV DNA greater than 7 $\log_{10}$ IU/ml, it was 85% for TAF versus 96% for TDF ($p = 0.23$, CI = −10% (23–9%)) [167]. In patients with e antigen positive chronic hepatitis B and serum HBV DNA less than 7–8 $\log_{10}$ IU/ml, risk difference for TAF-TDF was 77% versus 86% ($p = 0.009$, CI 10% (−20% to +2%), and in patients with HBV DNA greater than or equal to 8 $\log_{10}$ IU/ml, the risk difference between TAF and TDF was 43% versus 51% ($p = 0.14$, CI = −8% (−18% to +2%)) [168]. In the context of TAF, an analysis of genotypic resistance was conducted in patients in whom a virological breakthrough had been documented over the 48 weeks of treatment. The results did not reveal any specific resistance pathway, suggesting that breakthrough was due to intermittent changes in HBV replication and lack of adherence to medication. The tolerability of TAF was similar to that of TDF. Bone mineral density was documented to decrease by 5% in a smaller number of patients on TAF than in TDF, with a reported decrease of 6% and 3.2% for TAF in the lumbar spine and femoral neck, respectively, and 20% and 5.7%, respectively for TDF. There were no renal laboratory abnormalities in association with either one of these two drugs; however, renal function should be monitored in patients on long-term treatment with this type of drug (Tables 7.4 and 7.5).

The development of resistant variants to antiviral therapy manifest itself clinically by an increase in HBV DNA by more than 1 log from the lowest point during treatment and may be accompanied by hepatitis, evidenced by abnormal liver profile and even decompensation. Two patterns of mutations have been identified: (i) those that include codon rtM204, which is part of the catalytic domain of the polymerase enzyme, i.e., the methionine residue of the conserved tyrosine (Y), methionine (M), aspartate (D), aspartate (D) motif of RNA-dependent DNA polymerase (YMDD) and (ii) those that do not include this codon. rtM204I/V is selected by lamivudine, entecavir, and the combination of TDF and lamivudine, whereas rtN236T ± rtA181V is selected by adefovir.

The cumulative percentage of mutants was reported as 24–70% from year 1–5 for lamivudine, 3–29% for adefovir, and for telbivudine, 4 and 7% at years 1 and 2. These findings contrast to that of entecavir and TDF for which it was 1.2 to 0 percent over 5 years, respectively. These two drugs, and TAF, which also is not associated with the development of resistance [165, 170], are now the preferred drugs to treat chronic HBV infection.

Combination therapy with oral antiviral drugs has been considered for patients who have developed resistance; however, it is now standard to use TDF alone in patients who have developed resistance to lamivudine. Alone, TDF is as efficacious as its combination with emtricitabine, as reported from a 5-year study in patients with lamivudine resistance in which normalization of ALT activity and rates of HBV DNA suppression and e antigen seroconversion were similar [171].

Although treatment with lamivudine was associated with a decrease in HBV DNA below assay detection limits, the suppression was temporary. HBV DNA became detected in a third of the patients on treatment. In addition, up to 27% of patients exhibited an increase in serum ALT activity after discontinuation of lamivudine greater than that observed in patients treated with the placebo. Lamivudine is no longer the drug of choice to treat patients with chronic HBV because of its temporary effect and propensity to trigger mutant HBV variants; however, it is still used in some countries. YMDD-mutant variants emerged in 81 of 335 (24%) subjects treated with lamivudine 100 mg once daily for 52 weeks. The emergence of YMDD mutants increased over time on treatment to 69% at 5 years. Combination therapy with another nucleoside analogue, adefovir, decreased the proportion of patients in whom mutants were detected; however, combination therapy is not being proposed anymore, as it has not been associated with therapeutic advantages and has been associated with increased nephrotoxicity [172].

Combination therapy, especially on the basis of different mechanisms of actions between interferon and nucleosid(t)ides analogues has been studied. A meta-analysis of 14 studies that included 2829 subjects treated with pegylated interferon alpha in e antigen positive and e antigen negative patients documented that the combination of pegylated interferon and lamivudine was associated with improved virological and biochemical response compared to monotherapy with pegylated interferon alpha; in addition, the combination of pegylated interferon alpha with adefovir dipivoxil was associated with enhanced seroconversion compared to pegylated interferon alpha alone in HBe antigen positive patients [169]. Furthermore, the combination of TDF with pegylated interferon for 48 weeks was associated with a significant increase in s Ag loss (9%) at week 72 compared to the effect of other combinations that included TDF alone, TDF followed by pegylated interferon, and interferon alone. The use of combination therapy with interferon and nucleosid(t) ide analogues, however, has not been universally documented to improve suppression and seroconversion rates in the treatment of chronic hepatitis B [173–175]. At the time of this writing, therapy guidelines do not include combination therapy [141, 148].

In patients with e Ag + chronic hepatitis B, seroconversion to anti-HBs followed by 1 year of treatment consolidation with the same agent is considered acceptable to stop treatment. In e Ag negative patients, treatment can be for long periods, and discontinuation only recommended after the loss of sAg and development of anti-HBs, a definitive seroconversion, without recommendations regarding consolidation therapy.

The question of the duration of treatment with oral nucleosides/nucleotides analogues remains unanswered. Published studies have documented that after prolonged suppression of HBV replication, as measured by serum HBV DNA for at least 5 years, medications can be discontinued, and patients followed vigilantly to detect flares in association with viral replication and increased activity of ALT [176]. In this regard, it has been reported that loss of HBsAg is greater after discontinuation of therapy in patients who have exhibited a response on it than in patients who remain on treatment [177, 178]. In the reference cited [178], 1075 patients with e antigen negative chronic hepatitis B were treated with oral nucleosides/nucleotides for a median of three (1–8) years in Taiwan according to the guidelines of the Asian Pacific Association for the Study of Liver Disease; loss of surface antigen was rare on treatment (0.15%). Consistent with the stopping rules of the Association, 691, 44.6% of whom had been identified as having cirrhosis by histology, or inferred by indirect studies, had the medications stopped and were followed off therapy for a median period of 155 (2-614) weeks, during which time 42 patients lost HBsAg, with an estimated 6-year cumulative incidence of 13% and an estimated annual incidence of 1.78%. A time of fewer than 12 weeks to undetected HBV DNA while on treatment, the magnitude of reduction of HBsAg during therapy, i.e., greater than 1 log10, serum HBsAg less than 100 IU/ml, sustained response, and patients who relapsed and who were not restarted on therapy were factors associated with HBsAg clearance off treatment. These interesting results provide support for consideration to discontinue the treatment of oral therapy in patients with e antigen negative chronic hepatitis B under certain circumstances [178]. The author has observed loss of surface antigen and development of anti-HBs after discontinuation of treatment with nucleosides/nucleotides analogues that had gone on for 7 years in association with the absence of serum HBV DNA on treatment, as described in the case reported in this chapter.

Regardless of e antigen status, the use of hepatitis B surface antigen quantitation may be helpful in the care of patients with chronic hepatitis B. For example, in patients with chronic hepatitis B from genotypes B and C, low HBsAg (i.e., <1000 IU/ml) in serum 1 year after seroconversion from e to anti e was reported to portend sAg loss [179]. Conversely, lack of sAg decrease in association with suboptimal reduction of HBV DNA (<2 log) after 3 months of treatment in e antigen negative patients was reported as an indication to discontinue therapy, i.e., stopping rule, in patients infected with genotype D [147]. From results of a systematic review that included 1716 patients, it was reported that patients who had serum HBsAg <100 IU/ml at a time considered end of treatment had virological and clinical relapse rates that ranged from 9.1 to 19.6% and 15.4 to 29.4%, respectively, whereas those in patients with HBsAg > 100 IU/mL at the same treatment time point ranged from 31.4 to 86.8% and 48.1 to 63.6%, respectively, regardless of the e antigen status, at least 12 months after completion of treatment. In the e Ag negative patients, HBsAg loss rates ranged from 21.1 to 58.8% in the patients who at the end of the treatment point had HBsAg serum concentrations <100 IU/ml, and in those with >100 IU/ml, it ranged from 3.3 to 7.4% at more than 39 months off therapy. Although the measure of HBsAg during treatment is not used routinely in clinical practice because of lack of availability, it can be used in the decision to discontinue treatment, especially in e Ag negative patients in whom the duration of therapy remains uncertain.

The cure of chronic hepatitis B virus infection, which requires, based on current knowledge, the disappearance of HBsAg, and complete eradication of intrahepatic cccDNA and its integration in the host's DNA, has not been obtained with available pharmacological interventions. The development of drugs that block different pathways that perpetuate hepatitis B virus infection is an area of active investigation and includes: (i) blockage of viral entry into the hepatocyte, (ii) disruption of epigenetic regulation of transcription that would target cccDNA, (iii) RNA interference to eliminate viral transcripts, and (iv) capsid inhibitors that would prevent the assembly or the disassembly of the nucleocapsid particle and thus could prevent the entry of rcDNA into the nucleus and potential prevention of rcDNA conversion to cccDNA [180].

## Treatment of Chronic Delta Hepatitis

The treatment of chronic HDV infection is the off-label use of interferons, mostly pegylated interferons alpha 2a and 2b since the pegylation of the drug, for 1 year, at the standard doses used for chronic HVB infection [181–183]. It is recommended that treatment be given to patients with chronic HDV infection who have compensated cirrhosis with inflammatory activity, as suggested by high serum ALT activity and serum HDV RNA, which should be confirmed with more than one value, without a liver biopsy as a prerequisite; close follow-up to detect hepatic decompensation is required. Interferon is contraindicated in patients with decompensated liver disease. Co-treatment with oral antivirals is recommended [183].

From a retrospective review at Ankara University School of Medicine in Turkey, of 99 patients with chronic delta hepatitis who had been treated with interferon, standard or pegylated, it was reported that 35% of patients from the 99 who were treated exhibited virological response, defined as negative serum HDV RNA for

2 years after completion of treatment. The cumulative probability of maintained virological response increased in association with increased treatment duration, and it was reported as 50% in relationship with a treatment duration of 5 years. Maintained virological response was associated with a decrease in the probability of development of complications from liver disease and death from liver failure. Advanced liver disease and no response to therapy were predictors of adverse outcomes. Loss of HBsAg was reported in 37% of patients who experienced a maintained virological response [184]. It is important to identify patients in whom prolonged therapy may be beneficial. In this regard, patients who did not exhibit a decrease of more than 1 log10 IU/ml in serum HDV RNA by the sixth month of treatment were unlikely to respond to therapy; thus, extending treatment in those patients beyond what is recommended is not substantiated by the variable results available [183]. In contrast, in patients who exhibited at least a decrease in serum HDV RNA of 2 log10 IU/ml or undetected virus at the end of treatment, extending therapy may be considered, especially if the treatment has been tolerated, or if there has been relapse after its completion; thus, follow-up of patients over the following several years to restart therapy, as indicated, is necessary [183, 184].

Medications tested in early phase studies to treat delta hepatitis include the hepatocyte entry inhibitor myrcludex [185], the farnesyl transferase inhibitor lonafarnib, [186], nucleic acid polymers [187], and PegIFN lambda [188].

## Liver Transplantation in Patients with Chronic Hepatitis B and Chronic Delta Hepatitis

Liver transplantation is an option for treatment in patients with decompensated liver disease when pharmacological therapy fails or in acute liver failure [189, 190].

Recurrence of HBV infection in the transplanted graft was the limiting factor in the post transplant management of patients with chronic HBV infection. The use of hepatitis B immunoglobulin (HBIG) and antiviral therapy in the post transplant period has decreased the graft infection by HBV significantly and improved the survival of patients undergoing this procedure for this indication [191]. From the European Liver Transplant Registry the post transplant survival of patients with chronic HBV infection was reported as 83%, 78%, 75%, and 68%, and of their grafts, 80%, 74%, 71%, 64% at 1, 3, 5, and 10 years from 2006 to 2010 [191]. The standard management for patients with chronic HBV infection post liver transplantation consists of hepatitis B immunoglobulin (HBIG) and a high genetic barrier oral antiviral drug, associated with graft infection of less than 1% [192].

Patients with decompensated chronic liver disease or acute liver failure from HBV and HDV hepatitis can also be managed with liver transplantation and experienced good survival, which tends to depend on the survival of the graft free from HBV infection. A retrospective study from South America from May 2002 to December 2011 included patients with delta hepatitis and with hepatitis B virus infection alone. Patients with delta hepatitis, a group comprised of 29 subjects, men and women, and exclusively from the Brazilian Amazon region, had a survival of 95% at 4 years, compared to the 75% of the group of patients monoinfected with hepatitis B virus alone, comprised of 40 subjects, mostly men, and older than the coinfected group [193]. In a study from Europe that included 79 patients who underwent liver transplantation for end stage liver disease from chronic HDV infection from 1984 to 1990, the actuarial 5-year survival rate was 88%, with a recurrence of HBsAg in 10% of patients. The finding associated with a lack of HDV hepatitis recurrence was the inclusion of immunoprophylaxis against hepatitis B and the absence of HBsAg [194]. According to recent reviews, the reported recurrence of delta hepatitis post liver transplantation is less than 5% in association with immunoprophylaxis with HBIG and oral antiviral therapy. The latter is also given in the pre-transplant period for complete suppression of HBV viral replication [195].

In the post transplant care, antiviral therapy alone may be sufficient [196, 197] in some patients but not in those in whom serum HBV DNA is detected prior to transplant, delta hepatitis coinfection, and HCC with a high risk of recurrence [196].

## Hepatocellular Carcinoma in Chronic Hepatitis B

Chronic HBV virus infection can lead to hepatocellular carcinoma by causing inflammation with progression to fibrosis and cirrhosis, and by insertional mutations in the host DNA at sites that activate endogenous genes like retinoic acid $\beta$-receptor [198], cyclin A [199], and mevalonate kinase [200], the human telomerase reverse transcriptase (*hTERT*), and the inositol 1,4,5-triphosphate receptor (*IPR*) genes, the last two having been found to have site-specific HBV integrations in independent tumors [201–203], and by virus oncoproteins including HBx, which inactivates p53 dependent activities, including apoptosis [204]. Marked genetic changes and heterogeneity found in HCC tissues by sophisticated molecular studies have revealed deregulation of signaling pathways that include Wnt/$\beta$-catenin signaling [205], p14ARF/p53 pathway [206], transforming growth factor beta (TGF-$\beta$) signaling [207], Ras/MAPK signaling [208] and the PTEN/Akt [209], and mTOR pathways [6]. In addition, altered expression of growth factors, including hepatocyte growth factor [210], and insulin growth factor [211], and angiogenesis related genes may also participate in the development of HBV related HCC [212].

From a study in France with patients with HCC it was reported that chromosome instability in association with TP53 and *AXIN1* mutations and loss of chromosomes were related to HBV infection, the latter also documented in HCC in association with chronic HCV [213]. In addition, a decrease in losses in chromosome arms in 4q, 16q, and 17p was documented in non-HVB (or HCV related HCC) interpreted to suggest that certain specificity in chromosome gains or losses is related to HBV associated HCC [214].

Genetics may also play a role in the development of HCC in patients with chronic hepatitis B. By the use of genome-wide association study rs17401966, the intronic SNP in KIF1B on chromosome 1p36.22 was reported in association with HCC in patients with chronic HBV infection [215] as well as hepatitis B genotype C [216]. It is documented that the risk for HCC in patients with HBV genotype C is higher than that of those infected with genotype B. In concert, viral load, HBV genotypes, BCP A1762T/G1764A mutation, and pre S deletion are associated with HBV related liver disease progression and development of HCC [58]. Nomograms to predict the development of HCC in patients chronically infected with HBV have been developed with HBe antigen status, serum HBV DNA, and genotype C being the variables that scored the highest numbers consistent with the prediction of HCC development [217].

The diagnosis of HCC at an early stage for curative purposes is the goal of surveillance. In the context of chronic HVB infection, surveillance for HCC with liver ultrasound with or without alpha fetoprotein (AFP) should be conducted in all patients with cirrhosis, and in the absence of cirrhosis, in Asian men and women older than 40 and 50 years of age, respectively, in Black American and African subjects, even at ages younger than 40 [218], although specific guidance on age has not been provided for this group [219, 220], family history of HCC, and active disease as suggested by high serum ALT activity and or serum HBV DNA [219, 220]. Surveillance studies for HCC should be done every 6 months. If a mass smaller than 1 cm is identified, repeat studies (i.e., ultrasound with or without AFP) are recommended within 3 to 6 months. If a mass equal or greater than 1 cm is found, and the serum AFP is increased, a contrast enhanced computed tomography or magnetic resonance imaging studies should be done to confirm the diagnosis. The reader is referred to the current guidelines from the American Association for the Study of Liver Diseases for guidance regarding the approach to identified liver masses in the surveillance program [219].

There may never be a properly conducted study on the incidence of HCC in Hispanic patients with chronic HBV; in this regard, from a study that used the Surveillance, Epidemiology, and End Results (SEER) database as a source and that covered the period of 2004–2013, it was documented that Chinese patients presented with localized stage and absent vascular invation, and had the best survival compared to other Asian, non-Hispanic whites, Hispanic, and African American patients who had an increased mortality risk to 16.8, 35.1, 28.3, and 33.3%, respectively [221]. Although the underlying cause of liver disease in Hispanic patients was not chronic HBV, the findings of this and other studies tend to suggest that the diagnosis of HCC was made early and, thus, treatable. Although genetic factors cannot be excluded, screening subjects of Hispanic ethnicity with chronic HBV, especially after suspected prolonged infection or age 40, seems reasonable.

The incidence of HCC in veterans subjects with chronic hepatitis B without cirrhosis from the USA was documented as 9.5%, most commonly observed in African American and Asian subjects, reported from a group of 8539 patients, from whom 317 developed HCC in association with chronic HVB, with hypertension and family history being more common in that group [222].

From a retrospective study that included 1666 adult Caucasian patients with chronic HBV on entecavir or tenofovir for 3 and ¼ years, the cumulative probability of developing HCC was 1.3, 3.4, and 8.7%, at years 1, 3, and 5 post initiation of

treatment. Age older than 50 at the start of treatment and low platelet count suggestive of hypersplenism were predictors of development of HCC. Patients with decompensated liver disease had the estimated highest risk [223].

Treatments of HCC, which depend on the size of the tumor, comorbidities, and
degree of portal hypertension, include liver transplantation [224], hepatic resection
[225], various forms of locoregional therapy (LRT) such as radioembolization with
or without tyrosine-kinase inhibitors, e.g., transarterial chemoembolization (TACE)
in combination with radiofrequency ablation [226], TACE and chemotherapy with
sorafenib [227], TACE plus external beam radiotherapy [228], and LRT and immunotherapy, e.g., immune checkpoint inhibitors [229, 230]. In the context of chronic
hepatitis B, treatment with antiviral drugs in patients with cirrhosis, compensated,
or decompensated liver disease in patients with chronic HBV, is the standard.

**Acknowledgments** The author acknowledges Dr. Cesar del Rosario for having contributed
Figures 7.1 and 7.2.

# References

1. Blumberg BS, Alter HJ, Visnich S. A "new" antigen in leukemia sera. JAMA. 1965 Feb
   15;191:541–6.
2. Beck J, Nassal M. Hepatitis B virus replication. World J Gastroenterol WJG. 2007 Jan
   7;13(1):48–64.
3. Heermann KH, Goldmann U, Schwartz W, Seyffarth T, Baumgarten H, Gerlich WH. Large
   surface proteins of hepatitis B virus containing the pre-s sequence. J Virol. 1984
   Nov;52(2):396–402.
4. Garcia PD, Ou JH, Rutter WJ, Walter P. Targeting of the hepatitis B virus precore protein
   to the endoplasmic reticulum membrane: after signal peptide cleavage translocation can be
   aborted and the product released into the cytoplasm. J Cell Biol. 1988 Apr;106(4):1093–104.
5. Magnius LO, Espmark A. A new antigen complex co-occurring with Australia antigen. Acta
   Pathol Microbiol Scand B: Microbiol Immunol. 1972;80(2):335–7.
6. Yen CJ, Lin YJ, Yen CS, Tsai HW, Tsai TF, Chang KY, et al. Hepatitis B virus X protein
   upregulates mTOR signaling through IKKβ to increase cell proliferation and VEGF production in hepatocellular carcinoma. PLoS One. 2012;7(7):e41931.
7. Iwamoto M, Saso W, Sugiyama R, Ishii K, Ohki M, Nagamori S, Suzuki R, Aizaki H, Ryo
   A, Yun J-H, Park S-Y, Ohtani N, Muramatsu M, Shingo I. Epidermal growth factor receptor
   is a host-entry cofactor triggering hepatitis B virus internalization. Proc Natl Acad Sci U S
   A. 2019;116(17):8487–92.
8. Rabe B, Delaleau M, Bischof A, Foss M, Sominskaya I, Pumpens P, et al. Nuclear entry of
   hepatitis B virus capsids involves disintegration to protein dimers followed by nuclear reas-
   sociation to capsids. PLoS Pathog. 2009 Aug;5(8):e1000563.
9. Bock CT, Schwinn S, Locarnini S, Fyfe J, Manns MP, Trautwein C, et al. Structural organization of the hepatitis B virus minichromosome. J Mol Biol. 2001 Mar 16;307(1):183–96.
10. Levrero M, Pollicino T, Petersen J, Belloni L, Raimondo G, Dandri M. Control of cccDNA
    function in hepatitis B virus infection. J Hepatol. 2009 Sep;51(3):581–92.
11. Köck J, Rösler C, Zhang JJ, Blum HE, Nassal M, Thoma C. Generation of covalently closed
    circular DNA of hepatitis B viruses via intracellular recycling is regulated in a virus specific
    manner. PLoS Pathog. 2010 Sep 2;6(9):e1001082.

12. Ko C, Chakraborty A, Chou W-M, Hasreiter J, Wettengel JW, Stadler D, Bester R, Asen T, Zhang K, Wisskirchen J, McKeating JA, Ryu WS, Protzer U. Hepatitis B virus genome recycling and de novo secondary infection events maintain stable cccDNA levels. J Hepatol. 2018;69(6):1231–41.

13. Rall LB, Standring DN, Laub O, Rutter WJ, Rutter WJ. Transcription of hepatitis B virus by RNA polymerase II. Mol Cell Biol. 1983;10(3):1766–73.

14. Enders GH, Ganem D, Varmus HE. 5′-terminal sequences influence the segregation of ground squirrel hepatitis virus RNAs into polyribosomes and viral core particles. J Virol. 1987 Jan;61(1):35–41.

15. Summers J, Mason WS. Replication of the genome of a hepatitis B-like virus by reverse transcription of an RNA intermediate. Cell. 1982 Jun;29(2):403–15.

16. Kamimura T, Yoshikawa A, Ichida F, Sasaki H. Electron microscopic studies of Dane particles in hepatocytes with special reference to intracellular development of Dane particles and their relation with HBeAg in serum. Hepatology. 1981 Sep-Oct;1(5):392–7.

17. Roingeard P, Lu SL, Sureau C, Freschlin M, Arbeille B, Essex M, et al. Immunocytochemical and electron microscopic study of hepatitis B virus antigen and complete particle production in hepatitis B virus DNA transfected HepG2 cells. Hepatology. 1990 Feb;11(2):277–85.

18. Rost M, Mann S, Lambert C, Doring T, Thome N, Prange R. Gamma-adaptin, a novel ubiquitin-interacting adaptor, and Nedd4 ubiquitin ligase control hepatitis B virus maturation. J Biol Chem. 2006 Sep 29;281(39):29297–308.

19. Croagh CM, Lubel JS. Natural history of chronic hepatitis B: phases in a complex relationship. World J Gastroenterol WJG. 2014 Aug 14;20(30):10395–404.

20. Trepo C, Chan HL, Lok A. Hepatitis B virus infection. Lancet. 2014 Jun 18;384(9959):2053–63.

21. Dunn C, Peppa D, Khanna P, Nebbia G, Jones M, Brendish N, et al. Temporal analysis of early immune responses in patients with acute hepatitis B virus infection. Gastroenterology. 2009 Oct;137(4):1289–300.

22. Nguyen KB, Salazar-Mather TP, Dalod MY, Van Deusen JB, Wei XQ, Liew FY, et al. Coordinated and distinct roles for IFN-alpha beta, IL-12, and IL-15 regulation of NK cell responses to viral infection. J Immunol. 2002 Oct 15;169(8):4279–87.

23. Wang X, Li Y, Mao A, Li C, Li Y, Tien P. Hepatitis B virus X protein suppresses virus-triggered IRF3 activation and IFN-beta induction by disrupting the VISA-associated complex. Cell Mol Immunol. 2010 Sep;7(5):341–8.

24. Wei C, Ni C, Song T, Liu Y, Yang X, Zheng Z, et al. The hepatitis B virus X protein disrupts innate immunity by downregulating mitochondrial antiviral signaling protein. J Immunol. 2010 Jul 15;185(2):1158–68.

25. Wang H, Ryu WS. Hepatitis B virus polymerase blocks pattern recognition receptor signaling via interaction with DDX3: implications for immune evasion. PLoS Pathog. 2010 July 15;6(7):e1000986.

26. Zhang Z, Zhang S, Zou Z, Shi J, Zhao J, Fan R, et al. Hypercytolytic activity of hepatic natural killer cells correlates with liver injury in chronic hepatitis B patients. Hepatology. 2011 Jan;53(1):73–85.

27. Dunn C, Brunetto M, Reynolds G, Christophides T, Kennedy PT, Lampertico P, et al. Cytokines induced during chronic hepatitis B virus infection promote a pathway for NK cell-mediated liver damage. J Exp Med. 2007 Mar 19;204(3):667–80.

28. Stacey AR, Norris PJ, Qin L, Haygreen EA, Taylor E, Heitman J, et al. Induction of a striking systemic cytokine cascade prior to peak viremia in acute human immunodeficiency virus type 1 infection, in contrast to more modest and delayed responses in acute hepatitis B and C virus infections. J Virol. 2009 Apr;83(8):3719–33.

29. Hosel M, Quasdorff M, Wiegmann K, Webb D, Zedler U, Broxtermann M, et al. Not interferon, but interleukin-6 controls early gene expression in hepatitis B virus infection. Hepatology. 2009 Dec;50(6):1773–82.

30. Kumar M, Jung SY, Hodgson AJ, Madden CR, Qin J, Slagle BL. Hepatitis B virus regulatory HBx protein binds to adaptor protein IPS-1 and inhibits the activation of beta interferon. J Virol. 2011 Jan;85(2):987–95.

31. Hou F, Sun L, Zheng H, Skaug B, Jiang QX, Chen ZJ. MAVS forms functional prion-like aggregates to activate and propagate antiviral innate immune response. Cell. 2011 Aug 5;146(3):448–61.

32. Wu J, Meng Z, Jiang M, Pei R, Trippler M, Broering R, et al. Hepatitis B virus suppresses toll-like receptor-mediated innate immune responses in murine parenchymal and nonparenchymal liver cells. Hepatology. 2009 Apr;49(4):1132–40.

33. Visvanathan K, Skinner NA, Thompson AJ, Riordan SM, Sozzi V, Edwards R, et al. Regulation of toll-like receptor-2 expression in chronic hepatitis B by the precore protein. Hepatology. 2007 Jan;45(1):102–10.

34. Webster GJ, Reignat S, Maini MK, Whalley SA, Ogg GS, King A, et al. Incubation phase of acute hepatitis B in man: dynamic of cellular immune mechanisms. Hepatology. 2000 Nov;32(5):1117–24.

35. Fisicaro P, Valdatta C, Boni C, Massari M, Mori C, Zerbini A, et al. Early kinetics of innate and adaptive immune responses during hepatitis B virus infection. Gut. 2009 Jul;58(7):974–82.

36. Godfrey DI, MacDonald HR, Kronenberg M, Smyth MJ, Van Kaer L. NKT cells: what's in a name? Nat Rev Immunol. 2004 Mar;4(3):231–7.

37. Ferrari C, Penna A, Bertoletti A, Valli A, Antoni AD, Giuberti T, et al. Cellular immune response to hepatitis B virus-encoded antigens in acute and chronic hepatitis B virus infection. J Immunol. 1990 Nov 15;145(10):3442–9.

38. Xu D, Fu J, Jin L, Zhang H, Zhou C, Zou Z, et al. Circulating and liver resident CD4+CD25+ regulatory T cells actively influence the antiviral immune response and disease progression in patients with hepatitis B. J Immunol. 2006 Jul 1;177(1):739–47.

39. Asabe S, Wieland SF, Chattopadhyay PK, Roederer M, Engle RE, Purcell RH, et al. The size of the viral inoculum contributes to the outcome of hepatitis B virus infection. J Virol. 2009 Oct;83(19):9652–62.

40. Maini MK, Boni C, Lee CK, Larrubia JR, Reignat S, Ogg GS, et al. The role of virus-specific CD8(+) cells in liver damage and viral control during persistent hepatitis B virus infection. J Exp Med. 2000 Apr 17;191(8):1269–80.

41. Thursz MR, Kwiatkowski D, Allsopp CE, Greenwood BM, Thomas HC, Hill AV. Association between an MHC class II allele and clearance of hepatitis B virus in the Gambia. N Engl J Med. 1995 Apr 20;332(16):1065–9.

42. Hohler T, Gerken G, Notghi A, Lubjuhn R, Taheri H, Protzer U, et al. HLA-DRB1*1301 and *1302 protect against chronic hepatitis B. J Hepatol. 1997 Mar;26(3):503–7.

43. Ahn SH, Han KH, Park JY, Lee CK, Kang SW, Chon CY, et al. Association between hepatitis B virus infection and HLA-DR type in Korea. Hepatology. 2000 Jun;31(6):1371–3.

44. Almarri A, Batchelor JR. HLA and hepatitis B infection. Lancet. 1994 Oct 29;344(8931):1194–5.

45. Jiang YG, Wang YM, Liu TH, Liu J. Association between HLA class II gene and susceptibility or resistance to chronic hepatitis B. World J Gastroenterol WJG. 2003 Oct;9(10):2221–5.

46. Hohler T, Kruger A, Gerken G, Schneider PM, Meyer zum Buschenfelde KH, Rittner C. A tumor necrosis factor-alpha (TNF-alpha) promoter polymorphism is associated with chronic hepatitis B infection. Clin Exp Immunol. 1998 Mar;111(3):579–82.

47. Kim YJ, Lee HS, Yoon JH, Kim CY, Park MH, Kim LH, et al. Association of TNF-alpha promoter polymorphisms with the clearance of hepatitis B virus infection. Hum Mol Genet. 2003 Oct 1;12(19):2541–6.

48. Du T, Guo XH, Zhu XL, Li JH, Lu LP, Gao JR, et al. Association of TNF-alpha promoter polymorphisms with the outcomes of hepatitis B virus infection in Chinese Han population. J Viral Hepat. 2006 Sep;13(9):618–24.

49. Somi MH, Najafi L, Noori BN, Alizadeh AH, Aghah MR, Shavakhi A, et al. Tumor necrosis factor-alpha gene promoter polymorphism in Iranian patients with chronic hepatitis B. Indian J Gastroenterol. 2006 Jan–Feb;25(1):14–5.
50. Xu J, Zhang S, Zhang Z, Fu L, Zheng Q, Wang J, et al. TNF-alpha promoter region polymorphisms affect HBV virus clearance in southern Chinese. Clin Chim Acta. 2013 Oct 21;425:90–2.
51. Xia Q, Zhou L, Liu D, Chen Z, Chen F. Relationship between TNF-α gene promoter polymorphisms and outcomes of hepatitis B virus infections: a meta-analysis. PLoS One. 2011;6(5):e19606.
52. Frodsham AJ, Zhang L, Dumpis U, Taib NA, Best S, Durham A, et al. Class II cytokine receptor gene cluster is a major locus for hepatitis B persistence. Proc Natl Acad Sci U S A. 2006 June 13;103(24):9148–53.
53. Nishida N, Sawai H, Matsuura K, Sugiyama M, Ahn SH, Park JY, et al. Genome-wide association study confirming association of HLA-DP with protection against chronic hepatitis B and viral clearance in Japanese and Korean. PLoS One. 2012;7(6):e39175.
54. Norder H, Hammas B, Lee SD, Bile K, Couroucé AM, Mushahwar IK, et al. Genetic relatedness of hepatitis B viral strains of diverse geographical origin and natural variations in the primary structure of the surface antigen. J Gen Virol. 1993 July;74(Pt 7):1341–8.
55. Ozasa A, Tanaka Y, Orito E, Sugiyama M, Kang JH, Hige S, et al. Influence of genotypes and precore mutations on fulminant or chronic outcome of acute hepatitis B virus infection. Hepatology. 2006 Aug;44(2):326–34.
56. Suzuki Y, Kobayashi M, Ikeda K, Suzuki F, Arfase Y, Akuta N, et al. Persistence of acute infection with hepatitis B virus genotype A and treatment in Japan. J Med Virol. 2005 May;76(1):33–9.
57. Ito K, Yotsuyanagi H, Yatsuhashi H, Karino Y, Takikawa Y, Saito T, et al. Risk factors for long-term persistence of serum hepatitis B surface antigen following acute hepatitis B virus infection in Japanese adults. Hepatology. 2014 Jan;59(1):89–97.
58. Lin CL, Kao JH. The clinical implications of hepatitis B virus genotype: recent advances. J Gastroenterol Hepatol. 2011 Jan;26(Suppl 1):123–30.
59. Sarkar N, Pal A, Das D, Saha D, Biswas A, Bandopadhayay B, et al. Virological characteristics of acute hepatitis B in Eastern India: critical differences with chronic infection. PLoS One. 2015;10(11):e0141741.
60. van Houdt R, Bruisten SM, Speksnijder AG, Prins M. Unexpectedly high proportion of drug users and men having sex with men who develop chronic hepatitis B infection. J Hepatol. 2012 Sep;57(3):529–33.
61. Kamatani Y, Wattanapokayakit S, Ochi H, Kawaguchi T, Takahashi A, Hosono N, et al. A genome-wide association study identifies variants in the HLA-DP locus associated with chronic hepatitis B in Asians. Nat Genet. 2009 May;41(5):591–5.
62. Kim YJ, Kim HY, Lee JH, Yu SJ, Yoon JH, Lee HS, et al. A genome-wide association study identified new variants associated with the risk of chronic hepatitis B. Hum Mol Genet. 2013 Oct 15;22(20):4233–8.
63. Hu Z, Liu Y, Zhai X, Dai J, Jin G, Wang L, et al. New loci associated with chronic hepatitis B virus infection in Han Chinese. Nat Genet. 2013 Dec;45(12):1499–503.
64. Thio CL, Mosbruger T, Astemborski J, Greer S, Kirk GD, O'Brien SJ, et al. Mannose binding lectin genotypes influence recovery from hepatitis B virus infection. J Virol. 2005 Jul;79(14):9192–6.
65. http://www.cdc.gov/hepatitis/Statistics/SurveillanceGuidelines.htm. Division of Viral Hepatitis, National Center for HIV/AIDS, Viral Hepatitis, STD, and TB Prevention. 2018.
66. Cooke GS, Andrieux-Meyer I, Applegate TL, Atun R, Burry JR, Cheinquer H, et al. Accelerating the elimination of viral hepatitis: a Lancet Gastroenterology & Hepatology Commission. Lancet Gastroenterol Hepatol. 2019 Feb;4(2):135–84.

67. Nayagam S, Thursz M, Sicuri E, Conteh L, Wiktor S, Low-Beer D, et al. Requirements for global elimination of hepatitis B: a modelling study. Lancet Infect Dis. 2016 Dec;16(12):1399–408.
68. Hollinger BF, Purcell RH, Gerin JL, Ganem DE, Feinstone SM, Emerson SU, Major ME, Schneider RJ, Lian TJ, Casey JL, Rehermann B. Hepatitis B. Viral Hepatitis. Philadelphia: Lippincott Williams & Wilkins; 2002. p. 103–68.
69. Guillevin L, Mahr A, Callard P, Godmer P, Pagnoux C, Leray E, et al. Hepatitis B virus-associated polyarteritis nodosa: clinical characteristics, outcome, and impact of treatment in 115 patients. Medicine. 2005 Sep;84(5):313–22.
70. Johnson RJ, Couser WG. Hepatitis B infection and renal disease: clinical, immunopathogenetic and therapeutic considerations. Kidney Int. 1990 Feb;37(2):663–76.
71. Lai KN, Li PK, Lui SF, Au TC, Tam JS, Tong KL, et al. Membranous nephropathy related to hepatitis B virus in adults. N Engl J Med. 1991 May 23;324(21):1457–63.
72. Li SJ, Xu ST, Chen HP, Zhang MC, Xu F, Cheng SQ, et al. Clinical and morphologic spectrum of renal involvement in patients with HBV-associated cryoglobulinaemia. Nephrology (Carlton, VIC). 2017 June;22(6):449–55.
73. Tabor E. Guillain-Barré syndrome and other neurologic syndromes in hepatitis A, B, and non-A, non-B. J Med Virol. 1987 Mar;21(3):207–16.
74. Stübgen JP. Neuromuscular disorders associated with hepatitis B virus infection. J Clin Neuromuscul Dis. 2011 Sep;13(1):26–37.
75. Bao SP. Association between hepatitis B and hearing status. Eur Rev Med Pharmacol Sci. 2017 Mar;21(5):922–7.
76. Bertoletti A, Kennedy PT. The immune tolerant phase of chronic HBV infection: new perspectives on an old concept. Cell Mol Immunol. 2015 May;12(3):258–63.
77. Lok AS, McMahon BJ, Practice Guidelines Committee AAftSoLD. Chronic hepatitis B: update of recommendations. Hepatology. 2004 Mar;39(3):857–61.
78. Hoofnagle JH, Doo E, Liang TJ, Fleischer R, Lok AS. Management of hepatitis B: summary of a clinical research workshop. Hepatology. 2007 Apr;45(4):1056–75.
79. Livingston SE, Simonetti JP, Bulkow LR, Homan CE, Snowball MM, Cagle HH, et al. Clearance of hepatitis B e antigen in patients with chronic hepatitis B and genotypes A, B, C, D, and F. Gastroenterology. 2007 Nov;133(5):1452–7.
80. Hui CK, Leung N, Shek TW, Yao H, Lee WK, Lai JY, et al. Sustained disease remission after spontaneous HBeAg seroconversion is associated with reduction in fibrosis progression in chronic hepatitis B Chinese patients. Hepatology. 2007 Sep;46(3):690–8.
81. Liaw YF, Chu CM, Su IJ, Huang MJ, Lin DY, Chang-Chien CS. Clinical and histological events preceding hepatitis B e antigen seroconversion in chronic type B hepatitis. Gastroenterology. 1983 Feb;84(2):216–9.
82. Yu MW, Hsu FC, Sheen IS, Chu CM, Lin DY, Chen CJ, et al. Prospective study of hepatocellular carcinoma and liver cirrhosis in asymptomatic chronic hepatitis B virus carriers. Am J Epidemiol. 1997 June 1;145(11):1039–47.
83. Lok AS, Lai CL, Wu PC, Leung EK, Lam TS. Spontaneous hepatitis B e antigen to antibody seroconversion and reversion in Chinese patients with chronic hepatitis B virus infection. Gastroenterology. 1987 Jun;92(6):1839–43.
84. de Franchis R, Meucci G, Vecchi M, Tatarella M, Colombo M, Del Ninno E, et al. The natural history of asymptomatic hepatitis B surface antigen carriers. Ann Intern Med. 1993 Feb 1;118(3):191–4.
85. Martinot-Peignoux M, Boyer N, Colombat M, Akremi R, Pham BN, Ollivier S, et al. Serum hepatitis B virus DNA levels and liver histology in inactive HBsAg carriers. J Hepatol. 2002 Apr;36(4):543–6.
86. Zacharakis GH, Koskinas J, Kotsiou S, Papoutselis M, Tzara F, Vafeiadis N, et al. Natural history of chronic HBV infection: a cohort study with up to 12 years follow-up in North Greece (part of the Interreg I-II/EC-project). J Med Virol. 2005 Oct;77(2):173–9.

87. Kumar M, Sarin SK, Hissar S, Pande C, Sakhuja P, Sharma BC, et al. Virologic and histologic features of chronic hepatitis B virus-infected asymptomatic patients with persistently normal ALT. Gastroenterology. 2008 May;134(5):1376–84.

88. Saab S, Dong MH, Joseph TA, Tong MJ. Hepatitis B prophylaxis in patients undergoing chemotherapy for lymphoma: a decision analysis model. Hepatology. 2007 Oct;46(4):1049–56.

89. Perrillo RP. Acute flares in chronic hepatitis B: the natural and unnatural history of an immunologically mediated liver disease. Gastroenterology. 2001 Mar;120(4):1009–22.

90. Chang ML, Liaw YF. Hepatitis B flares in chronic hepatitis B: pathogenesis, natural course, and management. J Hepatol. 2014 Dec;61(6):1407–17.

91. Li YH, He YF, Jiang WQ, Wang FH, Lin XB, Zhang L, et al. Lamivudine prophylaxis reduces the incidence and severity of hepatitis in hepatitis B virus carriers who receive chemotherapy for lymphoma. Cancer. 2006 Mar 15;106(6):1320–5.

92. Idilman R, Arat M, Soydan E, Toruner M, Soykan I, Akbulut H, et al. Lamivudine prophylaxis for prevention of chemotherapy-induced hepatitis B virus reactivation in hepatitis B virus carriers with malignancies. J Viral Hepat. 2004 Mar;11(2):141–7.

93. Hwang JP, Suarez-Almazor ME, Cantor SB, Barbo A, Lin HY, Ahmed S, et al. Impact of the timing of hepatitis B virus identification and anti-hepatitis B virus therapy initiation on the risk of adverse liver outcomes for patients receiving cancer therapy. Cancer. 2017 Sep 1;123(17):3367–76.

94. McKenzie R, Fried MW, Sallie R, Conjeevaram H, Di Bisceglie AM, Park Y, Savarese B, Kleiner D, Tsokos M, Luciano C, Pruett T, Stotka JL, Straus SE, Hoofnagle JH. Hepatic failure and lactic acidosis due to fialuridine (FIAU), an investigational nucleoside analogue for chronic hepatitis B. N Engl J Med. 1995;333:1099–105.

95. Ishak K, Baptista A, Bianchi L, Callea F, De Groote J, Gudat F, et al. Histological grading and staging of chronic hepatitis. J Hepatol. 1995 Jun;22(6):696–9.

96. Tsai SL, Chen PJ, Lai MY, Yang PM, Sung JL, Huang JH, et al. Acute exacerbations of chronic type B hepatitis are accompanied by increased T cell responses to hepatitis B core and e antigens. Implications for hepatitis B e antigen seroconversion. J Clin Invest. 1992 Jan;89(1):87–96.

97. Takehara T, Hayashi N, Katayama K, Kasahara A, Fusamoto H, Kamada T. Hepatitis B core antigen-specific interferon gamma production of peripheral blood mononuclear cells during acute exacerbation of chronic hepatitis B. Scand J Gastroenterol. 1992 Sep;27(9):727–31.

98. Fukuda R, Ishimura N, Nguyen TX, Chowdhury A, Ishihara S, Kohge N, et al. The expression of IL-2, IL-4 and interferon-gamma (IFN-gamma) mRNA using liver biopsies at different phases of acute exacerbation of chronic hepatitis B. Clin Exp Immunol. 1995 Jun;100(3):446–51.

99. Feng IC, Koay LB, Sheu MJ, Kuo HT, Sun CS, Lee C, et al. HBcAg-specific CD4+CD25+ regulatory T cells modulate immune tolerance and acute exacerbation on the natural history of chronic hepatitis B virus infection. J Biomed Sci. 2007 Jan;14(1):43–57.

100. Tan AT, Koh S, Goh W, Zhe HY, Gehring AJ, Lim SG, et al. A longitudinal analysis of innate and adaptive immune profile during hepatic flares in chronic hepatitis B. J Hepatol. 2010 Mar;52(3):330–9.

101. Wenjin Z, Chuanhui P, Yunle W, Lateef SA, Shusen Z. Longitudinal fluctuations in PD1 and PD-L1 expression in association with changes in anti-viral immune response in chronic hepatitis B. BMC Gastroenterol. 2012 Aug 16;12:109.

102. Hoofnagle JH, Gerety RJ, Barker LF. Antibody to hepatitis-B-virus core in man. Lancet. 1973 Oct 20;2(7834):869–73.

103. Gerlich WH. Medical virology of hepatitis B: how it began and where we are now. Virol J. 2013;10:239.

104. Hoofnagle JH, Ponzetto A, Mathiesen LR, Waggoner JG, Bales ZB, Seeff LB. Serological diagnosis of acute viral hepatitis. Dig Dis Sci. 1985 Nov;30(11):1022–7.

105. http://www.cdc.gov/hepatitis/Statistics/SurveillanceGuidelines.htm. 2014.

106. Scheuer PF. Pathology of the liver. In: RNM MS, Anthony PP, Scheuer PJ, Burt AD, Portmann BC, editors. Pathology of the liver. Edinburgh: Churchill Livingston; 1994. p. 243–67.
107. Bianchi L, Gudat F. Chronic hepatitis. In: MacSween RNM, Anthony PP, Scheuer PJ, Burt AD, Portmann BC, editors. Pathology of the liver. Edinburgh: Churchill Livingston; 1994. p. 349–95.
108. Anthony PP, Vogel CL, Barker LF. Liver cell dysplasia: a premalignant condition. J Clin Pathol. 1973 Mar;26(3):217–23.
109. McMahon BJ, Holck P, Bulkow L, Snowball M. Serologic and clinical outcomes of 1536 Alaska natives chronically infected with hepatitis B virus. Ann Intern Med. 2001 Nov 6;135(9):759–68.
110. Yuen MF, Wong DK, Sablon E, Tse E, Ng IO, Yuan HJ, et al. HBsAg seroclearance in chronic hepatitis B in the Chinese: virological, histological, and clinical aspects. Hepatology. 2004 Jun;39(6):1694–701.
111. Chen CJ, Yang HI, Su J, Jen CL, You SL, Lu SN, et al. Risk of hepatocellular carcinoma across a biological gradient of serum hepatitis B virus DNA level. JAMA. 2006 Jan 4;295(1):65–73.
112. McMahon BJ. The natural history of chronic hepatitis B virus infection. Hepatology. 2009 May;49(5 Suppl):S45–55.
113. Sanchez-Tapias JM, Costa J, Mas A, Bruguera M, Rodes J. Influence of hepatitis B virus genotype on the long-term outcome of chronic hepatitis B in western patients. Gastroenterology. 2002 Dec;123(6):1848–56.
114. Yu MW, Yeh SH, Chen PJ, Liaw YF, Lin CL, Liu CJ, et al. Hepatitis B virus genotype and DNA level and hepatocellular carcinoma: a prospective study in men. J Natl Cancer Inst. 2005 Feb 16;97(4):265–72.
115. Yang HI, Yeh SH, Chen PJ, Iloeje UH, Jen CL, Su J, et al. Associations between hepatitis B virus genotype and mutants and the risk of hepatocellular carcinoma. J Natl Cancer Inst. 2008 Aug 20;100(16):1134–43.
116. Livingston SE, Simonetti JP, McMahon BJ, Bulkow LR, Hurlburt KJ, Homan CE, et al. Hepatitis B virus genotypes in Alaska native people with hepatocellular carcinoma: preponderance of genotype F. J Infect Dis. 2007 Jan 1;195(1):5–11.
117. Mahmoud D, Yerragorla P, Shady A, Shamian B, Bergasa NV. Characteristics of patient with chronic hepatitis b from a community hospital in North Brooklyn. Gastroenterol Hepatol Endosc 3: 2018. https://doi.org/10.15761/GHE.1000148.
118. Eloy AM, Moreira RC, Lemos MF, Silva JL, Coêlho MR. Hepatitis B virus in the state of Alagoas, Brazil: genotypes characterization and mutations of the precore and basal core promoter regions. Braz J Infect Dis. 2013 Nov–Dec;17(6):704–6.
119. Niederau C, Heintges T, Lange S, Goldmann G, Niederau CM, Mohr L, et al. Long-term follow-up of HBeAg-positive patients treated with interferon alfa for chronic hepatitis B. N Engl J Med. 1996 May 30;334(22):1422–7.
120. de Jongh FE, Janssen HL, de Man RA, Hop WC, Schalm SW, van Blankenstein M. Survival and prognostic indicators in hepatitis B surface antigen-positive cirrhosis of the liver. Gastroenterology. 1992 Nov;103(5):1630–5.
121. Di Marco V, Lo Iacono O, Camma C, Vaccaro A, Giunta M, Martorana G, et al. The long-term course of chronic hepatitis B. Hepatology. 1999 Jul;30(1):257–64.
122. Tokudome S, Ikeda M, Matsushita K, Maeda Y, Yoshinari M. Hepatocellular carcinoma among female Japanese hepatitis B virus carriers. Hepato-Gastroenterology. 1987 Dec;34(6):246–8.
123. Liaw YF, Lin DY, Chen TJ, Chu CM. Natural course after the development of cirrhosis in patients with chronic type B hepatitis: a prospective study. Liver. 1989 Aug;9(4):235–41.
124. Realdi G, Fattovich G, Hadziyannis S, Schalm SW, Almasio P, Sanchez-Tapias J, et al. Survival and prognostic factors in 366 patients with compensated cirrhosis type B: a multicenter study. The investigators of the European Concerted Action on Viral Hepatitis (EUROHEP). J Hepatol. 1994 Oct;21(4):656–66.
125. Fattovich G, Brollo L, Giustina G, Noventa F, Pontisso P, Alberti A, et al. Natural history and prognostic factors for chronic hepatitis type B. Gut. 1991 Mar;32(3):294–8.

126. Kew MC, Yu MC, Kedda MA, Coppin A, Sarkin A, Hodkinson J. The relative roles of hepatitis B and C viruses in the etiology of hepatocellular carcinoma in southern African blacks. Gastroenterology. 1997 Jan;112(1):184–7.

127. Kirk GD, Lesi OA, Mendy M, Akano AO, Sam O, Goedert JJ, et al. The Gambia Liver Cancer Study: infection with hepatitis B and C and the risk of hepatocellular carcinoma in West Africa. Hepatology. 2004 Jan;39(1):211–9.

128. Liaw YF, Tsai SL, Chang JJ, Sheen IS, Chien RN, Lin DY, et al. Displacement of hepatitis B virus by hepatitis C virus as the cause of continuing chronic hepatitis. Gastroenterology. 1994 Apr;106(4):1048–53.

129. Liaw YF, Chen YC, Sheen IS, Chien RN, Yeh CT, Chu CM. Impact of acute hepatitis C virus superinfection in patients with chronic hepatitis B virus infection. Gastroenterology. 2004 Apr;126(4):1024–9.

130. Donato F, Boffetta P, Puoti M. A meta-analysis of epidemiological studies on the combined effect of hepatitis B and C virus infections in causing hepatocellular carcinoma. Int J Cancer. 1998 Jan 30;75(3):347–54.

131. Chu CM, Yeh CT, Liaw YF. Fulminant hepatic failure in acute hepatitis C: increased risk in chronic carriers of hepatitis B virus. Gut. 1999 Oct;45(4):613–7.

132. Le Gal F, Brichler S, Drugan T, Alloui C, Roulot D, Pawlotsky JM, et al. Genetic diversity and worldwide distribution of the deltavirus genus: a study of 2,152 clinical strains. Hepatology. 2017 Dec;66(6):1826–41.

133. Su CW, Huang YH, Huo TI, Shih HH, Sheen IJ, Chen SW, et al. Genotypes and viremia of hepatitis B and D viruses are associated with outcomes of chronic hepatitis D patients. Gastroenterology. 2006 May;130(6):1625–35.

134. Pasetti G, Calzetti C, Degli Antoni A, Ferrari C, Penna A, Fiaccadori F. Clinical features of hepatitis delta virus infection in a northern Italian area. Infection. 1988;16(6):345–8.

135. Raimondo G, Smedile A, Gallo L, Balbo A, Ponzetto A, Rizzetto M. Multicentre study of prevalence of HBV-associated delta infection and liver disease in drug-addicts. Lancet. 1982 Jan 30;1(8266):249–51.

136. Negro F. Hepatitis D virus coinfection and superinfection. Cold Spring Harb Perspect Med. 2014;4(11):a021550.

137. Fattovich G, Giustina G, Christensen E, Pantalena M, Zagni I, Realdi G, et al. Influence of hepatitis delta virus infection on morbidity and mortality in compensated cirrhosis type B. The European Concerted Action on Viral Hepatitis (Eurohep). Gut. 2000 Mar;46(3):420–6.

138. Popper H, Thung SN, Gerber MA, Hadler SC, de Monzon M, Ponzetto A, et al. Histologic studies of severe delta agent infection in Venezuelan Indians. Hepatology. 1983 Nov–Dec;3(6):906–12.

139. Thio CL, Seaberg EC, Skolasky R Jr, Phair J, Visscher B, Munoz A, et al. HIV-1, hepatitis B virus, and risk of liver-related mortality in the Multicenter Cohort Study (MACS). Lancet. 2002 Dec 14;360(9349):1921–6.

140. European Association for the Study of the Liver. EASL 2017 clinical practice guidelines on the management of hepatitis B virus infection. J Hepatol. 2017 Aug;67(2):370–98.

141. Terrault NA, Lok ASF, McMahon BJ, Chang KM, Hwang JP, Jonas MM, et al. Update on prevention, diagnosis, and treatment of chronic hepatitis B: AASLD 2018 hepatitis B guidance. Hepatology. 2018 Apr;67(4):1560–99.

142. Hwang JP, Lok AS. Management of patients with hepatitis B who require immunosuppressive therapy. Nat Rev Gastroenterol Hepatol. 2014 Apr;11(4):209–19.

143. Choi J, Lim YS. Characteristics, prevention, and management of Hepatitis B Virus (HBV) reactivation in HBV-infected patients who require immunosuppressive therapy. J Infect Dis. 2017 Nov 16;216(suppl 8):S778–84.

144. Allen MI, Gauthier J, DesLauriers M, Bourne EJ, Carrick KM, Baldanti F, et al. Two sensitive PCR-based methods for detection of hepatitis B virus variants associated with reduced susceptibility to lamivudine. J Clin Microbiol. 1999 Oct;37(10):3338–47.

145. Bessesen M, Ives D, Condreay L, Lawrence S, Sherman KE. Chronic active hepatitis B exacerbations in human immunodeficiency virus-infected patients following development of resistance to or withdrawal of lamivudine. Clin Infect Dis. 1999 May;28(5):1032–5.

146. Buster EH, Hansen BE, Lau GK, Piratvisuth T, Zeuzem S, Steyerberg EW, et al. Factors that predict response of patients with hepatitis B e antigen-positive chronic hepatitis B to peginterferon-alfa. Gastroenterology. 2009 Dec;137(6):2002–9.

147. Lee JM, Ahn SH, Kim HS, Park H, Chang HY, Kim DY, et al. Quantitative hepatitis B surface antigen and hepatitis B e antigen titers in prediction of treatment response to entecavir. Hepatology. 2011 May;53(5):1486–93.

148. Terrault NA, Bzowej NH, Chang KM, Hwang JP, Jonas MM, Murad MH, et al. AASLD guidelines for treatment of chronic hepatitis B. Hepatology. 2016 Jan;63(1):261–83.

149. Chu CM, Liaw YF. Chronic hepatitis B virus infection acquired in childhood: special emphasis on prognostic and therapeutic implication of delayed HBeAg seroconversion. J Viral Hepat. 2007 Mar;14(3):147–52.

150. Pan CQ, Duan Z, Dai E, Zhang S, Han G, Wang Y, et al. Tenofovir to prevent hepatitis B transmission in mothers with high viral load. N Engl J Med. 2016 Jun 16;374(24):2324–34.

151. Brown RS Jr, McMahon BJ, Lok AS, Wong JB, Ahmed AT, Mouchli MA, et al. Antiviral therapy in chronic hepatitis B viral infection during pregnancy: a systematic review and meta-analysis. Hepatology. 2016 Jan;63(1):319–33.

152. Lampertico P, Maini M, Papatheodoridis G. Optimal management of hepatitis B virus infection - EASL special conference. J Hepatol. 2015 Nov;63(5):1238–53.

153. Vlachogiannakos J, Papatheodoridis GV. Hepatitis B: who and when to treat? Liver Int. 2018 Feb;38(Suppl 1):71–8.

154. Xu C, Guo H, Pan XB, Mao R, Yu W, Xu X, et al. Interferons accelerate decay of replication-competent nucleocapsids of hepatitis B virus. J Virol. 2010 Sep;84(18):9332–40.

155. Micco L, Peppa D, Loggi E, Schurich A, Jefferson L, Cursaro C, et al. Differential boosting of innate and adaptive antiviral responses during pegylated-interferon-alpha therapy of chronic hepatitis B. J Hepatol. 2013 Feb;58(2):225–33.

156. Belloni L, Allweiss L, Guerrieri F, Pediconi N, Volz T, Pollicino T, et al. IFN-alpha inhibits HBV transcription and replication in cell culture and in humanized mice by targeting the epigenetic regulation of the nuclear cccDNA minichromosome. J Clin Invest. 2012 Feb;122(2):529–37.

157. Lucifora J, Xia Y, Reisinger F, Zhang K, Stadler D, Cheng X, et al. Specific and nonhepatotoxic degradation of nuclear hepatitis B virus cccDNA. Science. 2014 Mar 14;343(6176):1221–8.

158. Bailon P, Palleroni A, Schaffer CA, Spence CL, Fung WJ, Porter JE, et al. Rational design of a potent, long-lasting form of interferon: a 40 kDa branched polyethylene glycol-conjugated interferon alpha-2a for the treatment of hepatitis C. Bioconjug Chem. 2001 Mar–Apr;12(2):195–202.

159. Perry CM, Jarvis B. Peginterferon-alpha-2a (40 kD): a review of its use in the management of chronic hepatitis C. Drugs. 2001;61(15):2263–88.

160. Lau GK, Piratvisuth T, Luo KX, Marcellin P, Thongsawat S, Cooksley G, et al. Peginterferon Alfa-2a, lamivudine, and the combination for HBeAg-positive chronic hepatitis B. The New England journal of medicine. 2005;352(26):2682–95.

161. Marcellin P, Lau GK, Bonino F, Farci P, Hadziyannis S, Jin R, et al. Peginterferon alfa-2a alone, lamivudine alone, and the two in combination in patients with HBeAg-negative chronic hepatitis B. The New England journal of medicine. 2004;351(12):1206–17.

162. Knodell RG, Ishak KG, Black WC, Chen TS, Craig R, Kaplowitz N, et al. Formulation and application of a numerical scoring system for assessing histological activity in asymptomatic chronic active hepatitis. Hepatology. 1981 Sep–Oct;1(5):431–5.

163. Hui AY, Chan HL, Cheung AY, Cooksley G, Sung JJ. Systematic review: treatment of chronic hepatitis B virus infection by pegylated interferon. Aliment Pharmacol Ther. 2005 Sep 15;22(6):519–28.

164. Clark DN, Flanagan JM, Hu J. Mapping of functional subdomains in the terminal protein domain of hepatitis B virus polymerase. J Virol. 2017 Feb;1:91(3).

165. Fung J, Lai CL, Seto WK, Yuen MF. Nucleoside/nucleotide analogues in the treatment of chronic hepatitis B. J Antimicrob Chemother. 2011 Dec;66(12):2715–25.

166. Marcellin P, Heathcote EJ, Buti M, Gane E, de Man RA, Krastev Z, et al. Tenofovir disoproxil fumarate versus adefovir dipivoxil for chronic hepatitis B. The New England journal of medicine. 2008;359(23):2442–55.

167. Buti M, Gane E, Seto WK, Chan HL, Chuang WL, Stepanova T, et al. Tenofovir alafenamide versus tenofovir disoproxil fumarate for the treatment of patients with HBeAg-negative chronic hepatitis B virus infection: a randomised, double-blind, phase 3, non-inferiority trial. Lancet Gastroenterol Hepatol. 2016 Nov;1(3):196–206.

168. Chan HL, Fung S, Seto WK, Chuang WL, Chen CY, Kim HJ, et al. Tenofovir alafenamide versus tenofovir disoproxil fumarate for the treatment of HBeAg-positive chronic hepatitis B virus infection: a randomised, double-blind, phase 3, non-inferiority trial. Lancet Gastroenterol Hepatol. 2016 Nov;1(3):185–95.

169. Kim V, Abreu RM, Nakagawa DM, Baldassare RM, Carrilho FJ, Ono SK. Pegylated interferon alfa for chronic hepatitis B: systematic review and meta-analysis. J Viral Hepat. 2016 Mar;23(3):154–69.

170. Matthews SJ. Entecavir for the treatment of chronic hepatitis B virus infection. Clin Ther. 2006;28(2):184–203.

171. Fung S, Kwan P, Fabri M, Horban A, Pelemis M, Hann HW, et al. Tenofovir disoproxil fumarate (TDF) vs. emtricitabine (FTC)/TDF in lamivudine resistant hepatitis B: a 5-year randomised study. J Hepatol. 2017 Jan;66(1):11–8.

172. Peng H, Liu J, Yang M, Tong S, Yin W, Tang H, et al. Efficacy of lamivudine combined with adefovir dipivoxil versus entecavir monotherapy in patients with hepatitis B-associated decompensated cirrhosis: a meta-analysis. J Clin Pharmacol. 2014 Feb;54(2):189–200.

173. Chang TT, Lai CL, Kew Yoon S, Lee SS, Coelho HS, Carrilho FJ, et al. Entecavir treatment for up to 5 years in patients with hepatitis B e antigen-positive chronic hepatitis B. Hepatology. 2010 Feb;51(2):422–30.

174. Chi H, Hansen BE, Guo S, Zhang NP, Qi X, Chen L, et al. Pegylated interferon alfa-2b add-on treatment in hepatitis B virus envelope antigen-positive chronic hepatitis B patients treated with Nucleos(t)ide analogue: a randomized, controlled trial (PEGON). J Infect Dis. 2017 Apr 1;215(7):1085–93.

175. Tenney DJ, Rose RE, Baldick CJ, Pokornowski KA, Eggers BJ, Fang J, et al. Long-term monitoring shows hepatitis B virus resistance to entecavir in nucleoside-naive patients is rare through 5 years of therapy. Hepatology. 2009 May;49(5):1503–14.

176. Hadziyannis SJ, Sevastianos V, Rapti I, Vassilopoulos D, Hadziyannis E. Sustained responses and loss of HBsAg in HBeAg-negative patients with chronic hepatitis B who stop long-term treatment with adefovir. Gastroenterology. 2012 Sep;143(3):629–36.

177. Berg T, Simon KG, Mauss S, Schott E, Heyne R, Klass DM, et al. Long-term response after stopping tenofovir disoproxil fumarate in non-cirrhotic HBeAg-negative patients - FINITE study. J Hepatol. 2017 Nov;67(5):918–24.

178. Jeng WJ, Chen YC, Chien RN, Sheen IS, Liaw YF. Incidence and predictors of hepatitis B surface antigen seroclearance after cessation of nucleos(t)ide analogue therapy in hepatitis B e antigen-negative chronic hepatitis B. Hepatology. 2018 Aug;68(2):425–34.

179. Tseng TC, Liu CJ, Su TH, Wang CC, Chen CL, Chen PJ, et al. Serum hepatitis B surface antigen levels predict surface antigen loss in hepatitis B e antigen seroconverters. Gastroenterology. 2011 Aug;141(2):517–25.e1-2.

180. Dusheiko G. Current and future directions for the management of hepatitis B. South Afr Med J. 2018 Aug 8;108(8b):22–30.

181. Niro GA, Ciancio A, Gaeta GB, Smedile A, Marrone A, Olivero A, et al. Pegylated interferon alpha-2b as monotherapy or in combination with ribavirin in chronic hepatitis delta. Hepatology. 2006 Sep;44(3):713–20.

182. Gheorghe L, Iacob S, Simionov I, Vadan R, Constantinescu I, Caruntu F, et al. Weight-based dosing regimen of peg-interferon alpha-2b for chronic hepatitis delta: a multicenter Romanian trial. J Gastrointestin Liver Dis JGLD. 2011 Dec;20(4):377–82.

183. Yurdaydin C, Tabak F, Kaymakoglu S, Akarsu M, Akinci EG, Akkiz H, et al. Diagnosis, management and treatment of hepatitis delta virus infection: Turkey 2017 clinical practice guidelines. Turk J Gastroenterol. 2017 Dec;28(Suppl 2):84–9.

184. Yurdaydin C, Keskin O, Kalkan C, Karakaya F, Caliskan A, Kabacam G, et al. Interferon treatment duration in patients with chronic delta hepatitis and its effect on the natural course of the disease. J Infect Dis. 2018 Mar 28;217(8):1184–92.

185. Blank A, Markert C, Hohmann N, Carls A, Mikus G, Lehr T, et al. First-in-human application of the novel hepatitis B and hepatitis D virus entry inhibitor myrcludex B. J Hepatol. 2016 Sep;65(3):483–9.

186. Yurdaydin C, Keskin O, Kalkan C, Karakaya F, Caliskan A, Karatayli E, et al. Optimizing lonafarnib treatment for the management of chronic delta hepatitis: The LOWR HDV-1 study. Hepatology. 2018 Apr;67(4):1224–36.

187. Bazinet M, Pântea V, Cebotarescu V, Cojuhari L, Jimbei P, Albrecht J, et al. Safety and efficacy of REP 2139 and pegylated interferon alfa-2a for treatment-naive patients with chronic hepatitis B virus and hepatitis D virus co-infection (REP 301 and REP 301-LTF): a non-randomised, open-label, phase 2 trial. Lancet Gastroenterol Hepatol. 2017 Dec;2(12):877–89.

188. Hamid SS, Etzion O, Lurie Y, Bader N, Yardeni D, Channa SM, Mawani M, Parkash O, Martins, EB, Gane EJ. A phase 2 randomized clinical trial to evaluate the safety and efficacy of pegylated interferon lambda monotherapy in patients with chronic hepatitis delta virus infection: interim results from the LIMT HDV Study. Hepatology. 2017, Abstract #927.

189. Reddy KR, Ellerbe C, Schilsky M, Stravitz RT, Fontana RJ, Durkalski V, et al. Determinants of outcome among patients with acute liver failure listed for liver transplantation in the United States. Liver Transpl. 2016 Apr;22(4):505–15.

190. Young K, Liu B, Bhuket T, Younossi Z, Saab S, Ahmed A, et al. Long-term trends in chronic hepatitis B virus infection associated liver transplantation outcomes in the United States. J Viral Hepat. 2017 Sep;24(9):789–96.

191. Burra P, Germani G, Adam R, Karam V, Marzano A, Lampertico P, et al. Liver transplantation for HBV-related cirrhosis in Europe: an ELTR study on evolution and outcomes. J Hepatol. 2013 Feb;58(2):287–96.

192. Cholongitas E, Papatheodoridis GV. High genetic barrier nucleos(t)ide analogue(s) for prophylaxis from hepatitis B virus recurrence after liver transplantation: a systematic review. Am J Transplant Off J Am Soc Transplant Am Soc Transplant Surg. 2013 Feb;13(2):353–62.

193. Lima DS, Murad Junior AJ, Barreira MA, Fernandes GC, Coelho GR, Garcia JHP. Liver transplantation in Hepatitis Delta: South America experience. Arq Gastroenterol. 2018 Jan–Mar;55(1):14–7.

194. Samuel D, Zignego AL, Reynes M, Feray C, Arulnaden JL, David MF, et al. Long-term clinical and virological outcome after liver transplantation for cirrhosis caused by chronic delta hepatitis. Hepatology. 1995 Feb;21(2):333–9.

195. Roche B, Samuel D. Liver transplantation in delta virus infection. Semin Liver Dis. 2012 Aug;32(3):245–55.

196. Fox AN, Terrault NA. The option of HBIG-free prophylaxis against recurrent HBV. J Hepatol. 2012 May;56(5):1189–97.

197. Fung J. Management of chronic hepatitis B before and after liver transplantation. World J Hepatol. 2015 Jun 8;7(10):1421–6.

198. de The H, Tiollais P, Dejean A. Hepatitis B virus and hepatocarcinoma: integration of HBV DNA in the gene coding for the receptor of retinoic acid. Pathologie-Biologie. 1989 Jan;37(1):5–6.

199. Wang J, Chenivesse X, Henglein B, Brechot C. Hepatitis B virus integration in a cyclin A gene in a hepatocellular carcinoma. Nature. 1990 Feb 8;343(6258):555–7.

200. Graef E, Caselmann WH, Wells J, Koshy R. Insertional activation of mevalonate kinase by hepatitis B virus DNA in a human hepatoma cell line. Oncogene. 1994 Jan;9(1):81–7.
201. Ferber MJ, Montoya DP, Yu C, Aderca I, McGee A, Thorland EC, et al. Integrations of the hepatitis B virus (HBV) and human papillomavirus (HPV) into the human telomerase reverse transcriptase (hTERT) gene in liver and cervical cancers. Oncogene. 2003 Jun 12;22(24):3813–20.
202. Horikawa I, Barrett JC. Transcriptional regulation of the telomerase hTERT gene as a target for cellular and viral oncogenic mechanisms. Carcinogenesis. 2003 Jul;24(7):1167–76.
203. Paterlini-Brechot P, Saigo K, Murakami Y, Chami M, Gozuacik D, Mugnier C, et al. Hepatitis B virus-related insertional mutagenesis occurs frequently in human liver cancers and recurrently targets human telomerase gene. Oncogene. 2003 June 19;22(25):3911–6.
204. Feitelson MA, Zhu M, Duan LX, London WT. Hepatitis B x antigen and p53 are associated in vitro and in liver tissues from patients with primary hepatocellular carcinoma. Oncogene. 1993 May;8(5):1109–17.
205. Kim SS, Cho HJ, Lee HY, Park JH, Noh CK, Shin SJ, et al. Genetic polymorphisms in the Wnt/beta-catenin pathway genes as predictors of tumor development and survival in patients with hepatitis B virus-associated hepatocellular carcinoma. Clin Biochem. 2016 Jul;49(10–11):792–801.
206. Peng CY, Chen TC, Hung SP, Chen MF, Yeh CT, Tsai SL, et al. Genetic alterations of INK4alpha/ARF locus and p53 in human hepatocellular carcinoma. Anticancer Res. 2002 Mar–Apr;22(2B):1265–71.
207. Liu N, Jiao T, Huang Y, Liu W, Li Z, Ye X. Hepatitis B virus regulates apoptosis and tumorigenesis through the microRNA-15a-Smad7-transforming growth factor beta pathway. J Virol. 2015 Mar;89(5):2739–49.
208. Wang F, Anderson PW, Salem N, Kuang Y, Tennant BC, Lee Z. Gene expression studies of hepatitis virus-induced woodchuck hepatocellular carcinoma in correlation with human results. Int J Oncol. 2007 Jan;30(1):33–44.
209. Ha HL, Yu DY. HBx-induced reactive oxygen species activates hepatocellular carcinogenesis via dysregulation of PTEN/Akt pathway. World J Gastroenterol WJG. 2010 Oct 21;16(39):4932–7.
210. Xie Q, Su Y, Dykema K, Johnson J, Koeman J, De Giorgi V, et al. Overexpression of HGF promotes HBV-induced hepatocellular carcinoma progression and is an effective Indicator for met-targeting therapy. Genes Cancer. 2013 Jul;4(7–8):247–60.
211. Kim SO, Park JG, Lee YI. Increased expression of the insulin-like growth factor I (IGF-I) receptor gene in hepatocellular carcinoma cell lines: implications of IGF-I receptor gene activation by hepatitis B virus X gene product. Cancer Res. 1996 Aug 15;56(16):3831–6.
212. Sarkar D. AEG-1/MTDH/LYRIC in liver cancer. Adv Cancer Res. 2013;120:193–221.
213. Laurent-Puig P, Legoix P, Bluteau O, Belghiti J, Franco D, Binot F, et al. Genetic alterations associated with hepatocellular carcinomas define distinct pathways of hepatocarcinogenesis. Gastroenterology. 2001 Jun;120(7):1763–73.
214. Marchio A, Pineau P, Meddeb M, Terris B, Tiollais P, Bernheim A, et al. Distinct chromosomal abnormality pattern in primary liver cancer of non-B, non-C patients. Oncogene. 2000 Aug 3;19(33):3733–8.
215. Zhang H, Zhai Y, Hu Z, Wu C, Qian J, Jia W, et al. Genome-wide association study identifies 1p36.22 as a new susceptibility locus for hepatocellular carcinoma in chronic hepatitis B virus carriers. Nat Genet. 2010 Sep;42(9):755–8.
216. Hakami A, Ali A, Hakami A. Effects of hepatitis B virus mutations on its replication and liver disease severity. Open Virol J. 2013;7:12–8.
217. Yang HI, Sherman M, Su J, Chen PJ, Liaw YF, Iloeje UH, et al. Nomograms for risk of hepatocellular carcinoma in patients with chronic hepatitis B virus infection. J Clin Oncol. 2010 May 10;28(14):2437–44.
218. Kew MC, Macerollo P. Effect of age on the etiologic role of the hepatitis B virus in hepatocellular carcinoma in blacks. Gastroenterology. 1988 Feb;94(2):439–42.

219. Marrero JA, Kulik LM, Sirlin CB, Zhu AX, Finn RS, Abecassis MM, et al. Diagnosis, staging, and Management of Hepatocellular Carcinoma: 2018 practice guidance by the American Association for the Study of Liver Diseases. Hepatology. 2018 Aug;68(2):723–50.

220. European Association for the Study of the Liver. EASL clinical practice guidelines: management of hepatocellular carcinoma. J Hepatol. 2018 Jul;69(1):182–236.

221. Ren F, Zhang J, Gao Z, Zhu H, Chen X, Liu W, et al. Racial disparities in the survival time of patients with hepatocellular carcinoma and intrahepatic cholangiocarcinoma between Chinese patients and patients of other racial groups: a population-based study from 2004 to 2013. Oncol Lett. 2018 Dec;16(6):7102–16.

222. Chayanupatkul M, Omino R, Mittal S, Kramer JR, Richardson P, Thrift AP, et al. Hepatocellular carcinoma in the absence of cirrhosis in patients with chronic hepatitis B virus infection. J Hepatol. 2017 Feb;66(2):355–62.

223. Papatheodoridis GV, Dalekos GN, Yurdaydin C, Buti M, Goulis J, Arends P, et al. Incidence and predictors of hepatocellular carcinoma in Caucasian chronic hepatitis B patients receiving entecavir or tenofovir. J Hepatol. 2015 Feb;62(2):363–70.

224. Mazzaferro V, Regalia E, Doci R, Andreola S, Pulvirenti A, Bozzetti F, et al. Liver transplantation for the treatment of small hepatocellular carcinomas in patients with cirrhosis. N Engl J Med. 1996 Mar 14;334(11):693–9.

225. Roayaie S, Jibara G, Tabrizian P, Park JW, Yang J, Yan L, et al. The role of hepatic resection in the treatment of hepatocellular cancer. Hepatology. 2015 Aug;62(2):440–51.

226. Iezzi R, Marsico VA, Guerra A, Cerchiaro E, Cassano A, Basso M, et al. Trans-arterial chemoembolization with irinotecan-loaded drug-eluting beads (DEBIRI) and capecitabine in refractory liver prevalent colorectal metastases: a phase II single-center study. Cardiovasc Intervent Radiol. 2015 Dec;38(6):1523–31.

227. Kudo M. Proposal of primary endpoints for TACE combination trials with systemic therapy: lessons learned from 5 negative trials and the positive TACTICS trial. Liver Cancer. 2018 Sep;7(3):225–34.

228. Yoon SM, Ryoo BY, Lee SJ, Kim JH, Shin JH, An JH, et al. Efficacy and safety of transarterial chemoembolization plus external beam radiotherapy vs Sorafenib in hepatocellular carcinoma with macroscopic vascular invasion: a randomized clinical trial. JAMA Oncol. 2018 May 1;4(5):661–9.

229. Nishida N, Kudo M. Immune checkpoint blockade for the treatment of human hepatocellular carcinoma. Hepatol Res. 2018 Jul;48(8):622–34.

230. Kudo M. Targeted and immune therapies for hepatocellular carcinoma: predictions for 2019 and beyond. World J Gastroenterol WJG. 2019 Feb 21;25(7):789–807.

# Chapter 8
# Alcohol Induced Liver Disease

Nora V. Bergasa

A 48-year-old man was evaluated in the hepatology clinic because of an abnormal liver profile. He had alcohol use disorder and had drunk excessively for many years, with four, 24 ounce beer cans per day for the last 20. He did not have a history of alcohol withdrawal. He was pleasant and a good historian. He had attempted to stop to drink alcohol by himself, with psychotherapy, by participation in peer chaired meetings, but nothing had worked for him. He had diabetes mellitus type 2, asthma, hypertension, and hyperlipidemia on treatment. Physical exam was notable for a flushed appearance and marked hepatomegaly. The liver panel revealed transaminases (AST and ALT) and gamma glutamyl transpeptidase (GGTP) serum activities of 267, 168, 1407 IU/ml, respectively, and normal bilirubin and serum albumin concentrations. Liver disease workup was notable for serum ferritin of 2729 ng/ml and transferrin saturation of 82%, and heterozygote for the C282Y mutation. A liver biopsy revealed steatosis, cirrhosis, and iron deposition on hepatocytes. After a rapport was established with the hepatologist, treatment of alcohol use disorder was initiated with naltrexone, 9 days after his last drink. On naltrexone, which he took for several months, he stopped drinking alcohol. In consultation with hematology, the patient underwent phlebotomy to a transferrin saturation of 28%. He has remained abstinent from alcohol for 9 years; no additional phlebotomies have been necessary.

N. V. Bergasa (✉)
Department of Medicine, H+H/Metropolitan, New York, NY, USA

New York Medical College, Valhalla, NY, USA

Hepatology, H+H/Woodhull, Brooklyn, NY, USA

N. V. Bergasa (ed.), *Clinical Cases in Hepatology*,
https://doi.org/10.1007/978-1-4471-4715-2_8

# Etiology

Alcohol can cause liver disease [1]. The National Institute of Alcohol Abuse and Alcoholism (NIAAA) defines binge drinking as a drinking pattern that brings blood alcohol concentration (BAC) levels to 0.08 g/dL, which typically occurs after four drinks for women and five drinks for men in about 2 h, with one drink having 14 g of alcohol [2]. The Substance Abuse and Mental Health Services Administration (SAMHSA) defines binge drinking as five or more alcoholic drinks for males or four or more alcoholic drinks for females on the same occasion (i.e., at the same time or within a couple of hours of each other) on at least 1 day in the past month (the month prior to when the question is being asked) [3]. SAMHSA defines heavy alcohol use as binge drinking on five or more days in the past month. NIAAA defines low risk drinking for women as no more than three drinks on any single day and no more than seven drinks per week and for men as no more than four drinks on any single day and no more than 14 drinks per week. NIAAA research has documented that only about two in 100 people who drink within these limits have alcohol use disorder (AUD) [3].

# Genetics

Fifteen percent of subjects who drink alcohol excessively develop cirrhosis, which suggests that unique features, including genetics, determine the susceptibility to this complication. Evidence in support of this idea has been provided from twin studies that have shown twin concordances for alcoholism and its complications by zygosity among male veterans from data from 15,924 male twin pairs registered in the National Academy of Sciences-National Research Council Twin Registry from which a prevalence for liver cirrhosis was reported as 14.2%, with case-wise twin concordance rates for cirrhosis of 14.6 and 5.4% in monozygotic and dizygotic twins, respectively [4].

It is reported that at low doses, most of the ingested alcohol is oxidized in the stomach, as first pass, by the activity of alcohol dehydrogenase (ADH) found in the mucosa, which has been suggested to provide a barrier against systemic toxicity of ethanol [5, 6]. In women, the ingestion of equivalent amounts of alcohol resulted in higher serum alcohol levels than in men. Also, women were reported to have reduced activity of gastric ADH compared to men and it was almost absent in women who drank alcohol excessively, which may have an impact on the higher vulnerability to develop liver disease in women versus men [7].

In the liver, alcohol is metabolized mostly by the action of ADH to form acetaldehyde, which is highly toxic, and by aldehyde dehydrogenase (ALDH) to acetate, subsequently broken down to water and carbon dioxide for elimination [8]. Single nucleotide polymorphisms in the genes that code for alcohol metabolizing enzymes change their function, affecting the production and elimination of ALDH. The single nucleotide polymorphism (SNP) rs1229984 or Arg48His in ADH1B was reported in a wide range of East Asian subjects, 19% to 91% [9] but was uncommon in other races [10]. The SNP rs671 in *ALDH* is associated with loss of function and decreased enzyme activity and accumulation of acetaldehyde; this SNP was documented in 30–50% of East Asians [8]. The ADH2-2 allele is reported in association with a decrease in the risk of alcohol dependence but with an increase in the risk of developing alcoholic liver disease (ALD) [11, 12].

In addition, alcohol is metabolized in the liver by the enzyme cytochrome P450IIE1 (CYP2E1), which may increase in chronic alcohol intake [13]. The rapidity with which alcohol is metabolized in the liver depends on catalytic enzymes' availability, which appears to be determined genetically.

*PNPLA3* has been consistently reported in association with non alcoholic fatty liver disease (NAFLD) and fibrosis in that condition [14–16]. NAFLD and ALD have common histological features, and, likely some of the mechanisms of fat-induced liver injury and susceptibility to the conditions are the same. In this regard, from a meta-analysis that included ten studies exploring a role of PNPLA3 in ALD, it was documented that the odds ratio (OR) for ALD was 2.09, 95% confidence interval (CI) of 1.79–2.44 for SNP rs738409 CG in heterozygotes and 3.37 (95% CI 2.49–4.58) for GG homozygotes [17], with an OR of 2.62 (95% CI 1.73–3.97) in association with alcohol associated cirrhosis versus OR of 8.45 (95% CI 2.52–28.37) for steatosis. *PNPLA3* codes adiponutrin, related to adipose triglyceride lipase (ATGL/PNPLA2), a triglyceride hydrolase in adipose tissue [18, 19]. Also, through genome-wide association studies (GWAS), the SNP rs626283 was identified in *MBOAT7* ($P = 1.03 \times 10(-9)$) and rs58542926 ($P = 7.89 \times 10^{-10}$) in *TM6SF2* both as genetic risks for the development of alcohol-related cirrhosis in subjects of European descent [20]. In addition to what has been stated above in reference to PNPLA3, the SNP identified in association with ALD (and NAFLD) contributes to the concentration of retinyl palmitate in the liver, suggesting a role in the steatosis aspect of fatty liver disease alcohol and non-alcohol related [21]. TM6SF2 regulates liver fat metabolism with opposing effects on triglyceride secretion and droplet lipid content in hepatocytes [22]. MBOAT7 specifically transfers polyunsaturated fatty acids, including arachidonoyl-CoA to lysophosphatidylinositol, other lysophospholipids· and associated metabolites of arachidonic acid that are involved in inflammation [23–25]. The mechanisms through which these SNPs mediate vulnerability to NAFLD or ALD are unknown; however, a role in the processing of fat and inflammation is plausible.

From a GWAS in patients with alcoholic hepatitis, a florid manifestation of ALD, it was reported in abstract form, the identification of an SNP in the Solute Carrier Family 38, Member A4 (SLC38A4) gene with OR 1.32 at a notable significance for this type of study; SLC38A4 is expressed mostly in the liver and is involved in amino acid transport [26].

In human beings, the expression of class mu glutathione-S-transferase in the liver is associated with liver disease [27]. The null phenotype GSTM1(0) was more common in alcoholic patients than in the controls and was associated with cirrhosis [27].

The role of genes including those associated with oxidative stress, endotoxin response, cytokine activity, activation of fibrosis mechanisms such as CD14, glutathione-S-transferase, interleukin 10, interleukin 1B, manganese superoxide dismutase, nuclear factor of kappa light polypeptide gene enhancer in B cells 1, Toll-like receptor 4, transforming growth factor β1, and tumor necrosis factor α have been reported to play a role in alcohol induced liver disease, but, robust and consistent information in support of their role has not been published [28].

Certain animal strains exhibit preference for or disinterest in alcohol. It was reported from a study of microarray analysis of brain gene expression from different mice strains that 3800 unique genes significantly and consistently changed between the models that differ in alcohol preference. Several functional groups that included mitogen-activated protein kinase signaling and transcription regulation pathways were documented as significantly overrepresented. Those pathways may play an important role in establishing a high voluntary alcohol drinking level in some mouse models. Further analysis was reported to identify an alcohol preference quantitative trait locus the candidate genes for an alcohol preference quantitative locus *Arhgef12*, *Carm1*, *Cryab*, *Cox5a*, *Dlat*, *Fxyd6*, *Limd1*, *Nicn1*, *Nmnat3*, *Pknox2*, *Rbp1*, *Sc5d*, *Scn4b*, *Tcf12*, *Vps11*, and *Zfp291*and four ESTs were identified in chromosome 9 [29]. This type of analysis may provide some clues to understand the genetic predisposition to liver disease from alcohol in human beings.

Increased GABAergic neurotransmission may contribute to the desirable mood effects of alcohol [30]. There have been inconsistent reports on the association between SNPs in the gene that codes gamma aminobutyric acid (GABA) and alcohol use disorders [31, 32] but not regarding risks for liver disease from alcohol yet.

Whether genetically modified or not, obesity and cigarette smoking have been identified in association with a risk to develop cirrhosis in patients who excessively drink alcohol. A large study from Scotland documented that obesity and excessive alcohol intake increase the relative rate of death from liver disease [33]. There was a significant interaction between obesity and excessive alcohol intake that increased the risk of death from liver disease. This study provided data from two prospective cohort studies from Scotland that included 9559 men over the years of 1965 and 1968 and 1970 to 1973 before the deluge of literature on NAFLD. The study documented that high mass body index (BMI) and alcohol intake were significantly associated with mortality due to liver disease. Individuals who drank 15 or more drinks per week regardless of the BMI and those who were obese and drank had a greater relative risk for liver disease versus those who were not obese or underweight who did not drink. The adjusted relative rate for mortality from liver disease in underweight and normal weight with 95% confidence interval (CI) for men was 3.16 (1.28 to 7.8), 7.01 (3.02 to 16.3) for overweight, and 18.9 (6.84 to 52.4) for obese men. The relative rate for obese men who consumed fewer than 15 drinks per week was reported as 5.3 (1.36 to 20.7) with a relative excess risk from interactions between BMI and alcohol consumption of 5.58 (1.09 to 10.1) [33]. A study from

California in the United States that included data from 128,934 subjects who had undergone health examinations between 1978 and 1985 documented that cigarette smoking was independently related to alcoholic cirrhosis. In addition, and consistent with recent writings [34], coffee was associated with a decrease in the risk of alcoholic cirrhosis, with drinking at least four cups of coffee per day being associated with one fifth of the risk for cirrhosis from alcohol of that of persons who did not drink coffee [35], an idea confirmed from another study that concluded that coffee but not other caffeine containing beverages might "inhibit" the development of alcoholic (and nonalcoholic) liver cirrhosis [36]. The role of coffee in society is important [37]. One wonders what the coffee drinking habits in women who drink alcohol excessively are. The author did not find a publication that specifically reported the relationship between coffee and ALD; however, from a relatively large European study, it was documented that "regular coffee but not espresso" was an independent factor protecting from liver fibrosis in severely obese women. The lack of protection is devastating for espresso drinkers; thus, no alcohol remains one's only option.

Women are more susceptible to ALD than men. From a study in Denmark that included 6152 people who drank alcohol, women and men had a 35 and 27 fold increase in mortality from cirrhosis, respectively, compared to the general population with five drinks per day, i.e., threshold, but not more, being associated with death from cirrhosis. This study added information supporting the idea of the alcohol threshold, at which there is liver injury, and beyond which there may not be significant differences in liver disease [38]. From a community hospital in New York City, New York, in the United States, a retrospective study that included 2002 to 2011 data revealed that patients of Hispanic ethnicity exhibited increased morbidity, as evidenced by admissions to the intensive care unit and mechanical ventilation requirements. There was a significant association between mortality and the Hispanic women group versus non-Hispanic patients ($p = 0.0007$); however, the 90 day mortality for Hispanic ($n = 6$) vs. non-Hispanic women ($n = 1$) was not significantly different ($p = 0.20$). This study, limited by its retrospective nature and the relatively small number of patients ($n = 165$), highlights the vulnerability of women, and of women of certain Hispanic ethnicity not only to develop ALD but to be gravely ill from it [39]. The perennial question of the susceptibility of women to develop ALD remains; in this regard, differences in the pharmacokinetics of alcohol between men and women, a role of estrogen and progesterone and their different availability in pre- and post-menopausal states, and the relationship between hormonal concentrations and intestinal permeability, which would increase the exposure of the liver and the whole system to bacterial products, including endotoxins, metabolism, and the physical volume where alcohol is distributed, smaller in women than in men that increases the concentration of alcohol to which the tissues are exposed have been proposed, and some investigated without the provision of unequivocal results [40–42].

## Epidemiology

In the United States, the prevalence of chronic liver disease from alcohol was reported from data extracted from Medicare claims between 1999 and 2012 among the fee-for-service participants, comprised of 106,458 subjects as the second most common cause, 21% in the whole group, and also, the most common cause of liver disease in Caucasians, 38.2% [43].

A study that reported data from the National Survey on Drug Data recorded information on drinking patterns in relation to socioeconomic and demographic characteristics and alcohol dependence, characterized by craving, increase tolerance to alcohol, withdrawal symptoms, and failed attempts to quit that can result in drinking even increased amounts [of alcohol] [3]. In this study, excessive drinking was defined as binge drinking according to the Substance Abuse and Mental Health Services Administration [3], heavy drinking, i.e., one drink per day on average for a woman, and more than two drinks per day on average for a man, any alcohol consumption by youth aged <21 years, and by pregnant women over the 30 days prior to the questions being asked [44]. The study documented that excessive drinking and alcohol dependence were most common among men from 18 to 24 years old, with binge drinking being the most usual pattern in individuals from families with an annual income of at least $75,000.00. Dependence was prevalent in individuals from families with an annual income of less than $25,000, with a prevalence of 10.5% in binge drinkers, 10.2% in excessive drinkers, and 1.3% in non-binge drinkers. The study results documented that most individuals who drink excessively do not meet the criteria for alcohol dependence; however, complications that result from intoxication happen independently from that diagnosis. Furthermore, although ALD develops only in 15% of persons who drink alcohol excessively, the global mortality attributed to cirrhosis from alcohol was reported as 156,900 deaths in women, and 336,400 in men in 2010, reported to represent 0.7% for women and 1.2% for men of all global deaths, respectively [45]. Indeed, studies have documented that one of the predicting variables of cirrhosis development from alcohol is drinking patterns [46, 47]. Decompensated liver disease from alcohol is relatively common in patients seen in the hospitals where the author works, and, notably, the number of patients considered for liver transplantation from this type of liver disease has increased; thus, it is useful for the clinician to be aware of the relevance of drinking patterns and their associations to refer patients for early treatment and preventive interventions [48, 49].

A vulnerability threshold beyond which there is a substantial risk of developing liver disease from alcohol has also been documented [50]. From the Dyonisos Study, a reputable source on the prevalence of chronic liver disease in Northern Italy, it was documented from 6534 participants that the threshold for the development of cirrhosis or non-cirrhotic liver damage was the intake of more than 30 g of alcohol per day in men and women. This group consisted of 1349 persons at risk from whom 5.5% had evidence of liver injury, with a prevalence of what the investigators defined as "pure" alcoholic cirrhosis of 0.43%, 30 from the whole cohort, which was 2.3% of the individuals at risk, with a ratio of nine men to one woman, versus 44 (3.3%) of the individuals at risk, who showed persistent signs of non-cirrhotic liver damage. After the age of 50 years, the cumulative risk for developing cirrhosis and non-cirrhotic liver damage was significantly higher in subjects who drank at separate times from eating food versus in those who reported drinking at mealtimes only, consistent with a recent study [51]. Thus, 30 g of alcohol per day, especially in various forms, and daily consumption over the years, increase the risk of developing alcohol induced liver damage as concluded from these data [50]. Along the idea of a threshold required for developing liver disease from alcohol was the publication with data from 1976 to 1978. Subjects aged 30–79 years were followed for 12 years from a group of 13,285 from whom complete clinical information was available. Two hundred sixty-one subjects had alcohol induced liver disease, and 124 had alcohol induced cirrhosis, which yielded an overall incidence of 0.2% per year in men and 0.03% per year in women with a sharp and significant increase in the relative risk to develop liver disease from alcohol at the intake of 7–13 drinks per week in women, and 14–27 in men. Notably, women were more vulnerable than men to develop liver disease at any given amount of alcohol consumed [52].

In summary, alcohol drinking patterns and a dose threshold beyond which liver disease develops itself contribute to the pathogenesis of liver disease, which appears to be modified by environmental factors and genetic backgrounds combined with the local toxic effects of alcohol in the liver, at least in part.

## Natural History of Alcoholic Liver Disease

A model that addressed the rate of decompensation of liver disease from a study that used data on clinical signs from general practices from 1987 to 2002 in the United Kingdom and that included 4537 patients with cirrhosis, 50.9% of whom had cirrhosis from alcohol, documented that the rate of decompensation overall was 11% per year but, higher, 31% (95% CI: 28.8%, 33.4%), in the first year post diagnosis of cirrhosis, and in patients with cirrhosis from alcohol, 37.6% (95% CI: 34.1%, 41.5%) compared with 25.2% (95% CI: 22.6%, 28.2%) for those with non-alcohol-related cirrhosis also in the first year; the rate of decompensation after the first year did not vary as per etiology of liver disease, being 7.3% per year (95% CI: 6.5%, 8.2%), adjusted for age and gender for patients with liver disease from alcohol, and 5.5% per year (95% CI: 4.8%, 6.2%) for those with non-alcohol-related cirrhosis [53]. Although the information on abstinence was not provided in the publication, abstinence likely was one of the most important factors that improved the survival after the first year, as reported from studies that had access to histological data and that assessed the progression of liver injury versus its degree [54–56]. A study of 100 consecutive patients with cirrhosis from alcohol followed from 1995 to 2000 documented that abstinence 1 month post diagnosis was associated with a 7-year survival of 72% versus 44% for the patients who did not abstain [55]. Another study was a retrospective review of 192 consecutive patients, 60 with compensated disease, in whom liver related mortality was documented as 13% at 5 years, and 43% in the 132 who were decompensated. Patients with severe fibrosis had a 10 year mortality of 45% versus no mortality in those with F0 to F2; mortality was reported as significantly lower in patients who abstained from alcohol than in those who did not by the use of the log-rank test, $p = 0.017$ [56].

An important study on the natural history of ALD from 88 patients with steatosis from alcohol followed for a median of 10.5 years from 1978 to 1985 revealed that nine (10%), eight of whom had continued to drink at least 40 units (one unit equals 8 g of pure alcohol) of alcohol per week, had developed cirrhosis. An additional seven had developed fibrosis, but there was no information regarding alcohol use in these seven patients. Mixed macro and microvesicular fat (Fig. 8.1), and the presence of giant mitochondria on liver histology at baseline independently predicted disease progression; these features identified patients at high risk for disease progression. Although alcohol abstinence is the pillar of the limited therapeutic interventions to treat alcoholism and prevent ALD or its progression, the findings provide a rationale for proposing a liver biopsy, which should always be individualized and strong collaboration with alcohol rehabilitation programs to facilitate abstinence. Pharmacological therapy, including naltrexone, an opioid antagonist, and baclofen, a gamma-aminobutyric acid (GABA)-B receptor agonist, is indicated [57]. A study from Denmark also identified alcoholic fatty liver disease as having a higher probability of progression to cirrhosis than NAFLD. Patients who had had liver biopsies from 1976 to 1987 were identified. Over 9 years (range 0.6 to 23), 22 of 106 (20%) patients with alcoholic fatty liver disease developed cirrhosis versus one of 109 (0.9%) over 16.7 years (range 0.2–21.9) in the NAFLD group. The death rate was

**Fig. 8.1** Microvesicular (top arrow) and macrovesicular steatosis (bottom arrow) in a patient with alcohol induced liver disease (Hematoxylin and Eosin stain, 40X)

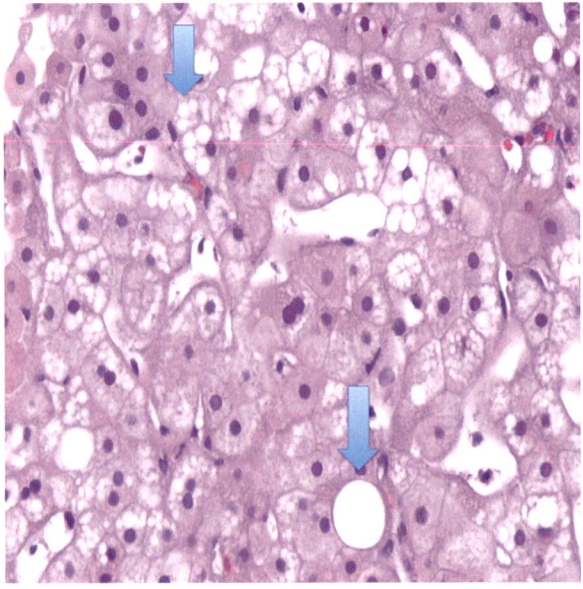

also higher in patients with ALD than in those with NAFLD [58]. Thus, ALD from the steatosis stage to the cirrhotic stage progresses faster than steatosis from nonalcoholic disease; however, there is no mention of the report of abstinence versus continuous alcohol intake over the follow-up period in that study. Another publication, from a retrospective review conducted in Iceland and that included patients who had had a liver biopsy from 1984 to 2009, identified 94 patients with steatosis from alcohol with a median of 20 year survival similar to the median survival of 24 years for patients with NAFLD. Seven percent of the group with NAFLD developed cirrhosis, significantly different from the 20% of patients with steatosis from alcohol; in addition, in 36% of patients in the latter group, the cause of death was liver related, versus cardiovascular disease in the NAFLD group. As previously reported, the degree of fibrosis, i.e., more, not less, was associated with risk of progression [59]. These data suggest that fat from alcohol induced liver injury is associated with a worse prognosis than fat from NAFLD.

Portal pressure has been proposed as the most important prognostic variable in cirrhosis; however, there was a lack of prognostic usefulness in the hepatic venous pressures. Hemodynamic measures were documented in a group of 87 patients with cirrhosis from alcohol prospectively studied from 1991 to 1993 at an index hospital admission and followed for a mean of 35 months (range of 1–76 months), during which 56 (64%) patients died at 5 years. Only age and bilirubin were significantly different from those who lived. Again, on Cox regression analysis, age and measures of liver function, e.g., Child–Pugh score, were the only prognostic factors for mortality [60]. Of much interest, and along the same line of interpretation from the data provided and as previously stated, the most significant predictive measure of survival at 5 years reported from a group of 122 hospitalized patients with cirrhosis and excessive intake of alcohol was the Child–Pugh class, with a 66%, 50%, and 25% for class A, B, and C, respectively [61]. In addition, the absence of alcoholic hepatitis, documented by histology, and continuous alcohol intake were significantly associated with increased risk ratios of death, the former results interpreted to suggest that the absence of a reversible condition, i.e., alcoholic hepatitis, was a poor prognostic factor, or, conversely, that the presence of alcoholic hepatitis, by virtue of its reversibility, was associated with a better prognosis than its absence [61].

The importance of relatively increased age and continuous alcohol use as independent predictors of a fatal outcome was supported by a study that followed 100 consecutively admitted patients with cirrhosis from alcohol for 15 years until death or year 2000. The group's mean age was 58 years, 35% of patients were women, 67 of whom had ascites, and 34% variceal bleeding on admission. Seventy-one percent and 90% died at 5 and 15 years, respectively, with bleeding and liver failure being the two most common causes of death [62]; however, Child–Pugh class was not identified as a prognostic factor for a bad outcome [62]. Furthermore, from an analysis that pooled 118 studies of the natural history of cirrhosis and that included 109 (46%) of patients with cirrhosis from alcohol, it was reported that alcohol as the etiology of cirrhosis was found independently predictive of survival in only one of the 48 studies (2%) in which it was included as a variable. Child–Pugh score, which was studied in 67 studies, was a predictor of survival in 42 (63%) [63]. Abstinence from alcohol significantly affected the natural history of the disease in 2 of the 12 (17%) studies in which it was included. Forty-six percent of the patients included in the analysis had cirrhosis from alcohol, and only 29% were classified as Child–Pugh class A [63]; thus, the majority had decompensated disease. Indeed, Child–Pugh and its components were the most common predictive variables identified across the studies. This result suggests that once cirrhosis is established, it is liver function that matters in survival. Thus, it can be inferred that, although with some variability according to the population studied, age, continuous alcohol use, and liver function are the most important prognostic factors of death in patients with cirrhosis from alcohol. In this regard, a study from Denmark that included 466 patients with a complication from cirrhosis due to alcohol examined the 1 year mortality, which was 64% for hepatic encephalopathy, 49% for ascites and variceal bleeding, 29% for ascites alone, and 17% for those who did not present with complications, the risk for which was 25% at 1 year, ascites being the complication in 12% of the patients, and 50% at five, with a risk of mortality at this point from 58% to 85% [64]. This publication, which reported the natural history of cirrhosis from alcohol more contemporaneously than previously cited studies, suggests that overall, the variables included in the Child–Pugh class calculation drive the prognosis of cirrhosis from alcohol. Thus, it can be inferred that, although with some variability according to the population studied, age, continuous alcohol use, and liver function are the most important prognostic factors of death in patients with cirrhosis from alcohol. Regarding liver function, the use of galactose elimination capacity (GEC) test is reported as a measure of hepatic metabolic capacity [65]. It is documented that in patients with cirrhosis of the liver, a decrease in the GEC is a predictor of short- and long-term mortality, suggesting the most important factor that determines the survival of patients with cirrhosis is liver function [65]. In this regard, investigators followed the patients from the cited study [64] to identify factors, labeled as patho-etiological, involved in developing complications, i.e., first-time hepatic encephalopathy, ascites, variceal bleeding, and mortality, in patients with cirrhosis from alcohol by the use of the GEC test. In addition, alcohol intake and plasma sodium, used as a measure of circulatory dysfunction, were assessed. It was reported that a low GEC increased the risk to develop hepatic encephalopathy; alcohol intake was associated with an increase in the risk to develop ascites, variceal bleeding, and mortality, with hyponatremia associated with an increased risk for all complications, as well as mortality. Although a reduction in GEC increased the risk of hepatic encephalopathy, the reduction of GED alone did not increase the risk of death in the absence of hepatic encephalopathy [66].

Bacterial infection affects the natural history of cirrhosis. Survival was examined in 501 patients, 48% of whom had ALD and a median Model of End-Stage Liver Disease (MELD) score of 17, e.g., meeting criteria for referral to liver transplant evaluation, who were admitted to the hospital because of complications of liver disease. The most common complication was bleeding from portal hypertension and ascites. The probability of survival was 50%, 46%, 41%, and 34% at 3, 6, 12, and 30 months in association with infections, 40% of which were nosocomial, compared to the 83%, 77%, 71%, and 62% without infection. The overall survival was independently associated with bacterial infections, with a hazard ratio of 2.226, with that of MELD and admissions to the intensive care unit of 1.099, and 1.967, respectively [67]. These data suggested that infection, irrespective of disease severity, affects long-term survival of patients with cirrhosis, including cirrhosis from alcohol [67].

## Clinical Manifestations

The most important part of the approach to a patient with liver disease is the history, and in the case of ALD, it is pivotal: drinking habits must be obtained; sometimes, this requires several visits, and the reader is encouraged to establish a relationship conducive to open communication regarding substance use, e.g., alcohol, in general towards a proper diagnosis, and treatment. In its statement of 2004, The U.S. Preventive Services Task Force (USPSTF) recommends that adult subjects, including pregnant women, be screened for alcohol misuse in the primary care setting [2, 68]. The use of the single question, "How many times in the past year have you had X or more drinks in a day?" X being five for men and four for women, and the response of at least one being considered positive, is a tool that the National Institute of Alcohol Abuse and Alcoholism has recommended for the use in primary care settings, where clinicians work under tremendous pressure to keep up with the limited time allotted in their *templates* to see their patients [69]. In addition, there are tools designed to screen for alcohol use disorder, including the Alcohol Disorder Use Identification Test (AUDIT) and its variations [2], and the CAGE questionnaire [70], an acronym derived from the keywords in the four questions that encompass the tool: have you ever felt you should *Cut* down on your drinking?, have people *Annoyed* you by criticizing your drinking?, have you ever felt bad or *Guilty* about your drinking?, have you ever had a drink first thing in the morning to steady your nerves or to get rid of a hangover (*Eye* opener), score as 0 for no, and 1 for yes, with a score of at least 2 highly suggestive of alcoholism, and a score of 4 diagnostic of such. The CAGE questionnaire has 93% sensitivity and 76% specificity for the identification of excessive drinking, and 91% sensitivity and 77% specificity for the identification of alcoholism [70, 71].

Patients with AUD with or without ALD can develop an alcohol withdrawal syndrome characterized by autonomic hyperactivity. The mechanism of alcohol withdrawal is considered to be mediated, at least in part, by decreased GABAergic type A and increased glutamatergic (N-methyl-D-aspartate) neurotransmission, respectively [72].

The manifestations of alcohol withdrawal tend to worsen with the length of time from decrease in alcohol intake or last alcoholic drink [73]. The timing of the alcohol withdrawal can be divided as follows: (i) from 6–12 h, mild alcohol withdrawal, characterized by tremors, diaphoresis, nausea and vomiting, hypertension, tachycardia, hyperthermia, and tachypnea, (ii) from 12 to 24 h, alcoholic hallucinosis, characterized by visual, e.g., animals in the surroundings, auditory, i.e., voices, and tactile, i.e., paresthesias often described as insects crawling on the skin, both associated with normal mental status, (iii) from 24 to 48 h, withdrawal seizures, typically generalized, tonic clonic, usually associated with a post ictal state, and (iv) from 48 to 72 h, delirium tremens (DT), the most severe manifestation of alcohol withdrawal, which can be fatal, and is characterized by delirium, psychosis, hallucinations, hyperthermia, hypertension, tachycardia, seizures, and coma [73]. Disorientation is typical of DT and absent in alcoholic hallucinosis.

Patients with ALD may be asymptomatic or report symptoms typical of liver disease, including fatigue and pruritus, the latter usually in patients with cholestasis from alcoholic hepatitis, or cirrhosis, and some right upper quadrant pain. The physical findings are a manifestation of the degree of liver disease and the state of compensation versus decompensation; thus, the physical exam may be normal or notable for cutaneous stigmata of chronic liver disease, including spider angiomata and palmar erythema, jaundice, parotid gland enlargement, Dupuytren's contractures, proximal muscle wasting, ascites, in cases of decompensation, and, in association with portal hypertension, a venous hum may be heard on the chest or superior abdomen. Patients with advanced liver disease tend to have pounding pulses, consistent with their hyperdynamic circulation, fetor hepaticus, jaundice, and any of the signs of hepatic encephalopathy, including somnolence and asterixis.

The presentation of alcoholic hepatitis is florid. Alcoholic hepatitis is a clinicopathological syndrome that can only be unequivocally diagnosed by liver histology. As described in the original series of seven cases, alcoholic hepatitis is usually associated with intensified drinking in chronic alcoholics. It is characterized by fever, anorexia, sometimes nausea and vomiting, jaundice, right upper quadrant abdominal pain, and hepatomegaly [74]. It is usually associated with tachycardia, warm skin, independent from body temperature because of the hyperdynamic state that characterizes this condition, and, depending on the severity, ascites, and hepatic encephalopathy.

## Associated Conditions

Alcohol can be toxic to organs other than the liver; however, there are conditions associated with ALD itself that include the heart and the nervous system. The treatment of primary liver disease or associated conditions starts with abstinence from alcohol.

The risk of extrahepatic malignancies was documented to be increased in patients with cirrhosis from alcohol for esophageal, colorectal, and pulmonary malignancies. This information is valuable because it should enhance vigilance in regard to symptoms that may alert the clinician to an investigation, and also because it emphasizes the importance of screening in the context of colorectal cancer [75].

From a prospective autopsy study from Mexico that explored cardiovascular complications from alcohol and that included 60 patients who had a history of alcohol abuse, there were no documented differences in age, nutritional status, gross and microscopic features, and frequency and degree of atherosclerosis versus a group of patients without a history of alcohol abuse [76]. Several years later, from a prospective study of 30 patients with a diagnosis of alcoholic cardiomyopathy (ACM), 13 (43%) had cirrhosis versus two from 30 "alcoholics" without a diagnosis of cardiomyopathy; in addition, 10 of 20 (50%) "active alcoholic" patients had dilated cardiomyopathy, with active alcohol use being associated with worse cardiac function compared with patients with cirrhosis who had been abstinent. These findings were in contrast to those of patients with cirrhosis not from alcohol who had a normal cardiac function. These data suggested an association between cirrhosis and cardiomyopathy in patients admitted to the hospital with the latter diagnosis, versus unselected patients with ALD without heart disease, with abstinence being related to normal function in patients with cirrhosis in contrast to those who were admitted with cirrhosis and who were actively drinking [77]. This study, which was from Barcelona, Spain, also contrasts with data from patients hospitalized because of cardiomyopathy in a community hospital in New York City, United States [78]. This retrospective study included 333 patients with heart failure, defined as ejection fraction lower than 40%, and identified over 5 years during which 817 with ALD had been admitted to the hospital. One hundred-seventeen of the 333 (35%) had ischemic cardiomyopathy, and 216 (64.8%) had nonischemic cardiomyopathy (NICM); of these, 53 (25%) had ACM, which is 6.4% of the 817 patients, i.e., a minority, admitted with ALD over the same period, with the only significant differences being a lower mean age, more men, and more black patients in the ACM group than in the NICM group [78]. It was concluded from these results that ACM was not common in the population studied, in contrast to the study from patients in Barcelona [77], in which most patients with ACM were reported to have cirrhosis, findings that have suggested that genetic predisposition [77, 78], race, and ethnicity may contribute to this complication of excessive alcohol use [78]. Indeed, susceptibility to developing ACM in patients with alcohol abuse disorder was reported in association with the angiotensin converting enzyme (ACE), DD genotype; however, this feature is not specific for ACM [79]. Also, miRNAs, including miR-138 [80], and other genes associated with alcohol metabolism, including ALDH2 (A/G or A/A), ADH1B (A/A), and CYP2E1(T/C or T/T) [81] have been implicated in this condition. Indeed, developing technologies to explore genetic risks will be useful in studying the ACM in ALD.

Wernicke's encephalopathy is a complication from thiamine deficiency. It is a complication from malnutrition in patients with hyperemesis gravidarum, bariatric surgery, hemodialysis, and most carefully studied, AUD, including those with liver disease. A retrospective study that included neuropsychological and neuropathological data from 28 patients concluded that two of four elements were required for the diagnosis of Wernicke's encephalopathy: (1) nutritional (B1) deficiency, (2) oculomotor abnormalities, (3) cerebellar dysfunction, and (4) altered mental status or mild memory impairment [82]. These findings were compared with autopsy reports from 106 "alcoholics." It was documented that neuropathological findings typical of Wernicke's (i.e., periventricular and brainstem hemorrhage) coexisted in patients with hepatic encephalopathy [82]. These findings further highlight the importance of considering Wernicke's encephalopathy in patients with ALD and hepatic encephalopathy as there is specific and necessary treatment for the former, i.e., thiamine replacement, which can prevent permanent short-term memory loss (Korsakoff syndrome) and death. The serum concentration of thiamine can be measured at baseline and in follow up but treatment should not be delayed while waiting for the results. It is recommended that thiamine be given intravenously before any carbohydrates, 200 mg three times a day. The practice of thiamine administration in the emergency rooms and intensive care units is recommended for all patients at risk of its deficiency [83].

Alcoholic neuropathy is considered to be secondary to the toxic effects of alcohol. From a series of 207 patients with cirrhosis, the prevalence of peripheral neuropathy was 53.6%; the odds ratio of having peripheral neuropathy in patients with cirrhosis from alcohol, who comprised 70% of the study group, was 2.27 (95% CI, 1.15–4.67, $p = 0.037$) [84]. A clinical study of patients with alcoholic neuropathy documented the sensory nature of this complication, characterized by burning pain, symmetrically affecting mostly the feet and distal part of the legs; small fiber axonal loss was documented in sural nerve specimen, typical of alcoholic neuropathy of short duration versus the presence of regeneration of small fibers in chronic cases, with segmental de/remyelination [85–87]. A meta-analysis of studies on the treatment of neuropathic pain reported the use of tricyclic antidepressants (TCAs), serotonin and norepinephrine reuptake inhibitors (SNRIs), pregabalin, and gabapentin as the first line of therapy [88]. Abstinence is needed to stop the neuropathic pain but may not help residual numbness.

Hepatic osteodystrophy is an entity characterized by osteoporosis or osteomalacia in patients with liver disease, the former being more prevalent than the latter [89–91]. The prevalence of bone disease in cirrhosis from alcohol was reported as 5 and 40% [92, 93]; however, in a study of 52 patients, it was reported that osteoporosis, the presence of which did not correlate with liver tests, was present in 78% of the subjects compared to the control group, in contrast to the absence of osteomalacia [94]. However, in a study that included 215 cirrhotic patients, a third of whom had osteoporosis, high liver stiffness, by transient elastography, was associated with bone disease [95]. There are some recommendations in regard to screening patients with cirrhosis for bone disease [96, 97]; however, guidelines for screening for osteoporosis in ALD, specifically, are not available, consistent with findings that suggest that the etiology of liver disease does not have a major impact on hepatic osteodystrophy [95], except in cases of primary biliary cholangitis, on which much literature, albeit controversial, has indicated an increased risk for bone disease [98].

The causes for bone disease in patients with ALD include the effects of alcohol on bone metabolism in association with low GLA protein, an index of bone formation [99], and high sclerostin, an endogenous inhibitor of the Wnt/β-catenin pathway, a central regulator of skeletal modeling and remodeling secreted by osteocytes [100, 101], malnutrition in association with vitamin D deficiency, hypogonadism, and alterations in the receptor activator of nuclear factor kappa B ligand (RANKL) and osteoprotegerin (OPG) mediated pathway of bone metabolism [102, 103].

A meta-analysis that included 15 studies of osteoporosis and bone fractures documented that in patients with ALD, the relative risk for bone fractures was 1.944, 95% CI = 1.354 to 2.791; however, it was 0.849 (95% CI = 0.523–1.380) for osteoporosis. In addition, bone mineral density (BMD) was similar between patients with ALD and the control group, although the BMD was lower in the former than in the latter. These results suggested that significant associations between bone fractures and ALD were independent of BMD and osteoporosis, suggesting the existence of extra osseous factors that affect the bone [104].

In the context of ALD and cirrhosis from alcohol, specifically, patients were reported to have had a decrease in bone mineral density and to have high serum concentrations of tumor necrosis factor (TNF)—R55, being significantly higher in patients with both cirrhosis and osteoporosis than in those with cirrhosis and no osteoporosis; in addition, there was a correlation between urinary excretion of deoxypyridinoline, a measure of bone resorption. Also, serum levels of IL-2 receptor, interpreted as a sign of immunological activation, were significantly higher in patients with cirrhosis and osteoporosis than in patients with cirrhosis alone, data interpreted to suggest that osteoporosis in patients with cirrhosis from alcohol was associated with activation of cellular immunity, and due to increased bone resorption [105].

Treatment of osteopenia and osteoporosis in patients with cirrhosis from alcohol is as recommended by guidelines to treat bone disease in the general population; however, specific considerations regarding risk versus benefits of treatment in regard to the risk of esophageal ulceration in patients with portal hypertension and esophageal varices must be considered [106]; collaboration with specialists in bone disease is advised regarding alternatives.

Intestinal dysbiosis is defined as an imbalance in the composition of the intestine's microbial entities with a disruption of symbiosis [107], and it has been reported in association with ALD [108]. In addition, endotoxemia, derived from intestinal bacteria, has been documented to be a factor as an initiator or perpetuator of ALD [109].

The reason for intestinal dysbiosis has been proposed as a combination of factors that include genetics, environment, bile flow (i.e., decreased in cirrhosis), dysmotility of the gastrointestinal tract, altered immune response to an increased population of different antigens, increased gastric pH, and metabolomic changes. The metabolome is the complete set of all low-molecular-weight metabolites (i.e., metabolic intermediates, hormones and other signaling molecules, and secondary metabolites) found in a biological sample, such as a single organism, which are the end products of gene expression [110, 111].

In support of a role of intestinal bacteria in ALD are the data from a study that documented, by the use of a breath analyzer in a controlled setting, intestinal bacterial overgrowth in 27 (30.3%) in a study that included 89 patients with alcoholic cirrhosis, significantly higher in patients with advanced or decompensated ALD than in those with compensated liver disease, in contrast to the findings in the control group, in which bacterial overgrowth was not documented. Twelve (17.1%) of the 70 patients with ascites had a documented episode of spontaneous bacterial peritonitis (SBP), the prevalence of which was higher in patients with bacterial overgrowth, data interpreted to support a role of bacterial overgrowth in the pathogenesis of SBP [108].

Exposure to intestinal bacteria and propensity to develop infections by patients with ALD may be related to the leaky gut, in part. In this regard, mucosal associated invariant T cells (MAIT) in blood from patients with cirrhosis from alcohol and those with severe alcoholic hepatitis were reported as depleted and to exhibit inadequate responses to bacterial exposure. These findings correlated with the increased expression of intrahepatic homing receptors and the preservation of mucosal associated invariant T cells (MAIT) within the liver in ALD. In vitro stimulation by fecal bacterial components was reported to result in impaired function of MAIT, comparable to that documented in these cells derived from patients with ALD, and depletion, selective towards MAIT. These results were interpreted in support of the idea of increased permeability in ALD, which may lead to MAIT dysfunction and increased infection in patients with ALD [112].

It was reported from a study that included alcoholic subjects with and without liver disease, that 8 of the 22 (36.7%) patients in the former group exhibited dysbiosis; however, there was no difference between this group and those characterized as alcoholics without liver disease, in which 5 of the 19 (26.3%) were dysbiotic [113]. Importantly, serum endotoxin concentrations were higher in the group of patients defined as alcoholics with or without liver disease than in the control group, but there was no difference between the first two groups. Patients from the group of alcoholics with dysbiosis had a decrease and an increase in the median abundance of Bacteroidetes and Proteobacteria, respectively; the group that included the patients defined as alcoholics had decreases in Bacteroidaceae. The lack of difference in taxa between the group with ALD and those without suggested that alcohol has an impact on the taxa of the gut microbiota but not the cirrhosis itself [113]. It was noted that the study was limited because of the sample size and inconsistent availability of histological data [113]. However, the results seem to support differences in the gut microbiome and interaction with endotoxemia in patients who drink alcohol excessively. In this regard, from a study that included 88 patients with cirrhosis from alcohol, endotoxemia was reported to be significantly more frequent, i.e., in 67.3% of patients, in patients with cirrhosis versus 45.5% in patients with cirrhosis from other etiologies [114]; however, the prevalence of endotoxemia was similar in patients with ascites and esophageal varices and patients without those features; in addition, in a group of 24 patients who were drinking alcohol actively, endotoxemia was documented in 11 (45.7%) on admission to the hospital but not in seven of the 11 subjects (64%) 5–8 days after hospitalization, a finding interpreted to suggest that heavy alcohol abuse is associated with transient endotoxemia even in the absence of liver disease [114]. The presence of endotoxemia was studied in 74 patients with ALD, 52 of whom had had a liver biopsy, and the rest had esophageal varices suggesting portal hypertension and who had been abstinent from alcohol for more than 6 months. It was reported that plasma levels of endotoxin were significantly higher in the group of patients with cirrhosis than in the group of healthy control subjects and that there was a correlation between the levels of endotoxin and degree of liver disease, being significantly higher in advanced disease. In addition, endotoxemia correlated with plasma concentrations of TNF-alpha and its soluble receptor form, strong promoters of inflammation [115]. Furthermore, it was documented that in patients with cirrhosis from alcohol, and with alcoholic hepatitis superimposed to cirrhosis, neutrophil activation and reduced phagocytic activity were associated with increased risk of infection, organ failure, and mortality; plasma from patients altered the function of normal neutrophils, also corrected by the addition of normal plasma. The removal of endotoxin, done ex vivo, from the patients' plasma was associated with a decrease in the resting burst and increased ability to phagocytose, i.e. improved neutrophil function [116]. These data provide support for a pathogenetic effect of endotoxin in the liver of patients with ALD.

A study of stool microbiome in 244 patients with liver disease documented that patients with cirrhosis from alcohol had a significantly higher amount of *Enterobacteriaceae* and *Halomonadaceae*, a lower amount of *Lachnospiraceae*, *Ruminococcaceae*, and Clostridialies XIV, high endotoxin levels, and lower cirrhosis dysbiosis ratio, i.e., the ratio of autochthonous to nonautochthonous taxa, a low number consistent with dysbiosis, despite a statistically similar degree of liver disease as compared to those with a liver disease not from alcohol [117]. As patients with cirrhosis from alcohol are reported to have an increase in infection rate and bacterial translocation [118], these findings were interpreted as an explanation for the increased infection rate and bacterial translocation in patients with cirrhosis from alcohol [117], as suggested from other studies [119, 120]. Furthermore, it was reported that patients with alcohol dependence had reduced intestinal fungal diversity and overgrowth of Candida. However, patients with cirrhosis from alcohol also had increased systemic exposure and immune response to mycobiota, measured by serum anti-*Saccharomyces cerevisiae* IgG antibodies, suggestive of translocation of fungal products, an additional factor beyond bacterial translocation in the pathogenesis of ALD, and a feature that correlated with mortality [121].

The fantastic, but plausible proposition of how metabolomic changes may lead to ALD states that a decrease in the synthesis of long-chain fatty acids by bacteria may result in a population decrease of organisms favorable to health, e.g., *Lactobacillus* spp., activation of inflammatory cells in the intestinal lamina propria, leading to TNF-alpha secretion, which binds to enterocytes disrupting tight junctions and increasing intestinal permeability, also in association with alcohol itself and its metabolite acetaldehyde. These factors may allow microbial products to translocate from the intestinal lumen to the portal system to activate hepatic stellate and Kupffer cells to cause hepatocellular injury, which adds to the injurious effects of alcohol, leading to progression of ALD [122].

# Laboratory and Radiological Exams

The hepatic panel in ALD is characterized by increased serum activities of transaminases in the low to mid hundreds IU/ml, and GGTP, which also increases from excessive alcohol intake [123]. The aspartate amino transferase (AST) activity is higher than that of alanine aminotransferase (ALT), usually at a ratio of 1.5 to less than 2 in alcohol abuse, and a 2:1 ratio in acute alcoholic hepatitis, i.e., the De Ritis ratio [124–127]; the reasons for this characteristic feature are reported to be: (1) from pyridoxal phosphate (vitamin B6) deficiency, which is required for AST and ALT to be active [128]; in this regard, the addition of pyridoxal to the assay increases transaminase activities but the ratio remains the same, and (2) because there is more AST than ALT as the former is located in the mitochondria and the cytoplasm, as co-enzymes, and the ALT is located only in the cytosol. The activity ratio of AST to ALT in the liver is 2.5, and in serum is 1 because the clearance of AST from the liver is twice as fast as that of ALT. In liver injury, there is more AST to be released (dual source) than ALT; thus, the 2:1 ratio. AST and ALT exist in the heart, muscle, and kidneys, where the predominant enzyme is the former [124]. Hyperbilirubinemia is typical of alcoholic hepatitis, usually equal to or greater than 5 mg/dl, but serum bilirubin may be normal or minimally raised. Regardless of the etiology, patients with cirrhosis can have low grade hemolysis. In this context, Zieve's syndrome, characterized by hemolysis, jaundice, and hyperlipidemia, in association with alcoholic fatty liver disease and cirrhosis, can present acutely, with an average hemoglobin decrease of 2 g, with recovery in association with supportive care and abstinence from alcohol [129]. In general, though, total serum bilirubin depends on the degree of decompensation, and it tends to be normal in steatosis (except as described above) and in compensated cirrhosis. Prothrombin time may be prolonged (high International Normalized Ratio) (INR), and albumin may be low, an expression of hepatic synthetic dysfunction. The hemogram may be normal or show macrocytosis, reported as secondary to an increase in unesterified serum cholesterol due to lecithin cholesterol acyl transferase deficiency, which results in the expansion of the lipid bilayer of the erythrocytes [130] and nutritional deficiencies, anemia, leukopenia, and thrombocytopenia, the last three from bone marrow suppression from alcohol in actively drinking patients, from liver disease itself, or in association with hypersplenism from portal hypertension. Serum immunoglobulins tend to be high in patients with cirrhosis, in part, because of the systemic exposure to bacterial products via portosystemic shunts; IgA, in particular, can be high in the serum of patients with ALD.

Ferritin and transferrin saturation tend to be high in patients with ALD. From a study that included 58 patients with ALD, it was reported that serum ferritin and necroinflammatory activity were significantly higher in active alcohol drinkers versus non-drinkers; the serum ferritin correlated with liver iron content, indirectly assessed by magnetic resonance imaging (MRI), the histological grade of iron stores, and necroinflammatory activity, with an odds ratio of 7.32, in association with active drinking of alcohol [131]. There are high iron content and indices of iron overload in association with ALD; decreased hepcidin from oxidative stress from

**Fig. 8.2** Iron deposition in hepatocytes (arrow) in a patient with alcohol induced liver disease and heterozygous mutation in C282Y (Prussian Blue, high power)

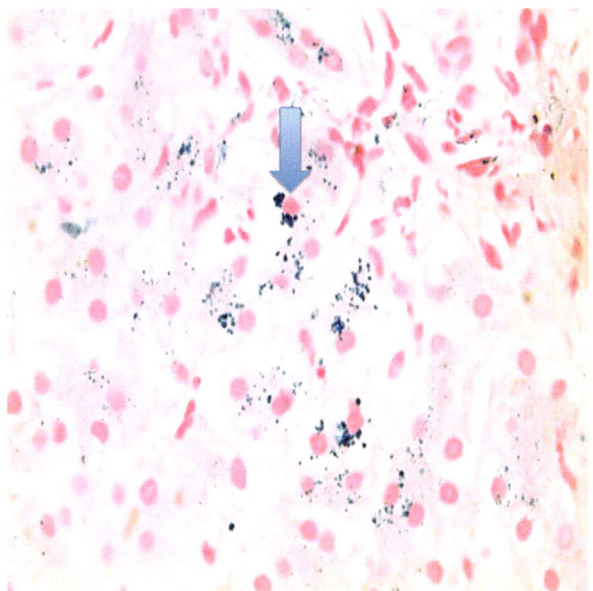

alcohol itself may also cause iron overload [132, 133]. The reason for this finding has not been unequivocally explained, but the reduction of hepcidin in association with oxidative stress from alcohol itself may be a cause of iron overload in patients with ALD [132, 133]. In regard to the patient presented in this chapter, he was heterozygote for the hemochromatosis gene mutation C282Y, surely contributing to his iron overload state (Fig. 8.2).

The use of non-invasive tests for the diagnosis of liver disease is desirable. The Fibrotest, Fibrometer A, and Hepascore are blood tests derived from laboratory values. They were reported to be accurate in diagnosing fibrosis and cirrhosis from alcohol [134]. As the definition of cirrhosis requires histology, in its absence, terms such as suggestive of, or consistent with cirrhosis, should be used for accuracy in medical documentation and patient care.

Imaging studies cannot discern the cause of fat; however, liver ultrasound can help to identify fat, which appears bright, in the liver, including that from ALD. Moderate to marked infiltration increases echogenicity. In addition, attenuation, the ultrasound beam's ability to traverse the liver, increases as the fat infiltration increases. A feature of angulation and geometric boundaries separating the normal and fatty liver parenchyma has been described as typical [135]. Liver ultrasound has been reported as the best test to identify liver nodularity, characteristic of cirrhosis [136]. In addition, the assessment of blood flow, hepatopedal versus hepatofugal, aids in the identification of portal hypertension, as does the appearance of collateral circulation [137].

Computed tomography is a valuable radiological test to identify fat; the greater the attenuation values, the lower the degree of fat. Attenuation values were reported to correlate with the degree of fat documented histologically [137, 138].

Several breath tests have been proposed to diagnose and determine disease severity of liver disease from alcohol, including the [13] C labeled breath tests, aminopyrine breath test, galactose breath test, methacetin breath test, and keto-isocaproic acid breath test, studies based on the quantification of volatile organic compounds. If confirmed, these tests can help the clinician identify patients in whom therapeutic and preventive measures may be started to prevent disease progression [139].

# Histology

Steatosis is the earliest finding in alcohol mediated liver injury [140]. Fat appears within hepatocytes giving the appearance of droplets that coalesce in the cytoplasm pusing the nucleus to the periphery. Fat tends to predominate in the pericentral, zone 3, of the liver lobule, continuing towards zones 2 and 1. In association with abstinence, fat can disappear from hepatocytes over several weeks, with some remnants in periportal macrophages. Fat filled hepatocytes can rupture stimulating an inflammatory response comprised of lymphocytes, macrophages, and eosinophils in the form of lipogranuloma, which disappear without fibrosis [140]. Alcoholic foamy degeneration is a complication of ALD characterized by microvesicular steatosis where fat appears in the cytoplasm as small droplets, and where the nucleus remains in the center of the hepatocyte; megamitochondria and bile pigment can be present, the latter in the perivenular hepatocytes and canaliculi. This type of liver injury, in which inflammation tends to be absent, is considered to be a degenerative process that can be complicated by jaundice and hepatomegaly, with a mixed liver profile and a prolonged picture of cholestasis. Hepatic decompensation was reported in less than 10% of the 20 patients in the original series, and resolved in association with abstinence from alcohol [141, 142]. Regarding cholestasis, loss of type 3 inositol 1,4,5-trisphosphate receptor (ITPR3) from biliary epithelial cells has been described in liver diseases characterized by bile duct injury, including primary biliary cholangitis and primary sclerosing cholangitis [143]. As the absence of ITPR3 in biliary epithelial cells is associated with decreased bicarbonate secretion, it has been suggested that loss of ITPR3 in this type of cell may be a common factor to conditions associated with cholestasis [144]. Biliary epithelial cells express Toll-like receptor 4 (TLR4), the LPS (i.e., endotoxin) receptor, the stimulation of which activates nuclear factor-κB (NF-κB), which subsequently downregulates ITPR3. Liver samples from seven patients out of 28 with alcoholic hepatitis and cholestasis, assessed by serum activity of alkaline phosphatase, had decreased expression of ITPR3, documented by immunohistochemistry [145]; thus, as endotoxemia is characteristic of excessive alcohol use, and is considered to contribute to ALD [109, 114], these findings provide a mechanism underlying cholestasis in alcoholic hepatitis, and lend support to the idea that endotoxin contributes to the pathogenesis of ALD.

Perivenular fibrosis consists of a rim of fibrous tissue covering at least two thirds of the perimeter of the terminal venule; in association with alcohol induced steatosis, it prognosticates the progression of liver disease in the absence of abstinence [140, 146].

**Fig. 8.3** Ballooned hepatocytes in a patient with alcohol induced liver disease (arrow) (Hematoxylin and eosin stain, 40X)

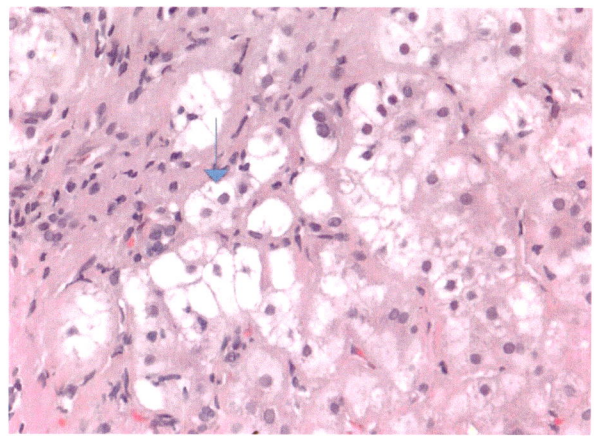

Alcoholic hepatitis is a clinicopathological syndrome that can only be unequivocally diagnosed by liver histology. Histologically it is characterized by steatosis, acidophilic necrosis of hepatocytes, i.e., apoptotic bodies, and an inflammatory infiltrate characterized by neutrophils. Mallory bodies, eosinophilic, irregularly shaped structures that have the appearance of a twisted rope (Cesar del Rosario, M.D., personal communication) and are located in the cytoplasm of the hepatocyte can be identified. Megamitochondria, appearing like needle-like cytoplasmic projections, can also be appreciated. The severity of the disease is associated with the degree of hepatocellular necrosis, with ballooned hepatocytes (Fig. 8.3) and Mallory bodies, around which the inflammatory infiltrate tends to be localized. Other features include bile stasis, bile ductular proliferation, and various degrees of fibrosis around hepatocytes and venules [140].

A role of interleukin 8 in the pathogenesis of alcoholic hepatitis was suggested from a study that reported marked expression of the cytokine in correlation with the neutrophil inflammatory infiltrate, a marker of severity, and in serum, significantly higher levels in patients who died from complications of the disease [147]. These findings were extended in a morphometric study in which neutrophils and T lymphocytes CD3+ infiltration, degree of apoptosis, expression of CXC and CC chemokines, protein levels of IL-8 and Gro-alpha, and serum concentrations of IL-8 and Gro-alpha were evaluated. The expression of CCL2 and CXCL10, IL-8, Gro-alpha, CXCL5, CXCL6 was enhanced in samples from patients with alcoholic hepatitis compared to that of samples in the control group, the latter four correlating with neutrophil infiltration, and with worse prognosis, with IL-8 protein levels identified as an independent predictor of 90 day mortality after the clinical presentation [148]. Some of the findings from a study that included 36 consecutive patients admitted to a hospital in Spain with a diagnosis of alcoholic hepatitis, supported by the clinical presentation and liver histology, concluded that transforming growth factor-beta1 (TGF-β1), a cytokine that plays a fundamental role in the development of hepatic fibrosis, was enhanced in the liver of patients with alcoholic hepatitis as well as other factors that mediate degradation of collagen in the liver, tissue inhibitor metalloproteinases (TIMP-1), matrix metalloproteinase-2 (MMP-2), and urokinase-type plasminogen activator (*ut*-PA), chemokine (C-X-C motif) ligand 1 (i.e., GrO-a), dual oxidase 1(DUOX-1), and monocyte chemoattractant protein 1(MCP-1), mediators of inflammation. In addition, important components of the phagocytic NADPH oxidase, which mediates neutrophil derived oxidant stress, was increased. The increase in TNF-alpha was mild, although, together with IL-6 correlated with infection. The results of this study identified potential treatment pathways and seemed to support documented histological findings of patients with alcoholic hepatitis, i.e. mediators of collagen deposition, collagen degradation, and the inflammatory consequences of the neutrophil invasion of the liver in alcoholic hepatitis [149].

Plasma levels of CCL2 were significantly higher in patients with alcoholic hepatitis than those without and correlated with disease severity, IL-8 expression, and degree of neutrophil infiltrate, with a predominance of the $-2518$ A $>$ G CCL2 polymorphism in patients with severe disease [150].

Patients with alcoholic hepatitis have been documented to have a dysregulated immune state as suggested by increased plasma concentrations of proinflammatory cytokines, including IL-8, a potent neutrophil chemotactic factor [148], but lower levels of the anti-inflammatory macrophage-derived chemokine (MDC), compared to the control groups, including a group of heavy alcohol drinkers without liver disease, the latter findings being consistent with a prior report [149]. In addition, CD4 T cells reacted poorly upon stimulation based on the low production of IFN-γ. Monocytes had a low expression of cluster of differentiation 38 (CD 38), a reflection of reduced leukocyte activation, in patients with alcoholic hepatitis, a finding that correlated with increased mortality, and which seems a paradox, as it is the migration of neutrophils to the liver that is believed to contribute to the pathogenesis of alcoholic hepatitis. Abstinence from alcohol was associated with the resolution of immunological dysregulation, emphasizing the importance of abstinence at any stage of ALD. CD38 and IL-8 were highlighted in this study as potentially relevant in the pathogenesis of alcoholic hepatitis thus identifying potential pathways towards drug development [151].

The lesion of sclerosing hyaline necrosis can be appreciated in cases of severe liver injury in alcoholic hepatitis, with hepatocellular necrosis around the terminal venules, occluded by fibrous tissue, which can be associated with portal hypertension, in the absence of cirrhosis, as it has been clinically described [152] (Fig. 8.4), and in patients with cirrhosis and superimposed alcoholic hepatitis with marked liver cell necrosis and neutrophilic infiltrate [153]. The lesion of sclerosing hyaline necrosis can progress, and fibrosis extends pericellularly; the bad prognostic features include fibrous septa, and general hepatocellular necrosis, occlusion of hepatic venules, which results from perivenular fibrosis, leading to luminal obstruction of venules [140]. In addition, lymphocytic phlebitis, characterized by an inflammatory infiltrate of the central and sublobular veins, and in as much as 52% of cases of alcoholic hepatitis in one series [154], veno-occlusive lesions, the degree of which correlate with the magnitude of portal hypertension [140, 154].

Alcoholic cirrhosis is the transformation of the liver architecture by regenerating nodules surrounded by fibrous septa (Fig. 8.5). The nodules tend to be small, i.e., micronodular, measuring 3 mm in diameter, although macronodules can also form,

**Fig. 8.4** Liver histology of a patient with sclerosing hyaline necrosis in a patient with alcoholic hepatitis. Strands of collagen (blue) extend from the central vein surrounding swollen hepatocytes, and sinusoids filled with collagen. (Masson stain, 500X) (published with permission [152])

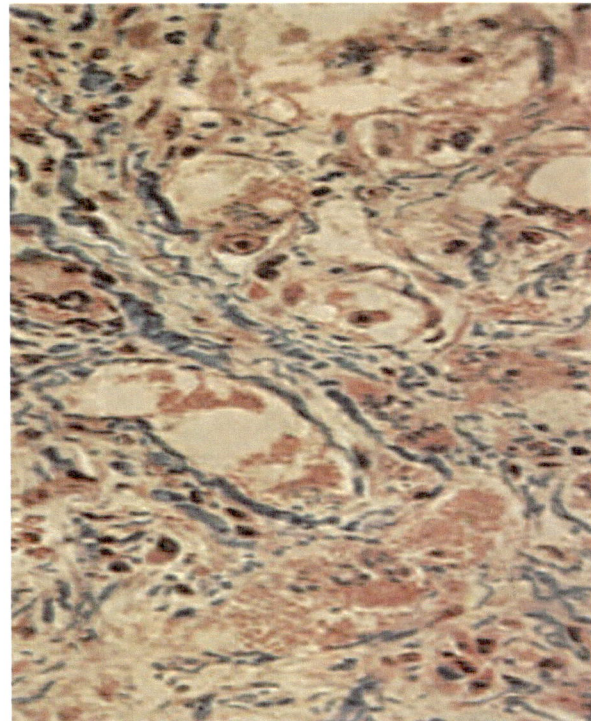

**Fig. 8.5** Cirrhosis in a patient with liver disease from alcohol use disorder; there is a nodule surrounded by collagen (Trichrome stain, high power)

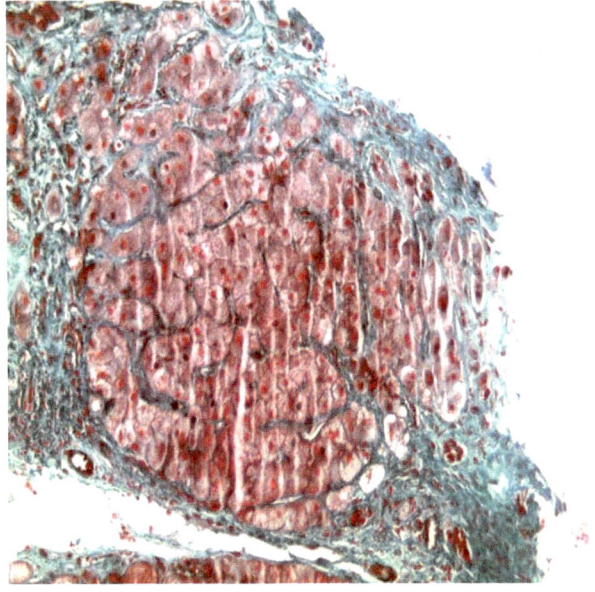

reportedly in association with alcohol abstinence. Features of inflammation characterized by neutrophils and plasma cells can be appreciated in the fibrous septa, usually when alcohol consumption has continued. Ductal metaplasia is noted in the periportal area. Alpha1 1-antitrypsin globules can be observed in the periphery of the nodules, suggesting impaired protein secretion by the hepatocytes [155], as well as Periodic Acid-Schiff (PAS)-positive granules identifying protein bound copper in the hepatocytes [140]. Hepatic oncocytes, characterized by a granular cytoplasm, can also be appreciated in the nodules' periphery [140, 156]. Portal fibrosis is not common in pure ALD; however, activated macrophages found in these areas have suggested that they may be the source of substances that mediate alcohol induced liver injury [140].

Iron metabolism in the context of excessive alcohol use and ALD has been discussed above. Siderosis is a feature in the liver histology of ALD, with iron detected in hepatocytes and Kupffer cells, modestly [140]. Intense iron staining in the liver of patients with ALD prompts the investigation of genetic forms of iron overload.

Characteristically, there is IgA deposition along the sinusoids in the liver of patients with ALD, a findings that has suggested a pathological role for the immunoglobulin [157]. In this regard, however, it was documented that B cells, isolated from human liver tissue, included IgA producing cells that reacted with commensal bacterial products, findings interpreted to suggest that the IgA originating from the liver could be involved in the clearance of intestinal antigens that get to the liver through the portal vein, and thus, protect the liver from injury due to gut-derived antigens in ALD [158].

## Treatment

The management of patients with AUD with or without liver disease is founded on abstinence; when AUD is associated with liver disease, in addition to abstinence, the treatment is aimed to stop the progression of the liver disease, and in cases of alcoholic hepatitis, to stop the acute inflammatory cascade that can result in liver failure and death.

Patients with AUD require collaborative management between substance abuse experts, internists, gastroenterologists, and hepatologists if they have liver disease, and support groups, including faith based organizations.

The Food and Drug Administration has approved several medications to manage AUD, including disulfiram, acamprosate, and naltrexone.

Disulfiram inhibits the enzyme mitochondrial aldehyde dehydrogenase; in the presence of alcohol, even small amounts of disulfiram produces unpleasant effects that include flushing, throbbing headache, nausea, vomiting, sweating, and thirst as well as respiratory and cardiovascular complications [159]. A meta-analysis of the results of clinical studies on disulfiram documented that in open label trials, the drug was more effective than the controls in maintaining abstinence; however, no efficacy was demonstrated in "blind trials." More side effects were reported in the disulfiram trials than in the control groups, with no difference in the number of deaths between them [160].

Naltrexone is an opioid antagonist that decreases the pleasant sensations associated with alcohol intake, and it has been reported to decrease craving [161, 162].

Acamprosate is a drug most effective in combination with psychosocial support in the treatment of AUD. The mechanisms of action of this drug in the treatment of AUD may include functional antagonism of the ionotropic glutamate N-methyl-d-aspartate (NMDA) receptor, but, as the binding between the drug and the receptor is weak, it is suggested that instead, the drug may modulate NMDA receptors via regulatory polyamine sites, or that it may act on metabotropic glutamate receptors [163].

Other drugs approved by the FDA for other indications have also been used to treat AUD, including fluoxetine, duloxetine, tiagabine, levitiracetam, gabapentin, pregabalin, sertraline, citalopram, ritanserin, aripiprazole, ondansetron, quetiapine, and topiramate [164].

Baclofen is a selective GABA-B receptor agonist used to treat AUD; the mechanism by which this drug helps in the management of alcoholism is unknown. Baclofen was documented to reduce the craving for alcohol and promote abstinence and prevent relapses after a period of sobriety in patients with and without liver disease [165], including cirrhosis [166]. However, the Cochrane Collaboration, which analyzed the clinical trials of baclofen for AUD, interpreted that the results of the studies, in general, were encouraging but that the evidence remained "uncertain" in support of the use of baclofen for the treatment of AUD [167].

In a randomized clinical trial, baclofen, at a dose of 10 mg orally three times a day, was associated with abstinence in 30 of 42 patients (71%) with a cumulative mean duration of 62.8 days versus placebo, associated with abstinence in 12 of 42 (29%) with a mean duration of 30.8 days in the absence of liver related side effects. The dropout rate was 14% for the drug, versus 31% for the placebo, reported as insignificant [165]. A study examined the effect of baclofen in 100 patients recruited over 3 years, 65 of whom had cirrhosis; after 1 year, 44 of the 86 patients being followed were abstinent, and the rest still drank up to 30 g per day on baclofen. The drug was associated with improved liver function and reduction of serum GGTP activity, a marker of excessive alcohol use [168]. In the author's experience, baclofen has been associated with abstinence of alcohol in patients with and without liver disease and not associated with complications.

A meta-analysis of results from 24 randomized controlled trials that included 2861 patients with AUD compared the effect of naltrexone to that of the placebo on the frequency of relapse, as a primary outcome, and time to first drink, drinking days, the number of standard drinks for a defined period, and craving over time. Naltrexone was associated with a significant decrease in the frequency of relapses but not on return to drinking, suggesting that it was an option for the treatment of AUD at short term. Of note, it was also reported that patients on naltrexone reported nausea, dizziness, and fatigue more frequently than those of placebo, effects that may be related to the opioid antagonism effect of the drug. The reader is referred to the FDA website for information regarding hepatotoxicity. A recent online update reported naltrexone to be associated with increased activity of ALT and AST in 13% and 10%, respectively, and of GGTP in 1%–10% [169, 170]; however, naltrexone had not been associated with hepatotoxicity [161, 171]. Based on these reports [161, 171] and the author's experience with the use of naltrexone in patients with pruritus from cholestasis [172], naltrexone was successfully used to treat the patient whose history is presented in this chapter without any complications.

## Alcohol Withdrawal

Patients with alcohol abuse disorder with or with liver disease can develop alcohol withdrawal and delirium tremens (DT), a dangerous condition associated with high mortality, in association with the discontinuation of alcohol use, and not infrequently during hospitalization. The clinician must be able to identify signs of alcohol withdrawal or DT to treat and prevent complications.

Risk factors for severe withdrawal syndrome include chronic heavy drinking and a history of generalized seizures and delirium tremens (DT) [173]. A history of DTs and baseline systolic blood pressure of at least 140 mmHg were associated with an increase in the risk of a severe alcohol withdrawal syndrome in an analysis of 530 studies. One thousand fifty-one of 1355 patients had documented DT, 53 had seizures and 251 DT. The Alcohol Withdrawal Severity Scale (PAWSS) [174] was most useful in the prediction of a severe alcohol withdrawal syndrome when patients were documented to have at least four individual findings with a likelihood ratio of 174 although, with a wide confidence interval (95%, 43–696, and specificity of 0.93), and a LR of 0.07 (95% CI, 0.02–0.26; sensitivity, 0.99) when there were only up to three findings [175].

Patients at risk for alcohol withdrawal must be treated to prevent it. The treatment of alcohol withdrawal concerns the provision of a quiet, controlled environment where the patient is attended by obtaining vital signs frequently, and providing hydration, and sedation, as needed to avoid symptoms (i.e., not a standard dose given without examining the patient). Patients with AUD can be malnourished and have multivitamin deficiencies, including pyridoxine and thiamine. Thiamine administration should always precede the administration of glucose to prevent Wernicke's encephalopathy [176]. The foundation of the treatment is benzodiazepines, including chlordiazepoxide, diazepam, lorazepam, and including oxazepam, which does not require further breakdown by the liver and hence, a decreased risk in metabolite accumulation. The treatment must be individualized; in this regard, anticonvulsants have been reported in association with a decrease in the symptoms of withdrawal. In addition, combination therapy with beta blockers, to reduce hyperautonomic states and craving, and alpha agonists, i.e., clonidine, to decrease the severity of withdrawal have been recommended [177].

## Delirium Tremens

The management of patients with DT includes supportive care, in the medical intensive care unit, when possible, in a quiet well lit room, with documented vital signs every 15–30 min with attention to keeping the patient oriented to self, time, and place. The use of thiamine is emphasized; a dose of 500 mg intravenously, once or twice a day, has been recommended. Pharmacotherapy with benzodiazepines intravenously is recommended to achieve some sedation but maintaining an arousable state until delirium resolves, which tends to occur in approximately 3 days after initiation of therapy. In patients with uncontrolled agitation and hallucination, antipsychotics, e.g., haloperidol, at low doses intravenously not to exceed 20 mg over 30–60 min, are useful. For patients who do not respond to sedation, ventilation support, management with propofol is recommended. The patient must be monitored in a controlled environment as the mortality associated with DT is high, and there are side effects of medications, such as respiratory depression and hypotension, which must be identified in a timely fashion. The reader is referred to a review and its commentaries published in 2015 [178].

## Treatment of Alcoholic Hepatitis

Malnutrition is common in patients with liver disease, and it is particularly problematic in patients with alcoholic hepatitis, in whom it can be associated with bad outcomes [179]. It is recommended that patients ingest a caloric intake of 35 kcal/kg and a daily protein intake of 1.2–1.5 g/kg. In patients unable to eat, feeding through a feeding tube is an option; it is recommended that it be placed by an experienced operator under direct endoscopic visualization. A study that examined the effect of tube feeding on patients who had bled from varices did not document complications related to prior variceal bleeding and its treatment with band ligation or sclerotherapy [180].

The beneficial effect of steroids on the treatment of severe AH has been documented at least in regard to short-term survival [181–186], although not without controversy [187]. Pentoxifylline, which inhibits tumor necrosis factor-$\alpha$ activity, considered to be involved in AH's pathogenesis, has been studied in its treatment; however, the level of evidence does not support its use in patients with severe AH [187]. Other medications that have been studied for AH treatment, including infliximab, propylthiouracil, N-acetylcysteine, silymarin, colchicine, insulin, glucagon, oxandrolone, testosterone, and polyunsaturated lecithin are not recommended and will not be discussed here [188].

A landmark placebo controlled study of 4 weeks duration examined the use of prednisolone, 40 mg/day, in 37 patients with alcoholic hepatitis, documented by liver histology. Patients exhibited a broad clinical spectrum from asymptomatic to hepatic encephalopathy, including coma and hepatic synthetic dysfunction.

Prednisolone was associated with an increase in caloric intake. Only one of the nine patients with hepatic encephalopathy randomized to prednisolone died versus six patients randomized to placebo. A rapid progression to cirrhosis was documented on liver histology during the follow-up period of 4 months, with five of the nine patients without cirrhosis at baseline exhibiting it on follow up, and with no documented benefit of prednisolone to deter progression to cirrhosis, i.e., four of the nine patients who had been randomized to placebo did not progress to cirrhosis [189]. The beneficial effect of prednisolone on short-term survival was strong and set the stage for clinical trials on the treatment of AH. In this regard, several controlled clinical trials have documented a beneficial effect of corticosteroids in alcoholic hepatitis, mostly in severe cases [184–186]; however, other studies have not documented a therapeutic effect of this type of drug [190]. The Maddrey discriminant function (DF) is a tool developed from a one month study that included 55 patients with AH treated in a randomized, double blind placebo controlled study of 40 mg per day of prednisolone for a period of 28 to 32 days, from which six of the 31 patients randomized to placebo died, versus one of the 24 randomized to the drug. From the 18 patients with hepatic encephalopathy, six (33%) from the placebo group died, versus one of the 13 from the prednisolone group; nevertheless, the difference was not significant. However, from a stepwise discriminant analysis, it was determined that hepatic encephalopathy, progressive renal insufficiency, prolonged prothrombin time, and serum bilirubin greater than 10 mg/dl predicted a bad outcome. The DF, calculated as $4.6 \times$ (prothrombin time in seconds) + serum bilirubin, when greater than 32, predicted mortality, and treatment with prednisolone improved survival during the duration of the study [183]. A follow-up study in which 66 patients with AH were enrolled within 7 days of admission to the hospital documented that two of the 35 patients (6%) treated with steroids (i.e., methylprednisolone) died versus 11 of the 31 (35%) patients treated with placebo, a significantly different advantage favoring the steroid. Hepatic encephalopathy was again identified as a factor that changed the natural history of AH in relationship with the use of steroids, i.e., nine of the 19 (47%) patients with hepatic encephalopathy randomized to placebo died, as compared to one of the 14 (7%) patients randomized to methylprednisolone, a significant difference. It was concluded from this study that methylprednisolone therapy decreases mortality in patients with AH complicated by hepatic encephalopathy or with a DF greater than 32 [184].

Many years after the important studies on steroids and alcoholic hepatitis, the early change in serum bilirubin level was reported as an important prognostic factor in severe alcoholic hepatitis treated with prednisolone. By the use of 6 month survival data in patients with AH, it was documented that an early change in serum bilirubin at 7 days, which happened in 73% of patients, was associated with continuous improvement in liver function and survival of 82.8% ± 3.3% as compared with 23% ± 5.8%, $p < 0.0001$, an analysis that opened a new pathway in the management of patients with AH: the use of the Lille score [191].

The Lille model was developed from a group of 320 patients with AH treated with steroids, prospectively, and validated from 118 patients. This study determined that a score of 0.45 at 7 days post initiation of treatment with steroids in patients with AH identified those who would not benefit from the treatment, i.e., non-responders, which comprised 40% of the patients. Statistical analysis was documented to show that the Lille score had a significantly higher area under the receiver operating curve (AUROC), 0.89 ± 0.02, higher than other predicting models, i.e., Child–Pugh and Maddrey scores, i.e. DF; in the validation study, the AUROC also significantly higher for the Lille score, 0.85 ± 0.04, higher than other scores, including the MELD and the Glasgow scores. A Lille score greater than 0.45 was associated with a significant decrease in the 6 months survival and predicted 75% of the deaths [192].

In combination with methylprednisolone, 40 mg per day, pentoxifylline, 400 mg, was not associated with a therapeutic advantage over prednisolone alone in a study that included 270 patients, with age that ranged from 18 to 70 years, and severe AH documented by liver histology, jaundice, exhibited 6 months prior to entry into the study, and a Maddrey DF of at least 32 followed for 6 months. Mortality was reported as not significantly different between the two groups, 69.9% (95% CI, 62.1%–77.7%) as compared to 69.2% (95% CI; 61.4%–76.9%), corresponding to 40 vs. 42 deaths, respectively, and no significant difference in the incidence of hepatorenal syndrome [193].

Conversion of prednisone to prednisolone is required for the effect of the latter; thus, because liver function may be impaired in patients with AH, it is preferable to use prednisolone for the treatment of AH. In addition, in a controlled study, prednisone's use to treat patients with AH was not associated with improved survival [194]. Patients are considered candidates for prednisolone therapy when the Maddrey DF is equal or greater than 32; it is prescribed at a dose of 40 mg per day for 28 days, at which time it can be tapered off and discontinued. Intravenous methylprednisolone at a dose of 32 mg per day is given to patients who cannot take medications orally. The decision to continue treatment with steroids is based on the response according to the Lille score, which supports their discontinuation if greater than 0.45 on day seven. A Lille score of 0.45 on day four of steroid therapy is now proposed as sufficient to discontinue treatment. Vigilance regarding the development of infections to which patients with alcoholic hepatitis are highly susceptible, prior, during, and in the immediate follow-up period post treatment is necessary. Liver transplantation is an option for patients with severe AH in whom steroid treatment is not associated with improvement [195]. A study that included 26 patients with a first episode of severe AH not responsive to steroid therapy reported that cumulative survival at 6 months in association with early liver transplantation was 77% versus the 23% for a historical control group. The benefit was notable during the first month post transplantation, and it was sustained over 2 years of follow up. Three patients went back to drinking alcohol post transplant, one at 720 days, one at 740 days, and one at 1140 days [195]. Thus, early referral to a liver transplant center is necessary.

Continuous follow up of patients with AH and any condition in the spectrum of ALD is fundamental to facilitate referral to addiction experts and to attend complications of liver disease that may develop over time. Patients with cirrhosis must be screened for the presence of esophageal varices to decide on prevention of index bleed either by band ligation or beta blockers, and to establish a screening schedule over time [196]. Of note, esophageal varices can regress in association with alcohol abstinence. In a population study from Denmark, hepatocellular carcinoma was reported to be of low incidence [197]; however, it is a complication of cirrhosis. Thus, patients with cirrhosis must be screened for this complication every 6 months with a liver sonogram and serum alpha fetoprotein [198]. Patients with decompensated liver disease from alcohol are candidates for liver transplantation.

**Acknowledgments** The author acknowledges Dr. Cesar del Rosario for having contributed Figures 8.1, 8.2, 8.3 and 8.5.

# References

1. Gao B, Bataller R. Alcoholic liver disease: pathogenesis and new therapeutic targets. Gastroenterology. 2011 Nov;141(5):1572–85.
2. Alcoholism NIoAAa. A pocket guide for alcohol screening and brief intervention 2001. Available from http://pubs.niaaa.nih.gov/publications/Practitioner/pocketguide/pocket_guide2.htm.
3. Newsletter NIAAA Drinking Levels Defined. In: Health NIo, editor, 2004.
4. Hrubec Z, Omenn GS. Evidence of genetic predisposition to alcoholic cirrhosis and psychosis: twin concordances for alcoholism and its biological end points by zygosity among male veterans. Alcohol Clin Exp Res. 1981 Spring;5(2):207–15.
5. Julkunen RJ, Di Padova C, Lieber CS. First pass metabolism of ethanol: a gastrointestinal barrier against the systemic toxicity of ethanol. Life Sci. 1985 Aug 12;37(6):567–73.
6. Lieber CS, Gentry RT, Baraona E. First pass metabolism of ethanol. Alcohol Alcohol Suppl. 1994;2:163–9.
7. Frezza M, di Padova C, Pozzato G, Terpin M, Baraona E, Lieber CS. High blood alcohol levels in women. The role of decreased gastric alcohol dehydrogenase activity and first-pass metabolism. N Engl J Med. 1990 Jan 11;322(2):95–9.
8. Edenberg HJ. The genetics of alcohol metabolism: role of alcohol dehydrogenase and aldehyde dehydrogenase variants. Alcohol Res Health. 2007;30(1):5–13.
9. Li D, Zhao H, Gelernter J. Strong association of the alcohol dehydrogenase 1B gene (ADH1B) with alcohol dependence and alcohol-induced medical diseases. Biol Psychiatry. 2011 Sep 15;70(6):504–12.
10. Goedde HW, Agarwal DP, Fritze G, Meier-Tackmann D, Singh S, Beckmann G, et al. Distribution of ADH2 and ALDH2 genotypes in different populations. Hum Genet. 1992 Jan;88(3):344–6.
11. Eng MY, Luczak SE, Wall TL. ALDH2, ADH1B, and ADH1C genotypes in Asians: a literature review. Alcohol Res Health. 2007;30(1):22–7.
12. Whitfield JB. Meta-analysis of the effects of alcohol dehydrogenase genotype on alcohol dependence and alcoholic liver disease. Alcohol Alcohol. 1997 Sep–Oct;32(5):613–9.
13. Koop DR, Tierney DJ. Multiple mechanisms in the regulation of ethanol-inducible cytochrome P450IIE1. BioEssays. 1990 Sep;12(9):429–35.
14. Sookoian S, Castano GO, Burgueno AL, Gianotti TF, Rosselli MS, Pirola CJ. A nonsynonymous gene variant in the adiponutrin gene is associated with nonalcoholic fatty liver disease severity. J Lipid Res. 2009 Oct;50(10):2111–6.
15. Rotman Y, Koh C, Zmuda JM, Kleiner DE, Liang TJ, Nash CRN. The association of genetic variability in patatin-like phospholipase domain-containing protein 3 (PNPLA3) with histological severity of nonalcoholic fatty liver disease. Hepatology. 2010 Sep;52(3):894–903.

16. Valenti L, Al-Serri A, Daly AK, Galmozzi E, Rametta R, Dongiovanni P, et al. Homozygosity for the patatin-like phospholipase-3/adiponutrin I148M polymorphism influences liver fibrosis in patients with nonalcoholic fatty liver disease. Hepatology. 2010 Apr;51(4):1209–17.
17. Salameh H, Raff E, Erwin A, Seth D, Nischalke HD, Falleti E, et al. PNPLA3 gene polymorphism is associated with predisposition to and severity of alcoholic liver disease. Am J Gastroenterol. 2015 Jun;110(6):846–56.
18. Zimmermann R, Strauss JG, Haemmerle G, Schoiswohl G, Birner-Gruenberger R, Riederer M, et al. Fat mobilization in adipose tissue is promoted by adipose triglyceride lipase. Science. 2004 Nov 19;306(5700):1383–6.
19. Romeo S, Huang-Doran I, Baroni MG, Kotronen A. Unravelling the pathogenesis of fatty liver disease: patatin-like phospholipase domain-containing 3 protein. Curr Opin Lipidol. 2010 Jun;21(3):247–52.
20. Buch S, Stickel F, Trepo E, Way M, Herrmann A, Nischalke HD, et al. A genome-wide association study confirms PNPLA3 and identifies TM6SF2 and MBOAT7 as risk loci for alcohol-related cirrhosis. Nat Genet. 2015 Dec;47(12):1443–8.
21. Kovarova M, Konigsrainer I, Konigsrainer A, Machicao F, Haring HU, Schleicher E, et al. The genetic variant I148M in PNPLA3 is associated with increased hepatic retinyl-palmitate storage in humans. J Clin Endocrinol Metab. 2015 Dec;100(12):E1568–74.
22. Mahdessian H, Taxiarchis A, Popov S, Silveira A, Franco-Cereceda A, Hamsten A, et al. TM6SF2 is a regulator of liver fat metabolism influencing triglyceride secretion and hepatic lipid droplet content. Proc Natl Acad Sci U S A. 2014 Jun 17;111(24):8913–8.
23. Gijon MA, Riekhof WR, Zarini S, Murphy RC, Voelker DR. Lysophospholipid acyltransferases and arachidonate recycling in human neutrophils. J Biol Chem. 2008 Oct 31;283(44):30235–45.
24. Yamashita A, Watanabe M, Sato K, Miyashita T, Nagatsuka T, Kondo H, et al. Reverse reaction of lysophosphatidylinositol acyltransferase. Functional reconstitution of coenzyme A-dependent transacylation system. J Biol Chem. 2003 Aug 8;278(32):30382–93.
25. Freigang S. The regulation of inflammation by oxidized phospholipids. Eur J Immunol. 2016 Aug;46(8):1818–25.
26. Atkinson S, Way M, McQuillin A, Morgan MY, Thursz M. A genome-wide association study identifies PNPLA3 and SLC38A4 as risk loci for alcoholic hepataitis. J Hepatol. 2016;64:S134.
27. Engracia V, Leite MM, Pagotto RC, Zucoloto S, Barbosa CA, Mestriner MA. Expression of class mu glutathione-S-transferase in human liver and its association with hepatopathies. Am J Med Genet A. 2003 Dec 15;123A(3):257–60.
28. Anstee QM, Daly AK, Day CP. Genetics of alcoholic liver disease. Semin Liver Dis. 2015 Nov;35(4):361–74.
29. Mulligan MK, Ponomarev I, Hitzemann RJ, Belknap JK, Tabakoff B, Harris RA, et al. Toward understanding the genetics of alcohol drinking through transcriptome meta-analysis. Proc Natl Acad Sci U S A. 2006 Apr 18;103(16):6368–73.
30. Banerjee N. Neurotransmitters in alcoholism: a review of neurobiological and genetic studies. Indian J Human Genetics. 2014 Jan;20(1):20–31.
31. Edenberg HJ, Dick DM, Xuei X, Tian H, Almasy L, Bauer LO, et al. Variations in GABRA2, encoding the alpha 2 subunit of the GABA(A) receptor, are associated with alcohol dependence and with brain oscillations. Am J Hum Genet. 2004 Apr;74(4):705–14.
32. Agrawal A, Edenberg HJ, Foroud T, Bierut LJ, Dunne G, Hinrichs AL, et al. Association of GABRA2 with drug dependence in the collaborative study of the genetics of alcoholism sample. Behav Genet. 2006 Sep;36(5):640–50.
33. Hart CL, Morrison DS, Batty GD, Mitchell RJ, Davey SG. Effect of body mass index and alcohol consumption on liver disease: analysis of data from two prospective cohort studies. BMJ. 2010 Mar 11;340:c1240.
34. Heath RD, Brahmbhatt M, Tahan AC, Ibdah JA, Tahan V. Coffee: the magical bean for liver diseases. World J Hepatol. 2017 May 28;9(15):689–96.

35. Klatsky AL, Armstrong MA. Alcohol, smoking, coffee, and cirrhosis. Am J Epidemiol. 1992 Nov 15;136(10):1248–57.
36. Corrao G, Zambon A, Bagnardi V, D'Amicis A, Klatsky A, Collaborative SG. Coffee, caffeine, and the risk of liver cirrhosis. Ann Epidemiol. 2001 Oct;11(7):458–65.
37. D'Costa K. Scientific America [Internet]2011. [cited 2019].
38. Kamper-Jorgensen M, Gronbaek M, Tolstrup J, Becker U. Alcohol and cirrhosis: dose--response or threshold effect? J Hepatol. 2004 Jul;41(1):25–30.
39. Sy AM, Ching R, Olivares G, Vinas C, Chang R, Bergasa NV. Hispanic ethnicity is associated with increased morbidity and mortality in patients with alcoholic liver disease. Ann Hepatol. 2017 Jan–Feb;16(1):169–71.
40. Marshall AW, Kingstone D, Boss M, Morgan MY. Ethanol elimination in males and females: relationship to menstrual cycle and body composition. Hepatology. 1983 Sep–Oct;3(5):701–6.
41. Baraona E, Abittan CS, Dohmen K, Moretti M, Pozzato G, Chayes ZW, et al. Gender differences in pharmacokinetics of alcohol. Alcohol Clin Exp Res. 2001 Apr;25(4):502–7.
42. Eagon PK. Alcoholic liver injury: influence of gender and hormones. World J Gastroenterol. 2010 Mar 21;16(11):1377–84.
43. Setiawan VW, Stram DO, Porcel J, Lu SC, Le Marchand L, Noureddin M. Prevalence of chronic liver disease and cirrhosis by underlying cause in understudied ethnic groups: the multiethnic cohort. Hepatology. 2016 Dec;64(6):1969–77.
44. Bouchery EE, Harwood HJ, Sacks JJ, Simon CJ, Brewer RD. Economic costs of excessive alcohol consumption in the U.S., 2006. Am J Prev Med. 2011 Nov;41(5):516–24.
45. Rehm J, Samokhvalov AV, Shield KD. Global burden of alcoholic liver diseases. J Hepatol. 2013 Jul;59(1):160–8.
46. Hatton J, Burton A, Nash H, Munn E, Burgoyne L, Sheron N. Drinking patterns, dependency and life-time drinking history in alcohol-related liver disease. Addiction. 2009 Apr;104(4):587–92.
47. Askgaard G, Gronbaek M, Kjaer MS, Tjonneland A, Tolstrup JS. Alcohol drinking pattern and risk of alcoholic liver cirrhosis: a prospective cohort study. J Hepatol. 2015 May;62(5):1061–7.
48. Esser MB, Hedden SL, Kanny D, Brewer RD, Gfroerer JC, Naimi TS. Prevalence of alcohol dependence among US adult drinkers, 2009-2011. Prev Chronic Dis. 2014 Nov 20;11:E206.
49. Tan CH, Hungerford DW, Denny CH, McKnight-Eily LR. Screening for alcohol misuse: practices among U.S. primary care providers, DocStyles 2016. Am J Prev Med. 2018 Feb;54(2):173–80.
50. Bellentani S, Saccoccio G, Costa G, Tiribelli C, Manenti F, Sodde M, The Dionysos Study Group, et al. Drinking habits as cofactors of risk for alcohol induced liver damage. Gut. 1997 Dec;41(6):845–50.
51. Simpson RF, Hermon C, Liu B, Green J, Reeves GK, Beral V, et al. Alcohol drinking patterns and liver cirrhosis risk: analysis of the prospective UK Million Women Study. Lancet Public Health. 2019 Jan;4(1):e41–e8.
52. Becker U, Deis A, Sorensen TI, Gronbaek M, Borch-Johnsen K, Muller CF, et al. Prediction of risk of liver disease by alcohol intake, sex, and age: a prospective population study. Hepatology. 1996 May;23(5):1025–9.
53. Fleming KM, Aithal GP, Card TR, West J. The rate of decompensation and clinical progression of disease in people with cirrhosis: a cohort study. Aliment Pharmacol Ther. 2010 Dec;32(11–12):1343–50.
54. Pares A, Caballeria J, Bruguera M, Torres M, Rodes J. Histological course of alcoholic hepatitis. Influence of abstinence, sex and extent of hepatic damage. J Hepatol. 1986;2(1):33–42.
55. Verrill C, Markham H, Templeton A, Carr NJ, Sheron N. Alcohol-related cirrhosis—early abstinence is a key factor in prognosis, even in the most severe cases. Addiction. 2009 May;104(5):768–74.

56. Lackner C, Spindelboeck W, Haybaeck J, Douschan P, Rainer F, Terracciano L, et al. Histological parameters and alcohol abstinence determine long-term prognosis in patients with alcoholic liver disease. J Hepatol. 2017 Mar;66(3):610–8.

57. Teli MR, Day CP, Burt AD, Bennett MK, James OF. Determinants of progression to cirrhosis or fibrosis in pure alcoholic fatty liver. Lancet. 1995 Oct 14;346(8981):987–90.

58. Dam-Larsen S, Franzmann M, Andersen IB, Christoffersen P, Jensen LB, Sorensen TI, et al. Long term prognosis of fatty liver: risk of chronic liver disease and death. Gut. 2004 May;53(5):750–5.

59. Haflidadottir S, Jonasson JG, Norland H, Einarsdottir SO, Kleiner DE, Lund SH, et al. Long-term follow-up and liver-related death rate in patients with non-alcoholic and alcoholic related fatty liver disease. BMC Gastroenterol. 2014 Sep 27;14:166.

60. Deltenre P, Rufat P, Hillaire S, Elman A, Moreau R, Valla D, et al. Lack of prognostic usefulness of hepatic venous pressures and hemodynamic values in a select group of patients with severe alcoholic cirrhosis. Am J Gastroenterol. 2002 May;97(5):1187–90.

61. Pessione F, Ramond MJ, Peters L, Pham BN, Batel P, Rueff B, et al. Five-year survival predictive factors in patients with excessive alcohol intake and cirrhosis. Effect of alcoholic hepatitis, smoking and abstinence. Liver Int. 2003 Feb;23(1):45–53.

62. Bell H, Jahnsen J, Kittang E, Raknerud N, Sandvik L. Long-term prognosis of patients with alcoholic liver cirrhosis: a 15-year follow-up study of 100 Norwegian patients admitted to one unit. Scand J Gastroenterol. 2004 Sep;39(9):858–63.

63. D'Amico G, Garcia-Tsao G, Pagliaro L. Natural history and prognostic indicators of survival in cirrhosis: a systematic review of 118 studies. J Hepatol. 2006 Jan;44(1):217–31.

64. Jepsen P, Ott P, Andersen PK, Sorensen HT, Vilstrup H. Clinical course of alcoholic liver cirrhosis: a Danish population-based cohort study. Hepatology. 2010 May;51(5):1675–82.

65. Jepsen P, Vilstrup H, Ott P, Keiding S, Andersen PK, Tygstrup N. The galactose elimination capacity and mortality in 781 Danish patients with newly-diagnosed liver cirrhosis: a cohort study. BMC Gastroenterol. 2009 Jun 30;9:50.

66. Jepsen P, Ott P, Andersen PK, Vilstrup H. The clinical course of alcoholic cirrhosis: effects of hepatic metabolic capacity, alcohol consumption, and hyponatremia--a historical cohort study. BMC Res Notes. 2012 Sep 18;5:509.

67. Dionigi E, Garcovich M, Borzio M, Leandro G, Majumdar A, Tsami A, et al. Bacterial infections change natural history of cirrhosis irrespective of liver disease severity. Am J Gastroenterol. 2017 Apr;112(4):588–96.

68. Force USPST. Screening and behavioral counseling interventions in primary care to reduce alcohol misuse: recommendation statement. Ann Intern Med. 2004 Apr 6;140(7):554–6.

69. Smith PC, Schmidt SM, Allensworth-Davies D, Saitz R. Primary care validation of a single-question alcohol screening test. J Gen Intern Med. 2009 Jul;24(7):783–8.

70. Ewing JA. Detecting alcoholism. The CAGE questionnaire. JAMA. 1984 Oct 12;252(14):1905–7.

71. O'Brien CP. The CAGE questionnaire for detection of alcoholism: a remarkably useful but simple tool. JAMA. 2008 Nov 5;300(17):2054–6.

72. Davis KM, Wu JY. Role of glutamatergic and GABAergic systems in alcoholism. J Biomed Sci. 2001 Jan-Feb;8(1):7–19.

73. Perry EC. Inpatient management of acute alcohol withdrawal syndrome. CNS Drugs. 2014 May;28(5):401–10.

74. Beckett AG, Livingstone AV, Hill KR. Acute alcoholic hepatitis. Br Med J. 1961 Oct 28;2(5260):1113–9.

75. Kalaitzakis E, Gunnarsdottir SA, Josefsson A, Bjornsson E. Increased risk for malignant neoplasms among patients with cirrhosis. Clin Gastroenterol Hepatol. 2011 Feb;9(2):168–74.

76. Salazar Salgado H, Ramos Martinez E, Lifshitz A. [Primary alcoholic cardiac disease and alcoholic liver disease. Anatomopathological study]. La Prensa medica mexicana. 1978 Sep–Oct;43(9–10):278–81. Enfermedad cardiaca alcoholica primaria y enfermedad hepatica alcoholica. Estudio anatomopatologico.

77. Estruch R, Fernandez-Sola J, Sacanella E, Pare C, Rubin E, Urbano-Marquez A. Relationship between cardiomyopathy and liver disease in chronic alcoholism. Hepatology. 1995 Aug;22(2):532–8.

78. Mene-Afejuku TO, Shady A, Akinlonu A, et al. Alcoholic cardiomyopathy and liver disease in a community hospital in east Harlem in New York City. Gastroenterol Hepatol Open Access. 2020;11(4):149–151. https://doi.org/10.15406/ghoa.2020.11.00431.

79. Fernandez-Sola J, Nicolas JM, Oriola J, Sacanella E, Estruch R, Rubin E, et al. Angiotensin-converting enzyme gene polymorphism is associated with vulnerability to alcoholic cardiomyopathy. Ann Internal Med. 2002 Sep 3;137(5 Part 1):321–6.

80. Jing L, Jin C, Lu Y, Huo P, Zhou L, Wang Y, et al. Investigation of microRNA expression profiles associated with human alcoholic cardiomyopathy. Cardiology. 2015;130(4):223–33.

81. Hung CL, Chang SC, Chang SH, Chi PC, Lai YJ, Wang SW, et al. Genetic polymorphisms of alcohol metabolizing enzymes and alcohol consumption are associated with asymptomatic cardiac remodeling and subclinical systolic dysfunction in large community-dwelling Asians. Alcohol Alcohol. 2017 Nov 1;52(6):638–46.

82. Caine D, Halliday GM, Kril JJ, Harper CG. Operational criteria for the classification of chronic alcoholics: identification of Wernicke's encephalopathy. J Neurol Neurosurg Psychiatry. 1997 Jan;62(1):51–60.

83. Galvin R, Brathen G, Ivashynka A, Hillbom M, Tanasescu R, Leone MA, et al. EFNS guidelines for diagnosis, therapy and prevention of Wernicke encephalopathy. Eur J Neurol. 2010 Dec;17(12):1408–18.

84. Jain J, Singh R, Banait S, Verma N, Waghmare S. Magnitude of peripheral neuropathy in cirrhosis of liver patients from central rural India. Ann Indian Acad Neurol. 2014 Oct;17(4):409–15.

85. Koike H, Iijima M, Sugiura M, Mori K, Hattori N, Ito H, et al. Alcoholic neuropathy is clinicopathologically distinct from thiamine-deficiency neuropathy. Ann Neurol. 2003 Jul;54(1):19–29.

86. Koike H, Sobue G. Alcoholic neuropathy. Curr Opin Neurol. 2006 Oct;19(5):481–6.

87. Koike H, Mori K, Misu K, Hattori N, Ito H, Hirayama M, et al. Painful alcoholic polyneuropathy with predominant small-fiber loss and normal thiamine status. Neurology. 2001 June 26;56(12):1727–32.

88. Finnerup NB, Attal N, Haroutounian S, McNicol E, Baron R, Dworkin RH, et al. Pharmacotherapy for neuropathic pain in adults: a systematic review and meta-analysis. Lancet Neurol. 2015 Feb;14(2):162–73.

89. Collier J. Bone disorders in chronic liver disease. Hepatology. 2007 Oct;46(4):1271–8.

90. Goel V, Kar P. Hepatic osteodystrophy. Trop Gastroenterol. 2010 Apr–June;31(2):82–6.

91. Marignani M, Angeletti S, Capurso G, Cassetta S, Delle FG. Bad to the bone: the effects of liver diseases on bone. Minerva Med. 2004 Dec;95(6):489–505.

92. Mobarhan SA, Russell RM, Recker RR, Posner DB, Iber FL, Miller P. Metabolic bone disease in alcoholic cirrhosis: a comparison of the effect of vitamin D2, 25-hydroxyvitamin D, or supportive treatment. Hepatology. 1984 Mar–Apr;4(2):266–73.

93. Lopez-Larramona G, Lucendo AJ, Gonzalez-Delgado L. Alcoholic liver disease and changes in bone mineral density. Revista Espanola de Enfermedades Digestivas. 2013 Nov–Dec;105(10):609–21.

94. Jorge-Hernandez JA, Gonzalez-Reimers CE, Torres-Ramirez A, Santolaria-Fernandez F, Gonzalez-Garcia C, Batista-Lopez JN, et al. Bone changes in alcoholic liver cirrhosis. A histomorphometrical analysis of 52 cases. Dig Dis Sci. 1988 Sep;33(9):1089–95.

95. Bansal RK, Kumar M, Sachdeva PR, Kumar A. Prospective study of profile of hepatic osteodystrophy in patients with non-choleastatic liver cirrhosis and impact of bisphosphonate supplementation. United European Gastroenterol J. 2016 Feb;4(1):77–83.

96. Loria I, Albanese C, Giusto M, Galtieri PA, Giannelli V, Lucidi C, et al. Bone disorders in patients with chronic liver disease awaiting liver transplantation. Transplant Proc. 2010 May;42(4):1191–3.

97. Lupoli R, Di Minno A, Spadarella G, Ambrosino P, Panico A, Tarantino L, et al. The risk of osteoporosis in patients with liver cirrhosis: a meta-analysis of literature studies. Clin Endocrinol. 2016 Jan;84(1):30–8.

98. Eastell R, Dickson ER, Hodgson SF, Wiesner RH, Porayko MK, Wahner HW, et al. Rates of vertebral bone loss before and after liver transplantation in women with primary biliary cirrhosis. Hepatology. 1991 Aug;14(2):296–300.

99. Peris P, Pares A, Guanabens N, Pons F, Martinez de Osaba MJ, Caballeria J, et al. Reduced spinal and femoral bone mass and deranged bone mineral metabolism in chronic alcoholics. Alcohol Alcohol. 1992 Nov;27(6):619–25.

100. Williams BO, Insogna KL. Where Wnts went: the exploding field of Lrp5 and Lrp6 signaling in bone. J Bone Mineral Res. 2009 Feb;24(2):171–8.

101. Gonzalez-Reimers E, Martin-Gonzalez C, de la Vega-Prieto MJ, Pelazas-Gonzalez R, Fernandez-Rodriguez C, Lopez-Prieto J, et al. Serum sclerostin in alcoholics: a pilot study. Alcohol Alcohol. 2013 May–June;48(3):278–82.

102. Moschen AR, Kaser A, Stadlmann S, Millonig G, Kaser S, Muhllechner P, et al. The RANKL/OPG system and bone mineral density in patients with chronic liver disease. J Hepatol. 2005 Dec;43(6):973–83.

103. Garcia-Valdecasas-Campelo E, Gonzalez-Reimers E, Santolaria-Fernandez F, De la Vega-Prieto MJ, Milena-Abril A, Sanchez-Perez MJ, et al. Serum osteoprotegerin and RANKL levels in chronic alcoholic liver disease. Alcohol Alcohol. 2006 May–June;41(3):261–6.

104. Bang CS, Shin IS, Lee SW, Kim JB, Baik GH, Suk KT, et al. Osteoporosis and bone fractures in alcoholic liver disease: a meta-analysis. World J Gastroenterol. 2015 Apr 7;21(13):4038–47.

105. Diez-Ruiz A, Garcia-Saura PL, Garcia-Ruiz P, Gonzalez-Calvin JL, Gallego-Rojo F, Fuchs D. Bone mineral density, bone turnover markers and cytokines in alcohol-induced cirrhosis. Alcohol Alcohol. 2010 Sep–Oct;45(5):427–30.

106. Gatta A, Verardo A, Di Pascoli M, Giannini S, Bolognesi M. Hepatic osteodystrophy. Clin Cases Mineral Bone Metab. 2014 Sep;11(3):185–91.

107. McLoughlin RM, Mills KH. Influence of gastrointestinal commensal bacteria on the immune responses that mediate allergy and asthma. J Allergy Clin Immunol. 2011 May;127(5):1097–107.

108. Casafont Morencos F, de las Heras Castano G, Martin Ramos L, Lopez Arias MJ, Ledesma F, Pons Romero F. Small bowel bacterial overgrowth in patients with alcoholic cirrhosis. Dig Dis Sci. 1996 Mar;41(3):552–6.

109. Rao R. Endotoxemia and gut barrier dysfunction in alcoholic liver disease. Hepatology. 2009 Aug;50(2):638–44.

110. Daviss B. Growing pains for metabolomics. Scientist. 2005;19(8):25–8.

111. Ellis DI, Dunn WB, Griffin JL, Allwood JW, Goodacre R. Metabolic fingerprinting as a diagnostic tool. Pharmacogenomics. 2007 Sep;8(9):1243–66.

112. Riva A, Patel V, Kurioka A, Jeffery HC, Wright G, Tarff S, et al. Mucosa-associated invariant T cells link intestinal immunity with antibacterial immune defects in alcoholic liver disease. Gut. 2018 May;67(5):918–30.

113. Mutlu EA, Gillevet PM, Rangwala H, Sikaroodi M, Naqvi A, Engen PA, et al. Colonic microbiome is altered in alcoholism. Am J Physiol Gastrointest Liver Physiol. 2012 May 1;302(9):G966–78.

114. Bode C, Kugler V, Bode JC. Endotoxemia in patients with alcoholic and non-alcoholic cirrhosis and in subjects with no evidence of chronic liver disease following acute alcohol excess. J Hepatol. 1987 Feb;4(1):8–14.

115. Hanck C, Rossol S, Bocker U, Tokus M, Singer MV. Presence of plasma endotoxin is correlated with tumour necrosis factor receptor levels and disease activity in alcoholic cirrhosis. Alcohol Alcohol. 1998 Nov–Dec;33(6):606–8.

116. Mookerjee RP, Stadlbauer V, Lidder S, Wright GA, Hodges SJ, Davies NA, et al. Neutrophil dysfunction in alcoholic hepatitis superimposed on cirrhosis is reversible and predicts the outcome. Hepatology. 2007 Sep;46(3):831–40.

117. Bajaj JS, Heuman DM, Hylemon PB, Sanyal AJ, White MB, Monteith P, et al. Altered profile of human gut microbiome is associated with cirrhosis and its complications. J Hepatol. 2014 May;60(5):940–7.
118. Rosa H, Silverio AO, Perini RF, Arruda CB. Bacterial infection in cirrhotic patients and its relationship with alcohol. Am J Gastroenterol. 2000 May;95(5):1290–3.
119. Fukui H, Brauner B, Bode JC, Bode C. Plasma endotoxin concentrations in patients with alcoholic and non-alcoholic liver disease: reevaluation with an improved chromogenic assay. J Hepatol. 1991 Mar;12(2):162–9.
120. Schafer C, Parlesak A, Schutt C, Bode JC, Bode C. Concentrations of lipopolysaccharide-binding protein, bactericidal/permeability-increasing protein, soluble CD14 and plasma lipids in relation to endotoxaemia in patients with alcoholic liver disease. Alcohol Alcohol. 2002 Jan-Feb;37(1):81–6.
121. Yang AM, Inamine T, Hochrath K, Chen P, Wang L, Llorente C, et al. Intestinal fungi contribute to development of alcoholic liver disease. J Clin Invest. 2017 June 30;127(7):2829–41.
122. Hartmann P, Seebauer CT, Schnabl B. Alcoholic liver disease: the gut microbiome and liver cross talk. Alcohol Clin Exp Res. 2015 May;39(5):763–75.
123. Salaspuro M. Use of enzymes for the diagnosis of alcohol-related organ damage. Enzyme. 1987;37(1–2):87–107.
124. De Ritis F, Coltorti M, Giusti G. An enzymic test for the diagnosis of viral hepatitis; the transaminase serum activities. Clin Chim Acta. 1957 Feb;2(1):70–4.
125. Cohen JA, Kaplan MM. The SGOT/SGPT ratio: an indicator of alcoholic liver disease. Dig Dis Sci. 1979 Nov;24(11):835–8.
126. Hietala J, Puukka K, Koivisto H, Anttila P, Niemela O. Serum gamma-glutamyl transferase in alcoholics, moderate drinkers and abstainers: effect on gt reference intervals at population level. Alcohol Alcohol. 2005 Nov-Dec;40(6):511–4.
127. Sharpe PC. Biochemical detection and monitoring of alcohol abuse and abstinence. Ann Clin Biochem. 2001 Nov;38(Pt 6):652–64.
128. Diehl AM, Potter J, Boitnott J, Van Duyn MA, Herlong HF, Mezey E. Relationship between pyridoxal 5'-phosphate deficiency and aminotransferase levels in alcoholic hepatitis. Gastroenterology. 1984 Apr;86(4):632–6.
129. Zieve L. Jaundice, hyperlipemia and hemolytic anemia: a heretofore unrecognized syndrome associated with alcoholic fatty liver and cirrhosis. Ann Intern Med. 1958 Mar;48(3):471–96.
130. Morse EE. Mechanisms of hemolysis in liver disease. Ann Clin Lab Sci. 1990 May–June;20(3):169–74.
131. Costa Matos L, Batista P, Monteiro N, Ribeiro J, Cipriano MA, Henriques P, et al. Iron stores assessment in alcoholic liver disease. Scand J Gastroenterol. 2013 Jun;48(6):712–8.
132. Harrison-Findik DD, Schafer D, Klein E, Timchenko NA, Kulaksiz H, Clemens D, et al. Alcohol metabolism-mediated oxidative stress down-regulates hepcidin transcription and leads to increased duodenal iron transporter expression. J Biol Chem. 2006 Aug 11;281(32):22974–82.
133. Pietrangelo A. Genetics, genetic testing, and management of hemochromatosis: 15 years since hepcidin. Gastroenterology. 2015 Oct;149(5):1240–51.
134. Chrostek L, Panasiuk A. Liver fibrosis markers in alcoholic liver disease. World J Gastroenterol. 2014 July 7;20(25):8018–23.
135. Quinn SF, Gosink BB. Characteristic sonographic signs of hepatic fatty infiltration. AJR Am J Roentgenol. 1985 Oct;145(4):753–5.
136. Berzigotti A, Abraldes JG, Tandon P, Erice E, Gilabert R, Garcia-Pagan JC, et al. Ultrasonographic evaluation of liver surface and transient elastography in clinically doubtful cirrhosis. J Hepatol. 2010 Jun;52(6):846–53.
137. Yeom SK, Lee CH, Cha SH, Park CM. Prediction of liver cirrhosis, using diagnostic imaging tools. World J Hepatol. 2015 Aug 18;7(17):2069–79.
138. Bydder GM, Chapman RW, Harry D, Bassan L, Sherlock S, Kreel L. Computed tomography attenuation values in fatty liver. J Comput Tomogr. 1981 Mar;5(1):33–5.

139. Furnari M, Ahmed I, Erpecum KJ, Savarino V, Giannini EG. Breath tests to assess alcoholic liver disease. Rev Recent Clin Trials. 2016;11(3):185–90.
140. Hall PDLM. Alcoholic liver disease. In: MacSween RNM, Anthony PP, Scheuer PJ, Burt AD, Portmann BC, editors. Pathology of the liver, vol. 1. 3rd ed. Edinburgh: Churchill Livingstone; 1994. p. 317–48.
141. Uchida T, Kao H, Quispe-Sjogren M, Peters RL. Alcoholic foamy degeneration: a pattern of acute alcoholic injury of the liver. Gastroenterology. 1983 Apr;84(4):683–92.
142. Roth N, Kanel G, Kaplowitz N. Alcoholic foamy degeneration and alcoholic fatty liver with jaundice: often overlooked causes of jaundice and hepatic decompensation that can mimic alcoholic hepatitis. Clin Liver Dis. 2015 Dec;6(6):145–8.
143. Shibao K, Hirata K, Robert ME, Nathanson MH. Loss of inositol 1,4,5-trisphosphate receptors from bile duct epithelia is a common event in cholestasis. Gastroenterology. 2003 Oct;125(4):1175–87.
144. Minagawa N, Nagata J, Shibao K, Masyuk AI, Gomes DA, Rodrigues MA, et al. Cyclic AMP regulates bicarbonate secretion in cholangiocytes through release of ATP into bile. Gastroenterology. 2007 Nov;133(5):1592–602.
145. Franca A, Carlos Melo Lima Filho A, Guerra MT, Weerachayaphorn J, Loiola dos Santos M, Njei B, et al. Effects of endotoxin on type 3 inositol 1,4,5-trisphosphate receptor in human cholangiocytes. Hepatology. 2019 Feb;69(2):817–30.
146. Nakano M, Worner TM, Lieber CS. Perivenular fibrosis in alcoholic liver injury: ultrastructure and histologic progression. Gastroenterology. 1982 Oct;83(4):777–85.
147. Sheron N, Bird G, Koskinas J, Portmann B, Ceska M, Lindley I, et al. Circulating and tissue levels of the neutrophil chemotaxin interleukin-8 are elevated in severe acute alcoholic hepatitis, and tissue levels correlate with neutrophil infiltration. Hepatology. 1993 July;18(1):41–6.
148. Dominguez M, Miquel R, Colmenero J, Moreno M, Garcia-Pagan JC, Bosch J, et al. Hepatic expression of CXC chemokines predicts portal hypertension and survival in patients with alcoholic hepatitis. Gastroenterology. 2009 May;136(5):1639–50.
149. Colmenero J, Bataller R, Sancho-Bru P, Bellot P, Miquel R, Moreno M, et al. Hepatic expression of candidate genes in patients with alcoholic hepatitis: correlation with disease severity. Gastroenterology. 2007 Feb;132(2):687–97.
150. Degre D, Lemmers A, Gustot T, Ouziel R, Trepo E, Demetter P, et al. Hepatic expression of CCL2 in alcoholic liver disease is associated with disease severity and neutrophil infiltrates. Clin Exp Immunol. 2012 Sep;169(3):302–10.
151. Li W, Amet T, Xing Y, Yang D, Liangpunsakul S, Puri P, et al. Alcohol abstinence ameliorates the dysregulated immune profiles in patients with alcoholic hepatitis: a prospective observational study. Hepatology. 2017 Aug;66(2):575–90.
152. Reynolds TB, Hidemura R, Michel H, Peters R. Portal hypertension without cirrhosis in alcoholic liver disease. Ann Intern Med. 1969 Mar;70(3):497–506.
153. Poynard T, Degott C, Munoz C, Lebrec D. Relationship between degree of portal hypertension and liver histologic lesions in patients with alcoholic cirrhosis. Effect of acute alcoholic hepatitis on portal hypertension. Dig Dis Sci. 1987 Apr;32(4):337–43.
154. Goodman ZD, Ishak KG. Occlusive venous lesions in alcoholic liver disease. A study of 200 cases. Gastroenterology. 1982 Oct;83(4):786–96.
155. Pariente EA, Degott C, Martin JP, Feldmann G, Potet F, Benhamou JP. Hepatocytic PAS-positive diastase-resistance inclusions in the absence of alpha-1-antitrypsin deficiency—high prevalence in alcoholic cirrhosis. Am J Clin Pathol. 1981 Sep;76(3):299–302.
156. Gerber MA, Thung SN. Hepatic oncocytes. Incidence, staining characteristics, and ultrastructural features. Am J Clin Pathol. 1981 Apr;75(4):498–503.
157. Brown WR, Kloppel TM. The liver and IgA: immunological, cell biological and clinical implications. Hepatology. 1989 May;9(5):763–84.
158. Moro-Sibilot L, Blanc P, Taillardet M, Bardel E, Couillault C, Boschetti G, et al. Mouse and human liver contain immunoglobulin A-secreting cells originating from Peyer's patches and directed against intestinal antigens. Gastroenterology. 2016 Aug;151(2):311–23.

159. NIH. ANTABUSE - disulfiram tablet In: Medicine NUNLo, editor. 2012.
160. Skinner MD, Lahmek P, Pham H, Aubin HJ. Disulfiram efficacy in the treatment of alcohol dependence: a meta-analysis. PLoS One. 2014;9(2):e87366.
161. Krystal JH, Cramer JA, Krol WF, Kirk GF, Rosenheck RA. Veterans affairs naltrexone cooperative study G. naltrexone in the treatment of alcohol dependence. N Engl J Med. 2001 Dec 13;345(24):1734–9.
162. Rosner S, Hackl-Herrwerth A, Leucht S, Vecchi S, Srisurapanont M, Soyka M. Opioid antagonists for alcohol dependence. Cochrane Database Syst Rev. 2010 Dec;8(12):CD001867.
163. Littleton JM. Acamprosate in alcohol dependence: implications of a unique mechanism of action. J Addict Med. 2007 Sep;1(3):115–25.
164. Akbar M, Egli M, Cho YE, Song BJ, Noronha A. Medications for alcohol use disorders: an overview. Pharmacol Ther. 2018 May;185:64–85.
165. Addolorato G, Leggio L, Ferrulli A, Cardone S, Vonghia L, Mirijello A, et al. Effectiveness and safety of baclofen for maintenance of alcohol abstinence in alcohol-dependent patients with liver cirrhosis: randomised, double-blind controlled study. Lancet. 2007 Dec 8;370(9603):1915–22.
166. Mosoni C, Dionisi T, Vassallo GA, Mirijello A, Tarli C, Antonelli M, et al. Baclofen for the treatment of alcohol use disorder in patients with liver cirrhosis: 10 years after the first evidence. Front Psych. 2018;9:474.
167. Minozzi S, Saulle R, Rosner S. Baclofen for alcohol use disorder. Cochrane Database Syst Rev. 2018 Nov 26;11:CD012557.
168. Barrault C, Lison H, Roudot-Thoraval F, Garioud A, Costentin C, Behar V, et al. One year of baclofen in 100 patients with or without cirrhosis: a French real-life experience. Eur J Gastroenterol Hepatol. 2017 Oct;29(10):1155–60.
169. drugs.com. Revia. 2018.
170. UNIVERSITY CC. FDA-approved medications.
171. Yen MH, Ko HC, Tang FI, Lu RB, Hong JS. Study of hepatotoxicity of naltrexone in the treatment of alcoholism. Alcohol. 2006 Feb;38(2):117–20.
172. Bergasa NV. Pruritus of cholestasis. In: Carstens E, Akiyama T, editors. Itch: mechanisms and treatment. Frontiers in neuroscience. Boca Raton, FL: CRC Press; 2014.
173. Alcohol withdrawal syndrome: how to predict, prevent, diagnose and treat it. Prescrire Int. 2007 Feb;16(87):24–31.
174. Maldonado JR, Sher Y, Ashouri JF, Hills-Evans K, Swendsen H, Lolak S, et al. The "prediction of alcohol withdrawal severity scale" (PAWSS): systematic literature review and pilot study of a new scale for the prediction of complicated alcohol withdrawal syndrome. Alcohol. 2014 Jun;48(4):375–90.
175. Wood E, Albarqouni L, Tkachuk S, Green CJ, Ahamad K, Nolan S, et al. Will this hospitalized patient develop severe alcohol withdrawal syndrome?: the rational clinical examination systematic review. JAMA. 2018 Aug 28;320(8):825–33.
176. Schabelman E, Kuo D. Glucose before thiamine for Wernicke encephalopathy: a literature review. J Emerg Med. 2012 Apr;42(4):488–94.
177. Kosten TR, O'Connor PG. Management of drug and alcohol withdrawal. N Engl J Med. 2003 May 1;348(18):1786–95.
178. Schuckit MA. Management of withdrawal delirium (delirium tremens). N Engl J Med. 2015 Feb 5;372(6):580–1.
179. Mendenhall CL, Moritz TE, Roselle GA, Morgan TR, Nemchausky BA, Tamburro CH, et al. A study of oral nutritional support with oxandrolone in malnourished patients with alcoholic hepatitis: results of a Department of Veterans Affairs cooperative study. Hepatology. 1993 Apr;17(4):564–76.
180. de Ledinghen V, Beau P, Mannant PR, Borderie C, Ripault MP, Silvain C, et al. Early feeding or enteral nutrition in patients with cirrhosis after bleeding from esophageal varices? A randomized controlled study. Dig Dis Sci. 1997 Mar;42(3):536–41.

181. Porter HP, Simon FR, Pope CE 2nd, Volwiler W, Fenster LF. Corticosteroid therapy in severe alcoholic hepatitis. A double-blind drug trial. N Engl J Med. 1971 Jun 17;284(24):1350–5.

182. Lesesne HR, Bozymski EM, Fallon HJ. Treatment of alcoholic hepatitis with encephalopathy. Comparison of prednisolone with caloric supplements. Gastroenterology. 1978 Feb;74(2 Pt 1):169–73.

183. Maddrey WC, Boitnott JK, Bedine MS, Weber FL Jr, Mezey E, White RI Jr. Corticosteroid therapy of alcoholic hepatitis. Gastroenterology. 1978 Aug;75(2):193–9.

184. Carithers RL Jr, Herlong HF, Diehl AM, Shaw EW, Combes B, Fallon HJ, et al. Methylprednisolone therapy in patients with severe alcoholic hepatitis. A randomized multicenter trial. Ann Intern Med. 1989 May 1;110(9):685–90.

185. Ramond MJ, Poynard T, Rueff B, Mathurin P, Theodore C, Chaput JC, et al. A randomized trial of prednisolone in patients with severe alcoholic hepatitis. N Engl J Med. 1992 Feb 20;326(8):507–12.

186. Phillips M, Curtis H, Portmann B, Donaldson N, Bomford A, O'Grady J. Antioxidants versus corticosteroids in the treatment of severe alcoholic hepatitis: a randomised clinical trial. J Hepatol. 2006 Apr;44(4):784–90.

187. Singal AK, Bataller R, Ahn J, Kamath PS, Shah VH. ACG clinical guideline: alcoholic liver disease. Am J Gastroenterol. 2018 Feb;113(2):175–94.

188. Teschke R. Alcoholic steatohepatitis (ASH) and alcoholic hepatitis (AH): cascade of events, clinical aspects, and pharmacotherapy options. Expert Opin Pharmacother. 2018 Jun;19(8):779–93.

189. Helman RA, Temko MH, Nye SW, Fallon HJ. Alcoholic hepatitis. Natural history and evaluation of prednisolone therapy. Ann Intern Med. 1971 Mar;74(3):311–21.

190. Depew W, Boyer T, Omata M, Redeker A, Reynolds T. Double-blind controlled trial of prednisolone therapy in patients with severe acute alcoholic hepatitis and spontaneous encephalopathy. Gastroenterology. 1980 Mar;78(3):524–9.

191. Mathurin P, Abdelnour M, Ramond MJ, Carbonell N, Fartoux L, Serfaty L, et al. Early change in bilirubin levels is an important prognostic factor in severe alcoholic hepatitis treated with prednisolone. Hepatology. 2003 Dec;38(6):1363–9.

192. Louvet A, Naveau S, Abdelnour M, Ramond MJ, Diaz E, Fartoux L, et al. The Lille model: a new tool for therapeutic strategy in patients with severe alcoholic hepatitis treated with steroids. Hepatology. 2007 June;45(6):1348–54.

193. Mathurin P, Louvet A, Duhamel A, Nahon P, Carbonell N, Boursier J, et al. Prednisolone with vs without pentoxifylline and survival of patients with severe alcoholic hepatitis: a randomized clinical trial. JAMA. 2013 Sep 11;310(10):1033–41.

194. Campra JL, Hamlin EM Jr, Kirshbaum RJ, Olivier M, Redeker AG, Reynolds TB. Prednisone therapy of acute alcoholic hepatitis. Report of a controlled trial. Ann Intern Med. 1973 Nov;79(5):625–31.

195. Mathurin P, Moreno C, Samuel D, Dumortier J, Salleron J, Durand F, et al. Early liver transplantation for severe alcoholic hepatitis. N Engl J Med. 2011 Nov 10;365(19):1790–800.

196. Garcia-Tsao G, Abraldes JG, Berzigotti A, Bosch J. Portal hypertensive bleeding in cirrhosis: risk stratification, diagnosis, and management: 2016 practice guidance by the American Association for the Study of Liver Diseases. Hepatology. 2017 Jan;65(1):310–35.

197. Jepsen P, Ott P, Andersen PK, Sorensen HT, Vilstrup H. Risk for hepatocellular carcinoma in patients with alcoholic cirrhosis: a Danish Nationwide Cohort Study. Ann Intern Med. 2012 June 19;156(12):841–7.

198. Heimbach JK, Kulik LM, Finn RS, Sirlin CB, Abecassis MM, Roberts LR, et al. AASLD guidelines for the treatment of hepatocellular carcinoma. Hepatology. 2018 Jan;67(1):358–80.

# Chapter 9
# Nonalcoholic Fatty Liver Disease

**Nora V. Bergasa**

A 35-year-old woman was referred to the hepatology clinic for evaluation of an abnormal liver profile. She did not have any symptoms. She did not have any comorbidities nor take any medications. She was of Hispanic ethnicity. Her physical examination was notable for obesity, with a BMI of 33. Her serum aspartate (AST) and alanine aminotransferase (ALT) activities were 125 IU/ml and 112 IU/ml, respectively. The liver disease workup was unrevealing, and the sonogram was normal. Liver histology revealed nonalcoholic steatohepatitis (NASH). She was treated with vitamin E for 96 weeks, associated with decreased transaminase serum activity but not normalization. She has been doing well, with no evidence of liver disease progression. She tries to exercise and eat as advised by the nutritionist.

Nonalcoholic fatty liver disease (NAFLD) is defined as the accumulation of fat, as lipid droplets, in the hepatocytes beyond 5% of the gland [1]. The spectrum of NAFLD is comprised of hepatic steatosis, steatohepatitis, fibrosis, and cirrhosis; the causes of fatty liver must be excluded in the purest sense of the definition. NAFLD receives much attention because of its reported high prevalence and presence in liver transplant centers as an important cause of end-stage liver disease and liver transplantation [2].

NAFLD is associated with central obesity, hypertension, diabetes mellitus, and hyperlipidemia, alone or in combination meeting the definition of metabolic syndrome [3–5]. The cause of fat accumulation in the liver is unknown; however, genetic predisposition is recognized as a permissive factor for NAFLD [6–10].

N. V. Bergasa (✉)
Department of Medicine, H+H/Metropolitan, New York, NY, USA

New York Medical College, Valhalla, NY, USA

Hepatology, H+H/Woodhull, Brooklyn, NY, USA

N. V. Bergasa (ed.), *Clinical Cases in Hepatology*,
https://doi.org/10.1007/978-1-4471-4715-2_9

# Epidemiology

Worldwide, NAFLD was recently reported to affect 25% of the population [2].

A study that used the National Health and Nutrition Examination Surveys (NHANES) as the source reported the prevalence rate for chronic liver disease as 11.78% from 1988 to 1994, 15.66% from 1999 to 2004, and 14.78% from 2005 to 2008. In contrast to the steady prevalence of hepatitis B and C and liver disease from alcohol, there was a progressive increase in NAFLD from 46.8% to 62.84%, to 75.1% over the periods examined. This increase coincided with an increase in obesity, type II diabetes, insulin resistance, and hypertension, the conditions associated with NAFLD, with obesity being an independent factor in the prediction of NAFLD [11].

From a meta-analysis that included a large number of subjects with NAFLD from 22 countries, the proportion of comorbidities that affected the subjects included in the various studies was reported as 51.34% (95% confidence interval (CI): 41.38–61.20) for obesity, 22.51% (95% CI: 17.92–27.89) for type 2 diabetes, 69.16% (95% CI: 49.91–83.46%) for hyperlipidemia, 39.34% (95% CI: 33.15–45.88) for hypertension, and 42.54% (95% CI: 30.06–56.05) for metabolic syndrome [3].

Data derived from the 6000 participants in the NHANES in the United States showed that 30% had NAFLD, of which 10.3% had advanced fibrosis, as per the NAFLD Fibrosis Score (NFS). In this group, the 5 and 8 year overall mortality was 18% and 35%, respectively, and significantly higher than the 2.6% and 5.5% from the subjects without NAFLD, in contrast with the percentage from subjects with NAFLD without fibrosis, which was 1.1% and 2.8% at 5 and 8 years as well. Advanced fibrosis was an independent predictor for mortality. In regard to ethnicity, Mexican Americans were reported to be at risk for NAFLD but not for advanced fibrosis or mortality [5].

By the use of proton magnetic resonance spectroscopy to determine the distribution of hepatic triglyceride content (HTGC), hepatic steatosis was documented in close to one third of the 2287 subjects included, with 45% being Hispanic, 33% white, and 24% black, with 42% being white men and 24% white women, suggesting an ethnic and racial predisposition to this condition [12]. In a study that examined liver histology of 105 patients who underwent bariatric surgery, a high risk group for fatty liver, 42% had advanced fibrosis, and 25% NASH for which insulin resistance, hypertension, and increased serum activity of ALT were independent predictors. Two or three of these factors, in combination, predicted the presence of NASH with high sensitivity and specificity [13].

These cumulative results from a large number of subjects support the prediction of 2011 [11] regarding the projected increase in the number of subjects with NAFLD, as it appears to be the case from subsequent studies [2, 3, 5].

# Etiology

Lipotoxicity concerns cellular damage that results from the accumulation of fat [14]. The metabolic syndrome or one or more of its components is associated with NAFLD. In obesity, the adipocyte is insulin resistant. In this milieu, this cell increases lipolysis and releases fatty acids (FA), adipokines, and inflammatory cytokines, which, combined with hepatocyte insulin resistance, is associated with NAFLD. The increased accumulation of triglycerides, mostly triacylglycerol, overcomes the liver's capacity to export triglycerides in the form of very low density lipoproteins (VLDL), and the beta-oxidation of free FA (FAA). The progression of liver disease to inflammation, i.e., steatohepatitis, fibrosis, and cirrhosis, concerns oxidation of fatty acid and oxidative stress, changes in the FA and phospholipid composition of cellular membranes, alterations in cellular cholesterol concentration, altered ceramide signaling pathway, and toxicity from FAA per se. The origin of liver fat was documented as nonesterified fatty acids, de novo lipogenesis, and diet [15].

Analysis of the hepatic lipid composition in NAFLD revealed a decrease in the concentration of hepatic phosphatidylcholine in both fatty liver and steatohepatitis, no changes in FFA, and a progressive increase in diacylglycerol (DAG), triacylglycerol (TAG), and free cholesterol (FC) in livers with steatosis and steatohepatitis as compared to normal livers. Arachidonic acid was decreased in FFA, TAG, and PC, and eicosapentanoic and docosahexanoic acids were reduced in TAG in steatohepatitis livers, where there was an increase in the n-6:n-3FFA ratio [16]. The mechanistic role of these findings in the pathogenesis of steatosis and nonalcoholic steatohepatitis is speculative; however, one conclusion derived from the study was support for n-3 fatty acid supplementation for the treatment of NASH [16]. A consensus supports that there is an increase in triacylglycerol in livers of patients with NAFLD and NASH and that circulating FFAs contribute to the hepatic deposition triacylglycerol [17].

In association with steatosis, apoptosis has been documented in NAFLD [18, 19]. In liver samples from patients with NAFLD, apoptosis, measured by the terminal deoxynucleotidyl transferase (Tdt) dUTp Nick-End Labeling (TUNEL) assay, was more prevalent in NASH than in steatosis; the Fas receptor was strongly expressed by hepatocytes in NASH, in reference to control liver samples and a positive correlation between hepatocyte apoptosis and hepatic inflammatory activity and fibrosis was documented [18]. To identify a peripheral marker of disease activity, fragments of cytokeratin 18, which are generated in apoptosis, were measured in vivo by an enzyme-linked immunosorbent assay, which documented marked increases in cytokeratin 18 fragments in blood, which independently predicted NASH [20].

The lipid profile in patients with NASH, in the absence of different diet composition compared to other NAFLD groups, was documented to have a reduction of polyunsaturated FA, n-3, and n-6; in addition, there was a reported decrease in the ratio of metabolites to essential FA precursors for both n-6 and n-3 FA, and an increase in liver lipid peroxides with decreased antioxidant ability versus patients with NAFLD and minimal histological activity, which suggested that the liver of patients with NASH is exposed to enhanced oxidative stress and decreased n-3 and n-6 polyunsaturated fatty acids (PUFA) [21]; however, PUFA have not been associated with apoptosis in NAFLD. In fact, it was reported from an in vitro model that unsaturated fatty acids protect from lipotoxicity by the enhanced accumulation of triglycerides [22]; it is the saturated FFA via the induction of c-jun N-terminal kinase (JNK) and activation of Bcl-2 proteins Bim and Bax that are considered instrumental in NAFLD apoptosis, i.e., via the mitochondrial pathway [23]. In this regard, in vitro studies have documented that the addition of FFA to hepatocyte preparations was associated with the translocation of the Bax protein to lysosomes, with their permeabilization and subsequent expression of TNF-alpha, by an NF-kB dependent manner via the activation of its canonical pathway, and release of cathepsin B, a lysosomal protease, into the cytoplasm, the importance of which was documented in hepatocytes from patients with NAFLD by the release of this protease into the cytoplasm and its correlation with disease severity [24].

The saturated fatty acids, palmitic acid, and stearic acid lead to JNK dependent activation of the proapoptotic protein Bax, leading to mitochondrial permeabilization with the release of cytochrome c, activation of effector caspases, and apoptosis. Palmitic acid can also activate the lysosomal pathway of apoptosis, via Bax activation and Bax-dependent lysosomal permeabilization; in addition, palmitic and stearic acids also activate protein phosphatase 2A (PP2A), followed by forkhead box3a (FoxO3a), and transcription of Bim, a proapoptosis protein. Monounsaturated FA, oleic acid, activates the extrinsic pathway by enhancing the sensitivity to the death receptor mediated extrinsic pathway of apoptosis, which sensitizes the steatotic hepatocyte to the binding of the Fas and TRAIL ligands to their receptors [17]. Other mechanisms have been proposed to participate in apoptosis in NAFLD, including endoplasmic reticulum stress, and failure to generate sXBP-1 [25].

It has been proposed that free cholesterol also contributes to steatohepatitis by the depletion of mitochondrial glutathione, which sensitizes the hepatocyte to TNF and Fas [26, 27].

Oxidative stress results from multiple processes that include oxidation of FFA, cytochrome P4502E1, iron overload, and inflammatory cytokines; there is consensus that oxidative stress contributes to the pathogenesis of NAFLD. Hepatic lipid peroxidation, assessed by immunohistochemical staining for 3-nitrotyrosine (3-NT), was documented in fatty liver, but the strongest expression was in NASH samples, which also showed loss of cristae in the mitochondria [28]; high systemic levels of products and in situ markers of lipid peroxidation have been documented in patients with NASH [29, 30].

An increase in circulating FFA that contributes to the accumulation of triacylglycerol (TAG) in livers of patients with NAFLD and NASH is an important etiologic factor of fatty liver [16, 31]. Sources of increased liver TAG include diet, hepatic synthesis from FA, increased intake of FA into the liver from lipolysis of adipose tissue and conversion to TAG, decreased export of triglycerides via VLDL, and decreased oxidation of FA.

Dietary intake of fat is considered important in NAFLD development [32]; however, hepatic steatosis extends beyond diet [33–35]. Peripheral FA and de novo lipogenesis (DNL) contribute to the accumulation of fat in NAFLD, as reported from a study that examined the source of hepatic and plasma lipoproteins in patients with NAFLD, all of whom were obese and had fasting hypertriglyceridemia and hyperinsulinemia [13]. The study documented that approximately 60% of TAG originated from nonesterified fatty acids, 26% from DNL, and 15% from the diet, that the liver used FA from adipose tissue and dietary sources equally, and that de novo lipogenesis was increased in fasting [15].

Most published studies that concern the genetic mechanisms of DNL have been derived from laboratory animals and in vitro molecular experiments. In this regard, the transcription factors reported to be involved in DNL in the liver include carbohydrate response element binding protein (ChREBP), and sterol responsive element binding protein-1c (SREBP-1c), the latter being mainly involved in insulin-mediated lipogenesis so that in a hyperinsulinemic state, there is increased hepatic lipogenesis by the activation of acetyl CoA carboxylase (ACC), fatty acid synthase (FASN), and stearoyl-CoA desaturase 1 (SCD1) genes, which are activated by SREBP-1c [36].

PPARs are nuclear receptors that participate in the transcriptional regulation of glucose and lipid metabolism; there are three PPAR isoforms: alpha ($\alpha$), beta/delta ($\beta/\delta$), and gamma ($\gamma$). PPAR$\alpha$ is expressed ubiquitously but is mostly present in the liver. PPAR$\beta/\delta$ is expressed mainly in skeletal muscle and, to some degree, in adipose tissue and skin. PPAR$\gamma$ is highly expressed in adipose tissue [33].

PPAR$\alpha$'s gene expression was reported to correlate negatively with histological severity in patients with NASH and improvement associated with an increase in the expression of peroxisome proliferator-activated receptor alpha (PPAR$\alpha$) [37]. PPAR $\delta$ is expressed by adipose tissue and skin but mostly in skeletal muscle; in laboratory animals, the activation of PPAR $\delta$ is associated with the induction of fatty acid beta-oxidation in skeletal muscle and attenuation of the metabolic syndrome [38]. In addition, these receptors have been implicated in fibrosis by activation of stellate cells suggesting a role in the mediation of the progression of liver disease in NAFLD [39].

PPAR$\gamma$ is highly expressed in adipose tissue; however, its expression is abundant in the liver of obese patients with NAFLD, thus facilitating fat accumulation by stimulating SREBP-1c [40]. In human beings, PPAR-$\gamma$, also involved in DNL, was documented most abundantly in adipose tissue. PPAR $\gamma$ 2 mRNA was reported to correlate with BMI, being downregulated by a low calorie diet in obese persons, and induced by insulin and corticosteroids in a background of human adipocytes, which has suggested that PPAR $\gamma$2 mRNA levels may contribute to the regulation of adipocyte development and function, including obesity [41]; thus, in an environment of hyperinsulinemia such as NAFLD, PPAR $\gamma$ 2 may contribute to DNL. In addition, weight loss was associated with reduced serum insulin and plasma TGA, and reduced adipose tissue PPARγ2, although only in the subcutaneous adipose tissue [42]. Furthermore, evaluation of fatty acid metabolism-related gene expression in NAFLD documented an increase in PPAR γ, further suggesting that increased de novo synthesis and decreased beta-oxidation in the mitochondria may lead to the accumulation of fatty acids in hepatic cells [43].

More than adipocytes, macrophages, which are proportionally increased with obesity in white adipose tissue in human beings, were documented to express high levels of the chemokines monocyte chemotactic protein 1, macrophage inflammatory protein 1alpha, IL-8, as well as resistin and visfatin, both adipokines, substances that participate in inflammatory mediation and energy control. Resistin was reported to induce lipolysis and re-esterification of triacylglycerol stores, and to increase cholesteryl ester deposition in human macrophages [44], to induce expression of FASN in adipocytes followed by an increase in cellular TAG and FFAs, and to stimulate adipocyte triglyceride lipolysis in in vitro cellular studies; thus, it has been proposed that this adipokine may increase the availability of FAAs that are taken up by the liver, which would lead to accumulation of TAG.

Impaired fatty acid oxidation may contribute to steatosis in NAFLD; the mechanisms postulated may be hypothetical at present or based on extrapolations from animal studies and await confirmation in the human condition [45].

Lipotoxicity occurs from the accumulation of fat in nonadipose tissue, a feature of metabolic syndrome and NAFLD; it leads to the activation of metabolic pathways via FA that result in apoptosis of lipid laden cells [46, 47]. Evidence from in vitro studies suggests that unsaturated fatty acids may protect against lipotoxicity by directing long-chain fatty acids, e.g., palmitic acid, towards triglyceride pools and away from apoptosis pathways [22]. Lipotoxicity may occur by dysfunction of mitochondria, leading to increased production of reactive oxygen species (ROS), lipid peroxidation, and oxidative stress [28, 48], associated with increased expression of CYP2E1 and subsequent increased activity of nicotinamide adenine dinucleotide phosphate-oxidase (NADPH). Also, a further increase in ROS production leads to increased hepatic CYP2E1 activity, which, interestingly, was predicted by the presence of nocturnal hypoxemia, a feature of some patients with NAFLD sometimes in association with metabolic syndrome [49]. Lysosomal dysfunction can be caused by chronic oxidative stress and the production of inflammatory cytokines and adipocytokine in adipose tissue. These products may act as proinflammatory and profibrogenic agents and alter the immune response in the setting of insulin resistance, which characterizes metabolic syndrome and its associated NAFLD. These many alterations are associated with increased peripheral lipolysis and FFA release, which can also be proinflammatory; this lipotoxic environment contributes to steatohepatitis [46, 47].

MicroRNAs (miRNAs) are endogenous RNAs, single stranded, of approximately 23 nucleotides that regulate protein coding genes by pairing to their mRNAs to direct their posttranscriptional repression [50]. It was reported that serum concentrations of miR-122, miR-34a, and miR-16 were significantly higher in patients with NAFLD than in control subjects. The first two correlated with steatosis and steatohepatitis; furthermore, miR-122 levels also correlated with serum lipids in NAFLD patients [51]. Whether these findings reflect a pathophysiological mechanism for NAFLD or whether serum microRNAs can be used to measure the disease stage remains to be confirmed [52–54].

Sarcopenia is prevalent in patients with cirrhosis, and it is being proposed as a risk factor for NAFLD. Results from a retrospective study that covered 5 years and included patients with histologically documented NAFLD versus a control group documented a significant decrease in muscle mass in the psoas and paraspinal muscles, consistent with sarcopenia. The mechanisms that mediate this potential association are proposed to be related to a cross talk between muscle and adipose tissue that involve adiponectin and myostatin [55].

# Genetics

The inference that genetic susceptibility contributes to NAFLD development derives itself from its associations, including type 2 diabetes, and cardiovascular disease, also considered to have a genetic influence. A genetic predisposition to NAFLD is supported by high prevalence in members of the same family [56–58], twin studies [59], and interethnic differences in susceptibility [12, 60].

Potential genetic modifiers to specific physiological and pathophysiological processes are glucose metabolism and insulin sensitivity, control of fatty acids and accumulation of TAG in the liver, and progression to NASH and fibrosis. By the use of large genome-wide association studies (GWAS), several genes have been identified in conglomerates of patients with suspected fat by imaging studies and by histologically documented NAFLD, including patatin-like phospholipase domain-containing 3 (PNPLA3) rs738409-G, glucokinase regulator (GCKR) rs780094-T, neurocan (NCAN) rs2228603-T and lysophospholipase-like 1 (LYPLAL1) [61], MBOAT7-TMC4 rs12137855-C [62].

Two genes, PNPLA3 and TM6SF2, have been consistently found in association with NAFLD in the largest GWAS [63].

PNPLA3, which has lipolytic and lipogenic activities, is expressed in human adipose and liver tissue, where it is found on the surface of the lipid droplets in the hepatocytes [64, 65]. PNPLA3 encodes a 481 amino acid protein similar to the adipose triglyceride hydrolase of adipose tissue. The I148M variant of this gene, reported in association with NAFLD, disrupts triglyceride hydrolysis [66].

PNPLA3-rs738409, TM6SF2-rs58542916, and glucokinase regulator gene [GCKR]-rs780094 or GCKR-rs1260326 regulate metabolic traits. Genetic variants have been identified in association with hepatic steatosis in individuals from European ancestries at variants in or near the PNPLA3, NCAN, LYPLAL1, GCKR, and PPP1R3B. Testing in a cohort of African American and of Hispanic individuals documented that hepatic steatosis was 0.20–0.34 heritable in African- and Hispanic-American families, a statistically significant finding per cohort. Variants in or near PNPLA3, NCAN, GCKR, PPP1R3B in African Americans, and PNPLA3 and

PPP1R3B in Hispanic Americans were significantly associated with hepatic steato-sis. Fine-mapping in African Americans identified missense variants at PNPLA3 and GCKR and confirmed the association region at LYPLAL1 [67].

From a study that included over 9000 Hispanic, African American, and European American patients, the allele PNPLA3 (rs738409[G], encoding I148M) was reported as strongly associated with increased fat hepatic content and inflammation; the allele was most commonly present in Hispanics, with a greater fat liver content in PNPLA3 rs738409[G] homozygotes than in those who did not carry the allele. In contrast, the allele PNPLA3 (rs6006460[T], encoding S453I) was associated with a decrease in fat content in African Americans, which is the group in which NAFLD is the least common [68]. In addition, an also protective from NAFLD was the splice variant (rs72613567:TA) in HSD17B13, which was associated with a decreased risk for NASH, but not in steatosis [69].

TM6SF2 encodes a protein of 351 amino acids with 7–10 predicted transmem-brane domains, reported in the endoplasmic reticulum (ER) and the ER-Golgi inter-mediate compartment of human liver cells. One variant in *TM6SF2*, coding p.Glu167Lys, was identified in an exome-wide association study in association with high-fat content, as well as in decreased concentrations of low-density lipoprotein cholesterol (LDL-C) and triglycerides in a large group of patients in support of a role of TM6SF2 activity in the secretion of VLDL and thus in NAFLD [70]. Studies performed in human hepatoma Huh7 and HepG2 cells confirmed that inhibition of TM6SF2 is associated with increased triglycerides in hepatocytes and increased lipid droplet content, and a decrease in the secretion of TG-rich lipoproteins. In contrast, overexpression of TM6SF2 was related to a reduction of fat [71], data interpreted to confirm a role of this gene in regulating the metabolism of hepatic fat [71].

MBOAT7, also known as lysophosphatidylinositol acyltransferase 1 (LPIAT1), catalyzes acyl-chain remodeling of phosphatidylinositols [72]. The rs641738 C > T variant of the membrane bound O-acyltransferase domain-containing 7 (*MBOAT7*) was reported to increase the risk of fatty liver disease in individuals of European descent, interpreted to result from changes in the hepatic phosphatidylinositol acyl-chain remodeling [73], and development of fibrosis [62].

Although animal models to explore the association between this gene and NAFLD have been developed [66, 74], inconsistencies between laboratory animals and human studies exist [74]; thus, expert consensus supports the need for addi-tional research to clarify the role of PNPLA3 and any of the other proposed genes in the pathogenesis of NAFLD.

The genetic component of NAFLD and NASH concerns variants in genes that control glucose and fat metabolism with overlap with those related to the metabolic syndrome, with the activation of adiponectin and STAT3, retinol O-fatty-acyltransferase, and beta adrenergic activity [75].

## Clinical Manifestations

Patients may present with or without symptoms and signs of chronic liver disease, e.g., fatigue, spider angiomata, or frank decompensation, e.g., ascites. Physical findings in patients with NAFLD can be very telling, and include, in addition to those of chronic liver disease, acanthosis nigricans (Fig. 9.1) and central obesity. Waist circumference was reported to predict the metabolic risk profile, and dorsocervical lipohypertrophy in association with the severity of the inflammatory component of NAFLD, i.e. steatohepatitis [76]; thus, documenting these findings from the clinical evaluation would help categorize patients regarding the anticipated course from the initial clinical encounter.

The laboratory findings are a hepatic panel suggestive of hepatocellular injury, usually modest, although the activities of alkaline phosphatase and gamma glutamyl transpeptidase may also be increased, also modestly. When NAFLD is suspected, glycosylated hemoglobin (HA1C) and lipid panel should be included in the laboratory investigation. Serum autoantibodies can be present in patients with NAFLD, and were reported in 21% of 182 patients studied [77]; histologically, however, there was no documented difference in disease severity between patients with and without autoantibodies [77].

Radiological investigations, which usually start with a liver sonogram, tend to reveal heterogeneous liver parenchyma consistent with fat; imaging studies such as computed tomography and magnetic resonance imaging can be incorporated in the workup depending on the clinical suspicion.

The diagnosis of NAFLD is made by histology. In the writer's opinion, the indication for a liver biopsy depends mostly on how the results would change the patient's management. Information regarding fibrosis is relevant to the patient, to determine follow up, e.g., screening for hepatocellular carcinoma when a diagnosis of cirrhosis is suspected; thus, the use of non-invasive measures to predict the degree

**Fig. 9.1** Neck of a patient displaying finding consistent with acanthosis nigricans in association withnonalcoholic fatty liver disease

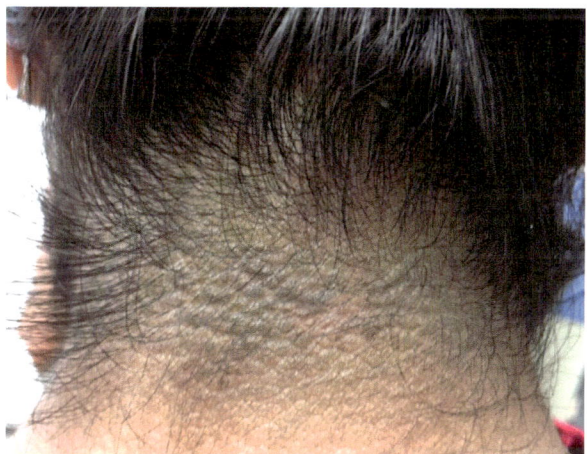

of fibrosis is useful. In this regard, transient elastography allows the indirect determination of steatosis and fibrosis, and its use has been incorporated in the evaluation of patients with NAFLD.

## Natural History

The progression from steatosis to cirrhosis has been documented in NAFLD; it tends to be slow, determined by fibrosis, and probably influenced by environmental factors and genetic predisposition [78–83]; in some patients, there is a regression of disease [80].

A study performed by an experienced group of investigators suggested that NAFLD be recognized as a cause of cryptogenic cirrhosis [84]. The study reported a slow disease progression in 42 patients, mostly women with metabolic syndrome features, followed over 21 years, with a median of 4.5 and a range of 1.5 to 21.5 [84]. Eighteen patients had fibrosis, one cirrhosis, and two severe fibrosis with altered architecture; on follow up, one patient exhibited progression from fibrosis to cirrhosis over five years, and those patients with marked fibrosis evolved to inactive cirrhosis devoid of fat and inflammation [84], finding reported in subsequent publications [85, 86].

A meta-analysis incorporated studies from 1985 to 2013 to assess the change from one stage to another on paired liver samples from biopsies performed at least 1 year apart [86]. Four hundred eleven patients, 150 with NAFLD and 261 with NASH, were identified. At baseline, the fibrosis stages were 0 for 35.8%, 1 for 32.5%, 2 for 16.7%, 3 in 9.3%, and 4 in 5.7%. Over 2145.5 person-years, the degree of fibrosis progressed in 33.6%, remained stable in 43.1%, and decreased in 22.3%. These findings were translated as progression by one stage over 14.3 years for patients with NAFLD, with a relatively wide CI of 9.1 to 50, and 7.1 years for patients with NASH, with a CI of 4.8 to 14.3 [86]. Collectively, the data tend to support that one third of patients with NAFLD progresses and that fibrosis is the predictor of such progression [86].

## Liver Histology

The histological components of NAFLD include: (i) steatosis (Fig. 9.2), usually starting in zone 3, (ii) inflammation, typically mild and comprised of lymphocytes, neutrophils, eosinophils, and Kupffer cells, (iii) ballooned hepatocytes (Fig. 9.2b), cells that have undergone disruption of their cytoskeleton, and exhibit aggregates of cytokeratins 8 and 18 dispersed to the periphery instead of their usual cytoplasmic presence [87, 88], and fibrosis that characteristically is perisinusoidal and, like steatosis, starts in zone 3 [87]. Mallory Denck bodies are irregular eosinophilic hyaline inclusions most commonly found in ballooned hepatocytes, usually in zone 3 [87,

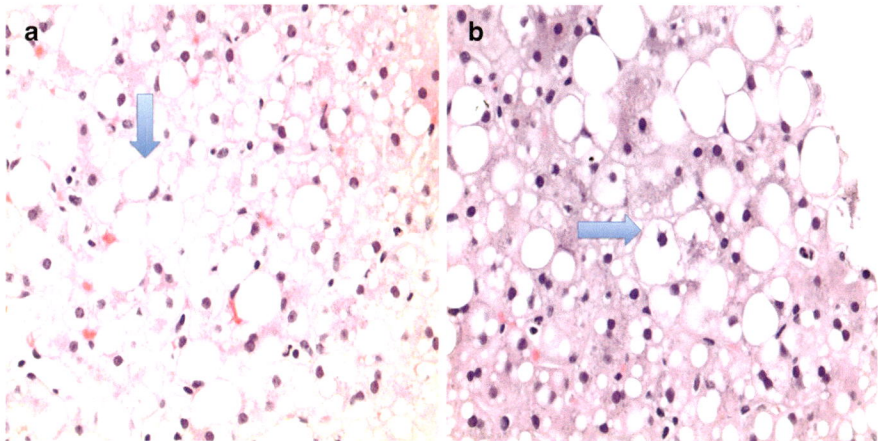

**Fig. 9.2** (**a**) Liver histology in a patient with nonalcoholic fatty liver disease exhibiting marked steatosis. Fat droplet (arrow) in a hepatocyte pushes the nucleus to the periphery of the cell. (**b**) Liver histology in a patient with nonalcoholic steatohepatitis and ballooning degeneration (arrow)

89]. Megamitochondria appear in all zones and hepatocytes with microvesicular fat [6]. Acidophilic bodies are hepatocytes that have undergone apoptosis and are typically found in NAFLD, usually in the sinusoids [90]. Glycogenated bodies are found in the liver in type 2 diabetes and are often found in NAFLD, which can differentiate NAFLD from alcoholic liver disease [91].

The NAFLD activity score (NAS), based on a revision from a prior score [92], was developed by the NAFLD research network and is comprised of the sum of semiquantitative scores, from 0 to 8. It consist of the following variables: 1) steatosis where 0 is <5% of fat in the sample, 1, 5–33%, 2, 34 to 66%, and 3 > 66%, 2) ballooning of hepatocytes where 0 is none, 1, mild and few, and 2 many, moderate, and marked, and 3) lobular inflammation, where 0 is none, 1 < 2 foci per 20× field, 2 is 2–4/20× field, 3 > 4/20× field [93, 94]. The stage of fibrosis is graded as: 0 for no significant fibrosis; 1a for delicate, perisinusoidal fibrosis in zone 3 where collagen stain is required for identification, 1b for dense perisinusoidal fibrosis in zone 3, and 1c for portal fibrosis only; 2 for zone 3 perisinusoidal fibrosis with periportal fibrosis; 3 for bridging fibrosis; and 4 for cirrhosis [93, 94]. A score of less than 3 and greater than 5 separates not NASH from NASH; however, when the score is greater than 5, the sensitivity and specificity of the NAS for the diagnosis of NASH is 57% and 95%, respectively, [95].

Histological information is of prognostic value; bad outcomes in patients with NAFLD occur more frequently in association with ballooning degeneration, Mallory bodies, and fibrosis than when these findings are absent [96]. Characteristically, NAFLD is devoid or associated with mild portal chronic inflammation, which, when more than mild, is related to increased age, female gender, high body mass index, high homeostasis model assessment of insulin resistance score (HOMA-IR), high insulin levels, diabetes, hypertension, and the use of medications to treat

NAFLD. Thus, it was concluded that more than mild portal chronic inflammation in NAFLD might be a marker of advanced disease [97]. The progression from NAFLD to NASH and fibrosis is variable; it was reported from a study that included 22 patients with NAFLD who had more than one liver biopsy over 5 years that a third increased in fibrosis score, the minority had a decrease, and the percentage of patients with fibrosis stages 3 and 4 doubled in follow up. In the minority, the disease progressed from fibrosis scores from 1 to 3 in less than 2 years, and from 2 to 4 in less than 3. The only test that correlated with histological progression was a high AST [78]; however, from a group of 106 patients with NASH, 22 underwent a repeat liver biopsy at least 3 years after the first one, in which fibrosis progression was documented in 32% of the patients, an outcome that correlated only with obesity and body mass index [79]. These series of observations helped to identify fibrosis as a prognostic factor for progression, for which evidence has been provided from a study that included 229 well-characterized patients with NAFLD who underwent follow up for an average of 26 years, and who exhibited increased mortality as compared to the reference population, with a hazard ratio (HR) of 1.29, CI: 1.04–1.59, $p = 0.020$, and increased risk for cardiovascular disease, hepatocellular carcinoma, and cirrhosis, all statistically significant. There was also an increase in mortality in patients with fibrosis stage 3 and 4, with HR 3.3, CI 2.27–4.76, $p < 0.001$, regardless of the NAS [98].

As reported above, liver histology is the gold standard to determine the state of disease, i.e., inflammation and fibrosis; however, the invasive nature of liver biopsy deters clinicians from the procedure in many cases; accordingly, efforts continue to establish the use of non-invasive tests for the diagnosis of NAFLD. In this regard, tests that include the NAFLD fibrosis score, the FIB-4, and FibroTest/Fibrosure have been adopted for clinical use and are available commercially. For example, the NAFLD fibrosis score is a measure that includes age, hyperglycemia, body mass index, platelet count, albumin, and AST/ALT ratio; a score of $-1.455$ excluded advanced fibrosis, and a score of 0.676 identified advanced fibrosis accurately [99]. These findings were confirmed in excluding advanced fibrosis in a study of patients from China [100]. The procedure of transient elastography concerns the measurement of a low frequency shear wave velocity transmitted via an ultrasound probe through the intercostal spaces over the liver area as an estimate of liver stiffness, measured in kilopaskals, which has been documented to correlate with fibrosis and cirrhosis [101–103]. Magnetic resonance elastography (MRE) in nonalcoholic fatty liver disease to assess liver fibrosis was reported to identify accurately the degree of fibrosis in patients with histologically proven NAFLD, independent from inflammation and obesity [103, 104]. In a study that included 58 patients with NAFLD, documented by liver histology, magnetic resonance elastography (MRE) was performed to assess liver stiffness, relative fat fraction, inflammatory activity, and fibrosis stage. Steatosis and inflammation without fibrosis had the significantly different scores of 2.5 and 3.24 kPa, respectively. Inflammation without fibrosis yielded a score lower than that of fibrosis, the latter being 4.16 kPa. A threshold of

2.74 kPa as a liver stiffness measures accurately differentiated patients with NASH from those with steatosis. These data supported the value of MRE to identify patients' inflammation before progression to fibrosis in NAFLD. This methodology is being explored widely as an alternative tool to assess liver disease from NAFLD [105].

## Inflammation: Its Potential Role in the Pathogenesis of NAFLD

Macrophage activation has been proposed as an initiator and perpetuator of NAFLD [106]. In the context of hepatic steatosis, from animal models, it is reported that hepatocytes release damage-associated molecular patterns (DAMPs) [107] and extracellular vesicles (EVs); in addition, diet components have an impact on the gut microbial environment [108, 109] and intestinal permeability, which, when increased [110], facilitates the vascular delivery of pathogen-associated molecular patterns (PAMPs) to the liver. This supportive hepatic microenvironment is associated with the release of inflammatory cytokines and chemokines, which can induce lipogenesis and recruit monocytes originating in the bone marrow, all of which can stimulate stellate cells and, thus, liver fibrosis [106]. Cluster of Differentiaion163 (CD163) is a macrophage specific protein with a soluble form, which, when activated, changes profile towards a participant in the inflammatory response [111]. The concentration of CD163 was reported to be significantly and independently associated with the degree of fibrosis in patients with NAFLD, findings that suggested a role of macrophages in fibrosis in association with this condition [112].

CD44 proteins are adhesion molecules [111] that may contribute to the pathogenesis of NAFLD. In obese patients, the soluble form of CD44 was increased in steatosis and NASH. CD44 liver expression was increased and correlated with features of NASH in obese patients. After bariatric surgery, "correction" of NASH was documented in association with decrease in the liver expression of CD-44. These findings suggested a role of CD44 in NASH and a therapeutic pathway [113].

## NAFLD Associated Diseases

Robust data to prove cause and effect between NAFLD and systemic complications appear to be lacking [114]; however, there is literature to support associations with several chronic conditions that render the individuals vulnerable to experience extrahepatic complications from the liver disease.

Cardiovascular disease is the most common association of NAFLD, which is an independent predictor of the former and informs the comorbidities that patients may experience. Data from a meta-analysis to quantify the association between NAFLD and events associated with cardiovascular disease documented from the 34,043 subjects included in the analysis, and of whom 36.3% had NAFLD that 2600 experienced a cardiovascular event, and over 70% of the group, death from cardiovascular disease over a period close to 7 years, with random effect odds ratio [OR] calculated as 1.64 (95% CI: 1.26–2.13). NAFLD was associated with a greater risk of experiencing a cardiovascular event, of a more severe impact if advanced liver disease was present (OR 2.58; 1.78–3.75) [115].

There is an association between type II DM and NAFLD; however, a genetic predisposition to support this association has not been unequivocally documented and, robust prospective studies in its support are lacking. In this context, the use of non-invasive indices to predict fatty liver, the fatty liver index, and the NAFLD fatty liver score (NAFLD-FLS) predicted the incidence of DM after 9 years of follow up, independently from glucose, family history, insulin, life style, smoking, and alcohol consumption, suggesting a screening measure to identify the development of DM in patients with NAFLD [116]. Also, in a prospective study from Europe that followed patients with histologically documented NAFLD for a mean of 13 years, 78% had diabetes or impaired glucose tolerance at follow up [81]. These studies support the idea that NAFLD is a predictor of insulin resistance and DM.

It was reported that NAFLD increases the risk of incident chronic kidney disease (CKD). The combination of nine observational studies that included 96,595 subjects, mostly Asian, 34% of whom had NAFLD, none histologically proven, documented that 4653 had incident CKD stage ≥3 over 5.2 years. In association with NAFLD, a significantly higher risk of incident CKD, especially in subjects with advanced liver disease, than in those without NAFLD was reported, with a random-effects HR of 1.37 (95% CI 1.20–1.53; $I^2$ = 33.5%). This analysis suggested that there is an approximately 40% increase in long-term incident CKD, although cause and effect could not be proven by the nature of the study [117].

The outcomes of eighteen cross-sectional studies that included 2183 subjects documented that the pooled OR for the presence of obstructive sleep apnea (OSA) and NAFLD diagnosed by histology was 2.01(95% CI: 1.36–2.97), with similar results for other indirect diagnostic means including radiographical and biochemical findings; in addition, the pooled ORs of OSA for NASH, fibrosis of any stage, or histologically documented advanced fibrosis were 2.37(1.59–3.51), 2.16(1.45–3.20), and 2.30(1.21–4.38), respectively, data that suggested that evaluation for the presence of NAFLD in patients with OSA is prudent [118]; in this regard, the importance of insulin resistance in association with OSA may be related to the reported occurrence [119].

Associations between polycystic ovarian syndrome (PCOS) and NAFLD have also been reported. A recent analysis of the world literature documented that the risk of NAFLD in patients with PCOS was significantly higher than that of controls when associated with hyperandrogenism [120].

Other associations with NAFLD have included cholelithiasis, psoriasis, and hypopituitarism [121].

# Lean Nonalcoholic Fatty Liver Disease

Some patients who are not obese and have insulin resistance are at risk for developing type 2 diabetes, hypertriglyceridemia, and early coronary artery disease [122]. This important and not small group of individuals also develop NAFLD in a lean body, i.e., lean NAFLD, as it is now termed, with a body mass index (BMI) within the ethnic-specific cutoff of 25 kg/m$^2$ in Caucasian and 23 kg/m$^2$ in Asian subjects.

The proportion of nonobese patients with NAFLD in epidemiological studies from Taiwan, Korea, and the United States comprised of Asian and Caucasian individuals ranged from 3.8 to 17% [12, 123–125].

Genetic polymorphisms have been identified in the genes PNPLA3, CETP, TMSF2, interferon lambda, and PENT as a predisposition for lean NAFLD. The pathophysiology of lean NAFLD includes an increase in the circulation of FFA, a decrease in adiponectin, insulin resistance, reduced mitochondrial function, increased de novo lipogenesis, decreased capacity to store fat in subcutaneous adipose tissue, decrease in muscle mass, and decreased Faecalibacterium and Ruminococcus and deficiency of lactobacillus. In this context, in mice, it was reported that the infusion of intestinal microbiota from lean donors to male recipients with metabolic syndrome was associated with an increase in insulin sensitivity in the latter and increased levels of intestinal microbiota that produce butyrate, which improves insulin sensitivity and increases energy expenditure [126].

From a study that used the NHANES III from 1988 to 1994 that included radiographic and laboratory data, and 11,613 subjects, of which 18.77% had NAFLD, and 11.78 of these, NASH, independent predictors of lean NAFLD were identified as relatively young age (i.e., median of 40 years), female gender, low probability of insulin resistance, and hypercholesterolemia, whereas Hispanic ethnicity, relatively young age, and components of the metabolic syndrome were independently associated with NASH, defined as suggestive imaging studies in association with type 2 DM, and with increased serum activity of transaminases [125]. From a European study, the relevance of lean NAFLD as a cause of cryptogenic liver disease was documented as 2.8% of a group of 1777 subjects all of whom had liver histology data, a contribution of 38% as a cause of cryptogenic liver disease [127]. Similar to the findings from the United States study [125], the patients were relatively young but, in contrast, most were men; fibrosis and steatohepatitis were present in more than 50% of the samples from patients with lean NAFLD [127].

There is limited information on the natural history of lean NAFLD. Published in abstract form, a study documented a follow up of 3 to 332 months of 1090 subjects, 11.5% of whom were reported as lean. The lean group was mostly comprised of men, non-Caucasian, and had a lower prevalence of diabetes, hypertension, hypertriglyceridemia, low-HDL cholesterol, central obesity, metabolic syndrome, less steatosis, lower levels of ALT, less advanced fibrosis, and less insulin resistance (HOMA) than the non-lean NAFLD group [128]. There was a significant difference in survival not in favor of lean subjects, even after statistical adjustment with only lean NAFLD and age, remaining significant, with HRs of 11.8 (95% CI: 2.8 to 50.1,

$p = 0.001$), and 1.05 (CI: 1.008 to 1.1, $p = 0.02$) [128]. In contrast, a study from Hong Kong that recruited 307 patients with NAFLD of whom 72 were nonobese, and who had less severe disease as suggested by lower NAS, and lower CAP score than their overweight counterparts were followed for a median of 49 months over which time, six from the group of obese patients died, two developed hepatocellular carcinoma, and one died of liver failure [129] suggesting that nonobese patients with NAFLD have a better prognosis than obese patients with NAFLD; however, in lean patients with NAFLD hypertriglyceridemia and a higher serum creatinine than the obese patients were factors associated with advanced disease [129]. Thus, the identification of these characteristics in lean patients with fatty liver may help in their follow up.

## Treatment

The treatment of NAFLD concerns the treatment of comorbidities and the search for specific treatment for its hepatic components, e.g., steatohepatitis and fibrosis.

Behavior modification is fundamental as an intervention, and has been associated with some improvement [130]; pharmacological interventions are expected to be identified for use in patients with advanced disease [131].

Lifestyle modification that included diet and exercise on NAFLD was associated with decreased inflammation and fibrosis. There was an improvement in glucose control and insulin sensitivity reported from most of the studies. These reports have supported the idea that behavior modification, i.e., diet and exercise associated with weight loss, could affect the histological lesions of fatty liver leading to improvement, in general [130]. The effects of an intensive lifestyle intervention program on portal hypertension in patients with compensated cirrhosis and obesity were recently reported from a prospective uncontrolled study. The study enrolled 60 patients, most of whom were men. The intervention was a behavior modification 16 week program that included low calorie and normal protein diet in association with supervised physical activity of 60 min/week. Fifty patients with a mean age of $56 \pm 8$ years old completed the study. Nonalcoholic steatohepatitis was reported in 24%, associated with hepatic venous pressure gradient (HVPG) $\geq 10$ mm Hg in 72% of the participants. The intervention was associated with a decrease in body weight by at least 5% and 10% in 52% and 16% of the subjects, a significant decrease in HVPG from $13.9 \pm 5.6$ to $12.3 \pm 5.2$ mm Hg; $p < 0.0001$) with a decrease of $\geq 10\%$ and $\geq 20\%$ in 42% and 24% of the participants, respectively. The decrease in HVPG was most substantial and significant in association with a weight loss of $\geq 10\%$, i.e. $-23.7 \pm 19.9\%$ vs. $-8.2 \pm 16.6\%$. The intervention was safe, and the weight loss documented at the end of the 16 week study period was sustained for six months [132]. This sophisticated study conducted by experts in the field of cirrhosis and portal hypertension remarkably revealed the importance of life style modification with a well delineated structure, and supports behavior modification as a fundamental aspect in the management of cirrhosis in association with obesity. This type of intervention should be considered in patients with NAFLD [84, 86].

Different medications according to the disease state and the mechanisms that can potentially influence the pathogenesis of NAFLD are being studied, including obeticholic acid, a farnesoid receptor agonist, the stimulation of which regulates lipogenesis and the conversion of cholesterol to bile acids in the steatosis phase, elafibranor, a PPAR alpha and beta agonist in steatosis and steatohepatitis phases, vitamin E, an antioxidant, liraglutide, a GLP 1 agonist, pioglitazone, a PPAR gamma agonist in steatohepatitis, selonsertib, an Ask-1 inhibitor, and ceniciviroc, a CCR2/CCR2 in the fibrosis stage [133].

In a prospective, randomized, placebo controlled, 96 week duration study of patients with NASH not associated with DM, vitamin E, an antioxidant [134], was associated with histological improvement related to inflammation but not in fibrosis as compared to placebo [135]. The effect of placebo was no different from that of pioglitazone, which was included in the study [135]. Pioglitazone is a nuclear receptor PPARγ agonist that increases insulin sensitivity [136]. Vitamin E is recommended for patients without DM with NASH at a dose of 800 IU per day.

In regard to vitamin E, and further to the study cited above [135], it was reported from a systematic review that vitamin E significantly decreased the degree of steatosis, hepatocyte ballooning, lobular inflammation, and fibrosis in patients with NASH, supporting its use in the treatment of this condition [137]. The guidelines from the American Association for the Study of Liver Disease (AASLD) state that vitamin E may be used in patients with NASH without DM and who do not exhibit cirrhosis on histology [138]. However, a retrospective study revealed that patients with advanced fibrosis and cirrhosis who took vitamin E at the dose stated above had a significantly higher adjusted transplant-free survival and a decrease in the rate of hepatic decompensation than those who did not take vitamin E, at a median follow-up up 5.62 (interquartile range [IQR], 4.3–7.5) and 5.6 (IQR, 4–6.9) years for those who took vitamin E versus those who did not. These findings applied to patients with and with DM [139]. Thus, considering the lack of adverse events in association with vitamin E, the use of this drug in patients with fibrosis and cirrhosis, irrespective of the presence of DM, may be a therapeutic option although data from robustly designed prospective studies are desired.

In a randomized, double blind, placebo controlled trial that included 101 patients with NASH and pre-diabetes, pioglitazone, at a dose of 45 mg/day in conjunction with a hypocaloric diet for a period of 18 months, was associated with a reduction of at least 2 points in the NAS in 58% of subjects, and resolution of NASH in 51%, and individual reductions in the fibrosis score, in contrast to placebo. In addition, hepatic triglyceride content decreased and adipose tissue, muscle, and hepatic insulin sensitivity were reported to have improved. The effects in association with pioglitazone persisted over 36 months of therapy, which was open label for an additional 18 months, and side effects were no different between the drug and placebo [140]. Consistent with the beneficial effects of pioglitazone, the AASLD indicates that this drug may be used to treat patients with NASH with or without type 2 DM; it is implicit in this recommendation that a liver histology is required prior to therapy [138].

Glucagon-like peptide 1 (GLP-1) is a peptide hormone produced in the intestinal epithelial endocrine cells and its function is to stimulate insulin secretion and to inhibit glucagon secretion thus contributing to modulated glucose excursions, to decrease gastrointestinal motility and secretion, and to regulate, in part, appetite [141]. In animal studies, GLP-1 analogues are associated with a reduction in liver steatosis, thus, the GLP-1 analogue liraglutide at doses of 1 and 8 mg subcutaneously once a week, was studied in a randomized, double blind, placebo controlled trial of 1 year duration in patients with steatohepatitis, from which it was reported that in patients who had a post treatment liver biopsy, 39% had resolution of NASH, versus those who were randomized to placebo. Fibrosis progressed in 9% of the patients on liraglutide versus 36% of those on placebo; diarrhea, constipation, and appetite loss were more common in the treatment group [142].

Obeticholic acid is a semi-synthetic bile acid analogue structured as 6α-ethyl-chenodeoxycholic that activates the farnesoid X nuclear receptor (FXR), a receptor that regulates genes involved in cholesterol catabolism and bile acids biosynthesis [143]. The activation of FRX is associated with the induction of Small Heterodimer Partner (SHP), a nuclear receptor that inhibits the production of bile acids, decreases the expression of Na+ taurocholate cotransport peptide (NTCP), a transporter of bile acids into the hepatocyte located in its sinusoidal side, and enhances the expression of the bile salt export pump (BSEP), the principal transporter of bile acids from the hepatocyte to the canalicular space, thus, protecting the liver from cholestasis induced liver injury. In animal models, obeticholic acid was reported to decrease steatosis and fibrosis. In a multicenter, double blind, placebo controlled, parallel group, randomized clinical trial of patients with NASH the administration of obeticholic acid at a dose of 25 mg per day was associated with improved liver histology, i.e., a decrease of two or more points in the total NAFLD activity score and no worsening in the fibrosis score, documented in 45% of the 110 subjects who had liver histology at baseline and 72 weeks, as planned, versus the improvement documented in the placebo group, which was in 21% of the 109 patients in whom liver biopsy was planned from that group. The findings on steatohepatitis, which were encouraging, were accompanied by an increase in total serum concentrations of cholesterol and LDL cholesterol, and a decrease in HDL cholesterol, posing concerns regarding cardiovascular health, a matter that remains under investigation. From A phase 3, double blind, randomized, placebo controlled multicenter study of obeticholic acid in patients with NASH and fibrosis stages 2 or 3 it was reported that the drug was associated with either improvement of fibrosis by equal or greater than one stage without worsening of NASH, or with its resolution without an increase in fibrosis, in 23.1% of 308 patients, randomized to a daily dose of 25 mg, versus, 17.6% of 312 randomized to 10 mg, both findings significantly different from placebo [144, 145]. Pruritus was a side effect documented in 23% of the patients [146], as reported in other studies with this medication [147].

PPARα receptor is at the center of all pathways related to fat metabolism; it has been characterized as the master regulator of hepatic lipid metabolism whereas its loss is associated with increased hepatic steatosis, and its activation with reduction of steatosis [148]. The activation of PPAR-δ is associated with a reduction of glucose use by skeletal muscle by switching the mitochondrial substrate preference from carbohydrates to lipids, increasing their combustion and exerting an antidiabetic effect in animals [149]. Elafibranor is an agonist of the PPAR-α and PPAR-δ. It was studied in doses of 80 and 120 mg/day in a randomized, double blind, placebo controlled study of 52 weeks duration in patients with NASH, which resolved without worsening of fibrosis in association with the highest dose of the drug in 19% of the patients versus 12% in the placebo group, with an OR of 2.31, and 95% CI: 1.02–5.24, and a $p = 0.045$ analysis provided as post hoc; however, the primary outcome, which was resolution of NASH without fibrosis worsening in an intention to treat analysis was not met as there was no significant difference between the treatment groups. Other improvements reported in association with elafibranor were lipids and glucose profiles. Of note, there was a significant, although reversible increase in serum creatinine in association with the drug [150]. A phase 3 study on the effect of elafibranor on steatohepatitis is being conducted [151].

Apoptosis contributes to the pathogenesis of NAFLD. In animal studies, inhibition of apoptosis through signal-regulating kinase 1, a serine/threonine kinase, has been reported to be associated with a decrease in inflammation and fibrosis [152]. In a human study, the safety and efficacy of selonsertib, a selective inhibitor of apoptosis signal-regulating kinase 1, alone or in combination with simtuzumab, a humanized monoclonal antibody that binds to LOX2, a molecule that interacts with collagen fibers, being studied for the treatment of fibrosis [153], was evaluated in a multicenter, phase 2 study of patients with NASH and stage 2 or 3 fibrosis. The results of this study were reported to document a decrease in the fibrosis by at least one stage in 43% and 30% of the 30 and 27 patients assigned to selonsertib 18 and 6 mg, respectively, findings confirmed by MRE, which was reported to show a decrease in liver stiffness, consistent with decreased fibrosis; in addition, liver collagen content and lobular inflammation decreased [154]. The lack of effect on fibrosis of simtuzumab in this study [154] was also reported in a subsequent publication [155]. A phase 3 trial on the effect of selonsertib for NASH has been completed [156].

Cenicriviroc is a dual antagonist of the chemokine receptors CCR5 and CCR2, the latter being a coreceptor involved in metabolic and cardiovascular diseases [157]. From a randomized, placebo controlled trial of cenicriviroc for treatment of NASH in patients with fibrosis it was reported that 150 mg of the drug was associated with a decrease in fibrosis by more than one stage in 20% of the 145 patients randomized to the drug in contrast to the 10% of the 144 randomized to placebo [158]. In follow up to this study, phase 3 studies are being conducted with cenicriviroc for the treatment of NAFLD and fibrosis [159, 160].

n-3 long-chain polyunsaturated fatty acids (LC-PUFAs) can prevent obesity, dyslipidemia, and insulin resistance in association with high-fat diet in animal models [161]. According to a meta-analysis, the use of n-3 LC-PUFAs, predominantly EPA and/or DHA supplementation, in patients with NAFLD was associated with a significant decrease in liver fat content, assessed by magnetic resonance imaging/

spectroscopy, and liver sonogram; however, no histological changes were reported in patients with NASH. These are encouraging findings and support the early identification of patients with steatosis for treatment with n-3 LC-PUFAs supplementation, however, the identification of factors that lead to progression from steatosis to steatohepatitis and to fibrosis remains a challenge in choosing patients who may benefit from that intervention. The investigators conclude that additional trials are necessary to understand the effects of LC-PUFAs on NAFLD [162].

Recently, from a prospective study over 2006 to 2015 that included 361 patients with NAFLD, daily use of aspirin was reported in association with a significant decrease in the risk for developing incident fibrosis versus nonaspirin users, effect that appeared to be related to the duration of aspirin use, with the highest benefit reported to be intake of aspirin for at least 4 years [163]. Surely, editorials and additional studies on this important observation will follow.

## Bariatric Surgery

The AASLD guidelines for the management of patients with NAFLD state that bariatric surgery can be considered in patients with obesity who meet criteria for the procedure [138].

From a prospective study that examined the effects of bariatric surgery on NAFLD in 381 patients without advanced disease, 56% of whom underwent gastric banding, 23%, biliointestinal bypass, and 21%, gastric bypass, it was reported that 5 years after the operation, the percentage of patients who had NASH decreased from 27.4% to 14.2%. The majority of patients exhibited significant increase in fibrosis, although assessed as equal or less than F1 [164], a finding that differs from that from a prospective study from which, at 1 year post surgery, the degree of fibrosis had decreased in 33.8% of the 109 patients [165]. The proportion of patients with steatosis decreased from 37.4% at baseline to 16 percent post surgery, with ballooning degeneration decreasing from 0.2 to 0.1, as per the NAFLD score [164]. The best predictor of persistence of steatosis and ballooning at 5 years post surgery was the presence of insulin resistance, which was suggested to be a good target for specific improvement post surgery in regard to liver disease [164]. From a systematic review and meta-analysis, it was reported that bariatric surgery was associated with a decrease in short-term mortality, and might be associated with long-term decrease in all-cause mortality, including cardiovascular disease and cancer [166]. However, from a review of the data in the Nationwide Inpatient Sample from patients who underwent bariatric surgery in the United States from 1998 to 2007 it was documented that patient without cirrhosis had a significantly lower mortality rate in association with the surgery, i.e. 0.3% than those with cirrhosis, compensated, 0.9% versus decompensated, 16.3%. Analysis after adjustment for covariates, the adjusted OR of mortality among patients with compensated cirrhosis was 2.17 (95% CI: 1.03–4.55) versus that of patients with decompensated cirrhosis, which was reported as 21.2% (95% CI: 5.39–82.9). As expected, the volume of surgery per center was associated with improved outcomes [167]. Accordingly, the decision to recommend bariatric surgery for the treatment of NAFLD requires a comprehensive assessment and collaboration with institutions with expertise in the procedures.

**Acknowledgments** The author acknowledges Dr. Cesar del Rosario for having contributed Figure 9.2.

# References

1. Neuschwander-Tetri BA, Caldwell SH. Nonalcoholic steatohepatitis: summary of an AASLD single topic conference. Hepatology. 2003 May;37(5):1202–19.
2. Younossi ZM, Marchesini G, Pinto-Cortez H, Petta S. Epidemiology of nonalcoholic fatty liver disease and nonalcoholic steatohepatitis: implications for liver transplantation. Transplantation. 2019 Jan;103(1):22–7.
3. Younossi ZM, Koenig AB, Abdelatif D, Fazel Y, Henry L, Wymer M. Global epidemiology of nonalcoholic fatty liver disease—meta-analytic assessment of prevalence, incidence, and outcomes. Hepatology. 2016 Jul;64(1):73–84.
4. Bellentani S. The epidemiology of non-alcoholic fatty liver disease. Liver Int. 2017 Jan;37(Suppl 1):81–4.
5. Le MH, Devaki P, Ha NB, Jun DW, Te HS, Cheung RC, et al. Prevalence of non-alcoholic fatty liver disease and risk factors for advanced fibrosis and mortality in the United States. PLoS One. 2017;12(3):e0173499.
6. Le TH, Caldwell SH, Redick JA, Sheppard BL, Davis CA, Arseneau KO, et al. The zonal distribution of megamitochondria with crystalline inclusions in nonalcoholic steatohepatitis. Hepatology. 2004 May;39(5):1423–9.
7. Wang AY, Dhaliwal J, Mouzaki M. Lean non-alcoholic fatty liver disease. Clin Nutr. 2019 Jun;38(3):975–81.
8. Dai G, Liu P, Li X, Zhou X, He S. Association between PNPLA3 rs738409 polymorphism and nonalcoholic fatty liver disease (NAFLD) susceptibility and severity: a meta-analysis. Medicine. 2019 Feb;98(7):e14324.
9. Zhu P, Lu H, Jing Y, Zhou H, Ding Y, Wang J, et al. Interaction between AGTR1 and PPARγ gene polymorphisms on the risk of nonalcoholic fatty liver disease. Genet Test Mol Biomarkers. 2019 Mar;23(3):166–75.
10. Liu J, Xing J, Wang B, Wei C, Yang R, Zhu Y, et al. Correlation between adiponectin gene rs1501299 polymorphism and nonalcoholic fatty liver disease susceptibility: a systematic review and meta-analysis. Med Sci Monit. 2019 Feb 8;25:1078–86.
11. Younossi ZM, Stepanova M, Afendy M, Fang Y, Younossi Y, Mir H, et al. Changes in the prevalence of the most common causes of chronic liver diseases in the United States from 1988 to 2008. Clin Gastroenterol Hepatol. 2011 June;9(6):524–30.
12. Browning JD, Szczepaniak LS, Dobbins R, Nuremberg P, Horton JD, Cohen JC, et al. Prevalence of hepatic steatosis in an urban population in the United States: impact of ethnicity. Hepatology. 2004 Dec;40(6):1387–95.
13. Dixon JB, Bhathal PS, O'Brien PE. Nonalcoholic fatty liver disease: predictors of nonalcoholic steatohepatitis and liver fibrosis in the severely obese. Gastroenterology. 2001 Jul;121(1):91–100.
14. Unger RH. Minireview: weapons of lean body mass destruction: the role of ectopic lipids in the metabolic syndrome. Endocrinology. 2003 Dec;144(12):5159–65.

15. Donnelly KL, Smith CI, Schwarzenberg SJ, Jessurun J, Boldt MD, Parks EJ. Sources of fatty acids stored in liver and secreted via lipoproteins in patients with nonalcoholic fatty liver disease. J Clin Invest. 2005 May;115(5):1343–51.
16. Puri P, Baillie RA, Wiest MM, Mirshahi F, Choudhury J, Cheung O, et al. A lipidomic analysis of nonalcoholic fatty liver disease. Hepatology. 2007 Oct;46(4):1081–90.
17. Malhi H, Barreyro FJ, Isomoto H, Bronk SF, Gores GJ. Free fatty acids sensitise hepatocytes to TRAIL mediated cytotoxicity. Gut. 2007 Aug;56(8):1124–31.
18. Feldstein AE, Canbay A, Angulo P, Taniai M, Burgart LJ, Lindor KD, et al. Hepatocyte apoptosis and fas activation are prominent features of human nonalcoholic steatohepatitis. Gastroenterology. 2003 Aug;125(2):437–43.
19. Ribeiro PS, Cortez-Pinto H, Sola S, Castro RE, Ramalho RM, Baptista A, et al. Hepatocyte apoptosis, expression of death receptors, and activation of NF-kappaB in the liver of nonalcoholic and alcoholic steatohepatitis patients. Am J Gastroenterol. 2004 Sep;99(9):1708–17.
20. Wieckowska A, Zein NN, Yerian LM, Lopez AR, McCullough AJ, Feldstein AE. In vivo assessment of liver cell apoptosis as a novel biomarker of disease severity in nonalcoholic fatty liver disease. Hepatology. 2006 Jul;44(1):27–33.
21. Allard JP, Aghdassi E, Mohammed S, Raman M, Avand G, Arendt BM, et al. Nutritional assessment and hepatic fatty acid composition in non-alcoholic fatty liver disease (NAFLD): a cross-sectional study. J Hepatol. 2008 Feb;48(2):300–7.
22. Listenberger LL, Han X, Lewis SE, Cases S, Farese RV Jr, Ory DS, et al. Triglyceride accumulation protects against fatty acid-induced lipotoxicity. Proc Natl Acad Sci U S A. 2003 Mar 18;100(6):3077–82.
23. Malhi H, Bronk SF, Werneburg NW, Gores GJ. Free fatty acids induce JNK-dependent hepatocyte lipoapoptosis. J Biol Chem. 2006 Apr 28;281(17):12093–101.
24. Feldstein AE, Werneburg NW, Canbay A, Guicciardi ME, Bronk SF, Rydzewski R, et al. Free fatty acids promote hepatic lipotoxicity by stimulating TNF-alpha expression via a lysosomal pathway. Hepatology. 2004 Jul;40(1):185–94.
25. Puri P, Mirshahi F, Cheung O, Natarajan R, Maher JW, Kellum JM, et al. Activation and dysregulation of the unfolded protein response in nonalcoholic fatty liver disease. Gastroenterology. 2008 Feb;134(2):568–76.
26. Mari M, Caballero F, Colell A, Morales A, Caballeria J, Fernandez A, et al. Mitochondrial free cholesterol loading sensitizes to TNF- and Fas-mediated steatohepatitis. Cell Metab. 2006 Sep;4(3):185–98.
27. Ioannou GN. The role of cholesterol in the pathogenesis of NASH. Trends Endocrinol Metab. 2016 Feb;27(2):84–95.
28. Sanyal AJ, Campbell-Sargent C, Mirshahi F, Rizzo WB, Contos MJ, Sterling RK, et al. Nonalcoholic steatohepatitis: association of insulin resistance and mitochondrial abnormalities. Gastroenterology. 2001 Apr;120(5):1183–92.
29. Chalasani N, Deeg MA, Crabb DW. Systemic levels of lipid peroxidation and its metabolic and dietary correlates in patients with nonalcoholic steatohepatitis. Am J Gastroenterol. 2004 Aug;99(8):1497–502.
30. Seki S, Kitada T, Sakaguchi H. Clinicopathological significance of oxidative cellular damage in non-alcoholic fatty liver diseases. Hepatol Res. 2005 Oct;33(2):132–4.
31. Malhi H, Gores GJ. Molecular mechanisms of lipotoxicity in nonalcoholic fatty liver disease. Semin Liver Dis. 2008 Nov;28(4):360–9.
32. Kong L, Lu Y, Zhang S, Nan Y, Qiao L. Role of nutrition, gene polymorphism, and gut microbiota in non-alcoholic fatty liver disease. Discov Med. 2017 Sep;24(131):95–106.
33. Videla LA, Pettinelli P. Misregulation of PPAR functioning and its pathogenic consequences associated with nonalcoholic fatty liver disease in human obesity. PPAR Res. 2012;2012:107434.
34. Lee J, Kim Y, Friso S, Choi SW. Epigenetics in non-alcoholic fatty liver disease. Mol Asp Med. 2017 Apr;54:78–88.

35. Chow MD, Lee YH, Guo GL. The role of bile acids in nonalcoholic fatty liver disease and nonalcoholic steatohepatitis. Mol Asp Med. 2017 Aug;56:34–44.
36. Wang Y, Viscarra J, Kim S-J, Sul HS. Transcriptional regulation of hepatic lipogenesis. Nat Rev Mol Cell Biol. 2015;16(11):678–89.
37. Francque S, Verrijken A, Caron S, Prawitt J, Paumelle R, Derudas B, et al. PPARα gene expression correlates with severity and histological treatment response in patients with non-alcoholic steatohepatitis. J Hepatol. 2015 Jul;63(1):164–73.
38. Tanaka T, Yamamoto J, Iwasaki S, Asaba H, Hamura H, Ikeda Y, et al. Activation of peroxisome proliferator-activated receptor delta induces fatty acid beta-oxidation in skeletal muscle and attenuates metabolic syndrome. Proc Natl Acad Sci U S A. 2003 Dec 23;100(26):15924–9.
39. Pawlak M, Lefebvre P, Staels B. Molecular mechanism of PPARalpha action and its impact on lipid metabolism, inflammation and fibrosis in non-alcoholic fatty liver disease. J Hepatol. 2015 Mar;62(3):720–33.
40. Pettinelli P, Videla LA. Up-regulation of PPAR-gamma mRNA expression in the liver of obese patients: an additional reinforcing lipogenic mechanism to SREBP-1c induction. J Clin Endocrinol Metab. 2011 May;96(5):1424–30.
41. Vidal-Puig AJ, Considine RV, Jimenez-Linan M, Werman A, Pories WJ, Caro JF, et al. Peroxisome proliferator-activated receptor gene expression in human tissues. Effects of obesity, weight loss, and regulation by insulin and glucocorticoids. J Clin Invest. 1997 May 15;99(10):2416–22.
42. Ribot J, Rantala M, Kesaniemi YA, Palou A, Savolainen MJ. Weight loss reduces expression of SREBP1c/ADD1 and PPARgamma2 in adipose tissue of obese women. Pflugers Arch. 2001 Jan;441(4):498–505.
43. Nakamuta M, Kohjima M, Morizono S, Kotoh K, Yoshimoto T, Miyagi I, et al. Evaluation of fatty acid metabolism-related gene expression in nonalcoholic fatty liver disease. Int J Mol Med. 2005 Oct;16(4):631–5.
44. Rae C, Robertson SA, Taylor JM, Graham A. Resistin induces lipolysis and re-esterification of triacylglycerol stores, and increases cholesteryl ester deposition, in human macrophages. FEBS Lett. 2007 Oct 16;581(25):4877–83.
45. Cheung O, Sanyal AJ. Abnormalities of lipid metabolism in nonalcoholic fatty liver disease. Semin Liver Dis. 2008 Nov;28(4):351–9.
46. Unger RH. Lipotoxic diseases. Annu Rev Med. 2002;53:319–36.
47. Montgomery MK, De Nardo W, Watt MJ. Impact of lipotoxicity on tissue "cross talk" and metabolic regulation. Physiology. 2019 Mar 1;34(2):134–49.
48. Wei Y, Rector RS, Thyfault JP, Ibdah JA. Nonalcoholic fatty liver disease and mitochondrial dysfunction. World J Gastroenterol. 2008 Jan 14;14(2):193–9.
49. Chalasani N, Gorski JC, Asghar MS, Asghar A, Foresman B, Hall SD, et al. Hepatic cytochrome P450 2E1 activity in nondiabetic patients with nonalcoholic steatohepatitis. Hepatology. 2003 Mar;37(3):544–50.
50. Bartel DP. MicroRNAs: target recognition and regulatory functions. Cell. 2009 Jan 23;136(2):215–33.
51. Cermelli S, Ruggieri A, Marrero JA, Ioannou GN, Beretta L. Circulating microRNAs in patients with chronic hepatitis C and non-alcoholic fatty liver disease. PLoS One. 2011;6(8):e23937.
52. Pirola CJ, Fernandez Gianotti T, Castano GO, Mallardi P, San Martino J, Mora Gonzalez Lopez Ledesma M, et al. Circulating microRNA signature in non-alcoholic fatty liver disease: from serum non-coding RNAs to liver histology and disease pathogenesis. Gut. 2015 May;64(5):800–12.
53. Szabo G, Csak T. Role of MicroRNAs in NAFLD/NASH. Dig Dis Sci. 2016 May;61(5):1314–24.
54. Liu CH, Ampuero J, Gil-Gomez A, Montero-Vallejo R, Rojas A, Munoz-Hernandez R, et al. miRNAs in patients with non-alcoholic fatty liver disease: A systematic review and meta-analysis. J Hepatol. 2018 Dec;69(6):1335–48.

55. Yerragorla P, Nepal P, Nekkalapudi D, et al. Prevalence of sarcopenia Access. 2020;11(4): 153–155. https://doi.org/10.15406/ghoa.2020.11.00432[page2image173863232].

56. Willner IR, Waters B, Patil SR, Reuben A, Morelli J, Riely CA. Ninety patients with non-alcoholic steatohepatitis: insulin resistance, familial tendency, and severity of disease. Am J Gastroenterol. 2001 Oct;96(10):2957–61.

57. Struben VM, Hespenheide EE, Caldwell SH. Nonalcoholic steatohepatitis and cryptogenic cirrhosis within kindreds. Am J Med. 2000 Jan;108(1):9–13.

58. Schwimmer JB, Celedon MA, Lavine JE, Salem R, Campbell N, Schork NJ, et al. Heritability of nonalcoholic fatty liver disease. Gastroenterology. 2009 May;136(5):1585–92.

59. Makkonen J, Pietilainen KH, Rissanen A, Kaprio J, Yki-Jarvinen H. Genetic factors contribute to variation in serum alanine aminotransferase activity independent of obesity and alcohol: a study in monozygotic and dizygotic twins. J Hepatol. 2009 May;50(5):1035–42.

60. Bambha K, Belt P, Abraham M, Wilson LA, Pabst M, Ferrell L, et al. Ethnicity and nonalcoholic fatty liver disease. Hepatology. 2012 Mar;55(3):769–80.

61. Speliotes EK, Yerges-Armstrong LM, Wu J, Hernaez R, Kim LJ, Palmer CD, et al. Genome-wide association analysis identifies variants associated with nonalcoholic fatty liver disease that have distinct effects on metabolic traits. PLoS Genet. 2011 Mar;7(3):e1001324.

62. Mancina RM, Dongiovanni P, Petta S, Pingitore P, Meroni M, Rametta R, et al. The MBOAT7-TMC4 variant rs641738 increases risk of nonalcoholic fatty liver disease in individuals of European descent. Gastroenterology. 2016 May;150(5):1219–30.

63. Spielman RSE, Ewens WJ. The TDT and other family-based tests for linkage disequilibrium and association. Am J Hum Genet. 1996;59(5):983–9.

64. Romeo S, Huang-Doran I, Baroni MG, Kotronen A. Unravelling the pathogenesis of fatty liver disease: patatin-like phospholipase domain-containing 3 protein. Curr Opin Lipidol. 2010 Jun;21(3):247–52.

65. Zimmermann R, Strauss JG, Haemmerle G, Schoiswohl G, Birner-Gruenberger R, Riederer M, et al. Fat mobilization in adipose tissue is promoted by adipose triglyceride lipase. Science. 2004 Nov 19;306(5700):1383–6.

66. He S, McPhaul C, Li JZ, Garuti R, Kinch L, Grishin NV, et al. A sequence variation (I148M) in PNPLA3 associated with nonalcoholic fatty liver disease disrupts triglyceride hydrolysis. J Biol Chem. 2010 Feb 26;285(9):6706–15.

67. Palmer ND, Musani SK, Yerges-Armstrong LM, Feitosa MF, Bielak LF, Hernaez R, et al. Characterization of European ancestry nonalcoholic fatty liver disease-associated variants in individuals of African and Hispanic descent. Hepatology. 2013 Sep;58(3):966–75.

68. Romeo S, Kozlitina J, Xing C, Pertsemlidis A, Cox D, Pennacchio LA, et al. Genetic variation in PNPLA3 confers susceptibility to nonalcoholic fatty liver disease. Nat Genet. 2008 Dec;40(12):1461–5.

69. Abul-Husn NS, Cheng X, Li AH, Xin Y, Schurmann C, Stevis P, et al. A protein-truncating HSD17B13 variant and protection from chronic liver disease. N Engl J Med. 2018 Mar 22;378(12):1096–106.

70. Kozlitina J, Smagris E, Stender S, Nordestgaard BG, Zhou HH, Tybjaerg-Hansen A, et al. Exome-wide association study identifies a TM6SF2 variant that confers susceptibility to non-alcoholic fatty liver disease. Nat Genet. 2014 Apr;46(4):352–6.

71. Mahdessian H, Taxiarchis A, Popov S, Silveira A, Franco-Cereceda A, Hamsten A, et al. TM6SF2 is a regulator of liver fat metabolism influencing triglyceride secretion and hepatic lipid droplet content. Proc Natl Acad Sci U S A. 2014 Jun 17;111(24):8913–8.

72. D'Souza K, Epand RM. Enrichment of phosphatidylinositols with specific acyl chains. Biochim Biophys Acta. 2014 Jun;1838(6):1501–8.

73. Luukkonen PK, Zhou Y, Hyotylainen T, Leivonen M, Arola J, Orho-Melander M, et al. The MBOAT7 variant rs641738 alters hepatic phosphatidylinositols and increases severity of non-alcoholic fatty liver disease in humans. J Hepatol. 2016 Dec;65(6):1263–5.

74. Lau JKC, Zhang X, Yu J. Animal models of non-alcoholic fatty liver diseases and its associated liver Cancer. Adv Exp Med Biol. 2018;1061:139–47.

75. Sookoian S, Pirola CJ. Genetics of nonalcoholic fatty liver disease: from pathogenesis to therapeutics. Semin Liver Dis. 2019 May;39(2):124–40.
76. Cheung O, Kapoor A, Puri P, Sistrun S, Luketic VA, Sargeant CC, et al. The impact of fat distribution on the severity of nonalcoholic fatty liver disease and metabolic syndrome. Hepatology. 2007 Oct;46(4):1091–100.
77. Vuppalanchi R, Gould RJ, Wilson LA, Unalp-Arida A, Cummings OW, Chalasani N, et al. Clinical significance of serum autoantibodies in patients with NAFLD: results from the nonalcoholic steatohepatitis clinical research network. Hepatol Int. 2012 Jan;6(1):379–85.
78. Harrison SA, Torgerson S, Hayashi PH. The natural history of nonalcoholic fatty liver disease: a clinical histopathological study. Am J Gastroenterol. 2003 Sep;98(9):2042–7.
79. Fassio E, Alvarez E, Dominguez N, Landeira G, Longo C. Natural history of nonalcoholic steatohepatitis: a longitudinal study of repeat liver biopsies. Hepatology. 2004 Oct;40(4): 820–6.
80. Adams LA, Sanderson S, Lindor KD, Angulo P. The histological course of nonalcoholic fatty liver disease: a longitudinal study of 103 patients with sequential liver biopsies. J Hepatol. 2005 Jan;42(1):132–8.
81. Ekstedt M, Franzen LE, Mathiesen UL, Thorelius L, Holmqvist M, Bodemar G, et al. Long-term follow-up of patients with NAFLD and elevated liver enzymes. Hepatology. 2006 Oct;44(4):865–73.
82. Wong VW, Wong GL, Choi PC, Chan AW, Li MK, Chan HY, et al. Disease progression of non-alcoholic fatty liver disease: a prospective study with paired liver biopsies at 3 years. Gut. 2010 Jul;59(7):969–74.
83. Pais R, Charlotte F, Fedchuk L, Bedossa P, Lebray P, Poynard T, et al. A systematic review of follow-up biopsies reveals disease progression in patients with non-alcoholic fatty liver. J Hepatol. 2013 Sep;59(3):550–6.
84. Powell EE, Cooksley WG, Hanson R, Searle J, Halliday JW, Powell LW. The natural history of nonalcoholic steatohepatitis: a follow-up study of forty-two patients for up to 21 years. Hepatology. 1990 Jan;11(1):74–80.
85. Caldwell SH, Lee VD, Kleiner DE, Al-Osaimi AM, Argo CK, Northup PG, et al. NASH and cryptogenic cirrhosis: a histological analysis. Ann Hepatol. 2009 Oct–Dec;8(4):346–52.
86. Singh S, Allen AM, Wang Z, Prokop LJ, Murad MH, Loomba R. Fibrosis progression in non-alcoholic fatty liver vs nonalcoholic steatohepatitis: a systematic review and meta-analysis of paired-biopsy studies. Clin Gastroenterol Hepatol. 2015 Apr;13(4):643–54.e1-9.
87. Brunt EM. Pathology of nonalcoholic fatty liver disease. Nat Rev Gastroenterol Hepatol. 2010 Apr;7(4):195–203.
88. Lackner C, Gogg-Kamerer M, Zatloukal K, Stumptner C, Brunt EM, Denk H. Ballooned hepatocytes in steatohepatitis: the value of keratin immunohistochemistry for diagnosis. J Hepatol. 2008 May;48(5):821–8.
89. Denk H, Stumptner C, Zatloukal K. Mallory bodies revisited. J Hepatol. 2000 Apr;32(4):689–702.
90. Feldstein AE, Gores GJ. Apoptosis in alcoholic and nonalcoholic steatohepatitis. Front Biosci. 2005 Sep 1;10:3093–9.
91. Pinto HC, Baptista A, Camilo ME, Valente A, Saragoca A, de Moura MC. Nonalcoholic steatohepatitis. Clinicopathological comparison with alcoholic hepatitis in ambulatory and hospitalized patients. Dig Dis Sci. 1996 Jan;41(1):172–9.
92. Brunt EM, Janney CG, Di Bisceglie AM, Neuschwander-Tetri BA, Bacon BR. Nonalcoholic steatohepatitis: a proposal for grading and staging the histological lesions. Am J Gastroenterol. 1999 Sep;94(9):2467–74.
93. Network CR. Nonalcoholic steatohepatitis clinical research network. Hepatology. 2003;37(2):244.
94. Kleiner DE, Brunt EM, Van Natta M, Behling C, Contos MJ, Cummings OW, et al. Design and validation of a histological scoring system for nonalcoholic fatty liver disease. Hepatology. 2005 Jun;41(6):1313–21.

95. Hjelkrem M, Stauch C, Shaw J, Harrison SA. Validation of the non-alcoholic fatty liver disease activity score. Aliment Pharmacol Ther. 2011 Jul;34(2):214–8.
96. Matteoni CA, Younossi ZM, Gramlich T, Boparai N, Liu YC, McCullough AJ. Nonalcoholic fatty liver disease: a spectrum of clinical and pathological severity. Gastroenterology. 1999 June;116(6):1413–9.
97. Brunt EM, Kleiner DE, Wilson LA, Unalp A, Behling CE, Lavine JE, et al. Portal chronic inflammation in nonalcoholic fatty liver disease (NAFLD): a histologic marker of advanced NAFLD-clinicopathologic correlations from the nonalcoholic steatohepatitis clinical research network. Hepatology. 2009 Mar;49(3):809–20.
98. Ekstedt M, Hagstrom H, Nasr P, Fredrikson M, Stal P, Kechagias S, et al. Fibrosis stage is the strongest predictor for disease-specific mortality in NAFLD after up to 33 years of follow-up. Hepatology. 2015 May;61(5):1547–54.
99. Angulo PH, Hui JM, Marchesini G, Bugianesi E, George J, Farrell GC, Enders F, Sushma S, Burt AD, Bida JP, Lindor K, Sanderson SO, Schuyler O, Lenzi M, Adams LA, Kench J, Therneau TM, Day CP. The NAFLD fibrosis score: a noninvasive system that identifies liver fibrosis in patients with NAFLD. Hepatology. 2007;45(4):846–54.
100. Wong VW, Wong GL, Chim AM, Tse AM, Tsang SW, Hui AY, et al. Validation of the NAFLD fibrosis score in a Chinese population with low prevalence of advanced fibrosis. Am J Gastroenterol. 2008 Jul;103(7):1682–8.
101. Sandrin L, Fourquet B, Hasquenoph JM, Yon S, Fournier C, Mal F, et al. Transient elastography: a new noninvasive method for assessment of hepatic fibrosis. Ultrasound Med Biol. 2003 Dec;29(12):1705–13.
102. Foucher J, Chanteloup E, Vergniol J, Castera L, Le Bail B, Adhoute X, et al. Diagnosis of cirrhosis by transient elastography (FibroScan): a prospective study. Gut. 2006 Mar;55(3):403–8.
103. Cheah MC, McCullough AJ, Goh GB. Current modalities of fibrosis assessment in non-alcoholic fatty liver disease. J Clin Transl Hepatol. 2017 Sep 28;5(3):261–71.
104. Singh S, Venkatesh SK, Loomba R, Wang Z, Sirlin C, Chen J, et al. Magnetic resonance elastography for staging liver fibrosis in non-alcoholic fatty liver disease: a diagnostic accuracy systematic review and individual participant data pooled analysis. Eur Radiol. 2016 May;26(5):1431–40.
105. Chen J, Talwalkar JA, Meng Y, Glaser KJ, Sanderson SO, Ehman RL. Early detection of nonalcoholic steatohepatitis in patients with nonalcoholic fatty liver disease by using MR elastography. Radiology. 2011;259(3):749–56.
106. Duarte N, Coelho IC, Patarrao RS, Almeida JI, Penha-Goncalves C, Macedo MP. How inflammation impinges on NAFLD: a role for Kupffer cells. Biomed Res Int. 2015;2015:984578.
107. Li L, Chen L, Hu L, Liu Y, Sun HY, Tang J, et al. Nuclear factor high-mobility group box1 mediating the activation of Toll-like receptor 4 signaling in hepatocytes in the early stage of nonalcoholic fatty liver disease in mice. Hepatology. 2011 Nov;54(5):1620–30.
108. Tremaroli V, Backhed F. Functional interactions between the gut microbiota and host metabolism. Nature. 2012 Sep 13;489(7415):242–9.
109. Leung C, Rivera L, Furness JB, Angus PW. The role of the gut microbiota in NAFLD. Nat Rev Gastroenterol Hepatol. 2016 Jul;13(7):412–25.
110. Tran CD, Grice DM, Wade B, Kerr CA, Bauer DC, Li D, et al. Gut permeability, its interaction with gut microflora and effects on metabolic health are mediated by the lymphatics system, liver and bile acid. Future Microbiol. 2015;10(8):1339–53.
111. Goodison S, Urquidi V, Tarin D. CD44 cell adhesion molecules. Mol Pathol. 1999 Aug;52(4):189–96.
112. Kazankov K, Barrera F, Moller HJ, Rosso C, Bugianesi E, David E, et al. The macrophage activation marker sCD163 is associated with morphological disease stages in patients with non-alcoholic fatty liver disease. Liver Int. 2016 Oct;36(10):1549–57.
113. Patouraux S, Rousseau D, Bonnafous S, Lebeaupin C, Luci C, Canivet CM, et al. CD44 is a key player in non-alcoholic steatohepatitis. J Hepatol. 2017 Aug;67(2):328–38.

114. Danford CJ, Yao ZM, Jiang ZG. Non-alcoholic fatty liver disease: a narrative review of genetics. J Biomed Res. 2018 Nov 20;32(5):389–400.

115. Targher G, Byrne CD, Lonardo A, Zoppini G, Barbui C. Non-alcoholic fatty liver disease and risk of incident cardiovascular disease: A meta-analysis. J Hepatol. 2016 Sep;65(3): 589–600.

116. Balkau B, Lange C, Vol S, Fumeron F, Bonnet F, Group Study DESIR. Nine-year incident diabetes is predicted by fatty liver indices: the French D.E.S.I.R. study. BMC Gastroenterol. 2010 June 7;10:56.

117. Mantovani A, Zaza G, Byrne CD, Lonardo A, Zoppini G, Bonora E, et al. Nonalcoholic fatty liver disease increases risk of incident chronic kidney disease: a systematic review and meta-analysis. Metab Clin Exp. 2018 Feb;79:64–76.

118. Musso G, Cassader M, Olivetti C, Rosina F, Carbone G, Gambino R. Association of obstructive sleep apnoea with the presence and severity of non-alcoholic fatty liver disease. A systematic review and meta-analysis. Obes Rev. 2013 May;14(5):417–31.

119. Almendros I, Garcia-Rio F. Sleep apnoea, insulin resistance and diabetes: the first step is in the fat. Eur Respir J. 2017 Apr;49(4):1700179.

120. Wu J, Yao XY, Shi RX, Liu SF, Wang XY. A potential link between polycystic ovary syndrome and non-alcoholic fatty liver disease: an update meta-analysis. Reprod Health. 2018 May 10;15(1):77.

121. Armstrong MJ, Adams LA, Canbay A, Syn WK. Extrahepatic complications of nonalcoholic fatty liver disease. Hepatology. 2014 Mar;59(3):1174–97.

122. Ruderman N, Chisholm D, Pi-Sunyer X, Schneider S. The metabolically obese, normal-weight individual revisited. Diabetes. 1998 May;47(5):699–713.

123. Das K, Das K, Mukherjee PS, Ghosh A, Ghosh S, Mridha AR, et al. Nonobese population in a developing country has a high prevalence of nonalcoholic fatty liver and significant liver disease. Hepatology. 2010 May;51(5):1593–602.

124. Chen CH, Huang MH, Yang JC, Nien CK, Yang CC, Yeh YH, et al. Prevalence and risk factors of nonalcoholic fatty liver disease in an adult population of Taiwan: metabolic significance of nonalcoholic fatty liver disease in nonobese adults. J Clin Gastroenterol. 2006 Sep;40(8):745–52.

125. Younossi ZM, Stepanova M, Negro F, Hallaji S, Younossi Y, Lam B, et al. Nonalcoholic fatty liver disease in lean individuals in the United States. Medicine. 2012 Nov;91(6):319–27.

126. Gao Z, Yin J, Zhang J, Ward RE, Martin RJ, Lefevre M, et al. Butyrate improves insulin sensitivity and increases energy expenditure in mice. Diabetes. 2009 Jul;58(7):1509–17.

127. Vos B, Moreno C, Nagy N, Fery F, Cnop M, Vereerstraeten P, et al. Lean non-alcoholic fatty liver disease (lean-NAFLD): a major cause of cryptogenic liver disease. Acta Gastro-Enterol Belg. 2011 Sep;74(3):389–94.

128. Dela Cruz AC, Bugianesi E, George J, Day CP, Liaquat H, Charatcharoenwitthaya P, Mills PR, Dam-Larsen S, Bjornsson ES, Haflidadottir S, Adams LA, Bendtsen F, Angulo P. Characteristics and long-term prognosis of lean patients with nonalcoholic fatty liver disease. Gastroenterology. 2014;146:S-909.

129. Leung JC, Loong TC, Wei JL, Wong GL, Chan AW, Choi PC, et al. Histological severity and clinical outcomes of nonalcoholic fatty liver disease in nonobese patients. Hepatology. 2017 Jan;65(1):54–64.

130. Thoma C, Day CP, Trenell MI. Lifestyle interventions for the treatment of non-alcoholic fatty liver disease in adults: a systematic review. J Hepatol. 2012 Jan;56(1):255–66.

131. Povsic M, Oliver L, Jiandani NR, Perry R, Bottomley J. A structured literature review of interventions used in the management of nonalcoholic steatohepatitis (NASH). Pharmacol Res Perspect. 2019 Jun;7(3):e00485.

132. Berzigotti A, Albillos A, Villanueva C, Genesca J, Ardevol A, Augustin S, Calleja JL, Bosch J. Effects of an intensive lifestyle intervention program on portal hypertension in patients with cirrhosis and obesity: the SportDiet study. Hepatology. 2017;65(4):1293–305.

133. Barritt IV SA. Abnormal liver enzymes in a patient with diabetes. American Association for the Study of Liver Diseases, annual meeting; November 10th, 2018, San Diego. Post Graduate Course, 2018.

134. Traber MG, Atkinson J. Vitamin E, antioxidant and nothing more. Free Radic Biol Med. 2007 July 1;43(1):4–15.

135. Sanyal AJ, Chalasani N, Kowdley KV, McCullough A, Diehl AM, Bass NM, et al. Pioglitazone, vitamin E, or placebo for nonalcoholic steatohepatitis. N Engl J Med. 2010 May 6;362(18):1675–85.

136. Soccio RE, Chen ER, Lazar MA. Thiazolidinediones and the promise of insulin sensitization in type 2 diabetes. Cell Metab. 2014 Oct 7;20(4):573–91.

137. Xu R, Tao A, Zhang S, Deng Y, Chen G. Association between vitamin E and non-alcoholic steatohepatitis: a meta-analysis. Int J Clin Exp Med. 2015;8(3):3924–34.

138. Chalasani N, Younossi Z, Lavine JE, Charlton M, Cusi K, Rinella M, et al. The diagnosis and management of nonalcoholic fatty liver disease: practice guidance from the American Association for the Study of Liver Diseases. Hepatology. 2018 Jan;67(1):328–57.

139. Gomez-Vilar E, Vuppalanchi R, Gawrieh S, Ghabril M, Saxena R, Cummings OW, Chalasani N. Vitamin E improves transplant-free survival and hepatic decompensation among patients with nonalcoholic steatohepatitis and advanced fibrosis. Hepatology. 2020;71(2):495–509.

140. Cusi K, Orsak B, Bril F, Lomonaco R, Hecht J, Ortiz-Lopez C, et al. Long-term pioglitazone treatment for patients with nonalcoholic steatohepatitis and prediabetes or type 2 diabetes mellitus: A randomized trial. Ann Intern Med. 2016 Sep 6;165(5):305–15.

141. Holst JJ. The physiology of glucagon-like peptide 1. Physiol Rev. 2007 Oct;87(4):1409–39.

142. Armstrong MJ, Gaunt P, Aithal GP, Barton D, Hull D, Parker R, et al. Liraglutide safety and efficacy in patients with non-alcoholic steatohepatitis (LEAN): a multicentre, double-blind, randomised, placebo-controlled phase 2 study. Lancet. 2016 Feb 13;387(10019):679–90.

143. Gioiello A, Macchiarulo A, Carotti A, Filipponi P, Costantino G, Rizzo G, et al. Extending SAR of bile acids as FXR ligands: discovery of 23-N-(carbocinnamyloxy)-3α,7α-dihydroxy-6α-ethyl-24-nor-5β-cholan-23-amine. Bioorg Med Chem. 2011 Apr 15;19(8):2650–8.

144. Randomized global phase 3 study to evaluate the impact on NASH with fibrosis of obeticholic acid treatment (REGENERATE) [Internet]. 2019.

145. Disease HGaL. "Watershed moment:" Ocaliva improves NASH 2019.

146. Neuschwander-Tetri BA, Loomba R, Sanyal AJ, Lavine JE, Van Natta ML, Abdelmalek MF, et al. Farnesoid X nuclear receptor ligand obeticholic acid for non-cirrhotic, non-alcoholic steatohepatitis (FLINT): a multicentre, randomised, placebo-controlled trial. Lancet. 2015 Mar 14;385(9972):956–65.

147. Nevens F, Andreone P, Mazzella G, Strasser SI, Bowlus C, Invernizzi P, et al. A placebo-controlled trial of Obeticholic acid in primary biliary cholangitis. N Engl J Med. 2016 Aug 18;375(7):631–43.

148. Kersten S. Integrated physiology and systems biology of PPARα. Mol Metab. 2014 Jul;3(4):354–71.

149. Brunmair B, Staniek K, Dorig J, Szocs Z, Stadlbauer K, Marian V, et al. Activation of PPAR-delta in isolated rat skeletal muscle switches fuel preference from glucose to fatty acids. Diabetologia. 2006 Nov;49(11):2713–22.

150. Ratziu V, Harrison SA, Francque S, Bedossa P, Lehert P, Serfaty L, et al. Elafibranor, an agonist of the peroxisome proliferator-activated receptor-alpha and -delta, induces resolution of nonalcoholic steatohepatitis without fibrosis worsening. Gastroenterology. 2016 May;150(5):1147–59.

151. Phase 3 study to evaluate the efficacy and safety of elafibranor versus placebo in patients with nonalcoholic steatohepatitis (NASH) [Internet]. 2019 [cited July 19, 2019].

152. Hattori K, Naguro I, Runchel C, Ichijo H. The roles of ASK family proteins in stress responses and diseases. Cell Commun Signal CCS. 2009 Apr 24;7:9.

153. Nishioka T, Eustace A, West C. Lysyl oxidase: from basic science to future cancer treatment. Cell Struct Funct. 2012;37(1):75–80.
154. Loomba R, Lawitz E, Mantry PS, Jayakumar S, Caldwell SH, Arnold H, et al. The ASK1 inhibitor selonsertib in patients with nonalcoholic steatohepatitis: a randomized, phase 2 trial. Hepatology. 2017 Sep;67:549–59.
155. Harrison SA, Abdelmalek MF, Caldwell S, Shiffman ML, Diehl AM, Ghalib R, et al. Simtuzumab is ineffective for patients with bridging fibrosis or compensated cirrhosis caused by nonalcoholic steatohepatitis. Gastroenterology. 2018 Oct;155(4):1140–53.
156. Safety and efficacy of selonsertib in adults with compensated cirrhosis due to nonalcoholic steatohepatitis (NASH) (STELLAR 4). 2019.
157. Baba M, Takashima K, Miyake H, Kanzaki N, Teshima K, Wang X, et al. TAK-652 inhibits CCR5-mediated human immunodeficiency virus type 1 infection in vitro and has favorable pharmacokinetics in humans. Antimicrob Agents Chemother. 2005 Nov;49(11):4584–91.
158. Friedman SL, Ratziu V, Harrison SA, Abdelmalek MF, Aithal GP, Caballeria J, et al. A randomized, placebo-controlled trial of cenicriviroc for treatment of nonalcoholic steatohepatitis with fibrosis. Hepatology. 2018 May;67(5):1754–67.
159. Safety, tolerability, and efficacy of a combination treatment of tropifexor (LJN452) and Cenicriviroc (CVC) in adult patients with nonalcoholic steatohepatitis (NASH) and Liver Fibrosis. (TANDEM) (TANDEM) [Internet]. 2019 [cited July 19th, 2019].
160. AURORA: Phase 3 Study for the efficacy and safety of CVC for the treatment of liver fibrosis in adults with NASH [Internet]. 2019 [cited July 19th, 2019].
161. Jelenik T, Rossmeisl M, Kuda O, Jilkova ZM, Medrikova D, Kus V, et al. AMP-activated protein kinase α2 subunit is required for the preservation of hepatic insulin sensitivity by n-3 polyunsaturated fatty acids. Diabetes. 2010 Nov;59(11):2737–46.
162. Musa-Veloso K, Venditti C, Lee HY, Darch M, Floyd S, West S, et al. Systematic review and meta-analysis of controlled intervention studies on the effectiveness of long-chain omega-3 fatty acids in patients with nonalcoholic fatty liver disease. Nutr Rev. 2018 Aug 1;76(8):581–602.
163. Simon TG, Henson J, Osganian S, Masia R, Chan AT, Chung RT, et al. Daily aspirin use associated with reduced risk for fibrosis progression in patients with nonalcoholic fatty liver disease. Clin Gastroenterol Hepatol. 2019 May;17(13):2776–2784.e4.
164. Mathurin P, Hollebecque A, Arnalsteen L, Buob D, Leteurtre E, Caiazzo R, et al. Prospective study of the long-term effects of bariatric surgery on liver injury in patients without advanced disease. Gastroenterology. 2009 Aug;137(2):532–40.
165. Lassailly G, Caiazzo R, Buob D, Pigeyre M, Verkindt H, Labreuche J, et al. Bariatric surgery reduces features of nonalcoholic steatohepatitis in morbidly obese patients. Gastroenterology. 2015 Aug;149(2):379–88.
166. Cardoso L, Rodrigues D, Gomes L, Carrilho F. Short- and long-term mortality after bariatric surgery: a systematic review and meta-analysis. Diabetes Obes Metab. 2017 Sep;19(9):1223–32.
167. Mosko JD, Nguyen GC. Increased perioperative mortality following bariatric surgery among patients with cirrhosis. Clin Gastroenterol Hepatol. 2011 Oct;9(10):897–901.

# Chapter 10
# Alpha-1-Antitrypsin Deficiency

Nora V. Bergasa

A 58-year-old man was evaluated because of dyspnea on exertion, with exercise tolerance of one and a half blocks. He was diagnosed with asthma at age 30 and had been an ex-smoker for 12 years. The physical examination was notable for the absence of stigmata of chronic liver disease and some wheezing on pulmonary auscultation. A chest X-ray exhibited hyperinflation of the lung fields associated with flattening of the diaphragm and prominence of pulmonary arteries suggestive of chronic obstructive pulmonary disease. Alpha-1-antitrypsin (A1AT) level was 34 mg/dl (normal 90–200 mg/dl), consistent with deficiency; the phenotype was ZZ. The liver profile revealed serum activities of aspartate (AST) and alanine (ALT) aminotransferases of 53 IU/ml for the former, and 144 IU/ml for the latter (normal 10–40 IU/ml, and 10–45 IU/ml, respectively). The sonogram revealed an echogenic liver. Pulmonary function tests documented severe obstructive lung defect consistent with marked air trapping and severe decrease in diffusing capacity of the lungs for carbon monoxide, associated with insignificant response to bronchodilators. The patient was referred for augmentation therapy with A1AT and to a geneticist for counseling.

In the seminal publication by Sharp et al. in 1969, the association between cirrhosis and alpha-1-antitrypsin (A1AT) deficiency was reported [1]. Three years before that publication, Laurell and Eriksonn had described the absence of alpha-1-globulin in a group of patients who had severe emphysema [2]. It is now established that A1AT deficiency is associated with lung and liver disease [3, 4].

N. V. Bergasa (✉)
Department of Medicine, H+H/Metropolitan, New York, NY, USA

New York Medical College, Valhalla, NY, USA

Hepatology, H+H/Woodhull, Brooklyn, NY, USA

© The Author(s), under exclusive license to Springer-Verlag London Ltd., part of Springer Nature 2022
N. V. Bergasa (ed.), *Clinical Cases in Hepatology*,
https://doi.org/10.1007/978-1-4471-4715-2_10

325

A1AT deficiency is an under-recognized condition for which there are no screening programs established; thus, the diagnosis depends on a clinician's inquisitive mind, after which measures to prevent early complications or disease progression, e.g., cigarette smoking cessation, screening for viral hepatitis, and vaccination, as appropriate, should be implemented.

In homeostasis, there is a balance between proteases, which participate in proteolytic processes, and their inhibitors, which inhibit the activity of the proteolytic enzymes. The predominant family of inhibitors is the serine proteinase inhibitors (serpins) to which A1AT belongs [5]. The serpins' mechanism of action concerns a conformational change, i.e., a change in the structure inhibits the protease and leads to its destruction. The protein enters the lung by diffusion, where it inhibits neutrophil elastase; the protease/inhibitor complex is internalized and degraded by lysosomes [6]; A1AT is also reported to exert anti-inflammatory effects, independent from elastase inhibition [7].

A1AT is molecularly characterized by three beta sheets, A, B, and C, and nine alpha helixes. Beyond the scaffold of the A1AT molecule protrudes the reactive center loop (RCL) in a highly stressed configuration with methionine 358-serine 359 at the active center, which ducks the target enzyme, i.e., neutrophil elastase, to form a substrate enzyme complex, i.e., Michaelis complex. After ducking at the receptive sequence of the RCL, the protease is inactivated and sprung to the bottom of the molecule where it hangs, after which the RCL inserts itself into the beta A sheet, as another strand. The process of inactivation has been described as a "mousetrap" with a spring-like shift from a metastable to a hyperstable state [8, 9]. The formation of the substrate–enzyme complex can lead to: (1) inactivation of the protease and (2) the formation of a fourth beta sheet by the RCL within the A1AT molecule, allowing the protease to escape, leaving it in the active state, with the serpin cleaved and inactive. Thus, in homeostasis, A1AT exists in: (1) a native inhibitory conformation, with the exposed reactive center loop, and (2) in a latent state with a partially inserted RCL and a non-inhibitory conformation. The non-inhibitory conformation occurs: (1) in the substrate–enzyme complex, i.e., A1AT and neutrophil elastase, which is removed from the circulation by the hepatocyte, (2) when the RCL is cleaved by non-target enzymes, (3) after oxidation by reactive oxygen species, and (4) polymerized as it happens with the A1AT variants, including Pi*ZZ, associated with lung and liver disease, which are also reported to exert a chemotactic action on neutrophils, thus triggering an inflammatory cascade, now considered part of the pathogenesis of emphysema in association with A1AT deficiency [10].

Mutations in a strand of the beta sheet allow the RCL to insert itself into the A beta sheet as a new strand, forming polymers, which can involve several molecules of A1AT (Fig. 10.1) [11] that are trapped in the hepatocyte's endoplasmic reticulum (ER) from where they cannot exit, leading to a deficiency of circulating levels of A1AT. In the ER, A1AT molecules interact with chaperones including Grp78/BiP, Grp94, Grp170, and calnexin [12], the role of which is to facilitate the folding of proteins required for translocation from the ER and to control the quality of the proteins being secreted, by ensuring that inappropriately folded proteins remain in the ER or are degraded by proteasomes, via a mechanism known as ER-associated

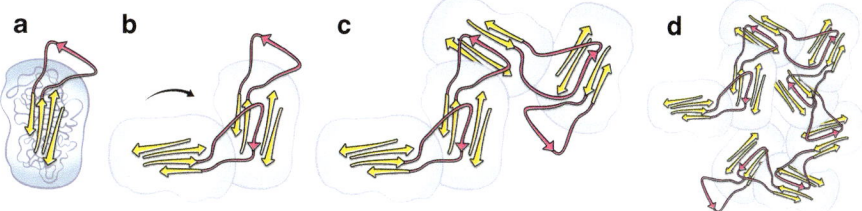

**Fig. 10.1** (**a**) Through (**d**) depict the polymerization of A1AT molecules. The amino acid substitution in the Z allele interferes with the folding and structure of the protein, changing the relationship between the reactive center loop (RCL (red ribbon)) and the beta sheet A (yellow ribbons), and allows for the opening of the latter to accept the partial insertion of RCL (**a** and **b**). Subsequently, the patent beta sheet A accepts the RCL of another A1AT molecule to form a dimer that extends by the insertion of another A1AT molecules forming chains of loop-sheet polymers (**c** and **d**). A1AT polymers accumulate in the cisterna of the rough endoplasmic reticulum, with a significant reduction of secretion, leading to the accumulation of the polymers in the hepatocytes that appear as periodic acid-Schiff-positive, diastase-resistant globules as shown in Fig. 10.2

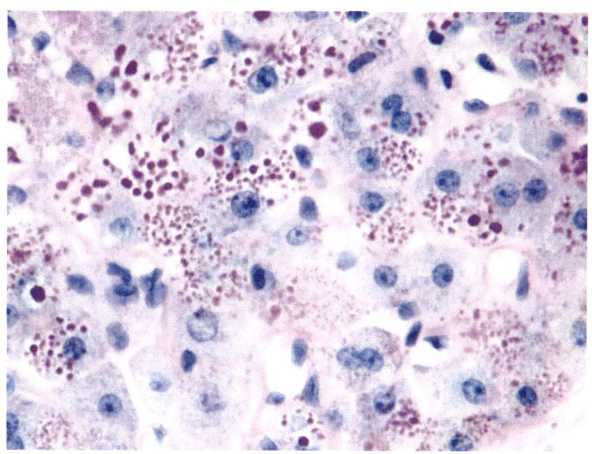

**Fig. 10.2** Histological study of a liver biopsy specimen from a patient with PI*ZZ alpha-1-antitrypsin deficiency. The eosinophilic inclusion bodies are periodic acid-Schiff-positive, diastase-resistant globules that contain polymerized, unsecreted Z-type alpha-1-antitrypsin (A1AT) (Courtesy of Dr. Maria Isabel Fiel, MD, FAASLD, Professor of Pathology, Icahn School of Medicine at Mount Sinai, New York, New York)

degradation (ERAD) [13]. In the ER, the interaction between the protein and the chaperones takes the form of soluble and conglomerate compounds, the latter identified by their characteristic stain features, i.e., peroxidase acid Schiff (PAS)-positive and diastase-resistant bodies that appear as magenta granules (Fig. 10.2). In the context of degradation, autophagy is a process identified as important in the elimination of A1AT polymers by the formation of autophagosomes. It is a mechanism being explored to develop treatments for A1AT deficiency-related liver disease. In this regard, drugs that increase autophagy, rapamycin, and carbamazepine, were reported to decrease A1AT ZZ polymers and liver fibrosis in a mouse model of the disease [14, 15].

Although A1AT deficiency has been traditionally viewed as a condition arising from a protease-antiprotease imbalance in the lungs, neutrophils' role as facilitators of inflammation in the pathogenesis of lung disease and other specific comorbidities is being recognized, adding an inflammatory component to the pathogenesis of the disease [16].

The plasma concentration of A1AT ranges from 0.9 to 2.0 g/L. A1AT is an acute phase reactant; thus, during inflammation, the concentrations increase by several folds [17]. In addition to neutrophil elastase (NE), A1AT inhibits other proinflammatory proteases, including proteinase 3 and cathepsin G [18].

# Genetics

The A1AT protein is encoded by the *SERPINA1* gene (also known as *PI*), located in chromosome 14q32.1,3–7. The disease is inherited in an autosomal recessive manner with codominant expression [19]. The two most common alleles found in A1AT deficiency-associated diseases are S and Z.

The Z variant contains a substitution of the amino acid glutamine for lysine in the 342 position. This mutation concerns an amino acid at the base of the center loop of the molecule [20], which can move in and out of the A-sheet that comprises the major feature of the molecule [21]. It was shown that by increasing the environment's temperature or under mild denaturing conditions, the center loop could move, and polymerization occur between A1AT molecules of the M, normal phenotype. The polymerization could be stopped by adding a synthetic-free peptide, which inserts itself into the A-sheet, forming a binary complex. The synthetic-free peptide was a 13-residue peptide derived from the reactive center loop of another serpin, antithrombin, and homologous to the amino acid sequence 345 to 357 of the center loop. The formation of the binary complex with A1AT was documented by the loss of the inhibitory activity, by features exhibited in electrophoresis, and by changes in physical properties [21]. It was further noted that the Z mutation at the hinge of the center loop enhanced polymerization, which spontaneously happened at 37 degrees, and that was accelerated at temperatures of 41 degrees; the synthetic-free peptide blocked polymerization regardless of the temperature used in the experiment. The polymerization rate also depended on the Z antitrypsin concentration, with an increased proportion of polymerization in association with increased concentrations of antitrypsin. The M antitrypsin did not polymerize itself under these conditions. The results of these experiments explained the accumulation of A1AT conglomerates in the hepatocytes of patients who were homozygotes for the Z mutation. Gel electrophoresis revealed findings to confirm that the inclusion bodies are bound together by non-covalent bonds and dissociate into monomers in the right experimental conditions; furthermore, electron microscopy revealed that the polymers were comprised of filaments identical to those observed in incubated isolated

Z antitrypsin. Loop-sheet polymerization is reported as equilibrium, and it occurs at a critical concentration of Z antitrypsin before it goes into the ER; 85% of the Z antitrypsin polymerizes itself, and the rest is secreted into the circulation as monomers, the concentration of which, however, is not adequate to protect the lungs from the proteolytic destruction by neutrophil elastase [22]. In addition to a low peripheral concentration, the Z allele is dysfunctional, as it has a decrease in the inhibitory activity of A1AT because of a diminished binding affinity to neutrophil elastase [23].

The S allele contains a substitution of glutamine for valine at the 264 position (Glu264Val). In homozygotes, this mutation results in a decrease in the plasma concentration by 40%, which does not result in major health problems; however, if inherited with the Z mutation, i.e., the substitution of glutamine for lysine at the 342 position (Glu342Lys), which results in 85% reduction in the plasma concentration of A1AT, it does. In summary, the low plasma concentration found with the ZZ homozygotes and with the SZ compound heterozygotes is associated with disease.

The M allele is encoded by the *A1AT* 2 gene and is associated with sufficient serum concentrations of A1AT to prevent disease. Other variants that include the M1, M2, G, X, C, and D alleles are not associated with health complications. Rare alleles have been reported in association with disease in case reports [24]. The alleles associated with intracellular accumulation of the protein related to liver and lung injury, as a result, are M Malton, Siiyama, and Z, with the latter being associated with impaired inhibition of NE as well. The alleles associated with lung disease related to intracellular degradation are M Heerlen, M procida, S, and M mineral springs, which are also related to impaired NE inhibition. The null alleles, which make very little amounts of A1AT, are $QO_{granite\ falls}$, characterized by a stop codon and absence of A1AT, and associated with emphysema, and $QO_{Ludwigshafen}$, characterized by abnormal mRNA, leading to inadequate protein, and associated with liver and lung disease, the $QO_{hongkong}$, associated with a stop codon from a frameshift, which results in a short protein and is associated with its intracellular accumulation, and development of emphysema at an early age, $QO_{isola\ di\ procida,}$ characterized by complete deletion without mRNA or protein, and associated with lung disease, $QO_{Bolton,}$ characterized by a stop codon and no mRNA or protein, and associated with lung disease [25]. The dysfunctional Pittsburgh allele is characterized by a substitution (358 met-to-arg) that results in the acquisition of antithrombin properties and is associated with bleeding diathesis [26] and F, which has defective binding to NE and that results in normal A1AT concentrations but abnormal anti-elastase functional activity [27, 28].

The mutant A1AT Z is synthesized appropriately and translocated to the ER of the hepatocyte where it binds to chaperone proteins, the role of which is to help in the folding of the molecule and to survey for abnormalities; as the mutant folds inefficiently, 85% of the molecules do not reach the conformation required for secretion and thus, they are retained in the hepatocyte, as stated above, where they appear as magenta granules (Fig. 10.2) [22]. The accumulation of these structures from the mutant Z molecule triggers liver injury in the individuals susceptible to disease, but not in all individuals with the mutation.

# Epidemiology

A1AT deficiency is under diagnosed, as screening guidelines are not strictly followed and the disease, in its full manifestation of early emphysema, tends to be diagnosed when preventive measures, e.g., smoking cessation, avoidance of environmental and occupational exposure, cannot be instituted; thus the prevalence has been calculated mostly by estimates. "AAT deficiency is probably one of the most common hereditary under-recognized disorders in the world, with only a small minority of subjects currently detected," as documented from a study that estimated the prevalence of A1AT in the world [29].

In the United States, the prevalence of A1AT deficiency in individuals of European extraction is 1 case per 3000 to 5000 persons [35]. It was concluded from a study that surveyed 4.4 billion people from 58 countries that there were at least 116 million carriers of A1AT Pi phenotypes PiMS and PiMZ and 3.4 million with deficiency allele combinations, phenotypes PiSS, PiSZ, and PiZZ, the latter two being the most prevalent. These results reiterate that A1AT deficiency may be one of the most common single-locus genetic diseases that have serious clinical consequences [30].

Reported per 1000 individuals in North and Central America, PI*S's prevalence ranged from 23 in the United States to 33–45 in Central America. The prevalence of PI*Z from 6 to 8 in Mexico and Central America to 10 and 13 in the United States and Canada; in the United States, the study documented an estimate of 14 million MS, 6 million MZ, 160,000 SS, 150,000 SZ, and 34,000 ZZ, which one can interpret as a result of its rich genetic pool [29].

Nineteen centers in the United States participated in a study that included 3152 subjects with fixed airflow obstruction who underwent pulmonary function tests; of these, 0.63% were characterized as Pi*ZZ and Pi*SZ, and 10.88% were carriers of mutations MS and MZ. However, pulmonary function test results did not allow the prediction of the phenotypic expression of the A1AT mutations [31]. These data support the measure of screening high-risk individuals prior to the establishment of irreversible airway disease.

The factors that have been associated with liver disease in adults are age greater than 50 years, male gender, abnormal liver profile, viral hepatitis, and components of the metabolic syndrome [25]. A consensus supports the idea that polymerization of the altered phenotype that results in the accumulation of AA1T globules is not sufficient to cause disease. Thus, environmental and other genetic and epigenetic influences are likely to be involved in the pathogenesis of A1AT deficiency-related liver disease [32–36]. In this regard, molecular epigenetic signatures have already been documented in a group of patients with the A1AT deficiency ZZ phenotype [37].

A study that included 262 patient cohorts from 71 countries, and 1,490,816 individuals with PiSZ phenotype of A1ATD, documented the prevalence of the disease as 708,792 in Europe, 582,984 in America and the Caribbean, 85,925 in Africa, 77,940 in Asia, and 35,176 in Australia and New Zealand [38].

## Natural History

A1AT deficiency can present in infancy with prolonged cholestatic hepatitis [39]. In a prospective study that screened 200,000 infants, 120 PiZ, 48 Pi SZ, two PI Z, and one Pi S were identified and followed under 6 months. Prolonged cholestasis was documented in 14 of the 120 (11.6%) infants, nine of whom had evidence of liver disease, with five exhibiting abnormal liver tests only. Twenty-two of the 120 (18.3%) infants with abnormal liver profile "seemed healthy" at 6 months of age; the other 98 did not have liver disease on clinical grounds, but liver tests were abnormal in some at 3 and 6 months of age. The number of small for gestational age infants increased in patients with clinical liver disease. The infants with PiSZ did not have liver disease; however, some had abnormal liver tests at 3 and 6 months of age. These data suggested that liver disease in children with the PiZ and PiSZ phenotypes presents itself by 3 months of life [40].

By the use of DEFI-ALPHA as a source, a French study, retrospective up to 2010 and prospective from 2017 that included 153 children who were born since 1989 with A1AT concentrations below 0.8 g/L and followed for 4.7 ± 2.1 years, documented a majority, 81.9%, with the PiZZ phenotype, with 8.1% being PiZZ, and 10% qualified as other, and a development of portal hypertension in 18.3%, at a mean age of 2.5 years (up to 11.6), with 15 children having a liver transplant, and one death in a 3-year-old child, with neonatal cholestasis being significantly associated with severe disease, defined as portal hypertension, liver failure, liver transplantation, or death; the diagnosis of A1AT deficiency was made before 2 months in 65.4% of patients, with PiZZ being the most common, 89.3%, and the rest being PiSZ, PiSZ, PiSZ, and PiM$_{like}$ Z, data interpreted to suggest that non PiZZ variants can be associated with liver disease, possibly related to other factors, which remain to be identified [41].

In the adult population, life expectancy is compromised in patients with A1AT deficiency. From a study conducted in Sweden that included 246 patients with severe PiZ A1ATD, diagnosed from 1963 to 1977, lung disease was present in 40% of the patients, with the majority of deaths being from this group [42]. Forty-seven patients (19%) had a diagnosis of liver cirrhosis by age 50 years; 13% of the deaths being from liver disease.

In regards to hepatic comorbidities, from 1184 subjects with nonalcoholic fatty liver disease (NAFLD) documented histologically, and from 2462 with alcohol use disorder, with appropriate control groups with and without cirrhosis, the calculated odds ratio (OR) to develop cirrhosis in association with the Pi*Z variant of A1AT in patients with NAFLD was reported as 7.3, with a 95% confidence interval (CI) between 2.2 and 24.8, with 13. 8% of the subjects with the abnormal phenotype having cirrhosis, versus the 2.4% of subjects without that variant. The PiZ* was present in 6.2% of subjects who had alcohol use disorder and cirrhosis, which was significantly higher than the 2.2% of patients with the same condition but without "significant liver injury," with a calculated adjusted OR of 5.8 (CI: 2.9 to 11.7) indicating that patients who drink excessively, and carry this A1AT phenotype were at risk to develop cirrhosis. The adjusted OR for the patients who had the Pi*S variant was 1.47 (95% CI: 0.99 to 2.19), a risk that, although small when compared to the Pi*Z variant, should be discussed in regards to preventive measures, e.g., stopping cigarette smoking, when evaluating carriers of Pi*S [43].

In this regard, a retrospective review also from Sweden identified 17 cases (one child and 16 adults) that had undergone an autopsy from 20 who had been diagnosed with A1AT deficiency between 1963 and 1982. From an analysis that matched the A1ATD cases with the non A1AT deficiency controls, a strong relationship between A1AT deficiency and cirrhosis and hepatocellular carcinoma was identified, with a Mantel-Haenszel odds ratio (ORmh) of 7.8, with a 95% confidence limits from 2.4 to 24.7, and 20, with a 95% confidence limits from 3.5 to 114.3, respectively, with significant association with male patients only, after data stratified for gender. These data suggested that in addition to A1AT deficiency, environmental, and possibly hormonal factors contribute to the development of HCC in patients with this genetic condition [44].

From a prospective study that included 94 adult patients with A1AT deficiency, Pi*ZZ, the prevalence of liver fibrosis, measured by transient elastography, was 35.1%, which was significantly associated with the presence of metabolic syndrome (OR 14.2; 95% CI 3.7–55; $p < 0.001$). Histologically, the typical hepatocellular A1AT globules and periportal inflammation were reported in association with significant fibrosis [25]. In addition to fibrosis, steatosis was documented in 39% out of 554 patients with A1AT deficiency PiZZ variant by the use of transient elastography, with controlled attenuation parameter $\geq 280$ dB/m, suggestive of severe steatosis, versus in 31% of the control subjects; in addition, patients with A1AT deficiency had lower concentrations of triglyceride and low- and very-low-density lipoprotein cholesterol as compared to those in the control group, data interpreted to suggest that impaired hepatic secretion of lipids is a feature of A1AT deficient PiZZ variant [45]. These results tend to support the findings of a prior study that documented some association between the A1AT deficiency PiMZ variant and NASH [46]; in this report, patients with both conditions had an increased risk for decompensation [46].

## Clinical Manifestations

In the absence of screening campaigns, patients tend to be diagnosed when they present with symptoms of pulmonary involvement, including COPD and asthma. Regarding subjects with liver disease, adult patients tend to be asymptomatic unless they have progressed to decompensation with all its complications or are referred for evaluation of an abnormal liver panel. In patients with compensated liver disease, the first clue to the diagnosis is increased serum activity of transaminases, which leads to a liver disease investigation that includes A1AT serum concentrations. If these are low, which can happen in the presence of rare alleles in addition to A1AT deficiency, it is recommended to check the genotype. In case of a discrepancy between A1AT concentration and genotype, phenotype analysis is advised [47]. Of note, in patients with PI*Null alleles, this method does not yield a result as the patients do not make circulating proteins. Also, rare genetic variants that result in low levels of A1AT, including PI*M $_{heerlen}$, or in normal levels of a dysfunctional protein (e.g., PI*F) may not be detected; thus, genotype testing can be added to the investigation [48]. Testing is recommended in siblings [27].

Environmental modifiers increase lung disease risk in patients with the Z protein phenotype, including cigarette smoking, male gender, and asthma [49, 50]. In a cross-sectional study, the heterozygous PiZ was not significantly more prevalent in patients with liver disease, 754, versus patients without, 651. From patients listed for liver transplantation, 10 of the 173 (5.7%) had PiMZ versus 10 of the 478 (2.1%) with liver disease considered to have "less severe" liver disease, which was reported as significantly different. In addition, there was an increased number of patients with the PiZ variant among patients with decompensated liver disease from chronic hepatitis C and nonalcoholic liver disease, 5.6%, and 5%, respectively, compared to those with "less severe" liver disease from chronic hepatitis C, 1.2%, and from NAFLD, 1.9%, reported as significantly different between the compensated and the "less severe" liver disease group. Cryptogenic cirrhosis was not associated with an increase in the percentage of PiMZ, as compared to liver disease in which the cause was known; thus, the presence of PiZ may accelerate the progression of liver disease in patients with chronic hepatitis C and NAFLD [46]. Although A1AT mutations have been reported in association with NAFLD, high serum ferritin concentrations, and an increase in the presence of sinusoidal siderosis, non-MM phenotypes were not associated with increased liver injury in NAFLD [51].

In regards to liver disease, in a retrospective study that explored liver disease in association with A1AT deficiency in children, and that included 6 girls and 14 boys, it was noted that the PiZZ phenotype was present in 8 (40%) of the children, and PiMZ in 12 (60%). The most common finding was an abnormal liver profile, with three patients having neonatal cholestasis and one compensated cirrhosis. Seven of the eight patients who underwent liver biopsy had typical histology of A1AT deficiency with PAS positive, diastase resistant conglomerates in the hepatocytes. PiZZ was associated with chronic hepatitis in all patients except one who had cirrhosis, over 12–101 months of follow-up versus only two of the patients who were PiMZ who had chronic hepatitis [52].

Transient elastograpy is a noninvasive technique that measures liver stiffness, which increases and correlates with fibrosis, expressed in kilopascals (kPa). In a study that included 29 patients with A1AT deficiency, ZZ phenotype, the median liver stiffness was 4.5 kPa (2.8–32.8), with an increase in patients with abnormal liver profile and ultrasound, but also, in patients with normal liver profile and ultrasound, albeit only 10% [53].

Patients with lung disease from A1AT deficiency should be referred to pulmonary medicine for evaluation and treatment that include bronchodilators, oxygen supplementation, and augmentation therapy.

Patients diagnosed with A1AT as part of the evaluation of abnormal liver tests should also be referred to pulmonary medicine to evaluate for lung disease.

## Laboratory Tests

The PI locus has approximately 123 single nucleotide polymorphisms; the difference in the migration rate that characterizes different protein variants is used to identify the phenotype. The M migrates at a medium rate, and the Z allele at the slowest rate. Null alleles can be inherited and are associated with no measurable concentration of A1AT in plasma. The phenotype PI Z defines subjects who have the Z pattern and include PIZZ and PIZ null variants. Although the phenotype refers to the pattern of movement in protein electrophoresis, in general, it concerns the clinical manifestations of the disease. PI Z phenotype is associated with plasma levels of A1AT less than 15% of PI MM and the development of COPD at a relatively early age. It was reported that the PI type is responsible for 72–92% of the variation in serum A1AT levels within families of known PI Z individuals, thus making the PI locus determinant of serum levels of AAT.

## Histology

The mechanism by which A1AT deficiency causes liver disease seems to be unknown; however, it is reported that liver injury correlates with the amount of A1AT protein, i.e., polymers, in the hepatocytes [54, 55]. Accumulated A1AT, the hallmark of A1AT deficiency, Z type, is exhibited by the PAS-positive, diastase resistant globules in the hepatocytes around the portal tracts. These globules are the polymerized A1AT molecules trapped in the ER, unable to exit and secreted into the circulation (Figs. 10.1 and 10.2). Other findings include bile stasis, steatosis, in zone 1, and hemosiderosis. Inflammation is not a dominant finding in A1ATD. Cirrhosis in this disease can be macro and micronodular; bile ductular proliferation may be present in cirrhosis [56].

## Hepatocellular Carcinoma

The mechanism through which A1AT deficiency causes HCC is unknown. It was hypothesized that hepatocytes laden with A1AT globules are growth suppressed, and elaborate "trans-acting regenerative signals" transduced by globules-devoid hepatocytes, which proliferate. Chronic regeneration in association with tissue injury, which results from the accumulation of A1AT, as interpreted from animal models [54, 55], leads to adenomata, which can degenerate into carcinoma [34].

In a study that included 675 patients with cirrhosis and end stage liver disease (ESLD) from a tertiary center where patients had been referred for liver transplantation from 2003 to 2014, A1AT deficiency was diagnosed in 47 (7%) patients, 14 of whom had the PI*ZZ phenotype, 8 PI*MZ, 10 had PI*MZ phenotype, and 14 did not have phenotype documented but were diagnosed by histology, with an incidence of HCC of 8.5% versus 31%, significantly different, in patients with cirrhosis from other causes (e.g., chronic hepatitis C, nonalcoholic steatohepatitis, and liver disease from alcohol), and a cumulative rate of 0.88% per year as compared to 2.7% in those with cirrhosis from chronic hepatitis C, 1.5% in those with NASH, and 0.9% in those with cirrhosis from alcohol abuse, from which it was concluded that HCC was relatively uncommon in patients from cirrhosis from AAT deficiency [57].

## Associated Conditions

Panniculitis is a rare condition associated with A1AT deficiency, usually with Pi*ZZ genotype, with an estimated prevalence of 1 in 1000 persons. It presents itself with painful ulcerating subcutaneous nodules that recur and leave a scar. Histologically, it is characterized by infiltrates of neutrophils deep in the dermis and connective tissue with secondary lobular panniculitis. This rare condition can be the only manifestation of A1AT deficiency, and thus, it is an indication to exclude the disease [58]. A1AT polymers were documented in the skin of a patient with panniculitis in association with A1AT deficiency PiZZ, which has suggested that these conglomerates of proteins exert proinflammatory effects [59]. The treatment of panniculitis is dapsone, and, if ineffective, augmentation therapy with human A1AT is indicated [60]. In cases of rapidly progressive disease, plasma exchange has been reported as an option [61].

Granulomatosis with polyangiitis (GPA) was also reported in association with A1AT deficiency Pi*Z, Pi*S, in addition to its association with PiZZ [62].

A retrospective study from Germany that included 4 million people identified 673 patients with A1AT deficiency yielding a prevalence of 23.73 per 100,000 subjects from all age groups and 29.36 per 100000 in individuals older than 30 years with an estimated 19,162 patients with A1AT deficiency over the study period. Hypertension, renal disease, and diabetes were more common in patients with A1AT deficiency than in the control group not affected by A1AT deficiency but who had asthma or emphysema. The patients with A1AT deficiency had higher utilization of health care services, findings that can be interpreted to suggest that comorbidities beyond lung disease complicate the natural history of A1AT deficiency [63].

A1AT deficiency has been considered a factor associated with arterial aneurysms. However, an increased number of A1AT deficiency alleles was not found among 173 patients with aortic aneurysms from the United States and England, nor among 72 patients with intracranial aneurysms [64].

A1AT deficiency has been reported in association with renal diseases, including glomerulonephritis [65] and antineutrophil cytoplasmic antibody-associated vasculitis, which may also be associated with renal disease [65]. In some publications, patients had liver and renal diseases, which may not have been related to their A1AT status [64].

## Treatment

The treatments of lung disease from A1AT deficiency in development are augmentation therapy, lung volume reduction surgery, and lung transplantation [27].

At present, there is no specific treatment for liver disease from A1AT deficiency. Patients with liver disease should be vaccinated to prevent viral hepatitis and should be encouraged to avoid alcohol. Patients with cirrhosis, or suggestion of cirrhosis by imaging studies, should be screened for hepatocellular carcinoma with a liver sonogram and serum alpha fetoprotein every 6 months, as per current guidelines [66]. Patients with end stage liver disease are candidates for liver transplantation.

A clinical trial, NCT01379469, to study the effects of carbamazepine in patients with severe liver disease secondary to A1AT deficiency is being conducted. Based on the mechanisms inferred to contribute to the pathogenesis of liver disease secondary to A1AT deficiency, areas that are being explored as potential treatments include gene correction, the use of chaperone proteins to enhance secretion of the mutated protein, acceleration of ERAD degradation, inhibition of polymerization, increased degradation by stimulating autophagy, inhibition of intracellular injury pathways, and drugs to decrease liver fibrosis [67].

## Liver Transplantation

The analysis from three liver transplantation databases from 1991 to 2012 revealed that 77% of 1677 transplants performed for liver disease from A1AT deficiency were in adult subjects aged 50–64 years, mostly men. Regarding phenotypes, it was documented that many patients who underwent liver transplantation for A1AT-related liver disease were heterozygotes and had comorbidities associated with liver disease, including obesity and excessive use of alcohol. In children, liver transplantation was performed in patients younger than 5 years. This analysis was interpreted to suggest that A1AT deficiency causes liver disease by mechanisms characterized as age-dependent degenerative diseases and more rarely in children by modifiers that include proteasomal and autophagic degradative pathways [32].

A pooled analysis of 35 published studies documented that cirrhosis had been reported in 7% of children, with 16.5% of patients diagnosed in childhood requiring liver transplantation. Ten percent of the subjects who made it to adulthood had cirrhosis, and 15% required liver transplantation. The 5-year survival post liver transplantation was over 90% in children and over 80% in adults [68].

Post liver transplantation survival in relation to A1AT variants at 1, 3, 5, and 10 years was reported as 86%, 83%, 80%, and 72%, respectively, for patients with the ZZ phenotype, and 91%, 86%, 79%, and 79%, respectively for those with SZ [69].

**Acknowledgments** The author acknowledges Dr. Maria Isabel Fiel for having contributed Figure 10.2.

# References

1. Sharp HL, Bridges RA, Krivit W, Freier EF. Cirrhosis associated with alpha-1-antitrypsin deficiency: a previously unrecognized inherited disorder. J Lab Clin Med. 1969 June;73(6):934–9.
2. Laurell C-BE S. The electrophoretic α 1-globulin pattern of serum in α 1-antitrypsin deficiency. Scand J Clin Lab Invest. 1963;15:132–40.
3. Torres-Duran M, Lopez-Campos JL, Barrecheguren M, Miravitlles M, Martinez-Delgado B, Castillo S, et al. Alpha-1 antitrypsin deficiency: outstanding questions and future directions. Orphanet J Rare Dis. 2018 Jul 11;13(1):114.
4. Karatas E, Di-Tommaso S, Dugot-Senant N, Lachaux A, Bouchecareilh M. Overview of alpha-1 antitrypsin deficiency-mediated liver disease. EMJ Hepatol. 2019;7(1):65–79.
5. Potempa J, Korzus E, Travis J. The serpin superfamily of proteinase inhibitors: structure, function, and regulation. J Biol Chem. 1994 June 10;269(23):15957–60.
6. Perlmutter DH, Joslin G, Nelson P, Schasteen C, Adams SP, Fallon RJ. Endocytosis and degradation of alpha 1-antitrypsin-protease complexes is mediated by the serpin-enzyme complex (SEC) receptor. J Biol Chem. 1990 Oct 5;265(28):16713–6.
7. Jonigk D, Al-Omari M, Maegel L, Muller M, Izykowski N, Hong J, et al. Anti-inflammatory and immunomodulatory properties of alpha1-antitrypsin without inhibition of elastase. Proc Natl Acad Sci U S A. 2013 Sep 10;110(37):15007–12.
8. Huntington JA, Read RJ, Carrell RW. Structure of a serpin-protease complex shows inhibition by deformation. Nature. 2000 Oct 19;407(6806):923–6.
9. Carrell RW, Lomas DA. Alpha1-antitrypsin deficiency - a model for conformational diseases. N Engl J Med. 2002 Jan 3;346(1):45–53.
10. Law RH, Zhang Q, McGowan S, Buckle AM, Silverman GA, Wong W, et al. An overview of the serpin superfamily. Genome Biol. 2006;7(5):216.
11. Nyon MP, Prentice T, Day J, Kirkpatrick J, Sivalingam GN, Levy G, et al. An integrative approach combining ion mobility mass spectrometry, X-ray crystallography, and nuclear magnetic resonance spectroscopy to study the conformational dynamics of alpha1-antitrypsin upon ligand binding. Protein Sci. 2015 Aug;24(8):1301–12.
12. Schmidt BZ, Perlmutter DH. Grp78, Grp94, and Grp170 interact with alpha1-antitrypsin mutants that are retained in the endoplasmic reticulum. Am J Physiol Gastrointest Liver Physiol. 2005 Sep;289(3):G444–55.
13. Hosokawa N, Wada I, Hasegawa K, Yorihuzi T, Tremblay LO, Herscovics A, et al. A novel ER alpha-mannosidase-like protein accelerates ER-associated degradation. EMBO Rep. 2001 May;2(5):415–22.

14. Kaushal S, Annamali M, Blomenkamp K, Rudnick D, Halloran D, Brunt EM, et al. Rapamycin reduces intrahepatic alpha-1-antitrypsin mutant Z protein polymers and liver injury in a mouse model. Exp Biol Med. 2010 Jun;235(6):700–9.
15. Hidvegi T, Ewing M, Hale P, Dippold C, Beckett C, Kemp C, et al. An autophagy-enhancing drug promotes degradation of mutant alpha1-antitrypsin Z and reduces hepatic fibrosis. Science. 2010 July 9;329(5988):229–32.
16. McCarthy C, Reeves EP, McElvaney NG. The role of neutrophils in Alpha-1 antitrypsin deficiency. Ann Am Thorac Soc. 2016 Aug;13(Suppl 4):S297–304.
17. Brantly ML, Wittes JT, Vogelmeier CF, Hubbard RC, Fells GA, Crystal RG. Use of a highly purified alpha 1-antitrypsin standard to establish ranges for the common normal and deficient alpha 1-antitrypsin phenotypes. Chest. 1991 Sep;100(3):703–8.
18. Janciauskiene SM, Bals R, Koczulla R, Vogelmeier C, Kohnlein T, Welte T. The discovery of alpha1-antitrypsin and its role in health and disease. Respir Med. 2011 Aug;105(8):1129–39.
19. Darlington GJ, Astrin KH, Muirhead SP, Desnick RJ, Smith M. Assignment of human alpha 1-antitrypsin to chromosome 14 by somatic cell hybrid analysis. Proc Natl Acad Sci U S A. 1982 Feb;79(3):870–3.
20. Huber R, Carrell RW. Implications of the three-dimensional structure of alpha 1-antitrypsin for structure and function of serpins. Biochemistry. 1989 Nov 14;28(23):8951–66.
21. Carrell RW, Evans DL, Stein PE. Mobile reactive Centre of serpins and the control of thrombosis. Nature. 1991 Oct 10;353(6344):576–8.
22. Lomas DA, Evans DL, Finch JT, Carrell RW. The mechanism of Z alpha 1-antitrypsin accumulation in the liver. Nature. 1992 June 18;357(6379):605–7.
23. Ogushi F, Fells GA, Hubbard RC, Straus SD, Crystal RG. Z-type alpha 1-antitrypsin is less competent than M1-type alpha 1-antitrypsin as an inhibitor of neutrophil elastase. J Clin Invest. 1987 Nov;80(5):1366–74.
24. Mahadeva R, Chang WS, Dafforn TR, Oakley DJ, Foreman RC, Calvin J, et al. Heteropolymerization of S, I, and Z alpha1-antitrypsin and liver cirrhosis. J Clin Invest. 1999 Apr;103(7):999–1006.
25. Clark VC, Marek G, Liu C, Collinsworth A, Shuster J, Kurtz T, et al. Clinical and histologic features of adults with alpha-1 antitrypsin deficiency in a non-cirrhotic cohort. J Hepatol. 2018 Dec;69(6):1357–64.
26. Owen MC, Brennan SO, Lewis JH, Carrell RW. Mutation of antitrypsin to antithrombin. alpha 1-antitrypsin Pittsburgh (358 Met leads to Arg), a fatal bleeding disorder. N Engl J Med. 1983 Sep 22;309(12):694–8.
27. American Thoracic Society, European Respiratory Society. American Thoracic Society/European Respiratory Society statement: standards for the diagnosis and management of individuals with alpha-1 antitrypsin deficiency. Am J Respir Crit Care Med. 2003 Oct 1;168(7):818–900.
28. Sinden NJ, Koura F, Stockley RA. The significance of the F variant of alpha-1-antitrypsin and unique case report of a PiFF homozygote. BMC Pulm Med. 2014 Aug 7;14:132.
29. de Serres FJ, Blanco I. Prevalence of alpha1-antitrypsin deficiency alleles PI*S and PI*Z worldwide and effective screening for each of the five phenotypic classes PI*MS, PI*MZ, PI*SS, PI*SZ, and PI*ZZ: a comprehensive review. Ther Adv Respir Dis. 2012 Oct;6(5):277–95.
30. de Serres FJ. Alpha-1 antitrypsin deficiency is not a rare disease but a disease that is rarely diagnosed. Environ Health Perspect. 2003 Dec;111(16):1851–4.
31. Rahaghi FF, Sandhaus RA, Brantly ML, Rouhani F, Campos MA, Strange C, et al. The prevalence of alpha-1 antitrypsin deficiency among patients found to have airflow obstruction. COPD. 2012 Aug;9(4):352–8.
32. Perlmutter DH. Alpha-1-antitrypsin deficiency: importance of proteasomal and autophagic degradative pathways in disposal of liver disease-associated protein aggregates. Annu Rev Med. 2011;62:333–45.
33. Volpert D, Molleston JP, Perlmutter DH. Alpha1-antitrypsin deficiency-associated liver disease progresses slowly in some children. J Pediatr Gastroenterol Nutr. 2000 Sep;31(3):258–63.

34. Perlmutter DH. Pathogenesis of chronic liver injury and hepatocellular carcinoma in alpha-1-antitrypsin deficiency. Pediatr Res. 2006 Aug;60(2):233–8.
35. Silverman EK, Sandhaus RA. Clinical practice. Alpha1-antitrypsin deficiency. N Engl J Med. 2009 Jun 25;360(26):2749–57.
36. Ghouse R, Chu A, Wang Y, Perlmutter DH. Mysteries of alpha1-antitrypsin deficiency: emerging therapeutic strategies for a challenging disease. Dis Model Mech. 2014 Apr;7(4):411–9.
37. Wang L, Marek GW 3rd, Hlady RA, Wagner RT, Zhao X, Clark VC, et al. Alpha-1 antitrypsin deficiency liver disease, mutational homogeneity modulated by epigenetic heterogeneity with links to obesity. Hepatology. 2019 Jul;70(1):51–66.
38. Blanco I, Bueno P, Diego I, Perez-Holanda S, Lara B, Casas-Maldonado F, et al. Alpha-1 antitrypsin Pi*SZ genotype: estimated prevalence and number of SZ subjects worldwide. Int J Chron Obstruct Pulmon Dis. 2017;12:1683–94.
39. Hussain M, Mieli-Vergani G, Mowat AP. Alpha 1-antitrypsin deficiency and liver disease: clinical presentation, diagnosis and treatment. J Inherit Metab Dis. 1991;14(4):497–511.
40. Sveger T. Liver disease in alpha1-antitrypsin deficiency detected by screening of 200,000 infants. N Engl J Med. 1976 June 10;294(24):1316–21.
41. Ruiz M, Lacaille F, Berthiller J, Joly P, Dumortier J, Aumar M, et al. Liver disease related to alpha1-antitrypsin deficiency in French children: the DEFI-ALPHA cohort. Liver Int. 2019 June;39(6):1136–46.
42. Larsson C. Natural history and life expectancy in severe alpha1-antitrypsin deficiency, Pi Z. Acta Med Scand. 1978;204(5):345–51.
43. Strnad P, Buch S, Hamesch K, Fischer J, Rosendahl J, Schmelz R, et al. Heterozygous carriage of the alpha1-antitrypsin Pi*Z variant increases the risk to develop liver cirrhosis. Gut. 2019 Jun;68(6):1099–107.
44. Eriksson S, Carlson J, Velez R. Risk of cirrhosis and primary liver cancer in alpha 1-antitrypsin deficiency. N Engl J Med. 1986 Mar 20;314(12):736–9.
45. Hamesch K, Mandorder M, Pereira VM, Moeller LS, Pons M, Dolman GE, Reichert MC. Liver fibrosis and metabolic alterations in adults with alpha-1-antitrypsin deficiency caused by the Pi*ZZ mutation. Gastroenterology. 2019;157(3):705–19.
46. Regev A, Guaqueta C, Molina EG, Conrad A, Mishra V, Brantly ML, et al. Does the heterozygous state of alpha-1 antitrypsin deficiency have a role in chronic liver diseases? Interim results of a large case-control study. J Pediatr Gastroenterol Nutr. 2006 Jul;43(Suppl 1):S30–5.
47. Snyder MR, Katzmann JA, Butz ML, Wiley C, Yang P, Dawson DB, et al. Diagnosis of alpha-1-antitrypsin deficiency: an algorithm of quantification, genotyping, and phenotyping. Clin Chem. 2006 Dec;52(12):2236–42.
48. Brantly M. Efficient and accurate approaches to the laboratory diagnosis of alpha1-antitrypsin deficiency: the promise of early diagnosis and intervention. Clin Chem. 2006 Dec;52(12):2180–1.
49. Janoff A, Carp H. Possible mechanisms of emphysema in smokers: cigarette smoke condensate suppresses protease inhibition in vitro. Am Rev Respir Dis. 1977 Jul;116(1):65–72.
50. Mayer AS, Stoller JK, Vedal S, Ruttenber AJ, Strand M, Sandhaus RA, et al. Risk factors for symptom onset in PI*Z alpha-1 antitrypsin deficiency. Int J Chron Obstruct Pulmon Dis. 2006;1(4):485–92.
51. Valenti L, Dongiovanni P, Piperno A, Fracanzani AL, Maggioni M, Rametta R, et al. Alpha 1-antitrypsin mutations in NAFLD: high prevalence and association with altered iron metabolism but not with liver damage. Hepatology. 2006 Oct;44(4):857–64.
52. Comba A, Demirbas F, Caltepe G, Eren E, Kalayci AG. Retrospective analysis of children with alpha-1 antitrypsin deficiency. Eur J Gastroenterol Hepatol. 2018 Jul;30(7):774–8.
53. Guillaud O, Dumortier J, Traclet J, Restier L, Joly P, Chapuis-Cellier C, et al. Assessment of liver fibrosis by transient elastography (Fibroscan®) in patients with A1AT deficiency. Clin Res Hepatol Gastroenterol. 2019 Feb;43(1):77–81.
54. Dycaico MJ, Grant SG, Felts K, Nichols WS, Geller SA, Hager JH, et al. Neonatal hepatitis induced by alpha 1-antitrypsin: a transgenic mouse model. Science. 1988 Dec 9;242(4884):1409–12.

55. Carlson JA, Rogers BB, Sifers RN, Finegold MJ, Clift SM, DeMayo FJ, et al. Accumulation of PiZ alpha 1-antitrypsin causes liver damage in transgenic mice. J Clin Invest. 1989 Apr;83(4):1183–90.

56. Ishak KG, Sharp HL. Metabolic errors and liver disease. In: MacSween RNM, Anthony PP, Scheuer PJ, Burt AD, Portmann BC, editors. Pathology of the liver. 3rd ed. Edinburgh: Churchill Livingstone; 1994. p. 123–218.

57. Antoury C, Lopez R, Zein N, Stoller JK, Alkhouri N. Alpha-1 antitrypsin deficiency and the risk of hepatocellular carcinoma in end-stage liver disease. World J Hepatol. 2015 June 8;7(10):1427–32.

58. Johnson EF, Tolkachjov SN, Gibson LE. Alpha-1 antitrypsin deficiency panniculitis: clinical and pathologic characteristics of 10 cases. Int J Dermatol. 2018 Aug;57(8):952–8.

59. Gross B, Grebe M, Wencker M, Stoller JK, Bjursten LM, Janciauskiene S. New findings in PiZZ alpha1-antitrypsin deficiency-related panniculitis. Demonstration of skin polymers and high dosing requirements of intravenous augmentation therapy. Dermatology. 2009;218(4):370–5.

60. Blanco I, Lipsker D, Lara B, Janciauskiene S. Neutrophilic panniculitis associated with alpha-1-antitrypsin deficiency: an update. Br J Dermatol. 2016 Apr;174(4):753–62.

61. Stone H, Pye A, Stockley RA. Disease associations in alpha-1-antitrypsin deficiency. Respir Med. 2014 Feb;108(2):338–43.

62. Hadzik-Blaszczyk M, Zdral A, Zielonka TM, Rozy A, Krupa R, Falkowski A, et al. SERPINA1 gene variants in granulomatosis with polyangiitis. Adv Exp Med Biol. 2018;1070:9–18.

63. Greulich T, Nell C, Hohmann D, Grebe M, Janciauskiene S, Koczulla AR, et al. The prevalence of diagnosed alpha1-antitrypsin deficiency and its comorbidities: results from a large population-based database. Eur Respir J. 2017 Jan;49(1):1600154.

64. St Jean P, Hart B, Webster M, Steed D, Adamson J, Powell J, et al. Alpha-1-antitrypsin deficiency in aneurysmal disease. Hum Hered. 1996 Mar-Apr;46(2):92–7.

65. Davis ID, Burke B, Freese D, Sharp HL, Kim Y. The pathologic spectrum of the nephropathy associated with alpha 1-antitrypsin deficiency. Hum Pathol. 1992 Jan;23(1):57–62.

66. Heimbach JK, Kulik LM, Finn RS, Sirlin CB, Abecassis MM, Roberts LR, et al. AASLD guidelines for the treatment of hepatocellular carcinoma. Hepatology. 2018 Jan;67(1):358–80.

67. Teckman JH. Emerging concepts and human trials in alpha-1-antitrypsin deficiency liver disease. Semin Liver Dis. 2017 May;37(2):152–8.

68. Townsend SA, Edgar RG, Ellis PR, Kantas D, Newsome PN, Turner AM. Systematic review: the natural history of alpha-1 antitrypsin deficiency, and associated liver disease. Aliment Pharmacol Ther. 2018;47(7):877–85. https://doi.org/10.1111/apt.14537.

69. Carey EJ, Iyer VN, Nelson ER, Nguyen JH, Krowka MJ. Outcomes for recipients of liver transplantation for alpha-1-antitrypsin deficiency–related cirrhosis. Liver Transpl. 2013;19(12):1370–6.

# Chapter 11
# Hemochromatosis

Nora V. Bergasa

A 26-year-old man was admitted to Behavioral Health for detoxification from heroin, which he had been using for 5 years. He had a history of polysubstance abuse since age fifteen. His physical exam was normal. His hepatic panel was notable for high serum activity of aspartate (AST) and alanine (ALT) amino transaminases, 128 IU/L (normal range: 10–40) and 437 IU/L (normal range: 10–45) IU/L, respectively, and alkaline phosphatase (AP) of 180 IU/L (normal range: 40–120), and normal serum concentration of bilirubin and albumin, and normal prothrombin time. The liver sonogram revealed hepatomegaly. Liver disease workup was notable for the presence of hepatitis C RNA, consistently documented, suggestive of chronic hepatitis C virus infection, a serum ferritin concentration of 4545 ng/ml (normal range 15–150) with a transferrin saturation of 96%. Hemochromatosis gene testing revealed two copies of C282Y consistent with primary hemochromatosis. The patient was referred to genetics and to the hepatology clinic to treat chronic hepatitis C and iron overload.

Hemochromatosis is a disease characterized by iron overload [1]. It results from mutations in the hemochromatosis gene (*HFE*), which codes HFE. There are non-*HFE* mutations that result in iron overload [1]. Hemochromatosis has been classified according to the gene where the mutation has been identified [1] (Table 11.1).

Hepcidin, a hormone made in the liver, controls iron absorption, which requires a normal functioning HFE [2]. The interaction between hepcidin and ferroportin (FPN) regulates the amount of iron in the bloodstream [3–5]. The development of progressive iron overload is more common in men than in women. It appears to be influenced by other genetic factors, the environment, blood loss, and alcohol consumption.

N. V. Bergasa (✉)
Department of Medicine, H+H/Metropolitan, New York, NY, USA

New York Medical College, Valhalla, NY, USA

Hepatology, H+H/Woodhull, Brooklyn, NY, USA

© The Author(s), under exclusive license to Springer-Verlag London Ltd., part of Springer Nature 2022
N. V. Bergasa (ed.), *Clinical Cases in Hepatology*,
https://doi.org/10.1007/978-1-4471-4715-2_11

**Table 11.1** Classification of hemochromatosis

| Type 1 *HFE*-hemochromatosis (*HFE*-related) | | Type 2 Hemochromatosis (non-*HFE*-related) | | Type 3 Mutated transferrin receptor | Type 4 Mutated ferroportin 1 gene, *SLC11A3* |
|---|---|---|---|---|---|
| Type 1 a | Cys282Tyr homozygosity | Type 2 a | Juvenile hemochromatosis (hemojuvelin mutations) | | |
| Type 1 b | Compound Cys282Tyr/His63Asp heterozygosity | Type 2 b | Juvenile hemochromatosis (hepcidin mutations) | | |
| Type 1 c | Ser65Cys, * Increased serum and ferritin concentration; iron overload has not been documented | | | | |

*and other HFE genotypes

# Iron Homeostasis

Iron is an essential element in human beings. Iron participates in energy generation reactions within the cytochrome p450 enzymatic group; when iron is complexed with protoporphyrins it forms heme, the major oxygen-binding molecule. Iron is transported in the circulation by transferrin, by haptoglobin in association with hemoglobin, and is stored in ferritin. Ferritin is a spherical protein comprised of 24 subunits of heavy or light types. The ferritin concentration reflects iron stores, although it is also an acute phase reactant. Ferrous iron is delivered to ferritin by Poly (rC)-binding protein 1 (PCBP1), a cytosolic iron chaperone, to be stored [6]; iron is released from ferritin, as documented in vitro, by lysosomal proteolysis [7].

Iron's only source to human beings is the diet. Dietary non-heme iron is absorbed through the apical membrane of the enterocyte in the ferrous form ($Fe^{++}$), which originates from the reduction of ferric iron ($Fe^{+++}$) by duodenal cytochrome b reductase 1 [8]; other ferric reductases may also be involved. Ferrous iron enters from the intestinal lumen through the brush border into the cytoplasm of the enterocyte through the divalent metal ion transporter-1 (DMT1) [9], whereas heme iron (i.e., from meat), which is more easily absorbed than ferrous iron, enters the enterocyte via the heme carrier protein-1 (HCP-1), which was subsequently identified as the folate transporter [10], formally named solute carrier family 46 *(SLC46A1)*. Ferrous iron is transported across the basolateral membrane of the enterocyte by FPN [5]; it is oxidized to ferric iron by hephaestin, a multi-copper oxidase located in the basolateral membrane, and binds to transferrin in the blood [11]. Alternatively, in the enterocyte, iron is incorporated into ferritin at the conversion of ferrous into ferric iron by the ferroxidase activity of the H chain of ferritin. Regardless of the iron's source entering the enterocyte, the exit to the blood is via the same route, i.e., FPN [3–5].

FPN is the only known exporter of iron [3–5]. It is expressed on the basolateral surface of the duodenal enterocytes [5, 12], membranes of macrophages [12], the sinusoidal surface of hepatocytes [13], and the placental surface facing the fetal circulation [4]. FPN is encoded by two tissue-specific differentially spliced transcripts, FPN1A and FPN1B, the latter being strongly expressed in the duodenum and erythroid cell precursors, and which differ between each other in the presence of 5'IRE (iron response element) in the former, and its absence in the latter, not being repressed in iron deficiency states [14].

The export of iron depends on copper-containing ferroxidases, including ceruloplasmin, hephaestin, and possibly zyklopen, which oxidize ferrous iron by the use of molecular oxygen [11, 15, 16]. Ceruloplasmin deficiency impairs iron absorption and its release from macrophages and is associated with liver and brain iron accumulation [15, 17]. The role of ferroxidases in the export of iron is proposed to be the facilitation of efflux of reduced iron by oxidizing it to its ferric form, thus allowing its uptake by apotransferrin and decreasing the concentration of ferrous iron on the cell surface, and maintaining a ferrous iron gradient to the extracellular face of FPN, which drives iron transport [18].

Iron travels bound to transferrin and is taken up by almost all cells by the transferrin receptor 1 (TFR1), to which diferric transferrin binds, being internalized by endosomes, where iron is released by endosomal acidification. Iron regulatory proteins 1 and 2 (IRP1 and IRP2) are cytoplasmic proteins that play a role in iron homeostasis by regulating ferritin translation and TfR1 mRNA stability, thus regulating the receptor expression central for iron uptake into the cell [19]. Ferric iron is reduced by STEASP3 and transported through the endosomal membrane by DMT1 [20]. In this form, iron is utilized by the cells or stored in ferritin. Apotransferrin (i.e., transferrin without iron) bound to TFR1 is recycled from the endosome to the surface of the cells where it is released from the bond at a neutral pH, making the receptor available to bind additional holotransferrin (i.e., diferric transferrin) [21]. The hepatocytes also express transferrin receptor 2 (TFR2); however, its affinity for holotransferrin is lower than that for TfR1, and is reported not to play a major role in the uptake of iron bound to transferrin, according to animal experiments [22].

Iron also circulates in relatively small amounts bound to proteins other than transferrin, i.e., nontransferrin bound iron (NTBI); however, when transferrin saturation increases, this type of iron also increases, being of pathological importance in iron overload conditions like hemochromatosis. NTBI is toxic and cleared by the hepatocytes by the transporters DMT1 [23] and Zrt-, Irt-like protein 14 (Zip14) [24].

Macrophages phagocytize senescent erythrocytes, digesting them and their hemoglobin, and releasing heme, which is subsequently degraded by the inducible oxygenase-1 (HO-1), making iron available for cytoplasmic storage, or export to plasma, also by the same route that iron leaves the enterocyte, i.e., via FPN. During hemolysis, heme may be exported in intact form by heme transporters bound to hemopexin, a plasma heme carrier, as an alternative pathway [18].

Hepcidin, a protein made in the liver, controls iron homeostasis in human beings [2]. The iron not transferred to plasma is stored in macrophages, hepatocytes, and possibly placenta. The iron not transferred from enterocytes to the plasma is lost by the sloughing intestinal epithelial cells every few days. In addition, iron is lost during menstruation.

# Hepcidin

The concentration of iron in human beings tends to be constant. It was reported from a study from the United States that in men, the distribution of iron stores is $9.82 \pm 2.82$ mg/kg and $5.5 \pm 3.35$ mg/kg in 93% of women, with the remaining 7% being deficient by $3.87 \pm 3.23$ mg/kg [25]. In iron deficiency, iron absorption increases, and in association with parenteral iron administration, it decreases [26]. It is the hormone hepcidin that controls iron homeostasis [2]. Hepcidin, encoded by *HAMP* in chromosome 19, is a peptide hormone produced by the hepatocytes. It is a negative regulator of iron absorption that exerts its function by binding to FPN, encoded by *FPN1 (SLC40A1)*. The binding of hepcidin to FPN leads to the internalization of the latter, with its final degradation, limiting the absorption of iron by the enterocyte, and its recycling by the macrophages to maintain a homeostatic transferrin saturation [27]. Low concentrations of hepcidin are associated with increased iron absorption versus high hepcidin concentrations, which are associated with low iron absorption [2].

Hepcidin is generated from an 84-amino acid prepropeptide that contains an $NH_2$-terminal 24-amino acid signal sequence cleaved to yield prohepcidin, which is cleaved by furin-like prohormone convertases at the COOH-terminal peptide bond after a polybasic sequence [28]. It circulates in plasma mostly free, with minimal binding to albumin and alpha 2-macroglobulin [29, 30]. Up to the residue nine of the terminal amino acids of hepcidin, including a single thiol cysteine, is required for its function [28, 31, 32], i.e., control of the expression of FPN, the iron exporter, by mediating its endocytosis and proteolysis by lysosomes, for which ubiquitination of lysines in the cytoplasmic loop of FPN may be required [33], and thus regulating the amount of iron that is delivered to plasma and all iron consuming tissues [27]. In regard to FPN, the extracellular FPN residue, C326, is essential for hepcidin binding [31]; in addition, some aromatic side chains, including phenylalanine and tyrosine, in the interacting segments of hepcidin and FPN, have been identified experimentally as important elements for their interaction [32].

The regulation of hepcidin is transcriptional and the major regulators of hepcidin synthesis are iron bound to transferrin (iron-transferrin), iron stores, inflammation, and erythroid activity [34]. It is reported that bone morphogenic proteins (BMP) receptors [35], likely Alk2 or Alk3 [36], as type I subunits, and ActRIIA, as type II subunits [37], and the SMAD pathway are pivotal in the regulation of hepcidin, the promoter of which has several BMP response elements. Hemojuvelin (HJV), a protein linked to glycophosphatidylinositol, is a coreceptor of BMP required for its activation in the context of iron homeostasis [38].

Extracellular iron sensors seem to be involved in iron homeostasis; however, the mechanisms have not been completely elucidated and may include transferrin receptor types 1 and 2 (TfR1 and TfR2), holotransferrin, and membrane serine protease mariptase-2 (TMPRSS6): (i) the disruption of transferrin receptor type 2 (TfR2) is associated with a loss of extracellular iron sensing [39, 40], (ii) holotransferrin and the protein involved in hemochromatosis, HFE, compete for binding with the TfR1, which has been interpreted to suggest that the HFE-TfR1 complex may be another sensor for holotransferrin, independent from TfR2, or via its interaction with TfR2 and with HJV [41], and (iii): TMPRSS6 cleaves BMP, an HJV agonist, thus inactivating the hepcidin-BMP signaling.

In regard to the effect of iron stores on hepcidin expression, it was documented that TfR2, HJV, BMP6, and HFE are involved in the response of hepcidin to acute iron overload but not in chronic iron overloading or BMP-6 expression [42]. Conditions that also regulate hepcidin include erythropoiesis [26], inflammation [43], and liver injury [44–46].

In high iron concentrations, the highly saturated transferrin stabilizes TfR2, disrupting the interaction between the HFE protein and TfR1 leading to increased BMP-6 secretion from nonparenchymal liver cells, which facilitates the formation of a complex comprised of BMP receptor/BMP6/HJV /neogenin/TfR2/HFE that induces the expression of hepcidin [47–49]. An increase in iron increases HAMP expression, and hence an increase in hepcidin, which prevents the transport of iron from the enterocyte and macrophage via FPN. Excess iron and inflammation both induce HAMP expression, which, in turn, results in decreased iron absorption and diminished iron release from macrophages.

Low iron hepatic concentrations decrease BMP6 secretion, which hampers the BMP signaling pathway, reducing the expression of hepcidin. In the presence of inflammation, interleukin 6 and activin B are induced in the liver, which activates hepcidin's transcription via the STAT3/JAK2 pathway and BMP signaling pathway, respectively.

A decrease in hepcidin may result from mutations in the HFE or TfR2 genes, leading to hemochromatosis in the adult. Mutations in the HJV or HAMP genes lead to juvenile hemochromatosis. Juvenile hemochromatosis is an autosomal recessive disorder resulting in iron overload at an early age, and high transferrin saturation, and ferritin concentrations [50].

A deficiency in hepcidin results in increased expression of ferroportin (FPN) at the cellular surface, mostly of enterocytes, and macrophages, which leads to an increase in the export of iron. Serum iron concentrations and transferrin saturation then increase, leading to increased iron uptake by the liver, pancreas, and heart resulting in iron overload, which characterizes hemochromatosis [1].

Mutations in FPN are also associated with iron overload due to resistance to hepcidin. A77D, V162del, and G490D mutations inhibit FPN activity, i.e., loss of function, associated with increased iron deposition in Kupffer cells, and normal transferrin saturation. The Y64N and C326Y variants are resistant to the inhibition by hepcidin. The N144D and N144H are partially resistant, i.e., gain of function, associated with high transferrin saturation, and increased deposition of iron in the liver parenchyma [51, 52].

## Iron Mediated Injury

It has been considered that iron, in its ferrous state, interacts with $H_2O_2$ to generate the highly injurious hydroxyl radical [53, 54]; it has been stated, however, that these experiments were not conducted in proper models of iron overload, nor experimental conditions analogous to the pathophysiology of iron overload in human beings [55]. Iron alone appears to be associated with limited hepatic inflammation and fibrosis but, in association with other toxic elements or hepatic comorbidities, and by stimulating hepatic stellate cells combined with cofactors to be identified, may drive liver injury and consequent cirrhosis [55].

## Genetics

The hemochromatosis gene (*HFE* (*H* for high and *FE* for iron)) is located on the short arm of chromosome 6 (6p22.1), within the extended HLA class I region [56]. *HFE* has six exons, with histone genes on each side; at least nine alternatively spliced forms have been documented. The product of *HFE* is HFE, a membrane associated beta 2-microglobulin protein, comprised of an alpha chain encoded by *HFE* and a beta 2-microglobulin, as the beta chain.

The most common mutations in *HFE* are substitutions of: (i) cysteine for tyrosine at position 282 (p.C282Y), (ii) histidine for aspartate at position 63 (p.H63D), and (iii) serine for cysteine at position 65 (p.S65C). C282Y is the most common mutation, considered to have originated in Northern Europe, with a frequency of one in 200 individuals [57]; most patients with hemochromatosis are homozygous for C282Y. H63D is geographically distributed more widely than C282Y [58]. Approximately 4% of patients with hemochromatosis are compound heterozygous for the mutations, i.e., C282Y/H63D. The evidence of iron overload in subjects with the S65C mutation is not strong; however, in combination with C282Y, there can be a phenotypic expression of the disease [59].

Experiments conducted in COS-7 cells revealed that HFE protein is expressed on the cell surface and that it binds beta 2-microglobulin; however, these characteristics disappear in the mutated C282Y, which was documented to remain in the endoplasmic reticulum and in the middle compartment of the Golgi apparatus, which does not process the protein normally, subsequently undergoing accelerated degradation [60]. The H63D and S65C mutations alter the α1 binding groove but do not prevent HFE presentation on cell surfaces.

Mutations can increase the phenotypic expression of C282Y in homozygosity in genes that concern iron homeostasis. The mutations pR59G, pG71D, or pR56X in the HAMP gene [61] and by the mutations S105L, E302K, N372D, R335Q L101P, and G320V in the HJV gene [62], both in the heterozygote state, in patients with homozygosity for C282Y result in marked iron overload, manifested relatively early [61]. Single nucleotide polymorphisms (SNP) may also influence the expression of C282Y homozygosity, including SNP in the haptoglobin (Hp) [63] and BMP2 genes [64]; however, the findings could not be reproduced [65].

Large genome-wide association studies (GWAS) identified three variants in serum transferrin, rs3811647, rs1799852, and rs2280673, in addition to the HFE C282Y mutation, which explained approximately 40% of the genetic variation in serum transferrin [66]. A subsequent GWAS confirmed rs3811647 in the TF gene as the only SNP associated with iron homeostasis through serum transferrin and iron concentrations [67]. Eleven genome-wide-significant loci that included HFE, SLC40A1, TF, TFR2, TFRC, TMPRSS6, and the newly identified ABO, ARNTL, FADS2, NAT2, TEX14 were documented, with SNPs at ARNTL, TF, and TFR2 that affect iron indices in patients homozygous for C282Y [68]. By the same methodology, the proprotein convertase subtilisin/kexin type 7 (PCSK7) rs236918 C allele was identified as a risk factor in patients homozygous for C282Y. These studies have helped to explain the variability of the C282Y homozygous phenotypic expression [69].

# Epidemiology

In 1990, important studies from Australia documented the prevalence of iron overload in patients with hemochromatosis. In homozygous, it was reported as 0.36% in a group of 1968 subjects, mostly Caucasian, translated as 1 in 300 subjects; a transferrin saturation greater than 45% along with high serum ferritin had a predictive value for accurate diagnosis of 64%, finding that suggested the use of this finding in screening programs [70].

Subsequent studies reported the frequency of the C282Y mutation in the general population to be 6.2% from a group of 127,613 participants included in an individual patient meta-analysis from 36 studies [71], four of which were from the United States, which documented from: (i) 100 randomly selected individuals, a prevalence of the C282Y homozygosity of 1% in Caucasians, and that of C282Y heterozygosity 8% in Caucasians, 3% in Hispanics, and 2% in African Americans, and of H63D homozygosity 4% in Caucasians and 1% in Hispanics, and heterozygosity in 24% in Caucasians, 15% in Hispanics, and 3.5% in African Americans [72], (ii) 10,198 adult subjects a frequency of the C282Y mutation of 0.063, of H63D 0.152 and of 0.016 for S65C mutation in whites [73], (iii) 5171 participants in the Third National Health and Nutrition Examination Survey conducted from 1992 to 1994 an estimated prevalence of the C282Y gene mutation of 0.26% (95% confidence interval (CI), 0.12%–0.49%), and 1.89% (95% CI, 1.48%–2.43%) for H63D homozygosity, with compound heterozygosity being 1.97% (95% CI, 1.54%–2.49%); an estimated prevalence of C282Y heterozygosity of 9.54% in non-Hispanic whites, 2.33% in non-Hispanic blacks, and 2.75% in Mexican-Americans [74], and (iv) 4865 subjects a frequency of C282Y of 0.0507 in whites, and 0.0067 in African Americans, and for H63D, 0.1512 in whites, and 0.0263 in African Americans [75]. It was concluded from the meta-analysis that a genotype frequency for C282Y could be calculated to be 0.38%, i.e., 1 in 260 subjects, with a wide geographic variation. However, it was documented from 41,038 subjects, from whom 152 were homozygous for the mutation, that only one patient had signs and symptoms suggestive of hemochromatosis, although a history of hepatitis and abnormal serum activity of serum aspartate aminotransferase, not correlated with iron burden or age, was more common in the subjects with the mutation than in those without it, suggesting that the penetrance of the mutation was low, with less than 1% of homozygous developing the clinical disease [76]. The biochemical expression of C282Y, i.e., high serum ferritin concentration and high transferrin saturation, is reported as 75% for men and 50% for women, as reported from studies that evaluated subjects of European descent [77, 78].

A meta-analysis that included 2802 European heritage subjects with hemochromatosis documented the proportion of homozygosity for C282Y as 80.6% and compound heterozygosity for C282Y and H63D as 5.3%. In the control subjects, the reported proportion of C282Y homozygosity was 0.6%, and compound heterozygosity was 1.3% [71].

In contrast to C282Y, H63D has less geographic variation, with a reported average allelic frequency of 14%. S65C, which can be associated with iron overload in association with C282Y, was documented to have a frequency of approximately 0.5%, most commonly found in Brittany, France [71].

From a study that included what was reported as a racially diverse group comprised of 99,711 subjects, 299 were documented as homozygous for the C282Y mutation, with an estimated prevalence of 0.44% in non-Hispanic whites, 0.11% in Native Americans, 0.027% in Hispanics, 0.014% in blacks, 0.012 in Pacific Islanders, and very uncommon in Asians, with a proportion of 0.000039% [77].

## Natural History

The natural history of hemochromatosis was documented from a group of patients with variable HFE genotypes known as the HealthIron cohort from a total of 31,192 of Northern European extraction subjects recruited from 1990 to 1994 in Australia. The study of serum iron indices in the 203 patients identified as homozygous for HFE C282Y and followed for a mean of 12 years documented that the predicted probability of having serum ferritin greater than 1000 mcg/ml was between 13% and 35% for men, and 16% to 22% for women. In patients with normal serum ferritin at baseline, the prediction to go over 1000 mcg/ml at follow up was less than 15% without any therapeutic interventions. These data were interpreted to indicate that sufficient iron to place patients at risk for complications would be accumulated by age 55. In addition, it was concluded that in men and not in women, a transferrin saturation greater than 95% at a mean age of 55 years increased the probability of having high serum ferritin by age 65 [79]. It was also concluded from the same group of subjects that 28.4% of men homozygous for C282Y had documented iron overload, versus 1.2% for women. There was an increase in reported symptoms, including fatigue and "use of arthritis medicine," and of liver disease in men versus women [78]; this difference was interpreted to result from blood loss from menstruation [78, 79]. One hundred and eighty patients, 84 of whom were men, were identified as compound heterozygotes, i.e., C282Y/ H63D, compared with 330 control subjects, 149 of whom were men in regard to iron studies, which revealed significantly increased serum concentration of serum ferritin and transferrin saturation in compound heterozygotes regardless of the gender, as compared to the normal genotype. Men and women, compound heterozygotes, had similar comorbidities related to iron overload as those with the wild type, with only one of 82 men and zero of 95 women with documented iron overload disease. These data were interpreted to indicate that although they may have abnormal iron indices in patients with compound heterozygosity, disease from iron overload is rare [80].

SNP have been identified in genes associated with iron metabolism, including *TF*, the gene that codes transferrin [78], and *DCYTB*, which codes cytochrome b reductase 1 [81] that likely modify the variable expression of iron overload disease [81]. In addition, an SNP in the gene TGF-beta1, which codes tumor growth factor-beta 1, was identified as associated with cirrhosis in patients with hemochromatosis [82]. Genetic factors also seem to protect from progressive disease, as reported by an increase in the survival of patients homozygous for C282Y identified as carrying HLA-A*03, B*14 [83].

Exogenous factors that include excessive alcohol use [84, 85], and hepatic comorbidities that include fatty liver [86], and chronic hepatitis C viral infection [87], have also been reported in association with an increase in the clinical expression of genetic hemochromatosis by accelerating liver injury from iron overload. Conversely, the C282Y mutation was reported in 44% of 27 patients with porphyria cutanea tarda (PCT) versus 12% in a control group of 12 patients; this finding has suggested that the mutation may be a triggering factor for the manifestations of the PTC [88].

## Clinical Manifestations

The classic clinical manifestations of hemochromatosis are cirrhosis, hyperpigmentation, and diabetes. They tend to become apparent in the fourth decade of life by which 15 to 40 g of iron have accumulated in the body.

Four states have been described in the disease: (I) genetic mutation and increased serum transferrin saturation, in some cases, (II) iron overload not associated with symptoms, (III) iron overload associated with symptoms of early disease, e.g., fatigue, and (IV) iron overload in association with end-organ damage including cirrhosis.

From a study conducted in Australia that included 251 patients with hemochromatosis enrolled from 1947 to 1991, most patients reported symptoms independent from the presence of cirrhosis [89]. Fatigue has been reported as the most common symptom in hemochromatosis [78, 90, 91]; however, most patients are asymptomatic at the time of diagnosis. Symptoms have been reported in association with serum ferritin greater than 1000 microg/L [1].

From a group of 251 patients [79], hepatomegaly was the most common finding in physical examination (81%), followed by hyperpigmentation (72%), body hair loss (16%), splenomegaly (10%), with less than 10% of patients having peripheral edema, jaundice, and ascites. Seven percent of men had gynecomastia. Except for hyperpigmentation and gynecomastia, all signs were significantly more common in patients with than in those without cirrhosis [79].

Serum activity of AST and ALT was abnormal in 60 to greater than 65% of patients [89, 92], especially in the presence of cirrhosis [92].

Cardiac complications from hemochromatosis were documented in 10% of patients with the disease in a study that investigated the relationship between iron overload, age, and clinical symptoms [90], with electrocardiogram changes being reported in 35% of patients in another study, found significantly more common in patients with cirrhosis (46%) than in those without (21%) [89].

Bronze diabetes was the name for hemochromatosis, diabetes being one of the most recognized complications of this disease. A quantitative immunohistochemical and ultrastructural study of human pancreas in hemochromatosis documented that in patients with the disease iron overload was prominent in the exocrine tissue, there was a reduced number of immunoreactive B cells, to which iron deposit was restricted, in association with a loss of their endocrine granules; the findings were reported to be different from those reported in type I and II diabetes and suggested a role of iron in the pathogenesis of diabetes in hemochromatosis [93]. The prevalence of diabetes in a study that included 410 patients with hemochromatosis from Canada and France was 14%, with a documented statistical association with iron overload [90]. It has been subsequently reported that the frequency of diabetes in patients with hemochromatosis was not higher in patients homozygous for C282Y versus those without *HFE* mutations [76, 77]; the screening nature of these studies might have decreased the prevalence of diabetes by not including patients with known hemochromatosis who might have had this complication of the disease [76, 77]. Also, the increased diabetes prevalence in the general population was proposed as a reason for the absence of diabetes as a more prevalent condition in patients with hemochromatosis than in those without the disease [78]. The interpretation of the risk of diabetes in hemochromatosis seems to be evolving as factors including increased iron entry into beta cells by mechanisms that include transferrin receptors, and DMT1, decreased insulin secretion due to pancreatic atrophy, islet cells inflammation, injury of beta cells, and genetic predisposition are identified [94].

Hypogonadotropic hypogonadism is a complication of hemochromatosis, which seems to be decreasing in incidence because of screening measures for hemochromatosis. The prevalence of hypogonadism in men was 14.6% from 1983 and 1995 [95, 96]. Hypogonadism significantly decreased to 3% from 1996 to 2003, [95], and to 6.4%, in a study that included subjects diagnosed from 1983 to the first half of the 2000 decade, with a reported prevalence of 5.2% in women [96]; however, the prevalence of hypogonadism in the latter referenced study was 89% in patients with cirrhosis and 33% in those with diabetes [96]. A study that assessed pituitary function in idiopathic hemochromatosis in 36 men documented that the pituitary deficiency associated with the disease is gonadotrophic [97]; however, another study reported abnormalities in both pituitary and end-organ function [98]. Impotence was documented in 40% of men [90]. A study that used mailed question-naires and that had the Dutch Hemochromatosis Association as a source docu-mented that some aspect of sexual function was impaired in 7% to 39% of the 69 participants, findings not different from that reported from studies from the general population [99]. The pathogenesis of hypopituitarism as a cause of hypogonadism in regard to iron overload has not been elucidated. In regard to testicular function, iron is required for spermatogenesis; it is considered that iron transport through the seminiferous tubules' basal membrane is independent and protects against iron overload associated with hemochromatosis [100]. Thus, a pituitary dysfunction that affects the hypophyseal–gonadal axis seems to be favored, although direct iron damage has not been unequivocally excluded [101].

The arthropathy associated with hemochromatosis is more common in men than in women and prevalent between 40 and 55 years of age; the most commonly involved joints are hips, knees, first carpometacarpal (CMC), proximal interphalan-geal (PIP), distal PIP, second and third metacarpophalangeal (MCP), and ankles [102]. With a specialty clinic in rheumatology from where 62 patients were included and the UK Haemochromatosis Society, with 470 patient survey respondents, as sources, a study reported that a diagnosis of hemochromatosis was made in the fifth decade of life, with 77% and 76% of subjects, respectively, having reported symp-toms related to joints for 8 years prior to the diagnosis, with the involvement of the MCP in 38.5% of patients, and ankles in 29.5%, followed by knees, hips, and PIP joints; at the time of clinical assessment or submission of the questionnaire for the study, the most commonly affected joints were PIP in 64.5% of subjects, knees in 64%, ankles in 61%, and MCP in 60%, in the group seen at the specialty clinic, versus CMC in 59%, wrists in 52%, PEP in 47%, MCP in 46%, knee in 42%, and ankle in 35% in the self-reporting group. It was concluded from this study that symptoms from arthropathy predate the diagnosis of hemochromatosis by almost 10 years and that arthropathy of MCP joints and ankles at a relatively early age in the absence of trauma, rare in osteoarthritis, is an indication to exclude hemochro-matosis [103].

A web-based cross-sectional study conducted in Australia in patients with hemo-chromatosis that included the assessment of the quality of life [104] revealed that patients who reported arthritis in association with the disease had lower mean utility (0.52: F(1,198) = 10.854, $p$ = 0.001), 0.66 as the reference value, utility being "...a measure of the strength of preference for a particular health state 'that, when combined with life years gained (LYG),'…the outcome reflects both morbidity and mortality: quality adjusted life years (QALYs)"[105]. This finding is consistent with the prior study that revealed that, although cirrhosis was the most important complication affecting survival, arthritis was the most important complication affecting the quality of life [106].

The pathogenesis of hemochromatosis related arthropathy has not been elucidated, although iron has been considered a relevant etiologic factor [107]. A study that examined the synovium and arthropathy radiographic changes in 27 patients with hemochromatosis documented the most prevalent findings as villus formation and iron deposition within synovial intimal cells [116]. Arthropathy did not correlate with histology but was present in 26% of cases with the above reported histological findings but did correlate with total body iron as per the differential ferrioxamine test [108]. Other histological studies of the synovium from patients with hemochromatosis have documented infiltration with mononuclear cells and lymphocytes, neovascularization, and hyperplasia, findings reported as prominent in association with hemosiderin deposition; although the type of cellular invasion in hemochromatosis was reported as similar to osteoarthritis, the neutrophil invasion was more pronounced in the former than in the latter, and it may contribute to the rapid progressive arthropathy of hemochromatosis [109]. Arthropathy is not reversed or its progression halted by iron removal [107, 108].

The prevalence of osteoporosis in patients with cirrhosis and hemochromatosis was 25% to 78% [110, 111], and osteopenia was 41% [112]. In a study that included 38 men with hemochromatosis, hypogonadism was documented in the minority of patients, and femoral neck bone mineral density was decreased in association with an increased degree of hepatic iron concentrations similar in patients with and without cirrhosis. These data were interpreted to suggest that factors, including iron itself, other than cirrhosis and hypogonadism, are involved in the pathogenesis of bone disease in hemochromatosis [111]. From a study that included 87 patients it was reported that osteoporosis and hypogonadism were associated with bone disease, findings related to the degree of iron overload [112]. An association between iron overload and osteoporosis was reported in a study of 304 patients with hemochromatosis, 23% of whom had been diagnosed with the bone complication. Also, wrist and vertebral fractures were prevalent in the latter group [113]. One mechanism in the development of bone disease in hemochromatosis involved the facilitation of osteoclasts' differentiation by iron [114], and the deterrence of the osteogenic differentiation of multipotent mesenchymal stem cells, from which osteoblasts derive themselves, and which are inhibited by iron, the latter by the inhibition of the osteogenic transcription factor runt-related transcription factor 2 (Runx2) [115]. Iron removal via phlebotomy was reported in association with improvement in bone density [116].

The most recognized dermatological manifestation of hemochromatosis is hyperpigmentation, characterized by a brown or gray slate color, most prominent on sun exposed areas. A retrospective study that included 22 patients documented hyperpigmentation in seventeen (77%) [117]; however, this study's retrospective nature may have overestimated the prevalence. Skin biopsies documented siderosis in eccrine sweat glands reported as specific for the disease, and melanin accumulation, in the epidermis' basal layers [118], the former associated with a decrease after phlebotomy but not the latter. In addition, ichthyosis and koilonychias are reported in patients with the disease [119].

## Laboratory Tests

The hallmark of hemochromatosis is high serum ferritin concentrations and transferrin saturation. Serum ferritin can be normal in the early stages of the disease. The increase in serum ferritin can result from a reaction to an acute event, i.e., ferritin being an acute phase reactant, and from hepatic comorbidities including alcoholic liver disease and chronic hepatitis C; thus, alone, it is not diagnostic of hemochromatosis. Transferrin saturation is the earliest laboratory evidence of hemochromatosis [120, 121]. It was documented that an unsaturated iron binding capacity equal or less than 25 micromoles/L confirmed C282Y homozygosity with 83% sensitivity and 99% specificity, indicating similar performance to transferrin saturation in the identification of patients with hemochromatosis [122]. The guidelines from the American College of Gastroenterology (ACG) recommend diagnostic workup that includes serum ferritin, iron, transferrin saturation, and unsaturated iron binding capacity [123]. The guidelines indicate that patients with hepatitis, suggested by serum activity of transaminases greater than 35 IU/ml with normal transferrin saturation and serum ferritin concentrations do not have hemochromatosis. Patients with hepatitis in association with either transferrin saturation of at least 45% or high serum ferritin, or both, should have hemochromatosis genetic testing. The guidelines recommend that: (i) patients who are homozygous for C282Y should have phlebotomy, (ii) for homozygous for C282Y with serum ferritin greater 1000 mg/dl or hepatitis, a liver biopsy can be considered to rule out cirrhosis. Serum ferritin concentration equal or greater than 1000 microg/L, a platelet count equal or lower than $200 \times 10(9)$/L, and serum activity of AST greater than the upper limit of normal were associated with the diagnosis of cirrhosis in 77% of patients in a study from Canada, and in 90% of patients in a study from France, findings that have been used to avoid a liver biopsy [124]. Serum hyaluronidase was reported to identify cirrhosis in patients with hemochromatosis and serum ferritin concentrations greater than 1000 micrograms/L [125]; however, in another study, the concentration of hyaluronic acid did not accurately predict severe fibrosis. The use of this marker in cirrhosis has not been incorporated into standard practice. For patients who are compound heterozygotes (i.e., C282Y/H63D), and who have non-C282Y hemochromatosis, evaluation of hepatic iron concentration should be done by liver biopsy or by magnetic resonance imaging (MRI); if increased tissue iron is documented, phlebotomy should be started if ferritin is greater than 1000 mg/dl [123].

Elevated serum ferritin concentration in association with high serum transferrin saturation can also result from mutations in hemojuvelin, hepcidin, and TfR2 genes, in contrast to patients with ferroportin disease with gain of function [126] or aceru-loplasminemia [15, 17] who have high serum ferritin concentrations but normal transferrin saturation. In this context, hepatic iron concentration assessment by liver biopsy or MRI is recommended; hepatic iron measure greater than 150 micromoles/g is consistent with ferroportin disease or aceruloplasminemia, between 50 and 150 micromoles/g with conditions of dysmetabolic iron overload syndrome [127], and less or equal to 50, is consistent with L ferritin disease [128]. The ACG guidelines suggest not to proceed with genetic testing in patients with iron indices suggestive of iron overload who are negative for the C282Y and H63D mutations [123].

In a study comprised of 182 patients with hemochromatosis from the United States, liver cirrhosis was absent in patients who are homozygous for C282Y and in compound heterozygous for C282Y/H63D whose serum ferritin was less than 1000 microgram/L; in combination with hepatitis, the probability of cirrhosis was 72%, and in patients with serum ferritin concentrations less than 1000 micrograms/L, it was 7.4%. These findings have suggested that a liver biopsy is not paramount in evaluating patients with hemochromatosis, as inferences regarding indications for phlebotomy and screening for hepatocellular carcinoma (HCC) can be made from non-invasive laboratory findings [124, 129].

The ACG practice guidelines suggest a non-invasive test, i.e., a non-contrast enhanced MRI in conjunction with the software used for the estimation of hepatic iron concentration (i.e., MRI T2*) in patients being investigated for iron overload in the absence of C282Y homozygosity. The use of transient elastography has not been sufficiently explored in patients with iron overload. One hundred and three consecutive subjects, 57 with hemochromatosis and 46 as control subjects, were prospectively evaluated and documented as having similar fibrosis measures, 5.20 kPa in the disease group and 4.9 kPa in the control group; however, 22.8% of patients had values greater than 7.1 kPa, suggesting significant fibrosis, in contrast to no subjects from the control group. There was no correlation reported between these measures and serum ferritin concentration. These findings were considered preliminary, identifying the need for additional studies [130]. A follow-up study from 2005 to 2013 included 77 patients homozygous for C282Y, with either serum ferritin greater than 1000 micrograms/L, who had hepatitis, or both who had a liver biopsy and transient elastography done. The transient elastography measure was 17.2 kPa in patients with severe fibrosis (F3-F4), comprised of 19.5% of the group, versus 4.9 kPa in patients without advanced fibrosis, with the ability to predict fibrosis stage in 77% of the patients accurately when the lower and upper thresholds of 6.4 kPa, no fibrosis, and 13.9 kPa, severe fibrosis, were used; however, intermediate kPa values were not useful in fibrosis determination. Validation studies have been recommended prior to inclusion in general practice [131]. A liver biopsy is the reliable method to determine the stage of fibrosis and to diagnose cirrhosis, and it is suggested as an option if this information is sought [123].

Early diagnosis allows for treatment in a timely fashion to prevent complications from the disease; in this regard, counseling and screening of family members must be followed. Population screening is not recommended; thus, the task of family screening falls on the clinician making the diagnosis. A study included 672 asymptomatic patients homozygous for C282Y identified as part of liver disease workup or screening after the diagnosis of a relative. In addition, a group of untreated patients who were homozygous for the mutation were followed for 24 years. Histologically, the amount of liver iron and fibrosis degree was similar in both groups, with diseases known to be associated with hemochromatosis more commonly documented in individuals identified during a liver disease workup, who were also older than those without symptoms. Fifty-six percent of liver samples from men had iron overload graded from 2 to 4, fibrosis staged from 2 to 4 in 18.4%, and cirrhosis in 5.6%; in women, the proportions were 34.5%, 18.8%, and 1.9% for the findings listed above. Hepatic iron concentration correlated with fibrosis and cirrhosis, with a 7.5 fold decrease in mean fibrosis score associated with phlebotomy. Of note, patients with cirrhosis did not report any symptoms. Thus, homozygous patients with C282Y identified by family screening or indicated liver disease workup had the same degree of iron and fibrosis. Importantly, both decreased substantially in association with phlebotomy [132]. In the absence of screening guidelines, it is reiterated that workup for iron overload conditions in patients with an abnormal liver profile is important. Genetic testing in children is not recommended before age 18. However, if there is a mutation in a parent, checking for mutations in the other parent allows inferring the children's genetic characteristics. If one parent is negative, the children are obligate heterozygotes, not at risk for developing clinical complications from the disease [133]. The exception in children concerns those with serum ferritin concentrations of 1000 micrograms/L seen in juvenile hemochromatosis and other uncommon forms of iron overload, which do require investigation when the condition is identified [134].

## Histology

Perls' Prussian blue stain is used to assess hemosiderin deposition in the liver. Early stages of iron overload in homozygous hemochromatosis are characterized by hemosiderin as small granules in hepatocytes in the periportal area in a "cruciate pattern". The iron stores tend to remain in zone one, with decreased expression in the perivenular zones. Fibrosis also develops from the portal tracts and subsequently evolves into irregular fibrosis and cirrhosis. Cirrhosis from hemochromatosis is described as exhibiting high amounts of iron stores in hepatocytes that outline the nodules with partial acini preservation. Cirrhosis in hemochromatosis is micronodular. In the late stages of the disease, after iron has accumulated itself in non-treated patients, iron can appear in Kupffer cells lining the sinusoids [135]. In addition, areas devoid or with minimal parenchymal iron accumulation appear surrounded by heavily hemosiderin laden hepatocytes in an appearance reminiscent of *glades in the forest;* the significance of these structures is not known [136]; however, it was reported that iron free foci are preneoplastic lesions and that, in a patient with hemochromatosis, may herald the development of HCC, and hence are an indication for screening for HCC [137].

In heterozygotes, iron overload can be modest; when notable, the hemosiderin appears in the hepatocytes in the portal areas and zone 1 of the liver acini. Fibrosis tends to be absent, and Kupffer cells are devoid of iron [135].

In association with iron depletion, iron stores disappear from the liver. It is documented that the changes in the iron expression in association with phlebotomy exhibit a pattern that is the reverse of the pattern of accumulation, i.e., the last cells noted to have large iron granules are in the portal areas, and zone 1 [135]. Decreased fibrosis has been reported in association with iron depletion over time, but regression from F4 was documented in a minority of patients [89].

## Treatment

The treatment of iron overload is the removal of iron by phlebotomy [123]. Survival of patients with hemochromatosis is decreased in comparison to that of individuals without the disease. Over 8.1 +/− 6.8 years (range, 0–31 years), seventeen patients from the group of 85 with hemochromatosis had died, with cirrhosis increasing the risk of death by 5.5 times over that of patients without cirrhosis. Patients who were not cirrhotic at the time of diagnosis had similar estimated survival to those from age- and sex-matched members of the normal population. These results were interpreted to indicate that the diagnosis and treatment of hemochromatosis prior to the development of cirrhosis could result in an improved long-term survival, similar to that of the general population; thus, it identified cirrhosis as the complication that marked the natural history of this disease associated with decreased survival in patients with hemochromatosis [138].

From a study that included 251 patients with hemochromatosis followed up for 14.1 +/− 6.8 years, the survival was reported as expected in patients without cirrhosis or diabetes or in patients diagnosed between 1982 and 1991, a period during which the identification of patients with hemochromatosis increased, as compared to prior decades. Survival was reduced in relation to iron overload. The number of deaths from HCC, cirrhosis, and diabetes was higher than expected, and an association between HCC and cirrhosis versus iron removed was reported. This important follow-up study documented that the prognosis of patients with hemochromatosis and the development of its complications depend on the amount and duration of exposure to excess iron and, thus, emphasized that early diagnosis and treatment prevent complications from iron overload [89]. The reader is referred to the excellent editorial [139] related to the publication cited above [89].

A study that included 672 asymptomatic homozygous for C282Y subjects screened because of family history or during general health assessments revealed a similar degree of hepatic iron and fibrosis, which was prevalent, and reversed in association with phlebotomy, except in cases of cirrhosis. This study further highlighted the importance of early diagnosis and treatment prior to cirrhosis development [132].

Clinical guidelines recommend starting treatment in C282Y homozygous subjects who have serum ferritin greater than 300 ng/ml for men, and more than 200 ng/mL in women and a transferrin saturation equal or greater than 45%. Five hundred (500) ml are removed once or twice a week, to decrease serum ferritin to 50 to 100 micrograms/L, with periodic phlebotomies to maintain the serum ferritin at that level, and hemoglobin between 11 and 12 g/dl. Compound heterozygotes, C282Y/H63D, or homozygous for H63D [140] tend not to develop iron overload in the absence of comorbidities including excessive alcohol drinking and chronic hepatitis C; in cases of uncertainty, a liver biopsy to determine hepatic iron index can be done to determine if phlebotomy is indicated [141]. A liver biopsy also allows for the calculation of hepatic iron index (HII) to differentiate C282Y from compound heterozygotes and as a prognostic factor for cirrhosis development. HII is calculated by dividing the hepatic iron content in micromoles per gram of dry liver weight by the patient age in years, with an index equal or greater than 1.9 and/or 71 micromoles/g dry liver weight distinguishing homozygous from compound heterozygotes and secondary iron overload [142].

In regard to fibrosis in association with phlebotomy, in a study that defined regression of fibrosis as a decrease in at least two METAVIR units, comprised of 36 patients homozygous for C282Y, regression was documented in nine of thirteen patients (69%) with baseline F3, and in eight of 23 (35%) with baseline F4 [143]. Although removal of iron may decrease the degree of fibrosis, patients with cirrhosis should continue to undergo screening tests for HCC, as the risk of this complication remains. Also in association with phlebotomy, a consensus report documented that "weakness," which may be similar to fatigue, was unchanged in 40% of patients, and arthralgias, unchanged in 50%, and even worsened in 20% [144].

In a study of survival and causes of death in cirrhotic and in non-cirrhotic patients with primary hemochromatosis that included 163 patients diagnosed between 1959 and 1983 and followed for an average of 10 years, the cumulative survival was calculated as 92% at 5 years, 76% at ten, 59% at 15, and 49% at 20; inadequate depletion of iron during the first eighteen months of therapy was associated with a significant decreased survival [89], supporting the recommendation of iron depletion in patients who meet criteria for such, as described [123]. In a hereditary hemochromatosis database 95 cirrhotic were identified. Sixty had undergone genetic testing, 87% of whom were homozygous for C282Y. The documented cumulative survival at one year was 88%, at five, 69%, and at 20, 56%. Advanced disease, determined by the Child-Pugh score, and HCC, which tended to be diagnosed between the ages of 48 and 79 years, were associated with death, on multivariate analysis. It was concluded that early diagnosis and treatment to prevent the development of cirrhosis may reduce the incidence of HCC in patients with hemochromatosis [145]. A study from France that included 1085 patients documented the overall mortality of patients with hemochromatosis similar to the general population;

however, deaths from liver disease were increased in the disease group, with death occurring in all the subjects between the ages of 53 and 81 years, and no difference between life span and diagnosis of hemochromatosis. Serum ferritin, however, was higher in patients who died from liver disease than in patients who died from other causes, $3816 \pm 1932$ µg/L and $2417 \pm 3723$ µg/L ($p = 0.11$), respectively. Iron depletion of at least 10 grams was not associated with a mortality rate different from the general population; however, removing 2 to 20 g of iron was associated with a standardized mortality rate (SMR) lower than that of the general population. Diabetes and arthropathy were not associated with increased mortality in patients with hemochromatosis. However, patients with cardiomyopathy of any kind had increased mortality with deaths from the cardiovascular disease being reported as fewer in patients with serum ferritin less than 1000 micrograms/L, and in those who had iron depletion characterized as low, i.e., 2 to 10 g total. The group of patients who died from liver disease was comprised of men, in the majority, who had mean serum ferritin of $3816 \pm 1932$ µg/L; however, excessive alcohol intake was documented in ten of 27 (37%); in this group, 20 of 27 (74%) died from complications of liver cancer, which represented an SMR of 15.96 (CI: 9.75–24.65). Cox proportional hazards models estimated that age of at least 56 years, diabetes, alcohol use, and liver fibrosis, at least F3, were independently associated with a risk of death, all of which carried a hazard ratio of at least 3. Of note, nine patients in the study group died from extrahepatic cancers compared to the 21.81 expected in the general population. Patients with serum ferritin levels less than 1000 microgram/L had lower mortality from extrahepatic malignancies than the general population [146].

Normalization of serum ferritin due to iron depletion was associated with fatigue improvement in patients with hereditary hemochromatosis and elevated serum ferritin levels [147]. A randomized, participant—blinded, placebo controlled trial conducted in Australia between 2012 and 2016 included patients aged 18 to 70 with hemochromatosis, homozygous for C282Y, to study the effect of iron depletion by erythrocytapheresis versus a sham intervention (i.e., plasmapheresis) performed every three weeks. Fatigue was the primary outcome, in association with a decrease in ferritin, which was aimed to decrease to less than 300 micrograms/L. At baseline, the serum ferritin was from 300–1000 µg/L, and the transferrin saturation was high. There was a significant improvement in the Modified Fatigue Impact Scale scores in association with erythrocytapheresis in the 50 patients who completed the study from the original 54 versus that of the 44 from the original 50 who had been randomized to the sham procedure; in addition, there was a significant improvement in the cognitive subcomponent of the tool in association with the therapeutic intervention versus the sham intervention, but not in the physical or psychosocial subcomponents [147]. This study indicated that iron depletion in patients with serum ferritin between 300 and 1000 micrograms/L should be considered.

Chelators are alternative therapies if phlebotomy is not tolerated or feasible. Deferasirox is a chelating agent approved for the treatment of iron overload. In a dose escalation trial in a group of patients homozygous for *HFE*-related hemochromatosis the daily administration of this drug for 48 weeks was associated with a decrease in the median serum ferritin concentrations by 63.5%, 74.8%, and 74.1% at doses of 5, 10, and 15 mg/kg, respectively, and to less than 250 ng/mL in all the doses studied. Significant side effects were increased ALT greater than three times the upper limit of normal in a few patients, and increased serum creatinine, both more common in the high than in the low dose. A second study, prospective and open label in ten patients with hemochromatosis in whom phlebotomy had been inadequate, or not tolerated, deferasirox at doses from 5 to 15 mg/kg per day was associated with a significant decrease in median serum ferritin, mean transferrin saturation, median iron concentration, and mean serum activity of ALT; in this study, the drug was not associated with increased serum creatinine [148]. Deferoxamine and deferiprone are chelators approved to treat secondary iron overload.

Erythrocytapheresis is a procedure through which red cells are exchanged [149]. A study that included 38 patients homozygous for C282Y newly diagnosed randomized to receive erythrocytapheresis versus phlebotomy documented that significantly fewer treatment sessions of erythrocytapheresis were required to reach target of serum ferritin concentration of 50 micrograms/L, nine versus 27 for phlebotomy [150]. A subsequent randomized crossover trial compared the number of sessions needed to reach a serum ferritin of 50 micrograms/L after one year of treatment with erythrocytapheresis versus phlebotomies, with subsequent crossover to the alternate treatment documented that significantly more sessions were necessary for phlebotomy versus erythrocytapheresis, 3.3 vs. 1.9 (mean difference, 1.4; 95% confidence interval, 1.1–1.7), with the time between treatment sessions 2.3 times longer for erythrocytapheresis than for phlebotomy. Although quality of life by the SF-36 was not significantly different in association with the two treatment modalities, joint swelling, an important complication of hemochromatosis, was substantially more common during the period of phlebotomy treatment versus that of erythrocytapheresis, which was the preferred treatment of the majority of patients. Erythrocytapheresis was more expensive than phlebotomy [151].

Proton pump inhibitors (PPI) decrease iron absorption; it has been reported that the use of PPI in patients with hemochromatosis required a reduced number of phlebotomy sessions to reach treatment targets. From a randomized controlled trial that included 30 homozygous for C282Y who underwent phlebotomies when serum ferritin was greater than 100 micrograms/L, it was documented that patients on PPIs required significantly fewer sessions than those not on PPIs, which suggested that PPIs can be used in combination with iron depletion therapy [152]; PPIs alone are not recommended as a treatment for iron overload in hemochromatosis [123].

It is recommended that patients being investigated for iron overload get a hormonal evaluation that includes testosterone, follicle stimulating hormone, luteinizing hormone, GnRH testing, and pituitary MRI, regardless of clinical manifestations. In patients younger than 40 years, weekly phlebotomy is proposed as treatment of hypogonadism combined with testosterone or gonado-tropin treatment in subjects older than 40 years; sperm cryopreservation is sug-gested [101].

## Liver Transplantation

Liver transplantation in patients with hemochromatosis is associated with normal-ization of hepcidin, thus preventing iron overload in the graft [153]. The indication for liver transplantation in patients with hemochromatosis is decompensated liver disease or hepatocellular carcinoma [123].

The survival post liver transplant in a study that included 260 patients with decompensated liver disease from iron overload and recruited from several centers in the United States was documented as 64%, 48%, and 34% at one, three, and 5 years, respectively, in homozygous for C282Y, which was lower than that for hetero-zygotes that included H63D. Iron overload not from hemochromatosis was associ-ated with a significant decreased survival versus that of the patients transplanted for other causes with an odds ratio of 1.4 (95% CI:1.15–1.61, $p < 0.001$) [154]. Subsequently, by the use of the United Network for Organ Sharing as a source, the survival of patients transplanted for hemochromatosis between 1990 and 1996 was documented as 79.1%, 71.8%, and 64.6%, at one, three, and 5 years, respectively. The survival improved for patients transplanted for hemochromatosis between 1997 and 2006, being 86.1%, 80.8%, and 77.3% as one, three, and 5 years, which was similar to that of patients transplanted for other conditions, with a hazard ratio for death of 0.89 (95% CI: 0.65–1.22) [155]. However, a retrospective review that included 22 patients with hemochromatosis transplanted for end-stage liver disease, for HCC, or for subacute liver failure documented a patient and graft survival of 80.7%, and 74%, at one and 5 years, respectively, with several deaths occurring over a median period of 46 months post transplantation from multiorgan failure or recur-rence of HCC; bacterial infections were the most common causes of complications, and iron removal prior to transplantation was reported to be associated with a decrease in cardiac complications and bacterial infections [156]. Thus, although there is a documented improvement in post transplant survival in patients with hemochromatosis, a complication that depends on the pathogenesis of the disease, i.e., iron overload, does have an impact on post surgical comorbidities. The finding that iron removal was associated with a decrease in infection rate support that early intervention is associated with improved general and post liver transplantation outcomes.

Diet changes include avoidance of iron supplements in any of their forms, vita-min C supplements because it increases iron absorption, alcohol, and raw fish and shellfish [157], the latter because of transmission of pathogens that thrive in iron laden conditions (e.g., *Listeria monocytogenes*, *Yersinia enterocolitica*, *Escherichia coli*, and *Vibrio vulnificus*) and because of impaired immune function in association with iron overload [158–161].

# Treatment of Other Genetic Iron Overload Conditions

In ferroportin disease, loss of function, serum ferritin is substantially increased. Iron depletion is the treatment to keep the serum ferritin between 50 and 100 micrograms/L; however, it is not well tolerated in general. Low transferrin saturation and anemia tend to develop quickly despite high serum ferritin. Chelation and erythropoietin have been reported to be a therapeutic option.

In aceruloplasminemia, phlebotomy is poorly tolerated; thus, chelation is the therapeutic alternative.

In juvenile hemochromatosis, the cardiac function from iron load may be seriously impaired for which aggressive and urgent iron removal may be necessary.

Hepcidin deficiency or resistance to the effects of hepcidin on FPN is associated with iron overload, the focus of this chapter. Mutations in TfR2 [162, 163], HJV [38], transferrin, and hepcidin [164] are associated with iron overload,

Ferroportin disease has high penetrance and results from a mutation with the autosomal dominant transmission in the SLC40A1 gene, which encodes ferroportin1/IREG1/MTP1 a product expressed in macrophages, enterocytes, and hepatocytes. This mutation results in decreased expression or decreased ability to transport iron. Phenotypically, it is characterized by high serum ferritin concentrations in association with low or normal transferrin saturation, accumulation of iron mostly in macrophages, anemia, and poor tolerability to phlebotomy [126]. Another form of ferroportin disease is characterized by loss of function, associated with hyperferritinemia, high transferrin saturation, and iron accumulation in the hepatocyte but low incidence of liver fibrosis and cirrhosis [165].

# Potential Pharmacological Treatment of Hepcidin-Ferroportin Disease

A decrease in hepcidin is associated with iron overload. A phase II clinical trial of LJPC-401, a synthetic human hepcidin, (ClinicalTrials.gov Identifier: NCT03395704), for the treatment of iron overload in adult patients with hereditary hemochromatosis was associated with a statistically significant reduction in change in transferrin saturation, the primary efficacy endpoint of the study, and frequency of phlebotomies, a key secondary efficacy endpoint of the study [166].

A decrease in iron absorption or export from duodenal cells into the circulation would decrease iron accumulation. Polyphenols have iron chelating properties and are present in the human diet. It was reported from an animal study that quercetin, a polyphenol, was associated with iron chelation in the intestinal lumen of rats. In the long term, it was associated with the regulation of FPN expression that resulted in a decrease of iron export [167]. A clinical trial on the Effects of Polyphenols on Iron Absorption in Iron Overload Disorders (POLYFER) is listed in ClinicalTrials.gov Identifier: NCT03453918; no published results were identified.

# References

1. Powell LW, Seckington RC, Deugnier Y. Haemochromatosis. Lancet. 2016 Aug 13;388(10045):706–16.
2. Nicolas G, Viatte L, Bennoun M, Beaumont C, Kahn A, Vaulont S. Hepcidin, a new iron regulatory peptide. Blood Cells Mol Dis. 2002 Nov-Dec;29(3):327–35.
3. Abboud S, Haile DJ. A novel mammalian iron-regulated protein involved in intracellular iron metabolism. J Biol Chem. 2000 Jun 30;275(26):19906–12.
4. Donovan A, Brownlie A, Zhou Y, Shepard J, Pratt SJ, Moynihan J, et al. Positional cloning of zebrafish ferroportin1 identifies a conserved vertebrate iron exporter. Nature. 2000 Feb 17;403(6771):776–81.
5. McKie AT, Marciani P, Rolfs A, Brennan K, Wehr K, Barrow D, et al. A novel duodenal iron-regulated transporter, IREG1, implicated in the basolateral transfer of iron to the circulation. Mol Cell. 2000 Feb;5(2):299–309.
6. Shi H, Bencze KZ, Stemmler TL, Philpott CC. A cytosolic iron chaperone that delivers iron to ferritin. Science. 2008 May 30;320(5880):1207–10.
7. Kidane TZ, Sauble E, Linder MC. Release of iron from ferritin requires lysosomal activity. Am J Physiol Cell Physiol. 2006 Sep;291(3):C445–55.
8. McKie AT, Barrow D, Latunde-Dada GO, Rolfs A, Sager G, Mudaly E, et al. An iron-regulated ferric reductase associated with the absorption of dietary iron. Science. 2001 Mar 2;291(5509):1755.
9. Gunshin H, Mackenzie B, Berger UV, Gunshin Y, Romero MF, Boron WF, et al. Cloning and characterization of a mammalian proton-coupled metal-ion transporter. Nature. 1997 Jul 31;388(6641):482–8.
10. Nakai Y, Inoue K, Abe N, Hatakeyama M, Ohta KY, Otagiri M, et al. Functional characterization of human proton-coupled folate transporter/heme carrier protein 1 heterologously expressed in mammalian cells as a folate transporter. J Pharmacol Exp Ther. 2007 Aug;322(2):469–76.
11. Vulpe CD, Kuo YM, Murphy TL, Cowley L, Askwith C, Libina N, et al. Hephaestin, a ceruloplasmin homologue implicated in intestinal iron transport, is defective in the sla mouse. Nat Genet. 1999 Feb;21(2):195–9.
12. Canonne-Hergaux F, Donovan A, Delaby C, Wang HJ, Gros P. Comparative studies of duodenal and macrophage ferroportin proteins. Am J Physiol Gastrointest Liver Physiol. 2006 Jan;290(1):G156–63.
13. Ramey G, Deschemin JC, Durel B, Canonne-Hergaux F, Nicolas G, Vaulont S. Hepcidin targets ferroportin for degradation in hepatocytes. Haematologica. 2010 Mar;95(3):501–4.
14. Zhang DL, Hughes RM, Ollivierre-Wilson H, Ghosh MC, Rouault TA. A ferroportin transcript that lacks an iron-responsive element enables duodenal and erythroid precursor cells to evade translational repression. Cell Metab. 2009 May;9(5):461–73.
15. Harris ZL, Durley AP, Man TK, Gitlin JD. Targeted gene disruption reveals an essential role for ceruloplasmin in cellular iron efflux. Proc Natl Acad Sci U S A. 1999 Sep 14;96(19):10812–7.
16. Cherukuri S, Potla R, Sarkar J, Nurko S, Harris ZL, Fox PL. Unexpected role of ceruloplasmin in intestinal iron absorption. Cell Metab. 2005 Nov;2(5):309–19.
17. Harris ZL, Takahashi Y, Miyajima H, Serizawa M, MacGillivray RT, Gitlin JD. Aceruloplasminemia: molecular characterization of this disorder of iron metabolism. Proc Natl Acad Sci U S A. 1995 Mar 28;92(7):2539–43.
18. Ganz T. Systemic iron homeostasis. Physiol Rev. 2013 Oct;93(4):1721–41.
19. Kuhn LC. Iron regulatory proteins and their role in controlling iron metabolism. Metallomics: Integrated Biometal Sci. 2015 Feb;7(2):232–43.
20. Ohgami RS, Campagna DR, Greer EL, Antiochos B, McDonald A, Chen J, et al. Identification of a ferrireductase required for efficient transferrin-dependent iron uptake in erythroid cells. Nat Genet. 2005 Nov;37(11):1264–9.

21. Chua AC, Graham RM, Trinder D, Olynyk JK. The regulation of cellular iron metabolism. Crit Rev Clin Lab Sci. 2007;44(5–6):413–59.
22. Chua AC, Delima RD, Morgan EH, Herbison CE, Tirnitz-Parker JE, Graham RM, et al. Iron uptake from plasma transferrin by a transferrin receptor 2 mutant mouse model of haemochromatosis. J Hepatol. 2010 Mar;52(3):425–31.
23. Shindo M, Torimoto Y, Saito H, Motomura W, Ikuta K, Sato K, et al. Functional role of DMT1 in transferrin-independent iron uptake by human hepatocyte and hepatocellular carcinoma cell, HLF. Hepatol Res. 2006 Jul;35(3):152–62.
24. Liuzzi JP, Aydemir F, Nam H, Knutson MD, Cousins RJ. Zip14 (Slc39a14) mediates non-transferrin-bound iron uptake into cells. Proc Natl Acad Sci U S A. 2006 Sep 12;103(37):13612–7.
25. Cook JD, Flowers CH, Skikne BS. The quantitative assessment of body iron. Blood. 2003 May 1;101(9):3359–64.
26. Finch C. Regulators of iron balance in humans. Blood. 1994 Sep 15;84(6):1697–702.
27. Nemeth E, Tuttle MS, Powelson J, Vaughn MB, Donovan A, Ward DM, et al. Hepcidin regulates cellular iron efflux by binding to ferroportin and inducing its internalization. Science. 2004 Dec 17;306(5704):2090–3.
28. Nemeth E, Preza GC, Jung CL, Kaplan J, Waring AJ, Ganz T. The N-terminus of hepcidin is essential for its interaction with ferroportin: structure-function study. Blood. 2006 Jan 1;107(1):328–33.
29. Krause A, Neitz S, Magert HJ, Schulz A, Forssmann WG, Schulz-Knappe P, et al. LEAP-1, a novel highly disulfide-bonded human peptide, exhibits antimicrobial activity. FEBS Lett. 2000 Sep 1;480(2–3):147–50.
30. Park CH, Valore EV, Waring AJ, Ganz T. Hepcidin, a urinary antimicrobial peptide synthesized in the liver. J Biol Chem. 2001 Mar 16;276(11):7806–10.
31. Fernandes A, Preza GC, Phung Y, De Domenico I, Kaplan J, Ganz T, et al. The molecular basis of hepcidin-resistant hereditary hemochromatosis. Blood. 2009 Jul 9;114(2):437–43.
32. Preza GC, Ruchala P, Pinon R, Ramos E, Qiao B, Peralta MA, et al. Minihepcidins are rationally designed small peptides that mimic hepcidin activity in mice and may be useful for the treatment of iron overload. J Clin Invest. 2011 Dec;121(12):4880–8.
33. Qiao B, Sugianto P, Fung E, Del-Castillo-Rueda A, Moran-Jimenez MJ, Ganz T, et al. Hepcidin-induced endocytosis of ferroportin is dependent on ferroportin ubiquitination. Cell Metab. 2012 Jun 6;15(6):918–24.
34. Ganz T, Olbina G, Girelli D, Nemeth E, Westerman M. Immunoassay for human serum hepcidin. Blood. 2008 Nov 15;112(10):4292–7.
35. Babitt JL, Huang FW, Wrighting DM, Xia Y, Sidis Y, Samad TA, et al. Bone morphogenetic protein signaling by hemojuvelin regulates hepcidin expression. Nat Genet. 2006 May;38(5):531–9.
36. Steinbicker AU, Bartnikas TB, Lohmeyer LK, Leyton P, Mayeur C, Kao SM, et al. Perturbation of hepcidin expression by BMP type I receptor deletion induces iron overload in mice. Blood. 2011 Oct 13;118(15):4224–30.
37. Xia Y, Babitt JL, Sidis Y, Chung RT, Lin HY. Hemojuvelin regulates hepcidin expression via a selective subset of BMP ligands and receptors independently of neogenin. Blood. 2008 May 15;111(10):5195–204.
38. Papanikolaou G, Samuels ME, Ludwig EH, MacDonald ML, Franchini PL, Dube MP, et al. Mutations in HFE2 cause iron overload in chromosome 1q-linked juvenile hemochromatosis. Nat Genet. 2004 Jan;36(1):77–82.
39. Goswami T, Andrews NC. Hereditary hemochromatosis protein, HFE, interaction with transferrin receptor 2 suggests a molecular mechanism for mammalian iron sensing. J Biol Chem. 2006 Sep 29;281(39):28494–8.
40. Johnson MB, Chen J, Murchison N, Green FA, Enns CA. Transferrin receptor 2: evidence for ligand-induced stabilization and redirection to a recycling pathway. Mol Biol Cell. 2007 Mar;18(3):743–54.

41. D'Alessio F, Hentze MW, Muckenthaler MU. The hemochromatosis proteins HFE, TfR2, and HJV form a membrane-associated protein complex for hepcidin regulation. J Hepatol. 2012 Nov;57(5):1052–60.

42. Ramos E, Kautz L, Rodriguez R, Hansen M, Gabayan V, Ginzburg Y, et al. Evidence for distinct pathways of hepcidin regulation by acute and chronic iron loading in mice. Hepatology. 2011 Apr;53(4):1333–41.

43. Maes K, Nemeth E, Roodman GD, Huston A, Esteve F, Freytes C, et al. In anemia of multiple myeloma, hepcidin is induced by increased bone morphogenetic protein 2. Blood. 2010 Nov 4;116(18):3635–44.

44. Fujita N, Sugimoto R, Takeo M, Urawa N, Mifuji R, Tanaka H, et al. Hepcidin expression in the liver: relatively low level in patients with chronic hepatitis C. Mol Med. 2007 Jan-Feb;13(1–2):97–104.

45. Girelli D, Pasino M, Goodnough JB, Nemeth E, Guido M, Castagna A, et al. Reduced serum hepcidin levels in patients with chronic hepatitis C. J Hepatol. 2009 Nov;51(5):845–52.

46. Harrison-Findik DD, Schafer D, Klein E, Timchenko NA, Kulaksiz H, Clemens D, et al. Alcohol metabolism-mediated oxidative stress down-regulates hepcidin transcription and leads to increased duodenal iron transporter expression. J Biol Chem. 2006 Aug 11;281(32):22974–82.

47. Huang FW, Pinkus JL, Pinkus GS, Fleming MD, Andrews NC. A mouse model of juvenile hemochromatosis. J Clin Invest. 2005 Aug;115(8):2187–91.

48. Meynard D, Kautz L, Darnaud V, Canonne-Hergaux F, Coppin H, Roth MP. Lack of the bone morphogenetic protein BMP6 induces massive iron overload. Nat Genet. 2009 Apr;41(4):478–81.

49. Andriopoulos B Jr, Corradini E, Xia Y, Faasse SA, Chen S, Grgurevic L, et al. BMP6 is a key endogenous regulator of hepcidin expression and iron metabolism. Nat Genet. 2009 Apr;41(4):482–7.

50. Camaschella C. Juvenile haemochromatosis. Baillieres Clin Gastroenterol. 1998 Jun;12(2):227–35.

51. Drakesmith H, Schimanski LM, Ormerod E, Merryweather-Clarke AT, Viprakasit V, Edwards JP, et al. Resistance to hepcidin is conferred by hemochromatosis-associated mutations of ferroportin. Blood. 2005 Aug 1;106(3):1092–7.

52. Schimanski LM, Drakesmith H, Merryweather-Clarke AT, Viprakasit V, Edwards JP, Sweetland E, et al. In vitro functional analysis of human ferroportin (FPN) and hemochromatosis-associated FPN mutations. Blood. 2005 May 15;105(10):4096–102.

53. Figueiredo MS, Baffa O, Barbieri Neto J, Zago MA. Liver injury and generation of hydroxyl free radicals in experimental secondary hemochromatosis. Res Exp Med. 1993;193(1):27–37.

54. Kadiiska MB, Burkitt MJ, Xiang QH, Mason RP. Iron supplementation generates hydroxyl radical in vivo. An ESR spin-trapping investigation. J Clin Invest. 1995 Sep;96(3):1653–7.

55. Bloomer SA, Brown KE. Iron-induced liver injury: a critical reappraisal. Int J Mol Sci. 2019 Apr;30:20(9).

56. Feder JN, Gnirke A, Thomas W, Tsuchihashi Z, Ruddy DA, Basava A, et al. A novel MHC class I-like gene is mutated in patients with hereditary haemochromatosis. Nat Genet. 1996 Aug;13(4):399–408.

57. Bacon BR, Olynyk JK, Brunt EM, Britton RS, Wolff RK. HFE genotype in patients with hemochromatosis and other liver diseases. Ann Intern Med. 1999 Jun 15;130(12):953–62.

58. Merryweather-Clarke AT, Pointon JJ, Shearman JD, Robson KJ. Global prevalence of putative haemochromatosis mutations. J Med Genet. 1997 Apr;34(4):275–8.

59. Asberg A, Thorstensen K, Hveem K, Bjerve KS. Hereditary hemochromatosis: the clinical significance of the S65C mutation. Genet Test. 2002 Spring;6(1):59–62.

60. Waheed A, Parkkila S, Zhou XY, Tomatsu S, Tsuchihashi Z, Feder JN, et al. Hereditary hemochromatosis: effects of C282Y and H63D mutations on association with beta2-microglobulin, intracellular processing, and cell surface expression of the HFE protein in COS-7 cells. Proc Natl Acad Sci U S A. 1997 Nov 11;94(23):12384–9.

61. Jacolot S, Le Gac G, Scotet V, Quere I, Mura C, Ferec C. HAMP as a modifier gene that increases the phenotypic expression of the HFE pC282Y homozygous genotype. Blood. 2004 Apr 1;103(7):2835–40.
62. Le Gac G, Scotet V, Ka C, Gourlaouen I, Bryckaert L, Jacolot S, et al. The recently identified type 2A juvenile haemochromatosis gene (HJV), a second candidate modifier of the C282Y homozygous phenotype. Hum Mol Genet. 2004 Sep 1;13(17):1913–8.
63. Van Vlierberghe H, Langlois M, Delanghe J, Horsmans Y, Michielsen P, Henrion J, et al. Haptoglobin phenotype 2-2 overrepresentation in Cys282Tyr hemochromatotic patients. J Hepatol. 2001 Dec;35(6):707–11.
64. Milet J, Dehais V, Bourgain C, Jouanolle AM, Mosser A, Perrin M, et al. Common variants in the BMP2, BMP4, and HJV genes of the hepcidin regulation pathway modulate HFE hemochromatosis penetrance. Am J Hum Genet. 2007 Oct;81(4):799–807.
65. Milet J, Le Gac G, Scotet V, Gourlaouen I, Theze C, Mosser J, et al. A common SNP near BMP2 is associated with severity of the iron burden in HFE p.C282Y homozygous patients: a follow-up study. Blood Cells Mol Dis. 2010 Jan 15;44(1):34–7.
66. Benyamin B, McRae AF, Zhu G, Gordon S, Henders AK, Palotie A, et al. Variants in TF and HFE explain approximately 40% of genetic variation in serum-transferrin levels. Am J Hum Genet. 2009 Jan;84(1):60–5.
67. de Tayrac M, Roth MP, Jouanolle AM, Coppin H, le Gac G, Piperno A, et al. Genome-wide association study identifies TF as a significant modifier gene of iron metabolism in HFE hemochromatosis. J Hepatol. 2015 Mar;62(3):664–72.
68. Benyamin B, Esko T, Ried JS, Radhakrishnan A, Vermeulen SH, Traglia M, et al. Novel loci affecting iron homeostasis and their effects in individuals at risk for hemochromatosis. Nat Commun. 2014 Oct 29;5:4926.
69. Stickel F, Buch S, Zoller H, Hultcrantz R, Gallati S, Osterreicher C, et al. Evaluation of genome-wide loci of iron metabolism in hereditary hemochromatosis identifies PCSK7 as a host risk factor of liver cirrhosis. Hum Mol Genet. 2014 Jul 15;23(14):3883–90.
70. Leggett BA, Halliday JW, Brown NN, Bryant S, Powell LW. Prevalence of haemochromatosis amongst asymptomatic Australians. Br J Haematol. 1990 Apr;74(4):525–30.
71. European Association For The Study Of The L. EASL clinical practice guidelines for HFE hemochromatosis. J Hepatol. 2010 Jul;53(1):3–22.
72. Marshall DS, Linfert DR, Tsongalis GJ. Prevalence of the C282Y and H63D polymorphisms in a multi-ethnic control population. Int J Mol Med. 1999 Oct;4(4):389–93.
73. Beutler E, Felitti V, Gelbart T, Ho N. The effect of HFE genotypes on measurements of iron overload in patients attending a health appraisal clinic. Ann Intern Med. 2000 Sep 5;133(5):329–37.
74. Steinberg KK, Cogswell ME, Chang JC, Caudill SP, McQuillan GM, Bowman BA, et al. Prevalence of C282Y and H63D mutations in the hemochromatosis (HFE) gene in the United States. JAMA. 2001 May 2;285(17):2216–22.
75. Phatak PD, Ryan DH, Cappuccio J, Oakes D, Braggins C, Provenzano K, et al. Prevalence and penetrance of HFE mutations in 4865 unselected primary care patients. Blood Cells Mol Dis. 2002 Jul-Aug;29(1):41–7.
76. Beutler E, Felitti VJ, Koziol JA, Ho NJ, Gelbart T. Penetrance of 845G--> a (C282Y) HFE hereditary haemochromatosis mutation in the USA. Lancet. 2002 Jan 19;359(9302):211–8.
77. Adams PC, Reboussin DM, Barton JC, McLaren CE, Eckfeldt JH, McLaren GD, et al. Hemochromatosis and iron-overload screening in a racially diverse population. N Engl J Med. 2005 Apr 28;352(17):1769–7.
78. Allen KJ, Gurrin LC, Constantine CC, Osborne NJ, Delatycki MB, Nicoll AJ, et al. Iron-overload-related disease in HFE hereditary hemochromatosis. N Engl J Med. 2008 Jan 17;358(3):221–30.
79. Gurrin LC, Osborne NJ, Constantine CC, McLaren CE, English DR, Gertig DM, et al. The natural history of serum iron indices for HFE C282Y homozygosity associated with hereditary hemochromatosis. Gastroenterology. 2008 Dec;135(6):1945–52.

80. Gurrin LC, Bertalli NA, Dalton GW, Osborne NJ, Constantine CC, McLaren CE, et al. HFE C282Y/H63D compound heterozygotes are at low risk of hemochromatosis-related morbidity. Hepatology. 2009 Jul;50(1):94–101.
81. Constantine CC, Anderson GJ, Vulpe CD, McLaren CE, Bahlo M, Yeap HL, et al. A novel association between a SNP in CYBRD1 and serum ferritin levels in a cohort study of HFE hereditary haemochromatosis. Br J Haematol. 2009 Oct;147(1):140–9.
82. Osterreicher CH, Datz C, Stickel F, Hellerbrand C, Penz M, Hofer H, et al. TGF-beta1 codon 25 gene polymorphism is associated with cirrhosis in patients with hereditary hemochromatosis. Cytokine. 2005 Jul 21;31(2):142–8.
83. Barton JC, Barton JC, Acton RT. Longer survival associated with HLA-A*03, B*14 among 212 hemochromatosis probands with HFE C282Y homozygosity and HLA-A and -B typing and haplotyping. Eur J Haematol. 2010 Nov;85(5):439–47.
84. Fletcher LM, Dixon JL, Purdie DM, Powell LW, Crawford DH. Excess alcohol greatly increases the prevalence of cirrhosis in hereditary hemochromatosis. Gastroenterology. 2002 Feb;122(2):281–9.
85. Adams PC, Agnew S. Alcoholism in hereditary hemochromatosis revisited: prevalence and clinical consequences among homozygous siblings. Hepatology. 1996 Apr;23(4):724–7.
86. Powell EE, Ali A, Clouston AD, Dixon JL, Lincoln DJ, Purdie DM, et al. Steatosis is a cofactor in liver injury in hemochromatosis. Gastroenterology. 2005 Dec;129(6):1937–43.
87. Diwakaran HH, Befeler AS, Britton RS, Brunt EM, Bacon BR. Accelerated hepatic fibrosis in patients with combined hereditary hemochromatosis and chronic hepatitis C infection. J Hepatol. 2002 May;36(5):687–91.
88. Stuart KA, Busfield F, Jazwinska EC, Gibson P, Butterworth LA, Cooksley WG, et al. The C282Y mutation in the haemochromatosis gene (HFE) and hepatitis C virus infection are independent cofactors for porphyria cutanea tarda in Australian patients. J Hepatol. 1998 Mar;28(3):404–9.
89. Niederau C, Fischer R, Purschel A, Stremmel W, Haussinger D, Strohmeyer G. Long-term survival in patients with hereditary hemochromatosis. Gastroenterology. 1996 Apr;110(4):1107–19.
90. Adams PC, Deugnier Y, Moirand R, Brissot P. The relationship between iron overload, clinical symptoms, and age in 410 patients with genetic hemochromatosis. Hepatology. 1997 Jan;25(1):162–6.
91. Delatycki MB, Allen KJ, Nisselle AE, Collins V, Metcalfe S, du Sart D, et al. Use of community genetic screening to prevent HFE-associated hereditary haemochromatosis. Lancet. 2005 Jul 23-29;366(9482):314–6.
92. Lin E, Adams PC. Biochemical liver profile in hemochromatosis. A survey of 100 patients. J Clin Gastroenterol. 1991 Jun;13(3):316–20.
93. Rahier J, Loozen S, Goebbels RM, Abrahem M. The haemochromatotic human pancreas: a quantitative immunohistochemical and ultrastructural study. Diabetologia. 1987 Jan;30(1):5–12.
94. Barton JC, Acton RT. Diabetes in HFE hemochromatosis. J Diabetes Res. 2017;2017:9826930.
95. Walsh CH, Wright AD, Williams JW, Holder G. A study of pituitary function in patients with idiopathic hemochromatosis. J Clin Endocrinol Metab. 1976 Oct;43(4):866–72.
96. McDermott JH, Walsh CH. Hypogonadism in hereditary hemochromatosis. J Clin Endocrinol Metab. 2005 Apr;90(4):2451–5.
97. Charbonnel B, Chupin M, Le Grand A, Guillon J. Pituitary function in idiopathic haemochromatosis: hormonal study in 36 male patients. Acta Endocrinol. 1981 Oct;98(2):178–83.
98. McNeil LW, McKee LC Jr, Lorber D, Rabin D. The endocrine manifestations of hemochromatosis. Am J Med Sci. 1983 May-Jun;285(3):7–13.
99. Van Deursen C, Delaere K, Tenkate J. Hemochromatosis and sexual dysfunction. Int J Impot Res. 2003 Dec;15(6):430–2.
100. Leichtmann-Bardoogo Y, Cohen LA, Weiss A, Marohn B, Schubert S, Meinhardt A, et al. Compartmentalization and regulation of iron metabolism proteins protect male germ cells from iron overload. Am J Physiol Endocrinol Metab. 2012 Jun 15;302(12):E1519–30.

101. El Osta R, Grandpre N, Monnin N, Hubert J, Koscinski I. Hypogonadotropic hypogonadism in men with hereditary hemochromatosis. Basic Clin Androl. 2017;27:13.
102. Kiely PD. Haemochromatosis arthropathy–a conundrum of the Celtic curse. J R Coll Physicians Edinb. 2018 Sep;48(3):233–8.
103. Richardson A, Prideaux A, Kiely P. Haemochromatosis: unexplained metacarpophalangeal or ankle arthropathy should prompt diagnostic tests: findings from two UK observational cohort studies. Scand J Rheumatol. 2017 Jan;46(1):69–74.
104. Hawthorne G, Richardson J, Osborne R. The assessment of quality of life (AQoL) instrument: a psychometric measure of health-related quality of life. Qual Life Res Int J Qual Life Asp Treat Care Rehab. 1999 May;8(3):209–24.
105. de Graaff B, Neil A, Sanderson K, Yee KC, Palmer AJ. Quality of life utility values for hereditary haemochromatosis in Australia. Health Qual Life Outcomes. 2016 Feb 29;14:31.
106. Adams PC, Speechley M. The effect of arthritis on the quality of life in hereditary hemochromatosis. J Rheumatol. 1996 Apr;23(4):707–10.
107. Ines LS, da Silva JA, Malcata AB, Porto AL. Arthropathy of genetic hemochromatosis: a major and distinctive manifestation of the disease. Clin Exp Rheumatol. 2001 Jan-Feb;19(1):98–102.
108. Walker RJ, Dymock IW, Ansell ID, Hamilton EB, Williams R. Synovial biopsy in haemochromatosis arthropathy. Histological findings and iron deposition in relation to total body iron overload. Ann Rheum Dis. 1972 Mar;31(2):98–102.
109. Heiland GR, Aigner E, Dallos T, Sahinbegovic E, Krenn V, Thaler C, et al. Synovial immunopathology in haemochromatosis arthropathy. Ann Rheum Dis. 2010 Jun;69(6):1214–9.
110. Sinigaglia L, Fargion S, Fracanzani AL, Binelli L, Battafarano N, Varenna M, et al. Bone and joint involvement in genetic hemochromatosis: role of cirrhosis and iron overload. J Rheumatol. 1997 Sep;24(9):1809–13.
111. Guggenbuhl P, Deugnier Y, Boisdet JF, Rolland Y, Perdriger A, Pawlotsky Y, et al. Bone mineral density in men with genetic hemochromatosis and HFE gene mutation. Osteoporos Int. 2005 Dec;16(12):1809–14.
112. Valenti L, Varenna M, Fracanzani AL, Rossi V, Fargion S, Sinigaglia L. Association between iron overload and osteoporosis in patients with hereditary hemochromatosis. Osteoporos Int. 2009 Apr;20(4):549–55.
113. Richette P, Ottaviani S, Vicaut E, Bardin T. Musculoskeletal complications of hereditary hemochromatosis: a case-control study. J Rheumatol. 2010 Oct;37(10):2145–50.
114. Ishii KA, Fumoto T, Iwai K, Takeshita S, Ito M, Shimohata N, et al. Coordination of PGC-1beta and iron uptake in mitochondrial biogenesis and osteoclast activation. Nat Med. 2009 Mar;15(3):259–66.
115. Balogh E, Tolnai E, Nagy B Jr, Nagy B, Balla G, Balla J, et al. Iron overload inhibits osteogenic commitment and differentiation of mesenchymal stem cells via the induction of ferritin. Biochim Biophys Acta. 2016 Sep;1862(9):1640–9.
116. Handzlik-Orlik G, Holecki M, Wilczynski K, Dulawa J. Osteoporosis in liver disease: pathogenesis and management. Ther Adv Endocrinol Metab. 2016 Jun;7(3):128–35.
117. Parkash O, Akram M. Hereditary hemochromatosis. J College Phys Surg Pakistan: JCPSP. 2015 Sep;25(9):644–7.
118. Schwartz RA. Dermatologic manifestations of hemochromatosis. Medscape. 2019 April;22:2019.
119. Chevrant-Breton J, Simon M, Bourel M, Ferrand B. Cutaneous manifestations of idiopathic hemochromatosis. Study of 100 cases. Arch Dermatol. 1977 Feb;113(2):161–5.
120. McLaren CE, McLachlan GJ, Halliday JW, Webb SI, Leggett BA, Jazwinska EC, et al. Distribution of transferrin saturation in an Australian population: relevance to the early diagnosis of hemochromatosis. Gastroenterology. 1998 Mar;114(3):543–9.
121. Olynyk JK, Cullen DJ, Aquilia S, Rossi E, Summerville L, Powell LW. A population-based study of the clinical expression of the hemochromatosis gene. N Engl J Med. 1999 Sep 2;341(10):718–24.

122. Adams PC, Bhayana V. Unsaturated iron-binding capacity: a screening test for C282Y hemochromatosis? Clin Chem. 2000 Nov;46(11):1870–1.
123. Kowdley KV, Brown KE, Ahn J, Sundaram V. ACG clinical guideline: hereditary hemochromatosis. Am J Gastroenterol. 2019 Aug;114(8):1202–18.
124. Beaton M, Guyader D, Deugnier Y, Moirand R, Chakrabarti S, Adams P. Noninvasive prediction of cirrhosis in C282Y-linked hemochromatosis. Hepatology. 2002 Sep;36(3):673–8.
125. Crawford DH, Murphy TL, Ramm LE, Fletcher LM, Clouston AD, Anderson GJ, et al. Serum hyaluronic acid with serum ferritin accurately predicts cirrhosis and reduces the need for liver biopsy in C282Y hemochromatosis. Hepatology. 2009 Feb;49(2):418–25.
126. Pietrangelo A. The ferroportin disease. Blood Cells Mol Dis. 2004 Jan-Feb;32(1):131–8.
127. Deugnier Y, Bardou-Jacquet E, Laine F. Dysmetabolic iron overload syndrome (DIOS). Presse Med. 2017 Dec;46(12 Pt 2):e306–e11.
128. Cadenas B, Fita-Torro J, Bermudez-Cortes M, Hernandez-Rodriguez I, Fuster JL, Llinares ME, et al. L-ferritin: one gene, five diseases; from hereditary Hyperferritinemia to Hypoferritinemia-report of new cases. Pharmaceuticals. 2019 Jan;23:12(1).
129. Morrison ED, Brandhagen DJ, Phatak PD, Barton JC, Krawitt EL, El-Serag HB, et al. Serum ferritin level predicts advanced hepatic fibrosis among U.S. patients with phenotypic hemochromatosis. Ann Intern Med. 2003 Apr 15;138(8):627–33.
130. Adhoute X, Foucher J, Laharie D, Terrebonne E, Vergniol J, Castera L, et al. Diagnosis of liver fibrosis using FibroScan and other noninvasive methods in patients with hemochromatosis: a prospective study. Gastroenterol Clin Biol. 2008 Feb;32(2):180–7.
131. Legros L, Bardou-Jacquet E, Latournerie M, Guillygomarc'h A, Turlin B, Le Lan C, et al. Non-invasive assessment of liver fibrosis in C282Y homozygous HFE hemochromatosis. Liver Int. 2015 Jun;35(6):1731–8.
132. Powell LW, Dixon JL, Ramm GA, Purdie DM, Lincoln DJ, Anderson GJ, et al. Screening for hemochromatosis in asymptomatic subjects with or without a family history. Arch Intern Med. 2006 Feb 13;166(3):294–301.
133. Adams PC. Implications of genotyping of spouses to limit investigation of children in genetic hemochromatosis. Clin Genet. 1998 Mar;53(3):176–8.
134. Delatycki MB, Powell LW, Allen KJ. Hereditary hemochromatosis genetic testing of at-risk children: what is the appropriate age? Genet Test. 2004 Summer;8(2):98–103.
135. Searle J, Kerr JFR, Halliday JW, Powell LW. Iron storage disease. In: MacSween PPA RNM, Scheuer PJ, Burt AD, Portmann BC, editors. Pathology of the liver. Edinburgh: Churchill Livingstone; 1994. p. 219–42.
136. Powell LW, Kerr JF. The pathology of the liver in hemochromatosis. Pathobiol Annu. 1975;5:317–37.
137. Deugnier YM, Charalambous P, Le Quilleuc D, Turlin B, Searle J, Brissot P, et al. Preneoplastic significance of hepatic iron-free foci in genetic hemochromatosis: a study of 185 patients. Hepatology. 1993 Dec;18(6):1363–9.
138. Adams PC, Speechley M, Kertesz AE. Long-term survival analysis in hereditary hemochromatosis. Gastroenterology. 1991 Aug;101(2):368–72.
139. Powell LW. Hemochromatosis: the impact of early diagnosis and therapy. Gastroenterology. 1996 Apr;110(4):1304–7.
140. Gochee PA, Powell LW, Cullen DJ, Du Sart D, Rossi E, Olynyk JK. A population-based study of the biochemical and clinical expression of the H63D hemochromatosis mutation. Gastroenterology. 2002 Mar;122(3):646–51.
141. Walsh A, Dixon JL, Ramm GA, Hewett DG, Lincoln DJ, Anderson GJ, et al. The clinical relevance of compound heterozygosity for the C282Y and H63D substitutions in hemochromatosis. Clin Gastroenterol Hepatol. 2006 Nov;4(11):1403–10.
142. Summers KM, Halliday JW, Powell LW. Identification of homozygous hemochromatosis subjects by measurement of hepatic iron index. Hepatology. 1990 Jul;12(1):20–5.
143. Falize L, Guillygomarc'h A, Perrin M, Laine F, Guyader D, Brissot P, et al. Reversibility of hepatic fibrosis in treated genetic hemochromatosis: a study of 36 cases. Hepatology. 2006 Aug;44(2):472–7.

144. Adams P, Brissot P, Powell LW. EASL international consensus conference on haemochromatosis. J Hepatol. 2000 Sep;33(3):485–504.

145. Beaton MD, Adams PC. Prognostic factors and survival in patients with hereditary hemochromatosis and cirrhosis. Can J Gastroenterol. 2006 Apr;20(4):257–60.

146. Bardou-Jacquet E, Morcet J, Manet G, Laine F, Perrin M, Jouanolle AM, et al. Decreased cardiovascular and extrahepatic cancer-related mortality in treated patients with mild HFE hemochromatosis. J Hepatol. 2015 Mar;62(3):682–9.

147. Ong SY, Gurrin LC, Dolling L, Dixon J, Nicoll AJ, Wolthuizen M, et al. Reduction of body iron in HFE-related haemochromatosis and moderate iron overload (mi-iron): a multicentre, participant-blinded, randomised controlled trial. Lancet Haematol. 2017 Dec;4(12):e607–e14.

148. Cancado R, Melo MR, de Moraes BR, Santos PC, Guerra-Shinohara EM, Chiattone C, et al. Deferasirox in patients with iron overload secondary to hereditary hemochromatosis: results of a 1-yr phase 2 study. Eur J Haematol. 2015 Dec;95(6):545–50.

149. Ullrich H, Fischer R, Grosse R, Kordes U, Schubert C, Altstadt B, et al. Erythrocytapheresis: do not forget a useful therapy! Transfus Med Hemother. 2008;35(1):24–30.

150. Rombout-Sestrienkova E, Nieman FH, Essers BA, van Noord PA, Janssen MC, van Deursen CT, et al. Erythrocytapheresis versus phlebotomy in the initial treatment of HFE hemochromatosis patients: results from a randomized trial. Transfusion. 2012 Mar;52(3):470–7.

151. Rombout-Sestrienkova E, Winkens B, Essers BA, Nieman FH, Noord PA, Janssen MC, et al. Erythrocytapheresis versus phlebotomy in the maintenance treatment of HFE hemochromatosis patients: results from a randomized crossover trial. Transfusion. 2016 Jan;56(1):261–70.

152. Vanclooster A, van Deursen C, Jaspers R, Cassiman D, Koek G. Proton pump inhibitors decrease phlebotomy need in HFE hemochromatosis: double-blind randomized placebo-controlled trial. Gastroenterology. 2017 Sep;153(3):678–80 e2.

153. Bardou-Jacquet E, Philip J, Lorho R, Ropert M, Latournerie M, Houssel-Debry P, et al. Liver transplantation normalizes serum hepcidin level and cures iron metabolism alterations in HFE hemochromatosis. Hepatology. 2014 Mar;59(3):839–47.

154. Kowdley KV, Brandhagen DJ, Gish RG, Bass NM, Weinstein J, Schilsky ML, et al. Survival after liver transplantation in patients with hepatic iron overload: the national hemochromatosis transplant registry. Gastroenterology. 2005 Aug;129(2):494–503.

155. Yu L, Ioannou GN. Survival of liver transplant recipients with hemochromatosis in the United States. Gastroenterology. 2007 Aug;133(2):489–95.

156. Dar FS, Faraj W, Zaman MB, Bartlett A, Bomford A, O'Sullivan A, et al. Outcome of liver transplantation in hereditary hemochromatosis. Transplant Int. 2009 Jul;22(7):717–24.

157. Aranda N, Viteri FE, Montserrat C, Arija V. Effects of C282Y, H63D, and S65C HFE gene mutations, diet, and life-style factors on iron status in a general Mediterranean population from Tarragona. Spain Ann Hematol. 2010 Aug;89(8):767–73.

158. Waterlot Y, Cantinieaux B, Hariga-Muller C, De Maertelaere-Laurent E, Vanherweghem JL, Fondu P. Impaired phagocytic activity of neutrophils in patients receiving haemodialysis: the critical role of iron overload. Br Med J. 1985 Aug 24;291(6494):501–4.

159. de Sousa M. Immune cell functions in iron overload. Clin Exp Immunol. 1989 Jan;75(1):1–6.

160. Pinto JP, Dias V, Zoller H, Porto G, Carmo H, Carvalho F, et al. Hepcidin messenger RNA expression in human lymphocytes. Immunology. 2010 Jun;130(2):217–30.

161. Porto G, Cruz E, Teles MJ, de Sousa M. HFE related hemochromatosis: uncovering the inextricable link between iron homeostasis and the immunological system. Pharmaceuticals. 2019 Aug;22:12(3).

162. Girelli D, Trombini P, Busti F, Campostrini N, Sandri M, Pelucchi S, et al. A time course of hepcidin response to iron challenge in patients with HFE and TFR2 hemochromatosis. Haematologica. 2011 Apr;96(4):500–6.

163. Worthen CA, Enns CA. The role of hepatic transferrin receptor 2 in the regulation of iron homeostasis in the body. Front Pharmacol. 2014;5:34.

164. Roetto A, Papanikolaou G, Politou M, Alberti F, Girelli D, Christakis J, et al. Mutant antimicrobial peptide hepcidin is associated with severe juvenile hemochromatosis. Nat Genet. 2003 Jan;33(1):21–2.

165. Mayr R, Janecke AR, Schranz M, Griffiths WJ, Vogel W, Pietrangelo A, et al. Ferroportin disease: a systematic meta-analysis of clinical and molecular findings. J Hepatol. 2010 Nov;53(5):941–9.
166. Jolla L. La Jolla Pharmaceutical Company Announces Positive Results from Pre-Specified Interim Analysis of Phase 2 Study of LJPC-401 in Patients with Hereditary Hemochromatosis 2019 [11/05/2019].
167. Lesjak M, Hoque R, Balesaria S, Skinner V, Debnam ES, Srai SK, et al. Quercetin inhibits intestinal iron absorption and ferroportin transporter expression in vivo and in vitro. PLoS One. 2014;9(7):e102900.

# Chapter 12
# Wilson's Disease

Nora V. Bergasa

A 29-year-old man presented to the hepatology clinic to establish care after moving to the area. The patient felt well. He had been diagnosed with Wilson's disease (WD) at age nine and was being managed with trientene, 500 mg orally twice a day, supplemented with pyridoxine. He had a history of rash in association with D-penicillamine (DPA). His comorbidities included type I diabetes since age four, managed via an insulin pump. His physical exam did not reveal any stigmata of chronic liver disease. Hepatic panel and hemogram were normal. Twenty-four hours urine for copper was ordered but not collected. The patient has continued his care at another institution.

In 1911, the British physician Samuel Alexander Kinnier Wilson presented his seminal monograph followed by a publication entitled "Progressive lenticular degeneration: a familial nervous disease associated with cirrhosis of the liver" [1–3].

The liver disease workup that we generate in the hepatology clinic includes the exclusion of Wilson's disease or hepatolenticular degeneration because the disease is treatable, as emphasized in the publication in the July 2019 issue of the Journal of Hepatology, "Wilson's disease: Fatal when overlooked, curable when diagnosed" [4].

N. V. Bergasa (✉)
Department of Medicine, H+H/Metropolitan, New York, NY, USA

New York Medical College, Valhalla, NY, USA

Hepatology, H+H/Woodhull, Brooklyn, NY, USA

© The Author(s), under exclusive license to Springer-Verlag London Ltd., part of Springer Nature 2022
N. V. Bergasa (ed.), *Clinical Cases in Hepatology*,
https://doi.org/10.1007/978-1-4471-4715-2_12

# Etiology

Wilson's disease (WD) is a genetic condition caused by mutations in the ATP7B gene, which codes for the transmembrane copper-transporting ATPase. Mutations associated with Wilson's disease lead to a dysfunctional ATP7B protein, which results in impaired biliary excretion of copper and its accumulation in organs, including the brain, liver, and heart [4].

# Copper Homeostasis

There are approximately 5 mg of copper in a regular diet, about which 40% is absorbed in the stomach and duodenum, and transported by the portal vein into the liver, which regulates copper homeostasis [5]. Foodstuffs are rich in copper; thus, a deficiency is rare. The liver is very efficient in extracting copper from the portal circulation. Within 24 h of its absorption, as documented by radioisotope studies, 6–8% of the copper appears in the circulation bound to the ferroxidase ceruloplasmin, which binds 95% of plasma copper [6, 7]. Although copper navigates in the blood bound to ceruloplasmin, the latter does not play a role in its transport through cell membranes; it is proposed that histidine and other amino acids bind copper and distribute it to various tissues.

Prior to absorption, dietary copper, i.e., $Cu^{2+}$, is reduced, likely by several reductases including DCYTB [8] and STEAP2 metalloreductase [9], to cuprous, $Cu^{1+}$ in which form is taken up by the copper transporter 1 (CTR1) [10], which is localized in the apical membrane and endosomes in the intestinal epithelial cells [11]. The copper concentration regulates the expression of CTR1, i.e., excess copper is associated with clathrin-mediated endocytosis of CTR1, and deficiency is associated with the recycling of CTR1 to the apical membrane of the intestinal epithelial cells [12, 13], where the copper chaperone antioxidant-1 (ATOX1) shuttles copper to the copper-transporting ATPase ATP7A, which exports copper into the portal circulation [14, 15]. ATP7A is essential for the transport of copper, for the biosynthesis of several secreted cuproenzymes and the efflux of copper from the basolateral membrane of the intestinal epithelial cells [14, 16].

ATP7A is not found in the liver. Mutations in the ATP7A gene, which codes for ATP7A, are associated with Menke's disease, an X-linked recessive disorder characterized by copper deficiency [17]. ATP7A is localized in the trans-Golgi network (TGN); when the concentration of intracellular copper increases, ATP7A relocates itself to the cytosolic vesicular compartment and is trafficked to the basolateral membrane [18–20], but it is unclear whether ATP7ase transports copper across the membrane [18–20]. It is proposed that ATP7A may mobilize copper into vesicles that fuse themselves with the basolateral membrane to release the metal for export; it may also be that ATP7A itself transports copper through the membrane [21]; however, how copper gets into the portal system is unknown [21].

Copper exported from intestinal epithelial cells binds to albumin or alpha 2 macroglobulin and is transported to the liver where it binds to ceruloplasmin [22, 23]. Ceruloplasmin binds over 95% of serum copper [7], a process mediated by ATP7B; as already stated, mutations in the ATP7B are associated with WD, a copper excess disease [1–4].

Intracellularly, chaperones transport copper to specific compartments. Cytochrome c oxidase (CcO) donates copper to superoxide dismutase, ATOX1 delivers copper to the secretory pathway by binding to the two ATPases, and COX17 takes copper to the mitochondria for the synthesis of cytochrome c oxidase [24]; COX17 is 1 of 30 assembly factors considered essential for the synthesis of CcO [25].

ATP7B is expressed in the liver; it is an efflux transporter also required in the TGN to deliver copper for the metallation of apoceruloplasmin, the major plasma cuproprotein, and the biliary excretion of the metal. Apoceruloplasmin refers to ceruloplasmin without copper. As the intracellular concentration of copper increases, ATP7B moves to a cytoplasmic compartment by the canalicular membrane, where copper accumulates itself into vesicles for biliary excretion. In WD, the dysfunctional ATPB7 cannot incorporate copper into ceruloplasmin; thus, what is secreted is apoceruloplasmin, which is rapidly degraded, leading to the typical finding of low ceruloplasmin in the diagnosis of WD [6, 26].

There are other intracellular hepatic binding proteins, including COMMD1 (copper metabolism MURR1 domain), XIAP (X-linked inhibitor of apoptosis protein), metallothionein, and amyloid precursor protein, which may also be involved in copper metabolism [24]. In this regard, it was reported that excess copper in the cytosol binds to the metallothionein, thus decreasing copper toxicity [27].

## Genetics of Wilson's Disease

WD is a monogenetic, autosomal recessive disease that results in mutations in the ATP7B gene, which codes the ATP7B protein, a P-type ATPase that transports copper out of the hepatocyte by biliary excretion [28–30]. Hundreds of mutations that include missense mutations, small deletions, insertions in the coding region, and promoter region mutations have been described [31]. Mutations in the ATP M645R in exon 6 are mutations identified in patients from Spain, versus the point mutation H1069Q, in exon 14, which is the most common in the rest of Europe, carried by over 50% of patients. In the south of Asia, the R778L in exon 8 mutation was reported in less than 50% of patients [32]. Truncating mutations in the WD gene ATP7B were reported in association with very low serum ceruloplasmin oxidase activity and an early onset of WD. Patients with two copies of what was labeled as severe protein-truncating ATP7B, i.e., mutations frameshift/nonsense/splice site mutations, had manifestations of disease at ages between 9 and 13 years. Also, a ceruloplasmin oxidase concentration of less or equal to 5 U/L was identified as a predictor of the presence of severe protein-truncating ATP7B mutations with high sensitivity and specificity [33]. A spectrum of mutations that completely disrupt the gene can result in liver disease in early childhood, alerting the clinician to consider WD in the differential diagnosis [34]. Although copper transporter activity can vary in association with variants of AT7PB, studies to define specific correlations between genotype and phenotype have not revealed consistent information [35]. For example, the case of a monozygote twin who presented with fulminant liver failure requiring liver transplantation was compared with the other twin who, despite having an identical genetic mutation to that of the twin with liver failure, was reported as having mild liver disease [36].

In regards to genetic variability, the methylenetetrahydrofolate reductase gene (MTHFR) was reported to affect the clinical expression of WD [37]. In addition, the presence of ApoE epsilon3/3 genotype was documented in association with a delay in the onset of neurological and hepatic manifestations of WD, although no modification of the disease phenotype was noted [38]. It was suggested that the mechanism that would support the extended asymptomatic period might be related to the antioxidant and membrane-stabilizing properties of the ApoE 3 protein [38]. In association with WD, a defect in oxidative-phosphorylation has been documented in studies of mitochondrial enzyme activity, which have suggested that free-radical formation and oxidative damage contribute to the pathogenesis of liver disease; a role of copper accumulation was suggested [39].

The dysfunction of the ATPase variant alters the intracellular handling of copper. Increased intracellular copper is associated with oxidative stress and free radical formation in addition to severe mitochondrial dysfunction. It was documented that the liver of patients with WD showed decreased enzymatic activity of complex I by 62%, complex II + III by 52%, complex IV by 33%, and aconitase by 71%, not reported to be associated with D-penicillamine use or to liver disease. These findings were interpreted to suggest that free radical formation and oxidative injury were possibly mediated by the accumulation of copper in the mitochondria, and provided a rationale for the study of antioxidants as treatment of WD [39].

# Epigenetics

Epigenetics in WD may explain, in part, its phenotypic expression. By the use of whole-genome bisulfite sequencing (WGBS) in a study that included liver tissue from patients with WD, normal and disease control samples, 969 hypermethylated and 871 hypomethylated differentially methylated regions (DMRs) specifically identified patients with WD, including 18 regions with genome-wide significance. The DMRs identified in WD were associated with genes related to folate and lipid metabolism and the acute inflammatory response. The WD-hypermethylated liver DMRs were enriched in liver specific enhancers, flanking active liver promoters, and binding sites of liver developmental transcription factors. DMRs found in the blood identified patients with WD versus control subjects. The DMRs differentiated patients with hepatic from those with neurological manifestations and were related to genes enriched for roles in mental dysfunction, abnormal B cell physiology, and as members of the polycomb repressive complex 1 (PRC1), which participate in the transcriptional regulation during development [40]. These findings were interpreted to suggest that the methylation changes identified in liver-specific enhancers and transcription factor binding sites indicate that WD is a condition affected by epigenetic changes, which may explain the disease's phenotypic expression including its progression and its pathogenesis.

# Epidemiology

The frequency of WD was estimated as 1:30,000 for WD with a heterozygous ATP7B mutation carrier frequency of 1:90 [41]. Subsequently, the estimated frequency of individuals predicted to carry two ATP7B pathogenic mutants was reported as 1 in 7026 [42], higher than the 1: 30,000 previously documented [41]. In Japan, screening studies from dry blood samples from 2789 children aged between 1 and 6 years identified two patients [43]. In Korea, screening tests on dried blood samples from 3667 identified one patient [44]. However, four recent clinical studies, which were considered high quality, noted that the prevalence estimates remain in the realm of 1:30,000, as previously reported [41], with a range of 1:29,000 to 1:40,000 [45]. Data from France and Sardinia suggested an estimated genetic prevalence three to four times higher than that of the disease's clinical manifestations, suggesting that penetrance may not be 100% [45].

# Natural History

The natural history of WD was deduced from a group of 55 patients with WD and neurological presentation, a group of 51 patients with only hepatic presentation, and a group of 11 patients considered asymptomatic with a median follow-up of 12 years, with a range of 1–41. The H1069Q ATP7B gene mutation was present in 54.3% of subjects, a finding not associated with neurological or hepatic manifestations. D-penicillamine was used for treatment in 81% of the patients, and zinc in 17%; three patients underwent liver transplantation. Most symptomatic patients improved or became asymptomatic during follow-up, i.e., 82% of the patients with hepatic manifestation versus 69% of patients with neurological manifestations. The documented long-term survival of the patients with WD did not differ from that of the general population from the Czech group, which comprised the study group [46]. In a study by the physician who introduced the use of D-penicillamine in the treatment of WD [47] and that included 67 patients, 34 of whom were women, from a total of 300 subjects seen from 1948 to 2000, Dr. John Walshe stated that the principal cause of death in WD was a diagnostic failure [48]. The importance of diagnosis and prompt treatment institution in patients with WD is clear; thus, its exclusion in evaluating patients with liver disease is warranted, regardless of hepatic comorbidities.

## Clinical Manifestations

Patients with WD may present without any signs or symptoms of liver disease. Most patients present after the age of three, considered to be due to the large capacity of the liver to accumulate copper. The most common presentation in children is liver disease, usually between ages from 10 to 13 years, much earlier than the age at which neurological manifestations become clinically apparent [49]. Ten percent of the patients present with psychiatric manifestations, 35% with neurological disease, and 45% with liver disease. Hemolytic anemia, cardiomyopathy, and altered thyroid function are some of the other manifestations of the disease. The hepatic abnormalities accompanying them should lead to the diagnosis [50].

Patients may exhibit physical findings of liver disease; azure lunulae, i.e., blue lunula due to copper deposition, in nails is described [51].

The Kayser–Fleischer (KF) ring is described as a dark band of pigment in the Descemet membrane of greenish yellow to golden brown color, which is comprised of copper [52]. In a study that included 55 patients with WD prior to treatment, KF rings were documented in 55%, with a proportion of 90% with neurological manifestations exhibiting this finding [53]. Sunflower cataracts is another ophthalmological manifestation of WD [54]; they were documented in 1.2% of 81 newly diagnosed patients with WD with a mean age of $32.3 \pm 11.8$ years 42% of whom had neurological manifestations [55]. This type of cataract is described as a thin, centralized opacification under the anterior capsule and occupying one-third to one-half of the anterior lens pole surface area, with opacifications emanating from the center that give the impression of sunflower [55].

A study that examined retrospectively the documented neurological examinations of a group of 119 patients reported that symptoms tended to start at a mean age of 19 years, with a range from 7 to 37, with dysarthria being the first one in 91% of patients, gait abnormalities in 75%, risus sardonicus in 72%, dystonia in 69%, rigidity in 66%, tremor in 60%, dysphagia in 50%, chorea in 16%, and athetosis in 14%; seizures and pyramidal signs were present in less than 5% of patients [56]. The clinician must be cognizant of WD's signs, labeled "A Great Masquerader" by the authors of a publication from a retrospective study of 50 patients referred to a university hospital and private clinic in Tehran from 1984 to 2004 [57]. The median age of onset of neurological symptoms or both hepatic and neurological manifestations ranged from 10 to 38 years, with a mean of 16, in contrast to patients with initial findings of liver disease, who exhibited neurological symptoms at a mean age of 18 years, with a range from 11 to 34, with dysarthria being the most common, i.e., in 80% of patients, as described in the prior study [56]. Drooling was present in 48% of patients, 44% had limb tremors, abnormal gait, alone or in combination with psychiatric and sleep alterations, and 42% had dystonia. Of note, a review of WD that included studies conducted over 66 years reported that 30–40% of patients have psychiatric manifestations at the time of diagnosis, and 20% had seen a psychiatrist prior to the diagnosis of WD [58]. As documented in these two studies, manifestations of WD tend to become apparent before age 40; however, late clinical presentations are well documented [59].

The clinical and genetic characterization of 46 of 1223 (3.8%) patients, 1053 of whom were index cases, and 170 siblings, who manifested clinically after the age of 40 was described [59]. Thirty-one (67.4%) patients presented with neurologic symptoms at a mean age of 44.5 years, with a range from 40 to 52; 15 (32.6%), 9 of whom were women, presented with liver disease at a mean age of 47 years, with a range from 40 to 58, and 2 (4.3%) were asymptomatic siblings. One patient's hepatic presentation was fulminant, with the rest having abnormal liver tests, hepatomegaly, or both. Of note, from the 13 patients from whom liver histology was available and who presented with liver test abnormalities, 10 had cirrhosis, 2 chronic hepatitis, 1 steatosis, and 1 did not have any histological abnormalities. Twenty-seven of the 46 index cases had mutations on both chromosomes and included H1069Q/H1069Q in 13, and in one chromosome in another 13. The authors concluded that WD could be "overlooked." The clinical characteristics of patients who presented after age 40 in this study were similar to those of the patients who present early in life, which suggested that other factors influence WD's clinical expression. Conversely, the case of a 9-month-old baby who exhibited abnormal liver panel was diagnosed with WD by genetic testing [60] and that of a 10-year-old boy who presented with a 3-month history of leg muscle cramps has been described. Again, as previously stated, "the principal cause of death in Wilson ('s) disease was diagnostic failure" [48].

## Acute Liver Failure

By definition, acute liver failure is the loss of liver function in patients without prior liver disease [61–64]; as inferred, it is characterized by hepatitis, associated with hepatic synthetic dysfunction, and hepatic encephalopathy developing over less than 8–12 weeks [64]. In WD, however, acute liver failure can be a presentation in patients with chronic liver disease, i.e., fibrosis and sometimes, cirrhosis. Acute liver failure from WD is fatal in the majority of patients without liver transplantation; accordingly, early recognition and transfer to a liver transplantation center are fundamental in the management of patients who present with this complication. Prognostic indeces to predict survival in patients with acute liver failure from WD have been developed [65, 66].

Five percent of the patients referred for liver transplantation because of acute liver failure have WD. The female-to-male ratio of patients with acute liver failure due to WD is 2:1 to 4:1. A study that included 140 patients with acute liver failure, 16 of whom had WD, 17 had treated chronic WD, and 29 other chronic liver diseases documented that a ceruloplasmin level of less than 20 mg/dl by the oxidase method had a diagnostic sensitivity of 21%, and specificity of 84%; when measured by nephelometry, the sensitivity was 56% and specificity 63%. Serum copper levels were higher than 200 micrograms/dl in all patients with acute liver failure from WD. A serum alkaline phosphatase to total bilirubin ratio less than 4, had a sensitivity of 94% and a specificity of 96%, while an AST-to-ALT ratio greater than 2.2 had a sensitivity of 94% and a specificity of 86% with the combination of all tests giving a diagnostic accuracy of 100% [67].

## Liver Histology

The liver histology in patients who present with acute hepatitis exhibits ballooned hepatocytes, acidophilic bodies, cholestasis, and scant lymphocytic infiltration. The pre-cirrhotic liver in WD shows anisonucleosis, focal necrosis, few sinusoidal acidophilic bodies, and moderate to marked steatosis. Glycogenated bodies, steatosis, moderate to marked copper accumulation, and Mallory bodies are seen in periportal hepatocytes [68]. In young, asymptomatic patients, copper accumulates itself in the cytoplasm of the hepatocytes. In contrast, in patients who present symptoms and signs of the disease, copper is widely distributed including inside the lysosomes. In the cirrhotic stage, copper is limited to the lysosomes. The p-dimethylaminobenzylidene rhodanine gives reproducible staining findings.

Cirrhosis in WD tends to be macronodular, but it can be mixed, with minimal bile ductular proliferation noted in the nodules' fibrous bands. Mallory bodies can be found in the periphery of the cirrhotic nodules.

Mitochondrial abnormalities were reported as distinctive in WD and included heterogeneity of size and shape, increased matrix density, separation of inner from outer membranes, and enlarged intercisternal spaces [68]. In association with chelating therapy with DPA for three to five years, mitochondrial abnormalities were documented to be less notable than at baseline or absent [69].

## Laboratory Findings

Patients can exhibit increased serum activity of transaminases or findings suggestive of portal hypertension from cirrhosis with or without hepatic synthetic dysfunction; typically, serum activity of alkaline phosphatase is low or in the low limits of normal.

## Diagnostic Investigations

The specific laboratory findings in WD are ceruloplasmin concentration less than 20 mg/dl, serum free or non-ceruloplasmin-bound copper less than 100 micrograms/dl, hepatic copper content greater than 250 micrograms/gram of dry weight, and urinary copper content greater than 100 micrograms per 24 h. Genetic testing is done to identify mutations in the ATP7B gene. Guidance on the diagnosis and treatment of WD is available from the American and the European Associations for the Study of Liver Diseases [70, 71].

## Imaging Studies

Magnetic resonance imaging (MRI) of the brain has provided the feature now recognized as typical of WD, the "face of the giant panda" sign. It has been recognized to distinguish WD from other early onset extrapyramidal disorders. A retrospective review that included images from 100 patients identified, specifically in patients with WD, the following findings: (1) "Face of giant panda" sign in 14.3%, (2) tectal plate hyperintensity in 75%, (3) central pontine myelinolysis-like abnormalities in 62.5%, and concurrent signal changes in basal ganglia, thalamus, and brainstem in 55.3%. The authors concluded that in addition to "Face of giant panda" sign, hyperintensities in the tectal-plate and central pons, and simultaneous involvement of basal ganglia, thalamus, and brainstem are "virtually pathognomonic" of WD [72]. Resolution of MRI findings in the globus and caudate regressed in association with liver transplantation over 2 years of follow-up in a 28-year-old patient [73].

## Transient Elastography

The experience in transient elastography with FibroScan® is still limited; however, a value of 6.6 kPa is considered suggestive of mild and moderate fibrosis, whereas a value higher than 8.4 is indicative of severe fibrosis. More studies are now necessary to confirm the usefulness of FibroScan® in managing chronic therapy for WD patients [74].

## Screening in Wilson's Disease

Siblings and first-degree relatives of patients with diagnosed WD must be screened for the disease.

Clinical manifestations of liver and neurological disease, alone or in combination should trigger suspicion for WD; in children, sudden poor school performance and behavioral problems should be considered indications for excluding the disease.

The clinical investigations include hepatic panel, hemogram, serum ceruloplasmin, 24-h urine for copper, serum copper, and referral to ophthalmology for slit lamp examination to exclude KF rings. Liver biopsy for copper quantitation and genetic testing can be included, according to published guidelines [70, 71]. In regards to liver histology, a biopsy is recommended when the combination of clinical signs and laboratory tests are not conclusive, or to exclude hepatic comorbidities [75]. The Leipzig score (Table 12.1) was developed to facilitate the diagnosis of WD; diagnostic algorithms have been derived from that score [70, 76, 77]. In patients with symptoms suggestive of WD, including extrapyramidal symptoms, KF rings, and low serum ceruloplasmin, a score between 0 and 3, should be followed by a 24-h urine collection of copper. If the urine copper concentration is greater than 1.6 micromols/24 hr. (100 microg/24 hr) (0.64 micromoles per day in children), a

**Table 12.1** Leipzig Score for the diagnosis of Wilson's Disease (WD) [76]

| Clinical findings suggestive of WD | Points | Additional Investigations | Points |
|---|---|---|---|
| **KF rings** | | **Liver copper concentration (in the absence of cholestasis)*** | |
| Present | 2 | > 4 micromol/g | 2 |
| Absent | 0 | 0.8–4 micromol/g | 1 |
| | | Normal (0.8 micromoles/g) | – 1 |
| | | *Rhodadine-positive granules | 1 |
| **Neurologic symptoms or typical brain magnetic resonance imaging findings** | | **24-hour urine for copper□** | |
| Severe | 2 | Normal | 0 |
| Mild | 1 | 1–2 x ULN | 1 |
| Absent | 0 | > 2 x ULN | 2 |
| | | Normal at baseline with an increase 5 X ULN after DPA | 2 |
| **Serum ceruloplasmin** | | **Genetic analysis** | |
| Normal (>0.2 g/L) | 0 | Mutations in 2 both chromosomes | 4 |
| 0.1–0.2 g/L | 1 | Mutations in 1 chromosome | 1 |
| < 0.1 g/ml | 2 | No mutations | 0 |
| **Hemolytic anemia, Coomb's negative** | | | |
| Present | 1 | | |
| Absent | 0 | | |

□: in the absence of acute hepatitis in regards to the urine collecdtion
DPA: D-penicillamine
*If the concentration of liver copper is not available
Summation of Scores
4 or more: diagnosis established
3: possible diagnosis; additional tests required (e.g., genetic testing, hepatic copper concentration)
2 or less: diagnosis is unlikely

liver biopsy for copper quantitation with a value of fewer than 4 micromoles per gram excluding WD in patients with a score of 0–1 but, in patients with a score equal or less than 3, mutation analysis is recommended for diagnosis. One of two mutations confirms the diagnosis, with an increase in the score to at least 4. In patients with a hepatic copper concentration greater than 4 micromols/g, a score increases to at least 4, which confirms the diagnosis.

Treatment for WD should be started immediately after diagnosis.

## Treatment

The American and European Associations for the Study of Liver Diseases have created guidelines for the treatment of WD [70, 71].

The starting dose of DPA is 250–500 mg/day, increased by 250 mg weekly, to a maximum of 1000 to 1500 mg per day in divided doses, taken 1 h before or 2 h after meals. The dose for children is 250 mg daily, with a maximum of 20 mg per kg, in divided doses. After the initial decoppering, which tends to occur between four to 6 months after initiation of treatment, a maintenance dose of 750–1000 mg per day in two divided doses is sufficient during the maintenance phase, usually after 4–6 months. The therapeutic response to changes in the maintenance dose usually will not become evident for 4–6 weeks [70, 71]. DPA can be administered during pregnancy. DPA can be associated with pyridoxine deficiency because of pyridoxine kinase inhibition; thus, pyridoxine is supplemented at doses of 25 to 50 mg orally per day during treatment [70, 71].

DPA can be associated with sensitivity reactions characterized by fever, rash, lymphadenopathy, bone marrow suppression, and proteinuria; follow-up is important to identify any side effects that can present after years of therapy. If these complications occur, the drug should be discontinued and the patient treated with an alternative medication.

Trientine (trimethylene tetramine dihydrochloride) is a chelating agent promoting urinary copper excretion; it also prevents intestinal absorption of copper by inducing metallothionein. Trientine is used at a starting dose of 20 mg/kg per day in children and adults, in divided doses, not to exceed 1500 mg per day, with a maintenance dose of 15 mg/kg also in divided doses, to be taken 1 h before or 2 h after meals. Side effects include hemorrhagic gastritis, dysgeusia, sideroblastic anemia, and rarely, hypersensitivity reactions and bone marrow suppression [70, 71].

Zinc acetate in children weighing less than 50 kg is given at a dose of 25 mg three times a day. In others, including adults, the recommended dose is 50 mg of elemental zinc three times a day. Zinc should be taken on an empty stomach, at least 1 h before or 2–3 h after meals, and separated from beverages, other than water, by at least 1 h [70, 71].

The use of DPA in pregnancy is accepted based on clinical experience [78]; however, zinc and trientine are also documented as safe [79, 80].

Maintenance doses are determined by measuring the excretion of copper in a 24-h urine collection, with a target of fewer than 0.6 micrograms per day [81].

In patients who present with liver disease, not in acute liver failure, the initial treatment is the pharmacological removal of copper from the blood and tissues and to increase its excretion [70, 71]. Maintenance therapy aims to prevent copper accumulation, which can be accomplished by the continuous use of DPA, and by the administration of zinc salts. In this regard, zinc interferes with the absorption of copper by inducing the synthesis of metallothionein in intestinal epithelial cells leading to increased preferential binding of dietary copper to the latter in these intestinal cells, which are shed subsequently as part of the rejuvenation process of the intestine. Although zinc prevents further copper accumulation, its capability to decopper is less than that of DPA, and thus, it does not mobilize copper from laden tissues [82].

The course of disease in patients on treatment with oral chelators for WD was examined retrospectively in a cohort study that included 405 patients, of whom 238 were women. Changes in medication were common, leading to the analysis of 471 chelator monotherapies, 326 on DPA, and 141 on trientine. Liver transplantation was performed in 9 of the 326 (2.8%) patients treated with DPA, and in 3 of the 141 (2.2%) treated with trientine. Adverse events were significantly more common in the patients receiving DPA than in those receiving trientine. After 4 years of therapy, 4 patients from the 333 (1.2%) who had been treated with oral chelators experienced worsening of liver function. Improvement of liver function was experienced by over 90% of patients. Eighty-eight of 143 patients (62%) exhibited neurological improvement after 4 years of treatment, with 38% not demonstrating any benefits, findings that may suggest that the neurological impairment was permanent. Of note, neurological deterioration was observed significantly less frequently in patients given DPA first (6 of 295) than in those given trientine first (4 of 38); $P = 0.018$. These findings suggest that chelating agents are effective therapies for most patients with WD [83].

Transient impairment of neurological function can be associated with the initial treatment with DPA in 20% of the patients at the beginning of the chelation period, which appears to be related to the copper bound to ceruloplasmin versus free copper, which is what causes toxicity, and which, as a result of oral chelators, changes in proportion, resulting in a relative increase of free copper. This idea is supported by studies documenting an association between high free copper pool and neurological deterioration; specifically, a study that included five patients with WD and who exhibited neurological worsening on trientine therapy over 8 weeks showed significant spikes in the concentration of free serum copper, in contrast to patients who did not worsen, in whom no free copper spikes were documented [84].

Long-term zinc monotherapy in symptomatic patients with WD was studied in 17 subjects with a mean age of 18 years, ranging from 13 to 26, whose clinical presentation was hepatic in 7, neurological in 5, and combined in another 5, followed up on treatment for a median of 14 years, with a range from 2 to 30. Zinc monotherapy was reported as good in patients with neurological complications; however, in patients with cirrhosis, it did not prevent decompensation of liver disease [85]. These findings contrast to those from a retrospective study in which 288 patients were followed for 17 years; it was documented that hepatic symptoms developed in 196 patients (68.1%) and neuropsychiatric in 99 (34.4%), with increased failure to improve liver disease in zinc monotherapy, i.e., in 14 of 88 (16%) versus 4 of 313 (1.3%). The actuarial survival, without transplantation, was calculated to favor chelating agents as compared to zinc. These data suggested that chelating agents are better than zinc in the prevention of deterioration of liver disease. Thus, monitoring the clinical course to determine if changes in therapy should be made is recommended for zinc managed patients with WD [86].

Patients diagnosed with WD should be started on chelating therapy. No studies comparing DPA versus zinc are available; thus, the choice of therapy depends on the clinician's experience and the patient's choice; however, monitoring the effect of decoppering is required. Adequate decoppering may take 1–3 years to change to maintenance therapy. On maintenance with DPA, the excretion of less than 0.6 mg per 24 h off medication is a practice followed by some investigators [81]. Of note, it is documented that 36% of children who have achieved acceptable decoppering with DPA or zinc have increased serum activity of transaminases [87].

Thirty-one percent of patients have been reported to discontinue DPA because of side effects, including nephrotoxicity, hematological abnormalities, and elastosis perforans serpiginosa [83]. In this regard, tetrathiomolybdate, which acts by forming a tripartite complex with copper and protein, preventing the absorption of endogenously secreted and dietary copper, is being studied for the management of WD and reported to be well tolerated versus trientine [88, 89].

Adherence to therapy is fundamental in managing patients with WD [90]; patients can regress to a copper-laden state and go into liver failure if the cessation of treatment occurs [91]. Unaffected relatives without findings of WD must also be treated lifelong [70].

The follow-up of stable patients consists of physical examination, hemogram, serum electrolytes, renal function, serum copper, and 24-h urine collection for copper every 6 months. Bone marrow suppression tends to suggest overtreatment, which required dose adjustment.

A considerable proportion of patients, i.e., 50.5% from a sample of 210 contacted by mail or identified retrospectively, still reported neurological symptoms; 31.3% were treated with anticholinergics and botulinum toxin to treat dystonia, and anticonvulsants to treat tremor [92].

Under maintenance therapy, the development of hepatic and neurological decompensation, or recurrence of clinical findings, including KF rings, suggest suboptimal control of copper accumulation for which reassessment is required.

It is recommended that patients avoid foodstuff rich in copper, for which referral to a nutritionist is encouraged.

The exclusion of WD in patients with liver disease is fundamental as the disease is treatable and dreadful complications can be prevented with treatment.

The reader is referred to ClinicalTrials.gov to identify clinical trials in WD.

# Hepatocellular Carcinoma

Hepatocellular carcinoma (HCC) is uncommon in WD. From a median follow-up of 15 years (range 0.1–51.2), a study that included 130 patients with WD documented that two patients from the sample developed HCC, one in spite of appropriate decoppering after 50 years of diagnosis, and another with newly diagnosed WD. Of the 74 patients with cirrhosis (57%), 64% compensated, and 36% decompensated, 20% improved, 46% remained stable, and 24% deteriorated, with no data presented in 10%. The estimated annual risk for HCC was reported as 0.09% (95% confidence interval [CI]: 0.01–0.28), with analysis of cirrhotic patients documenting an annual risk for HCC of 0.14% (95% CI: 0.02–0.46). The results of the meta-analysis were reported to show an annual risk for HCC of 0.04% (95% CI: 0.01–0.10) and a mortality rate of 2.6 per 10,000 person-years (95% CI: 0.7–7.0) [93]. These results coincide with those of a retrospective review that included 1186 patients, 14 of whom developed hepatobiliary malignancies including HCC in 8 and intrahepatic cholangiocarcinoma in 6, with a calculated prevalence of 1.2% and an incidence of 0.28 per 1000 person-years. Of note, the analysis of the tumor did not show abnormal copper concentration [94]. However, a retrospective study explored the incidence of intraabdominal malignancies in patients with WD, in two specialty clinics in the United Kingdom and Sweden. The study included 303 patients followed from 1955 to 2002. The frequency of HCC was 4.2% in patients followed between 10 and 19 years, 5.3% in patients followed between 20 and 29 years, and 15% in patients followed between 30 and 39 years, with no tumors identified after 40 years of follow-up. The types of malignancies included HCC, cholangiocarcinoma, and poorly differentiated adenocarcinomas of undetermined primary site. These authors did support the idea of screening patients with WD for malignancies, i.e., intraabdominal malignancies. In regards to HCC, screening in patients with cirrhosis is an established practice.

# Liver Transplantation

The indication for liver transplantation in WD is decompensated liver disease and acute liver failure, the latter mostly in children; however, liver transplantation in patients with neuropsychiatric involvement is controversial.

A retrospective multicenter study from liver transplant centers in Italy that covered the period of 2006–2016 documented a proportion of 0.4% of transplants done because of WD, comprised of 29 adult patients, 18 of whom were women, average aged 29 years, with a range from 19 to 60, with a median MELD score of 27, with a range of 6–49 at the time of transplantation. Seventeen patients (63%) had decompensated liver disease at the time of transplantation versus two (7%) who underwent transplantation for neurological complications. The documented survival post procedure was 88% at 1 year, and 83% at five, with the uncommon resolution of neuropsychiatric symptoms early post-transplant. These data were interpreted to indicate a low number of liver transplantation for patients with WD in Italy; uncertainty regarding the improvement of neuropsychiatric complications remains [95].

Long-term results from liver transplantation conducted in France from 1985 to 2009 for WD were documented in a retrospective review of 121 procedures, indicating that acute liver failure was a rare indication. Actuarial survival rates were 87% at 5, 10, and 15 years. The study group was comprised of 75 adult patients, with a median age of 29 years, a range from 18 to 66, and 46 children, with a median age of 14 years, and a range from 7 to 17. The indications for liver transplantation were fulminant liver failure in 64 (53%), with a median age of 16 years, range from 7 to 53, end-stage liver disease in 50 (41%), with a median age of 31.5 years and a range from 12 to 66, and severe neurological complications in seven (6%), with a median age of 21.5 years, and a range from 14 to 42, with a post transplantation follow-up ranging from 0 to 23.5 months, with a median of 72. The prognosis was worse in patients transplanted for fulminant and subfulminant liver failure, nonelective, pre-liver transplantation renal insufficiency, and liver transplantation prior to 2000 than liver transplantation for other indications. It was reported that there was improved renal function with no patient having stage III kidney disease. The results were interpreted to reflect good outcomes post liver transplantation in patients with WD, including those with renal insufficiency [96].

The large European experience with liver transplantation in children with WD was documented from a retrospective cohort study that included data from all patients transplanted for WD and enrolled in the European Liver Transplant Registry from January 1968 until December 2013. Three hundred and thirty-eight children, 57% of whom were girls, underwent LT at 80 different centers in Europe. The median age at liver transplantation was 14 years (interquartile range [IQR], 11.2–16.1 years) with a median post-liver transplantation follow-up of 5.4 years (IQR, 1.0–10.9 years). As documented in other studies, the survival rates were high, reported as 87%, 84%, and 81% at 1, 5, and 10 years post liver transplantation, respectively, with overall survival reported to have improved over the last decades [46]. Similar good post-liver transplantation outcomes were reported in the pediatric population [97]. A literature review from 1971 that concerned 290 patients documented that decompensated liver disease and acute liver failure were the main indications for LT, with a 1-year survival of 91.9% and 88.2% at 5 years, with a reported excellent quality of life. Retransplantation was done in 16 patients due to graft rejection [97].

# References

1. Wilson AAK. Progressive lenticular degeneration: a familial nervous disease associated with cirrhosis of the liver. Brain. 1912;34:295–509.
2. Barbosa ER, Machado AA, Cancado EL, Deguti MM, Scaff M. Wilson's disease: a case report and a historical review. Arq Neuropsiquiatr. 2009 Jun;67(2B):539–43.

3. Broussolle E, Trocello JM, Woimant F, Lachaux A, Quinn N. Samuel Alexander Kinnier Wilson. Wilson's disease, Queen Square and neurology. Rev Neurol. 2013 Dec;169(12):927–35.

4. Ferenci P, Ott P. Wilson's disease: fatal when overlooked, curable when diagnosed. J Hepatol. 2019 Jul;71(1):222–4.

5. Scheinberg IH, Sternlieb I. Wilson disease and idiopathic copper toxicosis. Am J Clin Nutr. 1996 May;63(5):842S–5S.

6. Sternlieb I, Scheinberg IH. Radiocopper in diagnosing liver disease. Semin Nucl Med. 1972 Apr;2(2):176–88.

7. Hellman NE, Gitlin JD. Ceruloplasmin metabolism and function. Annu Rev Nutr. 2002;22:439–58.

8. Knopfel M, Solioz M. Characterization of a cytochrome b(558) ferric/cupric reductase from rabbit duodenal brush border membranes. Biochem Biophys Res Commun. 2002 Feb 22;291(2):220–5.

9. Ohgami RS, Campagna DR, McDonald A, Fleming MD. The Steap proteins are metalloreductases. Blood. 2006 Aug 15;108(4):1388–94.

10. Lee J, Pena MM, Nose Y, Thiele DJ. Biochemical characterization of the human copper transporter Ctr1. J Biol Chem. 2002 Feb 8;277(6):4380–7.

11. Molloy SA, Kaplan JH. Copper-dependent recycling of hCTR1, the human high affinity copper transporter. J Biol Chem. 2009 Oct 23;284(43):29704–13.

12. Petris MJ, Smith K, Lee J, Thiele DJ. Copper-stimulated endocytosis and degradation of the human copper transporter, hCtr1. J Biol Chem. 2003 Mar 14;278(11):9639–46.

13. Clifford RJ, Maryon EB, Kaplan JH. Dynamic internalization and recycling of a metal ion transporter: cu homeostasis and CTR1, the human cu(+) uptake system. J Cell Sci. 2016 Apr 15;129(8):1711–21.

14. Lutsenko S, Barnes NL, Bartee MY, Dmitriev OY. Function and regulation of human copper-transporting ATPases. Physiol Rev. 2007 Jul;87(3):1011–46.

15. Harrison MD, Jones CE, Dameron CT. Copper chaperones: function, structure and copper-binding properties. J Biol Inorg Chem. 1999 Apr;4(2):145–53.

16. La Fontaine S, Mercer JF. Trafficking of the copper-ATPases, ATP7A and ATP7B: role in copper homeostasis. Arch Biochem Biophys. 2007 Jul 15;463(2):149–67.

17. Vairo FPE, Chwal BC, Perini S, Ferreira MAP, de Freitas Lopes AC, Saute JAM. A systematic review and evidence-based guideline for diagnosis and treatment of Menkes disease. Mol Genet Metab. 2019 Jan;126(1):6–13.

18. Greenough M, Pase L, Voskoboinik I, Petris MJ, O'Brien AW, Camakaris J. Signals regulating trafficking of Menkes (MNK; ATP7A) copper-translocating P-type ATPase in polarized MDCK cells. Am J Physiol Cell Physiol. 2004 Nov;287(5):C1463–71.

19. Nyasae L, Bustos R, Braiterman L, Eipper B, Hubbard A. Dynamics of endogenous ATP7A (Menkes protein) in intestinal epithelial cells: copper-dependent redistribution between two intracellular sites. Am J Physiol Gastrointest Liver Physiol. 2007 Apr;292(4):G1181–94.

20. Veldhuis NA, Gaeth AP, Pearson RB, Gabriel K, Camakaris J. The multi-layered regulation of copper translocating P-type ATPases. Biometals. 2009 Feb;22(1):177–90.

21. Kim BE, Nevitt T, Thiele DJ. Mechanisms for copper acquisition, distribution and regulation. Nat Chem Biol. 2008 Mar;4(3):176–85.

22. Liu N, Lo LS, Askary SH, Jones L, Kidane TZ, Trang T, et al. Transcuprein is a macroglobulin regulated by copper and iron availability. J Nutr Biochem. 2007 Sep;18(9):597–608.

23. Moriya M, Ho YH, Grana A, Nguyen L, Alvarez A, Jamil R, et al. Copper is taken up efficiently from albumin and alpha2-macroglobulin by cultured human cells by more than one mechanism. Am J Physiol Cell Physiol. 2008 Sep;295(3):C708–21.

24. Prohaska JR. Role of copper transporters in copper homeostasis. Am J Clin Nutr. 2008 Sep;88(3):826S–9S.

25. Carr HS, Winge DR. Assembly of cytochrome c oxidase within the mitochondrion. Acc Chem Res. 2003 May;36(5):309–16.

26. Schaefer M, Hopkins RG, Failla ML, Gitlin JD. Hepatocyte-specific localization and copper-dependent trafficking of the Wilson's disease protein in the liver. Am J Phys. 1999 Mar;276(3):G639–46.
27. Kelly EJ, Palmiter RD. A murine model of Menkes disease reveals a physiological function of metallothionein. Nat Genet. 1996 Jun;13(2):219–22.
28. Bull PC, Thomas GR, Rommens JM, Forbes JR, Cox DW. The Wilson disease gene is a putative copper transporting P-type ATPase similar to the Menkes gene. Nat Genet. 1993 Dec;5(4):327–37.
29. Petrukhin K, Fischer SG, Pirastu M, Tanzi RE, Chernov I, Devoto M, et al. Mapping, cloning and genetic characterization of the region containing the Wilson disease gene. Nat Genet. 1993 Dec;5(4):338–43.
30. Tanzi RE, Petrukhin K, Chernov I, Pellequer JL, Wasco W, Ross B, et al. The Wilson disease gene is a copper transporting ATPase with homology to the Menkes disease gene. Nat Genet. 1993 Dec;5(4):344–50.
31. Davies LP, Macintyre G, Cox DW. New mutations in the Wilson disease gene, ATP7B: implications for molecular testing. Genet Test. 2008;12(1):139–45.
32. Ferenci P. Regional distribution of mutations of the ATP7B gene in patients with Wilson disease: impact on genetic testing. Hum Genet. 2006 Sep;120(2):151–9.
33. Merle U, Weiss KH, Eisenbach C, Tuma S, Ferenci P, Stremmel W. Truncating mutations in the Wilson disease gene ATP7B are associated with very low serum ceruloplasmin oxidase activity and an early onset of Wilson disease. BMC Gastroenterol. 2010 Jan 18;10:8.
34. Thomas GR, Forbes JR, Roberts EA, Walshe JM, Cox DW. The Wilson disease gene: spectrum of mutations and their consequences. Nat Genet. 1995 Feb;9(2):210–7.
35. Shah AB, Chernov I, Zhang HT, Ross BM, Das K, Lutsenko S, et al. Identification and analysis of mutations in the Wilson disease gene (ATP7B): population frequencies, genotype-phenotype correlation, and functional analyses. Am J Hum Genet. 1997 Aug;61(2):317–28.
36. Kegley KM, Sellers MA, Ferber MJ, Johnson MW, Joelson DW, Shrestha R. Fulminant Wilson's disease requiring liver transplantation in one monozygotic twin despite identical genetic mutation. Am J Transplant. 2010 May;10(5):1325–9.
37. Gromadzka G, Rudnicka M, Chabik G, Przybylkowski A, Czlonkowska A. Genetic variability in the methylenetetrahydrofolate reductase gene (MTHFR) affects clinical expression of Wilson's disease. J Hepatol. 2011 Oct;55(4):913–9.
38. Schiefermeier M, Kollegger H, Madl C, Polli C, Oder W, Kuhn H, et al. The impact of apo-lipoprotein E genotypes on age at onset of symptoms and phenotypic expression in Wilson's disease. Brain. 2000 Mar;123(Pt 3):585–90.
39. Gu M, Cooper JM, Butler P, Walker AP, Mistry PK, Dooley JS, et al. Oxidative-phosphorylation defects in liver of patients with Wilson's disease. Lancet. 2000 Aug 5;356(9228):469–74.
40. Mordaunt CE, Kieffer DA, Shibata NM, Czlonkowska A, Litwin T, Weiss KH, et al. Epigenomic signatures in liver and blood of Wilson disease patients include hypermethylation of liver-specific enhancers. Epigenetics Chromatin. 2019 Feb 1;12(1):10.
41. Scheinberg IHaS, I. Wilson's disease. Philadelphia: W B Saunders; 1984.
42. Coffey AJ, Durkie M, Hague S, McLay K, Emmerson J, Lo C, et al. A genetic study of Wilson's disease in the United Kingdom. Brain. 2013 May;136(Pt 5):1476–87.
43. Ohura T, Abukawa D, Shiraishi H, Yamaguchi A, Arashima S, Hiyamuta S, et al. Pilot study of screening for Wilson disease using dried blood spots obtained from children seen at outpatient clinics. J Inherit Metab Dis. 1999 Feb;22(1):74–80.
44. Hahn SH, Lee SY, Jang YJ, Kim SN, Shin HC, Park SY, et al. Pilot study of mass screening for Wilson's disease in Korea. Mol Genet Metab. 2002 Jun;76(2):133–6.
45. Sandahl TD, Laursen TL, Munk DE, Vilstrup H, Weiss KH, Ott P. The prevalence of Wilson disease. An update. Hepatology. 2019 Aug 26.
46. Pfister ED, Karch A, Adam R, Polak WG, Karam V, Mirza D, et al. Predictive factors for survival in children receiving liver transplants for Wilson's disease: a cohort study using European liver transplant registry data. Liver Transpl. 2018 Sep;24(9):1186–98.

47. Walshe JM. Wilson's disease; new oral therapy. Lancet. 1956 Jan 7;270(6906):25–6.
48. Walshe JM. Cause of death in Wilson disease. Mov Disord. 2007 Nov 15;22(15):2216–20.
49. Walshe JM. Wilson's disease presenting with features of hepatic dysfunction: a clinical analysis of eighty-seven patients. Q J Med. 1989 Mar;70(263):253–63.
50. Gollan JL, Gollan TJ. Wilson disease in 1998: genetic, diagnostic and therapeutic aspects. J Hepatol. 1998;28(Suppl 1):28–36.
51. Bearn AG, Mc KV. Azure lunulae; an unusual change in the fingernails in two patients with hepatolenticular degeneration (Wilson's disease). J Am Med Assoc. 1958 Feb 22;166(8):904–6.
52. Harry J, Tripathi R. Kayser-Fleischer ring. A pathological study. Br J Ophthalmol. 1970 Dec;54(12):794–800.
53. Steindl P, Ferenci P, Dienes HP, Grimm G, Pabinger I, Madl C, et al. Wilson's disease in patients presenting with liver disease: a diagnostic challenge. Gastroenterology. 1997 Jul;113(1):212–8.
54. Litwin T, Langwinska-Wosko E, Dziezyc K, Czlonkowska A. Sunflower cataract: do not forget Wilson's disease. Pract Neurol. 2015 Oct;15(5):385–6.
55. Langwinska-Wosko E, Litwin T, Dziezyc K, Czlonkowska A. The sunflower cataract in Wilson's disease: pathognomonic sign or rare finding? Acta Neurol Belg. 2016 Sep;116(3):325–8.
56. Machado A, Chien HF, Deguti MM, Cancado E, Azevedo RS, Scaff M, et al. Neurological manifestations in Wilson's disease: report of 119 cases. Mov Disord. 2006 Dec;21(12):2192–6.
57. Soltanzadeh A, Soltanzadeh P, Nafissi S, Ghorbani A, Sikaroodi H, Lotfi J. Wilson's disease: a great masquerader. Eur Neurol. 2007;57(2):80–5.
58. Zimbrean PC, Schilsky ML. Psychiatric aspects of Wilson disease: a review. Gen Hosp Psychiatry. 2014 Jan-Feb;36(1):53–62.
59. Ferenci P, Czlonkowska A, Merle U, Ferenc S, Gromadzka G, Yurdaydin C, et al. Late-onset Wilson's disease. Gastroenterology. 2007 Apr;132(4):1294–8.
60. Kim JW, Kim JH, Seo JK, Ko JS, Chang JY, Yang HR, et al. Genetically confirmed Wilson disease in a 9-month old boy with elevations of aminotransferases. World J Hepatol. 2013 Mar 27;5(3):156–9.
61. Jones EA, Clain D, Clink HM, MacGillivray M, Sherlock S. Hepatic coma due to acute hepatic necrosis treated by exchange blood-transfusion. Lancet. 1967 Jul 22;2(7508):169–72.
62. Ritt DJ, Whelan G, Werner DJ, Eigenbrodt EH, Schenker S, Combes B. Acute hepatic necrosis with stupor or coma. An analysis of thirty-one patients. Medicine. 1969 Mar;48(2):151–72.
63. Jones EA, Bergasa NV. Fulminant hepatic failure. In: Taylor RW, Shoemaker WC, editors. Critical care state of the art Fullerton. Fullerton, CA: The Society of Critical Care Medicine; 1991. p. 509–39.
64. Lee WM, Squires RH Jr, Nyberg SL, Doo E, Hoofnagle JH. Acute liver failure: summary of a workshop. Hepatology. 2008 Apr;47(4):1401–15.
65. Nazer H, Ede RJ, Mowat AP, Williams R. Wilson's disease: clinical presentation and use of prognostic index. Gut. 1986 Nov;27(11):1377–81.
66. Dhawan A, Taylor RM, Cheeseman P, De Silva P, Katsiyiannakis L, Mieli-Vergani G. Wilson's disease in children: 37-year experience and revised King's score for liver transplantation. Liver Transpl. 2005 Apr;11(4):441–8.
67. Korman JD, Volenberg I, Balko J, Webster J, Schiodt FV, Squires RH Jr, et al. Screening for Wilson disease in acute liver failure: a comparison of currently available diagnostic tests. Hepatology. 2008 Oct;48(4):1167–74.
68. Ishak KG. Metabolic errors and liver disease. In: Roderick NM, MacSween PPA, Scheuer PJ, Burt AD, Portmann BC, editors. Pathology of the liver. Edinburgh: Churchill Livingstone; 1994. p. 123–218.
69. Sternlieb I, Feldmann G. Effects of anticopper therapy on hepatocellular mitochondria in patients with Wilson's disease: an ultrastructural and stereological study. Gastroenterology. 1976 Sep;71(3):457–61.
70. European Association for Study of L. EASL clinical practice guidelines: Wilson's disease. J Hepatol. 2012 Mar;56(3):671–85.

71. Roberts EA, Schilsky ML. American Association for Study of liver D. diagnosis and treatment of Wilson disease: an update. Hepatology. 2008 Jun;47(6):2089–111.
72. Prashanth LK, Sinha S, Taly AB, Vasudev MK. Do MRI features distinguish Wilson's disease from other early onset extrapyramidal disorders? An analysis of 100 cases. Mov Disord. 2010 Apr 30;25(6):672–8.
73. Litwin T, Dziezyc K, Poniatowska R, Czlonkowska A. Effect of liver transplantation on brain magnetic resonance imaging pathology in Wilson disease: a case report. Neurol Neurochir Pol. 2013 Jul-Aug;47(4):393–7.
74. Poujois A, Woimant F. Wilson's disease: a 2017 update. Clin Res Hepatol Gastroenterol. 2018 Dec;42(6):512–20.
75. Ludwig J, Moyer TP, Rakela J. The liver biopsy diagnosis of Wilson's disease. Methods in pathology. Am J Clin Pathol. 1994 Oct;102(4):443–6.
76. Ferenci P, Caca K, Loudianos G, Mieli-Vergani G, Tanner S, Sternlieb I, et al. Diagnosis and phenotypic classification of Wilson disease. Liver Int. 2003 Jun;23(3):139–42.
77. Nicastro E, Ranucci G, Vajro P, Vegnente A, Iorio R. Re-evaluation of the diagnostic criteria for Wilson disease in children with mild liver disease. Hepatology. 2010 Dec;52(6):1948–56.
78. Sternlieb I. Wilson's disease and pregnancy. Hepatology. 2000 Feb;31(2):531–2.
79. Brewer GJ, Johnson VD, Dick RD, Hedera P, Fink JK, Kluin KJ. Treatment of Wilson's disease with zinc. XVII: treatment during pregnancy. Hepatology. 2000 Feb;31(2):364–70.
80. Brewer GJ. Zinc and tetrathiomolybdate for the treatment of Wilson's disease and the potential efficacy of anticopper therapy in a wide variety of diseases. Metallomics. 2009;1(3):199–206.
81. Bandmann O, Weiss KH, Kaler SG. Wilson's disease and other neurological copper disorders. Lancet Neurol. 2015 Jan;14(1):103–13.
82. Nishito Y, Kambe T. Absorption mechanisms of iron, copper, and zinc: an overview. J Nutr Sci Vitaminol. 2018;64(1):1–7.
83. Weiss KH, Thurik F, Gotthardt DN, Schafer M, Teufel U, Wiegand F, et al. Efficacy and safety of oral chelators in treatment of patients with Wilson disease. Clin Gastroenterol Hepatol. 2013 Aug;11(8):1028–35 e1-2.
84. Brewer GJ, Askari F, Dick RB, Sitterly J, Fink JK, Carlson M, et al. Treatment of Wilson's disease with tetrathiomolybdate: V. control of free copper by tetrathiomolybdate and a comparison with trientine. Transl Res. 2009 Aug;154(2):70–7.
85. Linn FH, Houwen RH, van Hattum J, van der Kleij S, van Erpecum KJ. Long-term exclusive zinc monotherapy in symptomatic Wilson disease: experience in 17 patients. Hepatology. 2009 Nov;50(5):1442–52.
86. Weiss KH, Gotthardt DN, Klemm D, Merle U, Ferenci-Foerster D, Schaefer M, et al. Zinc monotherapy is not as effective as chelating agents in treatment of Wilson disease. Gastroenterology. 2011 Apr;140(4):1189–98 e1.
87. Iorio R, D'Ambrosi M, Marcellini M, Barbera C, Maggiore G, Zancan L, et al. Serum transaminases in children with Wilson's disease. J Pediatr Gastroenterol Nutr. 2004 Oct;39(4):331–6.
88. Brewer GJ, Dick RD, Yuzbasiyan-Gurkin V, Tankanow R, Young AB, Kluin KJ. Initial therapy of patients with Wilson's disease with tetrathiomolybdate. Arch Neurol. 1991 Jan;48(1):42–7.
89. Brewer GJ, Dick RD, Johnson V, Wang Y, Yuzbasiyan-Gurkan V, Kluin K, et al. Treatment of Wilson's disease with ammonium tetrathiomolybdate. I. Initial therapy in 17 neurologically affected patients. Arch Neurol. 1994 Jun;51(6):545–54.
90. Dziezyc K, Karlinski M, Litwin T, Czlonkowska A. Compliant treatment with anti-copper agents prevents clinically overt Wilson's disease in pre-symptomatic patients. Eur J Neurol. 2014 Feb;21(2):332–7.
91. Walshe JM, Dixon AK. Dangers of non-compliance in Wilson's disease. Lancet. 1986 Apr 12;1(8485):845–7.
92. Holscher S, Leinweber B, Hefter H, Reuner U, Gunther P, Weiss KH, et al. Evaluation of the symptomatic treatment of residual neurological symptoms in Wilson disease. Eur Neurol. 2010;64(2):83–7.

93. van Meer S, de Man RA, van den Berg AP, Houwen RH, Linn FH, van Oijen MG, et al. No increased risk of hepatocellular carcinoma in cirrhosis due to Wilson disease during long-term follow-up. J Gastroenterol Hepatol. 2015 Mar;30(3):535–9.

94. Pfeiffenberger J, Mogler C, Gotthardt DN, Schulze-Bergkamen H, Litwin T, Reuner U, et al. Hepatobiliary malignancies in Wilson disease. Liver Int. 2015 May;35(5):1615–22.

95. Ferrarese A, Morelli MC, Carrai P, Milana M, Angelico M, Perricone G, et al. Outcomes of liver transplant for adults with Wilson's disease. Liver Transpl. 2020 Jan;4

96. Guillaud O, Dumortier J, Sobesky R, Debray D, Wolf P, Vanlemmens C, et al. Long term results of liver transplantation for Wilson's disease: experience in France. J Hepatol. 2014 Mar;60(3):579–89.

97. Garoufalia Z, Prodromidou A, Machairas N, Kostakis ID, Stamopoulos P, Zavras N, et al. Liver transplantation for Wilson's disease in non-adult patients: a systematic review. Transplant Proc. 2019 Mar;51(2):443–5.

# Chapter 13
# Tumors of the Liver

Nora V. Bergasa

A 46-year-old man was referred to the hepatology clinic because of a liver mass found on a liver sonogram to investigate right upper quadrant pain. The patient did not have comorbidities. At the visit, the patient reported that the pain had resolved itself spontaneously. The physical exam and the hepatic panel were normal. Magnetic resonance imaging (MRI) to evaluate the mass further revealed findings consistent with a hemangioma (Fig. 13.1). The patient is doing well.

Patients may be referred to hepatology for the evaluation of liver tumors often found incidentally through liver imaging studies for indications not related to suspected liver disease [1]. This chapter introduces the general approach to patients with liver tumors, which may not include therapeutic intervention or may require aggressive diagnostic evaluation and treatment.

In the absence of liver disease, a liver lesion found in a patient incidentally has a high probability of being benign. The most common are liver cysts, hemangiomata, and focal nodular hyperplasia [2]. In contrast, in a patient with cancer, a liver mass may be a metastasis from extrahepatic malignancy, in a patient with cirrhosis, hepatocellular carcinoma (HCC) has to be excluded [3], in patients with primary sclerosing cholangitis, a mass may be from cholangiocarcinoma (CCA) [4]. Thus, knowing the context in which a mass develops in the liver is fundamental to creating an investigational plan.

The radiographic characteristics of liver lesions can help in developing an investigational plan. The fluid inside a liver lesion may be revealing of a cyst or abscess; the features of blood flow into the mass can be diagnostic for HCC [3].

N. V. Bergasa (✉)
Department of Medicine, H+H/Metropolitan, New York, NY, USA

New York Medical College, Valhalla, NY, USA

Hepatology, H+H/Woodhull, Brooklyn, NY, USA

N. V. Bergasa (ed.), *Clinical Cases in Hepatology*, https://doi.org/10.1007/978-1-4471-4715-2_13

**Fig. 13.1** An axial T2
weighted magnetic
resonance image from a 46
year old man showing a
lobular mass of increased
signal intensity in the right
hepatic lobe (arrow)
indicative of stagnant
blood flow consistent with
a hemangioma.

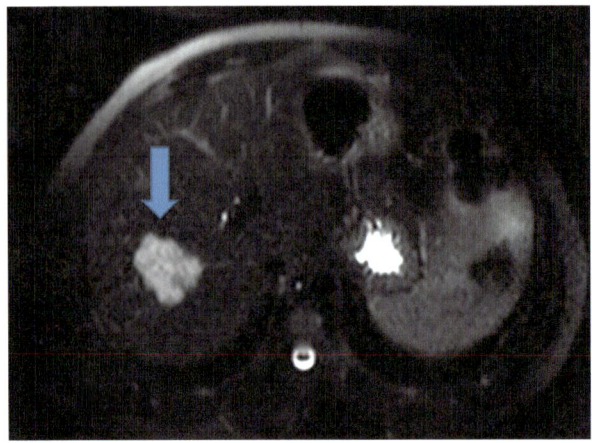

## Simple Hepatic Cysts

The prevalence of simple liver cysts in the general population has been reported in the range of 2.5–18% [5–8], and they are more common in women than in men. Although many hepatic cysts are not associated with symptoms, if they are large, abdominal pain, a palpable mass, and hepatomegaly are documented [9, 10]. Gamma-glutamyl transpeptidase (GGTP) has been reported as high in some series [11], but, in general, the serum liver profile tends to normal in association with liver cysts. On liver sonogram, simple cysts are seen as anechoic spaces, filled with fluid [5–8]. MRI reveals hepatic cysts as water-filled, well-defined lesions that do not enhance in association with intravenous gadolinium-based contrast agents. Congenital hepatic cysts tend to occur in the right hepatic lobe most commonly and arise from biliary ducts not communicating with the biliary system [11]. Histologically, the epithelium of hepatic cysts is most frequently cuboidal [9]. Most liver cysts are not associated with complications; however, serious complications have been documented from large cysts. They include hemorrhage, rupture into the abdominal cavity or bile duct, infection, and cholestasis from compression of bile ducts [11]. Treatment consists of aspiration, which is associated with recurrence of the cyst in most cases, or surgical resection, including cyst fenestration and excision.

## Polycystic Liver Disease

Patients with polycystic kidney disease may have liver cysts; however, isolated polycystic liver disease (PCLD) is a condition separate from polycystic kidney disease and is not associated with renal cysts or cerebral aneurysms [12].

PCLD is dominantly inherited. It is defined as the presence of more than 20 cysts in the liver [12].

PCLD is associated with germline mutations in the *PRKCSH* gene, which codes for hepatocystin. In association with the mutation, hepatocystin does not assemble with the glucosidase II alpha subunit, thus, it was suggested that altered endoplasmic reticulum processing in the regulation of cell proliferation may contribute to the pathogenesis of this disease [13].

Mutations in the *SEC63* gene, which codes for a component of the protein translocation machinery in the endoplasmic reticulum (ER) are also associated with PLD. These findings were interpreted to suggest that the cotranslational protein-processing pathways are fundamental in maintaining the epithelial luminal structure and implicate noncilial ER proteins in human polycystic disease [14].

Heterozygous loss-of-function mutations were identified in *ALG8, GANAB*, and *SEC61B*, which encode fundamental proteins in the biogenesis pathway of the endoplasmic reticulum. The inactivation of these genes in vitro was associated with defective maturation and trafficking of polycystin-1, considered a fundamental factor in cyst pathogenesis [15].

Liver cysts can grow leading to symptoms including pain, and early satiety, or may be complicated by infection or intraluminal bleeding, which are indications for treatment [12].

Somatostatin analogs decrease cAMP, suppressing bile duct proliferation, and inhibit the production of certain growth factors [12]. In this group, lanreotide was reported to reduce the volume of polycystic liver in a placebo-controlled study; however, the reduction was small and it is recommended for patients in whom risk factors impede surgical intervention [12]. Surgical treatment includes fenestration, usually done laparoscopically, and liver resection, which may be required in cases of multiple small cysts difficult to fenestrate [12]. The combination of cyst fenestration and hepatic resection was associated with improvement in the quality of life in a prospective study from the United States between 2014 and 2018 that included eighteen patients [16]. In extreme cases, liver transplantation is an alternative, if liver function is predicted to be poor from resection [12]. The reported estimated survival at 1 and 5 years was calculated as 93% and 92%, respectively, for patients undergoing liver transplantation [12].

## Hydadtic Cysts

Echinococcal infection is a cause of hepatic cysts. Echinococcosis is a zoonotic infection caused by the ingestion of the larvae of the cestode species of the genus Echinococcus [17, 18]. The liver is one of the most commonly affected organs, in which it manifests as cystic lesions.

The incidence of human disease has been reported to exceed 50 per 100,000 person-years in areas where it is endemic, with a prevalence of 5–10% reported in Peru, Argentina, east Africa, and China [19]. The prevalence of echinococcosis increases with age, and the disease is more prevalent in women than in men.

Cystic echinococcosis tends to occur in rural areas where sheep and other herbivores live in proximity with dogs, which, like other carnivores, are definitive hosts. Close contact between dogs and human beings is the reason for transmission, which is fecal-oral by the accidental ingestion of eggs from dogs' feces, e.g., contaminated foodstuff [20]. Human beings are considered accidental or aberrant hosts, and they are highly unlikely to be involved in disease transmission [18].

Carnivores, including dogs, are the definitive hosts, and herbivores, including sheep, goats, and cattle, are intermediate hosts. They maintain the parasite by harboring the larval stage of the parasite named metacestode. The egg-producing stage of the cestode happens in the small intestine of the definitive host, which carries hundreds of egg-producing worms. The eggs are excreted in the stool of the definitive host and are infective upon release. In the target organ, a hydatid cyst or metacestode develops and from it, protoscolices bud from the germinal layer and grow within the cyst. When the definitive host ingests these, they evaginate, attach themselves to the intestinal mucosae, and evolve to adults over weeks. Thousands of protoscolices can bud from a single cyst, and each protoscolex can turn into an adult worm when ingested by a definitive host. Secondary echinococcosis can occur when fluid from a cyst is spilled into a cavity, e.g., the abdominal cavity, leading to new cyst formation. All mammals in which metacestodes develop act as intermediate hosts; however, not all intermediate hosts can sustain the life cycle (Fig. 13.2). Human beings are considered accidental hosts and are not considered to be able to transmit the infection [18].

Most echinococcal cysts are single and tend to be located in the right lobe. Most patients are asymptomatic and are often diagnosed incidentally by radiographic studies (Fig. 13.3). Rupture of this type of cyst can be associated with anaphylaxis, stressing the importance of not aspirating liver cysts' contents, in the absence of absolute exclusion of an echinococcal etiology. Documented complications from echinococcal cysts include communication of the hydatid cyst with luminal structures including the biliary tract [21], intestine, and bronchial tree, or compression of their compression in cases of large cysts [18].

Diagnostic serology, the most common being ELISA, is reported as positive in 70% of the patients, with subsequent testing used for confirmation [22, 23].

Surgical excision is the standard treatment for hydatid cysts; medical therapy with mebendazole or albendazole is an alternative. Small cysts and those not associated with complications can be watched over time. It is recommended to consult local experts or liver centers prior to any intervention.

## Liver Abscess

Liver abscesses tend to occur in the right lobe of the liver, from streaming via the portal vein from intra-abdominal infections including appendicitis and diverticulitis; however, a recent retrospective review reported that nearly half of the patients identified did not have any comorbidities in association with their liver abscesses

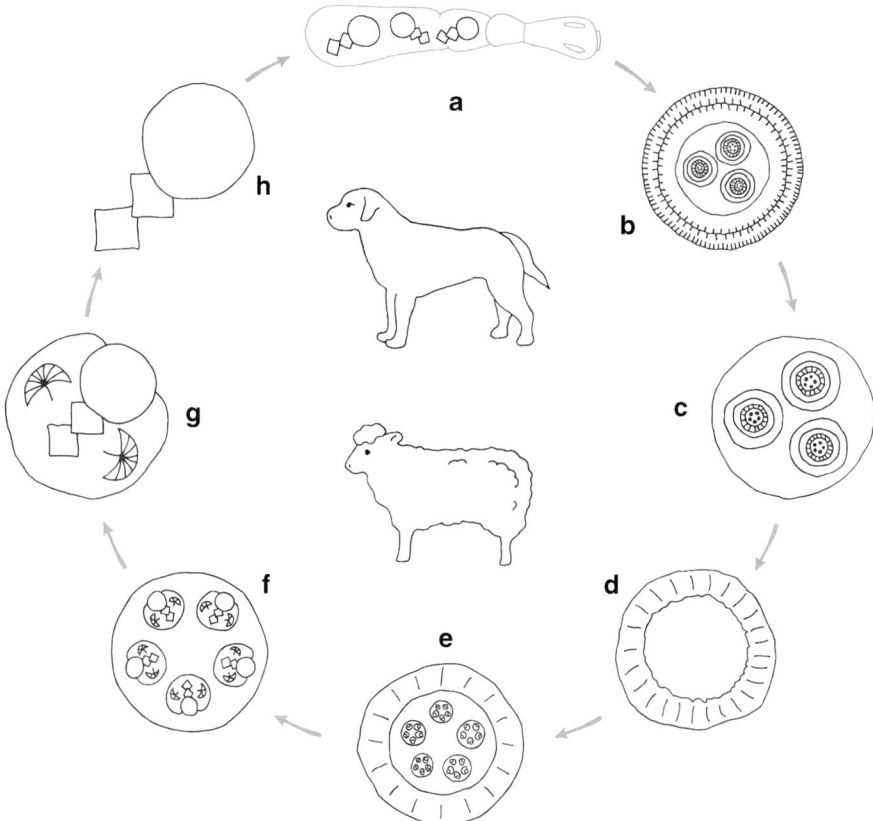

**Fig. 13.2** The adult Echinococcus granulosus (**a**) lives in the small intestine of the definitive host (dog). Gravid proglottids release eggs (**b**), which are infectious, and are fecally excreted. Eggs hatch in the intestine of the intermediate host (i.e. human beings, cattle, sheep) and release six-hooked oncospheres (**c**) that pierce the intestinal wall traveling through the vascular system to various organs including liver and lungs, where the oncospheres develop into a thick-walled hydatid cyst (**d**), which enlarges itself producing protoscolices and daughter cysts that occupy the cavity of the the cyst (**e** and **f**). The definitive host is infected by ingesting the cyst-containing organs of an infected intermediate host. After ingestion, the protoscolices with invaginated heads (**g**) evaginate (**h**) and attach to the intestinal mucosa and mature to adulthood (**a**) in 32 to 80 days. Human beings are aberrant intermediate hosts who get infected by ingesting eggs. Oncospheres are released in the intestine and hydatid cysts develop in several organs, including the liver (Fig. 13.3). Protoscolices create secondary cysts in other parts of the body if the main cyst ruptures (Illustration by Martha M. Dao, Graphic (+WEB) Design MMD).

[24]. Bacteremia and direct extension from the biliary tree in cholangitis can also result in liver abscesses. A history of travel to areas where amebiasis is common is fundamental in the diagnosis, as radiological features do not offer specific findings to differentiate bacterial versus amebic abscesses, for which specific antibiotic treatment is required.

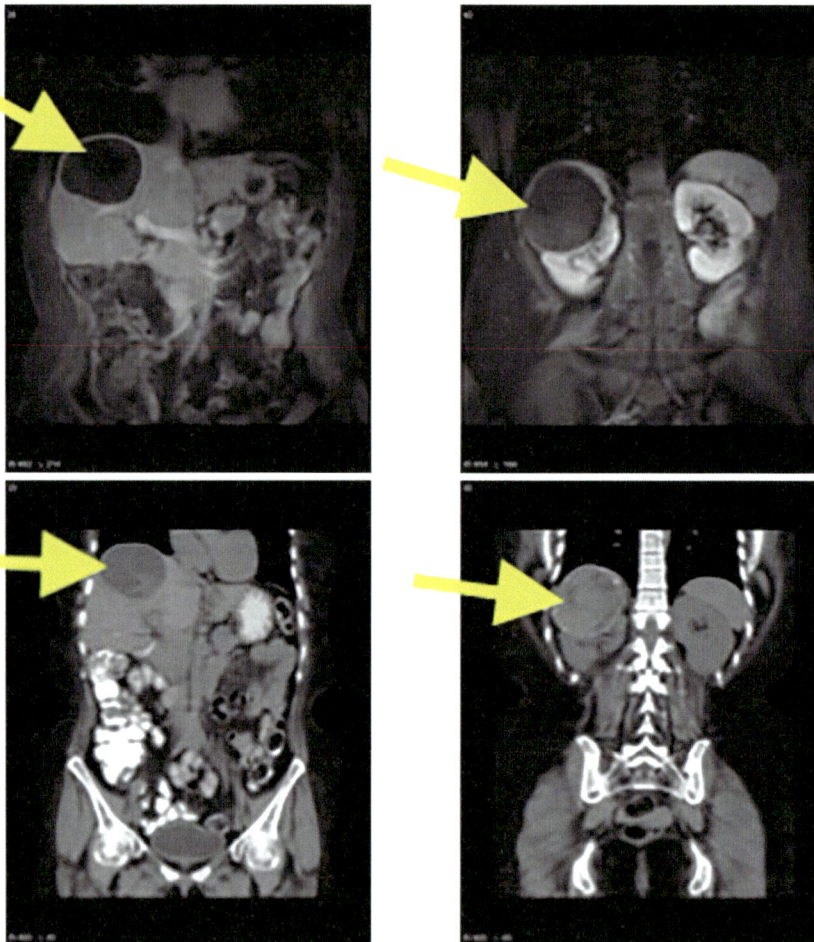

**Fig. 13.3** Coronal images from gadolinium enhanced magnetic resonance images (top row) and unenhanced computed tomography (bottom row) show two large complex cystic non enhancing masses in the right hepatic lobe compatible with echinococcal cysts (arrows).

The "crude annual incidence" of liver abscesses was reported from a retrospective study from the United Kingdom to be 2.3 per 100,000 per year [25].

Fever and abdominal pain, usually localized to the right upper quadrant, are the most common clinical manifestations in liver abscesses [26, 27]. An abnormal liver profile is common, with increased serum alkaline phosphatase activity being the most notable abnormality due to a space-occupying lesion.

Abdominal ultrasound and computed tomography (CT) are diagnostic in the majority of the cases [25, 28].

Aspiration of abscess content yields the pathogen(s), which tend to be enteric Gram-negative bacilli, *Streptococci*, and *Staphylococcus aureus*. Liver abscesses from which *Klebsiella pneumoniae* is isolated tend to be associated with a syndrome described in Asia; in this context, a publication from New York City reported that *Klebsiella pneumoniae* was identified in 41% of cases, which included 50% of the patients of Asian ethnicity [29]; this type of abscess has been reported in association with colorectal cancer in Asia.

Treatment consists of percutaneous drainage with needle aspiration or catheter insertion, especially for large abscesses (i.e., >5 cm). Large abscesses may require surgical drainage, a decision that should be made when the size does not decrease in association with nonsurgical treatment or when there is no clinical improvement. The aspirate should be sent for Gram stain and culture. Drainage is used concomitantly with intravenous antibiotics, beta-lactams being preferred, based on a study that documented an increase in the proportion of patients that was readmitted within 30 days post discharge when patients were transitioned to oral antibiotics for movement from inpatient to outpatient care [30]; metronidazole should be included to cover empirically for ameba until serology confirms its absence. The duration of antibiotics is 4–6 weeks; the radiographical resolution was reported within 18 weeks of diagnosis and treatment [31].

## Hepatic Hemangiomata

Hepatic hemangiomata are the most common benign tumors of the liver, reported to have a prevalence that ranges from 0.4% to 24% [32, 33]. They are more common in women than in men [34, 35], tend to be asymptomatic, and are diagnosed incidentally by the use of abdominal imaging. They are usually found in the right lobe of the liver and are generally solitary, although more than one hemangioma can be found. The liver profile is normal.

Giant hemangioma is a term reserved for tumors greater than 10 cm, which can be associated with symptoms, which tend to be right upper quadrant pain and early satiety. Pain secondary to thrombosis [36] and hemobilia due to the rupture of the tumor into the bile ducts has been documented [37] in cases of large hemangiomata.

Vascular malformations are considered to be the etiology of these lesions, which, histologically, have been described as tumors having an irregular interface with the liver parenchyma. Collagen, elastic fibers, and smooth muscle comprised the vessels' walls, with low proliferation rate and absence of estrogen or progesterone receptors [38]. However, an increase in size in association with exposure to female hormones has been reported [39].

Radiographically, liver hemangiomata appear like well-defined hyperechoic lesions on ultrasound [40]. In contrast-enhanced computed tomography and MRI studies contrast material fills the lesion irregularly from the periphery (Fig. 13.1).

Tumors with the typical appearance of hemangiomata by radiographic studies that are not associated with symptoms do not require intervention [32]. A giant hemangioma may require surgical treatment. Enucleation was reported to be associated with fewer complications than surgical resection [41, 42]. Institutional expertise is fundamental in the management of patients who required surgery [36].

## Focal Nodular Hyperplasia

Focal nodular hyperplasia (FNH) is a benign tumor of the liver, reported as having a prevalence that ranges between 0.4% and 3% in the general population [32, 43].

FNH is mostly diagnosed in individuals aged between 20 and 50 years, with a higher prevalence in women than men. The lesions are single in 80% of the cases and range between 0.5 and 8 cm in diameter [32, 43, 44].

The etiology of FNH is considered to be a proliferative cell response to an aberrant dystrophic artery [44]. Conditions of vascular etiology that can be associated with FNH are hereditary hemorrhagic telangiectasia or previously treated solid tumors in children, suggesting that a disturbance in blood flow may be relevant in the pathogenesis of FNH [32]. The nodule is not encapsulated. Macroscopically, it is characterized by a central, stellate fibrovascular zone comprised of dystrophic arterial vessels, making the diagnosis by radiographic means possible [45]. However, a histological study documented scars in 49% of cases [46], which has suggested that mechanisms different from vascular processes may play a role in the formation of FNH; in this regard, the idea of clonality as an etiological factor was supported by a study that showed a uniform pattern of X chromosome inactivation [45]. It has also been documented that signaling pathways mediated by transforming growth factor β and Wnt/β-catenin are overexpressed [47]. The overexpression of Wnt/β--catenin results in the activation of the genes it targets, including GLUL, coding for glutamine synthase, which results in a typical glutamine synthetase expression by immunostaining described as a "map-like" pattern in the hepatocytes that comprise the lesion, usually located around hepatic veins [48].

Patients with FNH tend not to have symptoms from the tumor. Physical examination does not provide any diagnostic clues.

On liver ultrasound, FNHs have been described as inhomogeneous nodules with poorly delineated borders, as isoechoic lesions, in reference to the surrounding parenchyma, and as having a rim surrounding the mass and displaying a central fibrous scar. The use of conventional, color, and power Doppler may highlight the presence of arteries that radiate toward the periphery in a spoke-wheel pattern, and that of a hypertrophic hepatic artery consistent with the feeding vessel [49]. MRI offers the best diagnostic option [50].

On computed tomography, the typical FNH tends to have a lobulated contour, hypoattenuated or isoattenuated with respect to the surrounding liver tissue. In association with intravenous contrast, the lesion becomes hyperattenuated in the arterial phase, except for the central scar. In the portal and following phases, there is isoattenuation, compared to the parenchymal contour, and central scar enhancement may be appreciated [51].

On MRI, FNH is isointense or hypointense on T1-weighted images, with hyperintensity in T-2 with a hyperintense central scar in 80% of the cases [52]. In association with gadolinium, FNH exhibits intense homogeneous enhancement in the arterial phase, enhancing the central scar in subsequent phases [51].

Patients in whom a diagnosis of FNH is confirmed, as described above, do not require diagnostic interventions [53]. If imaging studies cannot ascertain the diagnosis of FNH, referral to a center with expertise in biopsy and resection is recommended [32].

## Hepatocellular Adenomata

Hepatocellular adenomata (HCA) are rare tumors with a reported prevalence of 0.001 and 0.004%, more common in women than in men, usually diagnosed between 35 and 40 years [32, 54]. There is an association between oral contraceptive pill use (OCP) and anabolic steroids use and a reported increase in their incidence in relationship with obesity [54]. Other rare associations include familial HCA associated with maturity-onset diabetes type 3 (MODY3), iron overload disorders, McCune–Albright syndrome, and glycogen storage disease [32].

Mutations characterize specific subtypes of HCA: (i) *HNF1α* mutated (HA-H), with somatic mutations of *TCF1* (*HNF1A*) gene and heterozygous germline mutations of *CYP1B1* gene, which lead to increase in lipogenesis by enhancement of fatty acid synthesis and by downregulation of liver type fatty acid-binding protein [55]; (ii) β catenin mutated hepatocellular adenoma (HA-B), with mutations in the β catenin gene and increased or transient activation of the Wnt /β catenin signaling pathway, reported to have an increased risk of malignant transformation [56]; (iii) inflammatory hepatocellular adenoma (HA-I), with gain of function mutations of the *IL6ST* gene, activation of STAT3 signaling pathway, and acute-phase inflammatory response [57]; and (iv) sonic hedgehog (*SHH*) hepatocellular adenoma (HA-sh), associated with activation of the sonic hedgehog pathway via fusion of promoter of *INHBE* with *GLI1* [58], and by upregulation of argininosuccinate synthase 1, which were reported in association with increased risk of bleeding [59, 60].

Histologically, HCAs are characterized by thickened plates of hepatocytes with preserved reticulin network and arteries not accompanied by bile ducts. Other features include steatosis, inflammatory cells, and dilated sinusoids. Fat can be appreciated [61].

HCAs can be complicated by hemorrhage, especially from lesions greater than 5 cm, and those protruding from the liver surface, and by malignant transformation. In men, regardless of the adenoma size, resection is recommended because of the risk for malignant transformation [32]. In women, lesions less than 5 cm tend not to rupture or convert into malignant tumors; however, it is recommended to discontinue OCP and implement behavior modification in obese subjects [62].

In contrast-enhanced ultrasound (CEUS), HCA demonstrates homogeneous contrast enhancement in the arterial phase, associated with rapid centripetal filling. HCAs become isoechoic in reference to the surrounding liver parenchyma in the early portal phase, although in some cases, there may be hyperechogenicity [63]. On CT scan, tumors are well demarcated and isoattenuating with respect to the surrounding liver parenchyma, and after contrast administration, they exhibit transient homogenous enhancement with a return to baseline isodensity in the portal and delayed phases [64]. HCAs appear hyperattenuating in association with recent hemorrhage, and hypoattenuating if they contain fat. On magnetic resonance imaging, HCAs are bright on T1-weighted images and hyperintense, versus the surrounding liver tissue, on T2-weighted images [64]; MRI is the preferred diagnostic modality.

Follow-up of patients with HCAs is recommended with a contrast-enhanced MRI at 6 months after the diagnosis. A lesion greater than 5 cm and those that grow 20% of its diameter should be considered for resection because of the risks of hemorrhage and malignant transformation. A biopsy is recommended only for lesions that cannot be characterized radiologically or for those in which malignancy cannot be excluded [32].

Follow up with annual liver ultrasound up to 10 years from diagnosis, and twice a year beyond 10 years is recommended to assess growth and decide on definitive treatment [32].

Special attention is required for pregnant women with HCAs, with liver sonograms recommended every 6–12 weeks to assess growth. Lesions smaller than 5 cm in size, not protruding, nor growing do not require that a cesarean section at the time of delivery be performed [32]. In women with large tumors, surgical resection may be recommended [32, 65]. Management, in collaboration with the obstetrical team, is required [32, 65].

## Hepatocellular Carcinoma

Hepatocellular carcinoma (HCC) is a malignant tumor of the liver. Cirrhosis is a risk factor for HCC secondary to several types of liver diseases, including chronic hepatitis C and B, and those with genetic diseases including porphyria [66], iron overload in association with hemochromatosis [67], and alpha-1 antitrypsin deficiency [68]. Patients with chronic hepatitis B, in the absence of cirrhosis, are also at risk of developing this type of cancer. Exposure to aflatoxin B1 through contaminated foodstuff via mutations in tumor-suppressor gene p53 is a risk factor for HCC [69–71]. The mortality from liver cancer was reported to have decreased in women and to be stable in men [72]. Most cases of HCC are in Africa and East Asia; however, the incidence of HCC in the United States and Europe has increased. In general, viral hepatitis has been the driving cause of liver disease; however, it is reported that cirrhosis from nonalcoholic fatty liver disease has become an important risk factor for this type of cancer [73].

The tumor is more prevalent in men than in women [74], with estrogens being proposed as protective in the latter [75].

HCC is a vascular tumor. The physical examination may reveal a bruit on an enlarged liver or one in which a mass can be palpated. The rest of the physical exam may be notable for stigmata of chronic liver disease. Many times, the exam is non-contributory; hence, the importance of imaging studies as part of a surveillance program or as part of the liver disease workup initiated in a patient referred for evaluation of possible liver disease.

The liver profile can be predominantly cholestatic or mixed. Serum concentration of alfa-fetoprotein (AFP) can be in hundreds or thousands.

Imaging studies reveal a mass, which, in a cirrhotic liver, HCC has to be considered. On liver sonogram, the mass is hypo or hyperechoic. The characteristic features of HCC on CT scan or MRI are arterial enhancement versus the surrounding liver tissue, and hypodensity also compared to the surrounding liver tissue, known as wash out in the venous phase [76].

The treatment of HCC includes resection, local ablation, liver transplantation, or a combination of the three, depending on the characteristics of the tumor and the patient's comorbidities. Systemic therapy is an alternative for patients who are not eligible for invasive and surgical interventions or who progressed after local therapy and includes sorafenib, regorafenib, nivolumab, and lenvatinib [77].

Screening measures are pivotal in managing patients at risk for HCC with a liver sonogram and AFP every 6 months, as suggested by the guidelines [78].

## Fibrolamellar Carcinoma

Fibrolamellar carcinoma (FLC) is an uncommon malignant tumor most prevalent in teenagers and patients in their 30s, with no gender preference [79].

FLC is associated with activation of protein kinase A, reported to occur from a DNAJB1-PRKACA fusion transcript, secondary to somatic intrachromosomal deletion on chromosome 19 [79].

Patients may present with weight loss, abdominal pain, and a palpable liver mass [80], confirmed by imaging studies (see HCC above). The liver profile may be suggestive of cholestasis or mixed, and an AFP is usually normal and rarely over 200 ng/ml [81]. Histologically, the neoplastic hepatocytes are deeply eosinophilic, associated with fibrosis arranged in a lamellar fashion, which gives it its name, around the neoplastic hepatocytes [80].

In regards to enhancement features on CT scans, a retrospective study of 37 patients indicated arterial enhancement in 81%, with 96% exhibiting heterogeneity. On MRI, 62% of the tumors were hypointense on T1-weighted imaging and hyperintense on T2-weighted imaging [82].

Treatment of FLC is resection or liver transplantation [83]. Chemotherapy with a combination of cisplatin, epirubicin, and fluorouracil has not been associated with substantial benefits [84]. Sorafenib similarly has not been associated with favorable response [84, 85]. A clinical trial that included mTOR inhibitors was not associated with a therapeutic advantage [86]. The reader is referred to clinicaltrials.org for information regarding study availability.

A retrospective review that identified 95 patients from three institutions identified female gender, macroinvasion, lymph node involvement, advanced stage, and unresectability as poor prognostic features [84].

## Intrahepatic Cholangiocarcinoma

Intrahepatic cholangiocarcinoma (ICC) originates from the intrahepatic biliary epithelial cells, comprising 20% of the cholangiocarcinomas, which most commonly emerge from extrahepatic bile ducts [87]. The risk factors that have been identified in association with ICC include primary sclerosing cholangitis, hepatobiliary flukes, hepatolithiasis, and biliary malformations, or patients may not have risk factors for ICC.

Patients may be asymptomatic or present with right upper quadrant pain and an associated mass. The liver profile is suggestive of cholestasis [88]. Cancer antigen 19–9 (CA 19–9), with a value greater than 1000 U/ml, suggests metastatic disease [89].

Radiographically, peripheral tumors tend to be associated with bile duct dilatation, with retraction of the liver capsule noted in 36% of cases in a series of 24 patients, which included 25 tumors. In the portal phase, the tumors were hypodense, with hyperattenuation in delayed phases. It was noted that rim-like contrast enhancement was the most common feature in the arterial or portal phases, with portal encasement in 40% of the cases [90, 91]. However, the definitive diagnosis is made histologically.

The treatment of choice is the resection of the tumor [92]. Liver transplantation has not been associated with a favorable prognosis because of the high recurrence rate [93]. For patients with unresectable tumors, locoregional therapies are proposed and include transarterial chemoembolization, radioembolization, and high-dose, conformal external-beam radiation [94].

## Hepatic Angiosarcoma

Hepatic angiosarcoma is uncommon. It originates from the sinusoidal lining. It tends to be more common in men than in women at least 50 years old [95]. The risk factors identified in this type of tumor are thorium dioxide, vinyl chloride, arsenic, and radiation exposure [96]. In addition, hemochromatosis and von Recklinghausen disease have been reported in association with hepatic angiosarcoma [96].

Patients tend to present with fatigue, abdominal pain, hepatomegaly, ascites, and hemoperitoneum from tumor hemorrhage [97].

Histologically, the tumor is comprised of dilated cavernous vascular spaces lined by pleomorphic neoplastic cells and spindle cells [98]. It is a highly aggressive tumor at risk for spontaneous bleeding and in association with biopsy.

Imaging studies with CT and MRI are reported to exhibit tumor enhancement in different phases of the dynamic post-contrast study, with heterogeneous hyperenhancement on the first post-contrast phase that progressively expands on the subsequent phases, and typically follow blood pool with regards to CT attenuation and magnetic resonance signal intensity [99].

The prognosis of hepatic angiosarcoma is dismal, with a reported survival period of 5 months [100]. Surgical resection is the optimal treatment for patients with localized disease [101]. Several chemotherapeutic regimens have been used, but a therapeutic benefit has not been demonstrated [101]. Hepatic angiosarcoma is an aggressive liver tumor for which treatment is suboptimal in the absence of curative resection [102].

## Hepatic Epithelioid Hemangioendothelioma

Hepatic epithelioid hemangioendothelioma (HEHE) is a hepatic tumor of endothelial origin characterized by an unpredictable behavior [103], more common in women, and reported to occur in 1 per one million persons [104].

Patients present with abdominal pain associated with a mass, or masses, and weight loss [105]. The liver profile tends to be mixed, with a predominance of cholestasis, reflecting the space-occupying effect of the liver masses.

Histologically, the tumors have dendritic and epithelioid cells with vacuoles that represent intracellular lumina. The stroma is fibrous. The tumorous cells are positive for endothelial markers, including factor VIII-related antigen, CD34, and/or CD31 [106].

Radiographic findings from contrast-enhanced CT and MRI include multiple hypoattenuating lesions in both hepatic lobes that merge into large hypoattenuating regions in a peripheral or subcapsular distribution, with a halo or target pattern of enhancement in large lesions. There may be capsular retraction associated with peripheral lesions. A typical finding known as *lollipop sign* is the tapering of hepatic or portal veins to terminate at the end or within the masses' edge. MRI reveals hypointense lesions versus the surrounding parenchyma on unenhanced T1 with heterogeneously increased signal intensity on T2-weighted images. Contrast enhancement with gadolinium shows a peripheral halo or what has been described as a target-type enhancement pattern with a peripheral hypointense rim [107].

The treatment of HEHE depends on the clinical status of the patient and includes liver transplantation, resection, and chemotherapy with agents that include doxorubicin, vincristine, interferon-$\alpha$, 5-fluorouracil, thalidomide, and monoclonal antibodies against vascular endothelial growth factor, with the first two being associated with the best prognosis. After liver transplantation, the 5-year survival rate is 55% to 75%, and with resection, 75% [108].

# Hepatic Mucinous Cystic Neoplasm

Hepatic mucinous cystic neoplasms comprise less than 5% of hepatobiliary tumors [109].

The tumors have been reported mostly in middle-aged women, in the case of cystadenomata, and in men, cystadenocarcinoma, with associated right upper quadrant pain, usually in association with large masses [110, 111].

In a study that characterized this type of tumor, the lesions were identified radiologically as measuring 25–250 mm in diameter, the majority intrahepatic in location, unilocular, multicystic, and multilocular, the latter being the most common, with the absence of papillary mural nodule in 25 of 26 tumors [112].

Cystadenocarcinomas are characterized by cellular pleomorphism, anaplasia, and infiltration of fibrous stroma. It has been suggested that cystadenocarcinomas evolve from cystadenomata [110]. The tumors are now defined as cyst-forming epithelial neoplasms that usually do not communicate with the bile ducts, characterized by cuboidal to columnar epithelial cells, with various degrees of mucin production, and associated with ovarian-type subepithelial stroma [112].

It is difficult to determine the nature of these tumors [113]; thus, malignancy must be considered when the tumors appear as described above. In those cases, surgical resection is a definitive treatment, associated with good outcomes [113]. We recommend referral to centers with expertise in hepatobiliary surgery for an optimal approach.

**Acknowledgments** The author acknowledges Dr. Anatole Sladen for having contributed Fig. 13.1.

# References

1. Reddy KR, Schiff ER. Approach to a liver mass. Semin Liver Dis. 1993 Nov;13(4):423–35.
2. Ros PR, Davis GL. The incidental focal liver lesion: photon, proton, or needle? Hepatology. 1998 May;27(5):1183–90.
3. Bruix J, Ayuso C. Diagnosis of hepatic nodules in patients at risk for hepatocellular carcinoma: LI-RADS probability versus certainty. Gastroenterology. 2019 Mar;156(4):860–2.
4. Lee JJ, Schindera ST, Jang HJ, Fung S, Kim TK. Cholangiocarcinoma and its mimickers in primary sclerosing cholangitis. Abdominal Radiol. 2017 Dec;42(12):2898–908.
5. Gaines PA, Sampson MA. The prevalence and characterization of simple hepatic cysts by ultrasound examination. Br J Radiol. 1989 Apr;62(736):335–7.
6. Horton KM, Bluemke DA, Hruban RH, Soyer P, Fishman EK. CT and MR imaging of benign hepatic and biliary tumors. Radiographics. 1999 Mar-Apr;19(2):431–51.
7. Fulcher AS, Sterling RK. Hepatic neoplasms: computed tomography and magnetic resonance features. J Clin Gastroenterol. 2002 Apr;34(4):463–71.
8. Carrim ZI, Murchison JT. The prevalence of simple renal and hepatic cysts detected by spiral computed tomography. Clin Radiol. 2003 Aug;58(8):626–9.
9. Sanfelippo PM, Beahrs OH, Weiland LH. Cystic disease of the liver. Ann Surg. 1974 Jun;179(6):922–5.

10. Bahirwani R, Reddy KR. Review article: the evaluation of solitary liver masses. Aliment Pharmacol Ther. 2008 Oct 15;28(8):953–65.
11. Rawla P, Sunkara T, Muralidharan P, Raj JP. An updated review of cystic hepatic lesions. Clin Exp Hepatol. 2019 Mar;5(1):22–9.
12. Drenth JP, Chrispijn M, Nagorney DM, Kamath PS, Torres V. Medical and surgical treatment options for polycystic liver disease. Hepatology. 2010;52(6):2223–30.
13. Drenth JPH, te Morsche RHM, Smink R, Bonifacino JS, Jansen JBMJ. Germline mutations in PRKCSH are associated with autosomal dominant polycystic liver disease. Nat Genet. 2003;33:345–7.
14. Davila S, Furu L, Gharavi AG, Tian X, Tamenhito O, Qian Q, Li A, Cai Y, Kamath PS, King BF, Azurmendi PJ, Tahvanainen P, Kääriäinen H, Höckerstedt K, Devuyst O, Pirson I, Martin RS, Lifton RP, Tahvanainen E, Torres VE, Somlo S. Mutations in SEC63 cause autosomal dominant polycystic liver disease. Nat Genet. 2004;36(6):575–7.
15. Besse W, Dong K, Choi J, Punia S, Fedeles SV, Choi M, Gallagher A-R, Huand EB, Gulati A, Knight J, Mane S, Tahvanainen E, Tahvanainen P, Sanna-Cherchi S, Lifton RP, Watnick T, Pei YP, Torres VE, Somlo S. Isolated polycystic liver disease genes define effectors of polycystin-1 function. J Clin Invest. 2017;127(5):1772–85.
16. Bernts LHP, Neijenhuis MK, Edwards ME, Sloan JA, Fischer J, Smoot RL, Nagorney DM, Drenth JP, Hogan MC. Symptom relief and quality of life after combined partial hepatectomy and cyst fenestration in highly symptomatic polycystic liver disease. Surgery. 2020;168(1):25–32.
17. Shaw JM, Bornman PC, Krige JE. Hydatid disease of the liver. S Afr J Surg. 2006;44(2):70–2. 4-7
18. Agudelo Higuita NI, Brunetti E, McCloskey C. Cystic echinococcosis. J Clin Microbiol. 2016 Mar;54(3):518–23.
19. Craig PS, McManus DP, Lightowlers MW, Chabalgoity JA, Garcia HH, Gavidia CM, et al. Prevention and control of cystic echinococcosis. Lancet Infect Dis. 2007 Jun;7(6):385–94.
20. Craig PS, Li T, Qiu J, Zhen R, Wang Q, Giraudoux P, et al. Echinococcosis and Tibetan communities. Emerg Infect Dis. 2008 Oct;14(10):1674–5.
21. Demircan O, Baymus M, Seydaoglu G, Akinoglu A, Sakman G. Occult cystobiliary communication presenting as postoperative biliary leakage after hydatid liver surgery: are there significant preoperative clinical predictors? Canadian J Surg J Canadien De Chirurgie. 2006 Jun;49(3):177–84.
22. Manzano-Roman R, Sanchez-Ovejero C, Hernandez-Gonzalez A, Casulli A, Siles-Lucas M. Serological diagnosis and follow-up of human cystic echinococcosis: a new Hope for the future? Biomed Res Int. 2015;2015:428205.
23. Sarkari B, Rezaei Z. Immunodiagnosis of human hydatid disease: where do we stand? World J Methodol. 2015 Dec 26;5(4):185–95.
24. Osman K, Srinivasa S, Koea J. Liver abscess: contemporary presentation and management in a Western population. N Z Med J. 2018 Feb 23;131(1470):65–70.
25. Mohsen AH, Green ST, Read RC, McKendrick MW. Liver abscess in adults: ten years experience in a UK centre. QJM. 2002 Dec;95(12):797–802.
26. Rubin RH, Swartz MN, Malt R. Hepatic abscess: changes in clinical, bacteriologic and therapeutic aspects. Am J Med. 1974 Oct;57(4):601–10.
27. Huang CJ, Pitt HA, Lipsett PA, Osterman FA Jr, Lillemoe KD, Cameron JL, et al. Pyogenic hepatic abscess. Changing trends over 42 years. Ann Surg. 1996;223(5):600–7. Discussion 7–9
28. Bachler P, Baladron MJ, Menias C, Beddings I, Loch R, Zalaquett E, et al. Multimodality imaging of liver infections: differential diagnosis and potential pitfalls. Radiographics. 2016 Jul-Aug;36(4):1001–23.
29. Rahimian J, Wilson T, Oram V, Holzman RS. Pyogenic liver abscess: recent trends in etiology and mortality. Clin Infect Dis. 2004 Dec 1;39(11):1654–9.

30. Giangiuli SE, Mueller SW, Jeffres MN. Transition to Oral versus continued intravenous anti-biotics for patients with pyogenic liver abscesses: a retrospective analysis. Pharmacotherapy. 2019 Jul;39(7):734–40.

31. Sudhamshu KC, Sharma D. Long-term follow-up of pyogenic liver abscess by ultrasound. Eur J Radiol. 2010 Apr;74(1):195–8.

32. European Association for the Study of the L. EASL clinical practice guidelines on the management of benign liver tumours. J Hepatol. 2016 Aug;65(2):386–98.

33. Rungsinaporn K, Phaisakamas T. Frequency of abnormalities detected by upper abdominal ultrasound. J Med Assoc Thailand = Chotmaihet Thangphaet. 2008 Jul;91(7):1072–5.

34. Farges O, Daradkeh S, Bismuth H. Cavernous hemangiomas of the liver: are there any indications for resection? World J Surg. 1995 Jan-Feb;19(1):19–24.

35. Gandolfi L, Leo P, Solmi L, Vitelli E, Verros G, Colecchia A. Natural history of hepatic haemangiomas: clinical and ultrasound study. Gut. 1991 Jun;32(6):677–80.

36. Tait N, Richardson AJ, Muguti G, Little JM. Hepatic cavernous haemangioma: a 10 year review. Aust N Z J Surg. 1992 Jul;62(7):521–4.

37. Mikami T, Hirata K, Oikawa I, Kimura M, Kimura H. Hemobilia caused by a giant benign hemangioma of the liver: report of a case. Surg Today. 1998;28(9):948–52.

38. Kim GE, Thung SN, Tsui WM, Ferrell LD. Hepatic cavernous hemangioma: underrecognized associated histologic features. Liver Int. 2006 Apr;26(3):334–8.

39. Glinkova V, Shevah O, Boaz M, Levine A, Shirin H. Hepatic haemangiomas: possible association with female sex hormones. Gut. 2004 Sep;53(9):1352–5.

40. Perkins AB, Imam K, Smith WJ, Cronan JJ. Color and power Doppler sonography of liver hemangiomas: a dream unfulfilled? J Clin Ultrasound: JCU. 2000 May;28(4):159–65.

41. Kuo PC, Lewis WD, Jenkins RL. Treatment of giant hemangiomas of the liver by enucleation. J Am Coll Surg. 1994 Jan;178(1):49–53.

42. Miura JT, Amini A, Schmocker R, Nichols S, Sukato D, Winslow ER, et al. Surgical management of hepatic hemangiomas: a multi-institutional experience. HPB (Oxford). 2014 Oct;16(10):924–8.

43. Dimitroulis D, Charalampoudis P, Lainas P, Papanikolaou IG, Kykalos S, Kouraklis G. Focal nodular hyperplasia and hepatocellular adenoma: current views. Acta Chir Belg. 2013 May-Jun;113(3):162–9.

44. Buscarini E, Danesino C, Plauchu H, de Fazio C, Olivieri C, Brambilla G, et al. High prevalence of hepatic focal nodular hyperplasia in subjects with hereditary hemorrhagic telangiectasia. Ultrasound Med Biol. 2004 Sep;30(9):1089–97.

45. Gaffey MJ, Iezzoni JC, Weiss LM. Clonal analysis of focal nodular hyperplasia of the liver. Am J Pathol. 1996 Apr;148(4):1089–96.

46. Nguyen BN, Flejou JF, Terris B, Belghiti J, Degott C. Focal nodular hyperplasia of the liver: a comprehensive pathologic study of 305 lesions and recognition of new histologic forms. Am J Surg Pathol. 1999 Dec;23(12):1441–54.

47. Nault JC, Bioulac-Sage P, Zucman-Rossi J. Hepatocellular benign tumors-from molecular classification to personalized clinical care. Gastroenterology. 2013 May;144(5):888–902.

48. Bioulac-Sage P, Laumonier H, Rullier A, Cubel G, Laurent C, Zucman-Rossi J, et al. Overexpression of glutamine synthetase in focal nodular hyperplasia: a novel easy diagnostic tool in surgical pathology. Liver Int. 2009 Mar;29(3):459–65.

49. Uggowitzer MM, Kugler C, Ruppert-Kohlmayr A, Groell R, Raith J, Schreyer H. [Current status of diagnostic imaging of focal nodular hyperplasia of the liver]. RoFo: Fortschritte auf dem Gebiete der Rontgenstrahlen und der Nuklearmedizin. 2000 Sep;172(9):727–38. Aktueller Stand der bildgebenden Diagnostik der fokalen nodularen Hyperplasie der Leber.

50. Venturi A, Piscaglia F, Vidili G, Flori S, Righini R, Golfieri R, et al. Diagnosis and management of hepatic focal nodular hyperplasia. J Ultrasound. 2007 Sep;10(3):116–27.

51. Hussain SM, Terkivatan T, Zondervan PE, Lanjouw E, de Rave S, Ijzermans JN, et al. Focal nodular hyperplasia: findings at state-of-the-art MR imaging, US, CT, and pathologic analysis. Radiographics. 2004;24(1):3–17. Discussion 8–9

52. Mortele KJ, Praet M, Van Vlierberghe H, Kunnen M, Ros PR. CT and MR imaging findings in focal nodular hyperplasia of the liver: radiologic-pathologic correlation. AJR Am J Roentgenol. 2000 Sep;175(3):687–92.

53. Mezhir JJ, Fourman LT, Do RK, Denton B, Allen PJ, D'Angelica MI, et al. Changes in the management of benign liver tumours: an analysis of 285 patients. HPB (Oxford). 2013 Feb;15(2):156–63.

54. Chang CY, Hernandez-Prera JC, Roayaie S, Schwartz M, Thung SN. Changing epidemiology of hepatocellular adenoma in the United States: review of the literature. Int J Hepatol. 2013;2013:604860.

55. Bluteau O, Jeannot E, Bioulac-Sage P, Marques JM, Blanc JF, Bui H, et al. Bi-allelic inactivation of TCF1 in hepatic adenomas. Nat Genet. 2002 Oct;32(2):312–5.

56. Zucman-Rossi J, Jeannot E, Nhieu JT, Scoazec JY, Guettier C, Rebouissou S, et al. Genotype-phenotype correlation in hepatocellular adenoma: new classification and relationship with HCC. Hepatology. 2006 Mar;43(3):515–24.

57. Rebouissou S, Amessou M, Couchy G, Poussin K, Imbeaud S, Pilati C, et al. Frequent in-frame somatic deletions activate gp130 in inflammatory hepatocellular tumours. Nature. 2009 Jan 8;457(7226):200–4.

58. Nault JC, Couchy G, Balabaud C, Morcrette G, Caruso S, Blanc JF, et al. Molecular classification of hepatocellular adenoma associates with risk factors, bleeding, and malignant transformation. Gastroenterology. 2017 Mar;152(4):880–94 e6.

59. Henriet E, Abou Hammoud A, Dupuy JW, Dartigues B, Ezzoukry Z, Dugot-Senant N, et al. Argininosuccinate synthase 1 (ASS1): a marker of unclassified hepatocellular adenoma and high bleeding risk. Hepatology. 2017 Dec;66(6):2016–28.

60. Nault JC, Couchy G, Caruso S, Meunier L, Caruana L, Letouze E, et al. Argininosuccinate synthase 1 and periportal gene expression in sonic hedgehog hepatocellular adenomas. Hepatology. 2018 Sep;68(3):964–76.

61. Dhingra S, Fiel MI. Update on the new classification of hepatic adenomas: clinical, molecular, and pathologic characteristics. Arch Pathol Lab Med. 2014 Aug;138(8):1090–7.

62. van der Windt DJ, Kok NF, Hussain SM, Zondervan PE, Alwayn IP, de Man RA, et al. Case-orientated approach to the management of hepatocellular adenoma. Br J Surg. 2006 Dec;93(12):1495–50.

63. D'Onofrio M, Crosara S, De Robertis R, Canestrini S, Mucelli RP. Contrast-enhanced ultrasound of focal liver lesions. AJR Am J Roentgenol. 2015 Jul;205(1):W56–66.

64. Grazioli L, Federle MP, Brancatelli G, Ichikawa T, Olivetti L, Blachar A. Hepatic adenomas: imaging and pathologic findings. Radiographics. 2001;21(4):877–92. Discussion 92–4

65. Noels JE, van Aalten SM, van der Windt DJ, Kok NF, de Man RA, Terkivatan T, et al. Management of hepatocellular adenoma during pregnancy. J Hepatol. 2011 Mar;54(3):553–8.

66. Linet MS, Gridley G, Nyren O, Mellemkjaer L, Olsen JH, Keehn S, et al. Primary liver cancer, other malignancies, and mortality risks following porphyria: a cohort study in Denmark and Sweden. Am J Epidemiol. 1999 Jun 1;149(11):1010–5.

67. Elmberg M, Hultcrantz R, Ekbom A, Brandt L, Olsson S, Olsson R, et al. Cancer risk in patients with hereditary hemochromatosis and in their first-degree relatives. Gastroenterology. 2003 Dec;125(6):1733–41.

68. Eriksson S, Carlson J, Velez R. Risk of cirrhosis and primary liver cancer in alpha 1-antitrypsin deficiency. N Engl J Med. 1986 Mar 20;314(12):736–9.

69. Soini Y, Chia SC, Bennett WP, Groopman JD, Wang JS, DeBenedetti VM, et al. An aflatoxin-associated mutational hotspot at codon 249 in the p53 tumor suppressor gene occurs in hepatocellular carcinomas from Mexico. Carcinogenesis. 1996 May;17(5):1007–12.

70. Yan RQ, Su JJ, Huang DR, Gan YC, Yang C, Huang GH. Human hepatitis B virus and hepatocellular carcinoma. II. Experimental induction of hepatocellular carcinoma in tree shrews exposed to hepatitis B virus and aflatoxin B1. J Cancer Res Clin Oncol. 1996;122(5):289–95.

71. Chu YJ, Yang HI, Wu HC, Liu J, Wang LY, Lu SN, et al. Aflatoxin B1 exposure increases the risk of cirrhosis and hepatocellular carcinoma in chronic hepatitis B virus carriers. Int J Cancer. 2017 Aug 15;141(4):711–20.

72. Siegel RL, Miller KD, Jemal A. Cancer statistics, 2020. CA Cancer J Clin. 2020 Jan;70(1):7–30.

73. Singal AG, Lampertico P, Nahon P. Epidemiology and surveillance for hepatocellular carcinoma: new trends. J Hepatol. 2020 Feb;72(2):250–61.

74. Global Burden of Disease Liver Cancer C, Akinyemiju T, Abera S, Ahmed M, Alam N, Alemayohu MA, et al. The burden of primary liver cancer and underlying etiologies from 1990 to 2015 at the global, regional, and National Level: results from the global burden of disease study 2015. JAMA Oncol. 2017 Dec 1;3(12):1683–91.

75. Naugler WE, Sakurai T, Kim S, Maeda S, Kim K, Elsharkawy AM, et al. Gender disparity in liver cancer due to sex differences in MyD88-dependent IL-6 production. Science. 2007 Jul 6;317(5834):121–4.

76. Ayuso C, Rimola J, Vilana R, Burrel M, Darnell A, Garcia-Criado A, et al. Diagnosis and staging of hepatocellular carcinoma (HCC): current guidelines. Eur J Radiol. 2018 Apr;101:72–81.

77. Bteich F, Di Bisceglie AM. Current and future systemic therapies for hepatocellular carcinoma. Gastroenterol & Hepatol. 2019 May;15(5):266–72.

78. Heimbach JK, Kulik LM, Finn RS, Sirlin CB, Abecassis MM, Roberts LR, et al. AASLD guidelines for the treatment of hepatocellular carcinoma. Hepatology. 2018 Jan;67(1):358–80.

79. Graham RP, Torbenson MS. Fibrolamellar carcinoma: a histologically unique tumor with unique molecular findings. Semin Diagn Pathol. 2017 Mar;34(2):146–52.

80. Craig JR, Peters RL, Edmondson HA, Omata M. Fibrolamellar carcinoma of the liver: a tumor of adolescents and young adults with distinctive clinico-pathologic features. Cancer. 1980 Jul 15;46(2):372–9.

81. Ward SC, Huang J, Tickoo SK, Thung SN, Ladanyi M, Klimstra DS. Fibrolamellar carcinoma of the liver exhibits immunohistochemical evidence of both hepatocyte and bile duct differentiation. Modern Pathol. 2010 Sep;23(9):1180–90.

82. Do RK, McErlean A, Ang CS, DeMatteo RP, Abou-Alfa GK. CT and MRI of primary and metastatic fibrolamellar carcinoma: a case series of 37 patients. Br J Radiol. 2014 Aug;87(1040):20140024.

83. Atienza LG, Berger J, Mei X, Shah MB, Daily MF, Grigorian A, et al. Liver transplantation for fibrolamellar hepatocellular carcinoma: a national perspective. J Surg Oncol. 2017 Mar;115(3):319–23.

84. Ang CS, Kelley RK, Choti MA, Cosgrove DP, Chou JF, Klimstra D, et al. Clinicopathologic characteristics and survival outcomes of patients with fibrolamellar carcinoma: data from the fibrolamellar carcinoma consortium. Gastrointestinal Cancer Res: GCR. 2013 Jan;6(1):3–9.

85. Bauer U, Mogler C, Braren RF, Algul H, Schmid RM, Ehmer U. Progression after immunotherapy for Fibrolamellar carcinoma. Visceral Med. 2019 Mar;35(1):39–42.

86. El Dika I, Mayer RJ, Venook AP, Capanu M, LaQuaglia MP, Kobos R, et al. A multicenter randomized three-arm phase II study of (1) Everolimus, (2) estrogen deprivation therapy (EDT) with leuprolide + Letrozole, and (3) Everolimus + EDT in patients with Unresectable Fibrolamellar carcinoma. Oncologist. 2020 May;12

87. Saha SK, Zhu AX, Fuchs CS, Brooks GA. Forty-year trends in cholangiocarcinoma incidence in the U.S.: intrahepatic disease on the rise. Oncologist. 2016 May;21(5):594–9.

88. Nakeeb A, Pitt HA, Sohn TA, Coleman J, Abrams RA, Piantadosi S, et al. Cholangiocarcinoma. A spectrum of intrahepatic, perihilar, and distal tumors. Ann Surg. 1996;224(4):463–73. Discussion 73–5

89. Patel AH, Harnois DM, Klee GG, LaRusso NF, Gores GJ. The utility of CA 19-9 in the diagnoses of cholangiocarcinoma in patients without primary sclerosing cholangitis. Am J Gastroenterol. 2000 Jan;95(1):204–7.

90. Valls C, Guma A, Puig I, Sanchez A, Andia E, Serrano T, et al. Intrahepatic peripheral cholangiocarcinoma: CT evaluation. Abdom Imaging. 2000 Sep-Oct;25(5):490–6.
91. Iavarone M, Piscaglia F, Vavassori S, Galassi M, Sangiovanni A, Venerandi L, et al. Contrast enhanced CT-scan to diagnose intrahepatic cholangiocarcinoma in patients with cirrhosis. J Hepatol. 2013 Jun;58(6):1188–93.
92. El-Diwany R, Pawlik TM, Ejaz A. Intrahepatic cholangiocarcinoma. Surg Oncol Clin N Am. 2019 Oct;28(4):587–99.
93. Pascher A, Jonas S, Neuhaus P. Intrahepatic cholangiocarcinoma: indication for transplantation. J Hepato-Biliary-Pancreat Surg. 2003;10(4):282–7.
94. Rizvi S, Khan SA, Hallemeier CL, Kelley RK, Gores GJ. Cholangiocarcinoma - evolving concepts and therapeutic strategies. Nat Rev Clin Oncol. 2018 Feb;15(2):95–111.
95. Gaballah AH, Jensen CT, Palmquist S, Pickhardt PJ, Duran A, Broering G, et al. Angiosarcoma: clinical and imaging features from head to toe. Br J Radiol. 2017 Jul;90(1075):20170039.
96. Young RJ, Brown NJ, Reed MW, Hughes D, Woll PJ. Angiosarcoma. Lancet Oncol. 2010 Oct;11(10):983–91.
97. Bhatia K, Shiels MS, Berg A, Engels EA. Sarcomas other than Kaposi sarcoma occurring in immunodeficiency: interpretations from a systematic literature review. Curr Opin Oncol. 2012 Sep;24(5):537–46.
98. Buetow PC, Buck JL, Ros PR, Goodman ZD. Malignant vascular tumors of the liver: radiologic-pathologic correlation. Radiographics. 1994;14(1):153–66. quiz 67-8
99. Pickhardt PJ, Kitchin D, Lubner MG, Ganeshan DM, Bhalla S, Covey AM. Primary hepatic angiosarcoma: multi-institutional comprehensive cancer Centre review of multiphasic CT and MR imaging in 35 patients. Eur Radiol. 2015 Feb;25(2):315–22.
100. Zheng YW, Zhang XW, Zhang JL, Hui ZZ, Du WJ, Li RM, et al. Primary hepatic angiosarcoma and potential treatment options. J Gastroenterol Hepatol. 2014 May;29(5):906–11.
101. Mokutani Y, Hata T, Miyake Y, Kuroda H, Takahashi H, Haraguchi N, et al. Metastasis from a primary hepatic angiosarcoma to the colon: a case report and literature review. Oncol Lett. 2017 Apr;13(4):2765–9.
102. Chen N, Aidan Y, Jung J. Primary hepatic Angiosarcoma: a brief review of the literature. EMJ Hepatol. 2018;6(1):64–71.
103. Weiss SW, Enzinger FM. Epithelioid hemangioendothelioma: a vascular tumor often mistaken for a carcinoma. Cancer. 1982 Sep 1;50(5):970–81.
104. Treska V, Daum O, Svajdler M, Liska V, Ferda J, Baxa J. Hepatic epithelioid Hemangioendothelioma - a rare tumor and diagnostic dilemma. In Vivo. 2017 Jul-Aug;31(4):763–7.
105. Lauffer JM, Zimmermann A, Krahenbuhl L, Triller J, Baer HU. Epithelioid hemangioendothelioma of the liver. A rare hepatic tumor. Cancer. 1996 Dec 1;78(11):2318–27.
106. Makhlouf HR, Ishak KG, Goodman ZD. Epithelioid hemangioendothelioma of the liver: a clinicopathologic study of 137 cases. Cancer. 1999 Feb 1;85(3):562–82.
107. Lyburn ID, Torreggiani WC, Harris AC, Zwirewich CV, Buckley AR, Davis JE, et al. Hepatic epithelioid hemangioendothelioma: sonographic, CT, and MR imaging appearances. AJR Am J Roentgenol. 2003 May;180(5):1359–64.
108. Mehrabi A, Kashfi A, Fonouni H, Schemmer P, Schmied BM, Hallscheidt P, et al. Primary malignant hepatic epithelioid hemangioendothelioma: a comprehensive review of the literature with emphasis on the surgical therapy. Cancer. 2006 Nov 1;107(9):2108–21.
109. Caremani M, Vincenti A, Benci A, Sassoli S, Tacconi D. Ecographic epidemiology of non-parasitic hepatic cysts. J Clin Ultrasound: JCU. 1993 Feb;21(2):115–8.
110. Ishak KG, Willis GW, Cummins SD, Bullock AA. Biliary cystadenoma and cystadenocarcinoma: report of 14 cases and review of the literature. Cancer. 1977 Jan;39(1):322–38.
111. Regev A, Reddy KR, Berho M, Sleeman D, Levi JU, Livingstone AS, et al. Large cystic lesions of the liver in adults: a 15-year experience in a tertiary center. J Am Coll Surg. 2001 Jul;193(1):36–45.

112. Zen Y, Pedica F, Patcha VR, Capelli P, Zamboni G, Casaril A, et al. Mucinous cystic neo-
     plasms of the liver: a clinicopathological study and comparison with intraductal papillary
     neoplasms of the bile duct. Modern Pathol. 2011 Aug;24(8):1079–89.
113. Fragulidis GP, Vezakis AI, Konstantinidis CG, Chondrogiannis KK, Primetis ES, Kondi-
     Pafiti A, et al. Diagnostic and therapeutic challenges of intrahepatic biliary cystadenoma
     and cystadenocarcinoma: a report of 10 cases and review of the literature. Int Surg. 2015
     Jul;100(7–8):1212–9.

# Chapter 14
# Drug Induced Liver Injury

Nora V. Bergasa

A 60 year old man was seen in the hepatology clinic for follow up prior to initiating treatment of chronic hepatitis C. The patient reported pruritus, which had started over several days prior to the second visit. On exam, he had scleral icterus, excoriations from chronic scratching, and hepatomegaly at the expense of the left lobe of the liver.

On the index visit, which had taken place eight weeks prior to the second visit, no risk factors for viral hepatitis had been identified. The patient's comorbidities included hypertension, type 2 diabetes, and a remote cerebrovascular accident that had left him emotionally labile without gross sensory or motor neurological deficits. He had been born outside the United States and was unemployed.

His medications included amlodipine and insulin. Three weeks prior to the index visit, the patient had been treated for Helicobacter pylori infection with pantoprazole, clarithromycin, and metronidazole for fourteen days. The patient had not taken any over the counter medications or herbal remedies.

A liver disease workup had not revealed any causes of liver disease other than chronic hepatitis C. The liver sonogram was normal. The APRI score was 0.96, consistent with advanced fibrosis.

Drug-induced liver injury (DILI) from clarithromycin was suspected. A summary of the liver profile over the course of his acute illness is shown in Table 14.1.

The patient suffered from pruritus, which was treated with cholestyramine and naloxone infusions in the hospital and subsequently managed with naltrexone and pregabalin. Antipruritic medications were tapered and discontinued as pruritus decreased. The serum activity (SA)s of AST, ALT, and AP and the serum bilirubin

N. V. Bergasa (✉)
Department of Medicine, H+H/Metropolitan, New York, NY, USA

New York Medical College, Valhalla, NY, USA

Hepatology, H+H/Woodhull, Brooklyn, NY, USA

© The Author(s), under exclusive license to Springer-Verlag London Ltd., part of Springer Nature 2022
N. V. Bergasa (ed.), *Clinical Cases in Hepatology*,
https://doi.org/10.1007/978-1-4471-4715-2_14

**Table 14.1** Laboratory exams of the patient described over the course of illness

| Liver Profile Hepatitis C Viral Load and genotype | T minus 21 | T0 | T12 | T16 | T20 (HCV Rx started) | T32 | T48 | T144 |
|---|---|---|---|---|---|---|---|---|
| | Treatment of HP with pantoprazole, clarithromycin, and metronidazole started | | | | | | | |
| AST (IU/ml) | | 70 | 101 | 86 | 78 | 45 | 24 | 25 |
| ALT(IU/ml) | | 64 | 60 | 42 | 38 | 26 | 25 | 36 |
| AP (IU/ml) | | 159 | 449 | 560 | 556 | 410 | 168 | 235 |
| TB (mg/dl) | | 0.7 | 5.5 | 10.7 | 2.5 | 0.3 | 0.4 | 0.4 |
| Albumin 9 g/dl) | | 3.9 | 3.0 | 2.7 | 2.5 | 2.7 | 4.0 | 3.8 |
| PT (seconds)/INR | | 10.9/1.05 | 10.9 | 10.6 | 10.7 | 11.5/1.12 | 11.5 | |
| HCV RNA IU/ml/Genotype | | 100,921/1a | 101 | 86 | 78 | Not detected | Not detected | Not Detected |

T minus 21: 21 days prior to the index visit to the clinic

T0: index visit

T12-T144: twelve to 144 weeks post index visit

*AST* aspartate aminotransferase, *ALT* alanine aminotransferase, *AP* alkaline phosphatase, *HCV* hepatitis C, *INR* international normalized ratio

concentration decreased gradually over eight weeks. He was started on sofosbuvir/velpatasvir for the treatment of his HCV eight weeks after the first documentation of DILI.

The treatment of HCV was associated with a cure. He is enrolled in a surveillance program for hepatocellular carcinoma. He has developed diabetic nephropathy, which explains the increase in AP SA, which likely has a component of bone origin.

# Etiology

Hepatotoxicity is defined as toxic damage to the liver. The spectrum of hepatotoxicity includes the nature of the hepatotoxic agent, the type and mechanism of liver injury, the circumstances of the exposure, and the medical and social importance [1]

Hepatotoxic agents can be inorganic and organic. The inorganic agents include metals, hydrazine derivatives, and iodides. The organic agents include plant toxins such as pyrrolizidines and tannic acid, mycotoxins such as aflatoxin, bacterial endotoxins and exotoxins, and synthetic compounds including nonmedicinal agents such as organic amines and azo compounds, and medicinal agents used for diagnostic and treatment purposes [1].

Hepatotoxicity can be associated with necrosis, steatosis, cirrhosis, and carcinoma. Other forms of hepatotoxicity concern impaired bile flow and bilirubin excretion. Vascular and degenerative lesions can also result from hepatotoxicity [1].

The mechanisms of liver injury can be true hepatotoxicity or secondary to the host susceptibility to an agent. True hepatotoxicity refers to an agent's ability to cause liver injury in most recipients of different species. An idiosyncratic reaction is mediated by the host's immune or metabolic response to an agent. There is a mix of host susceptibility and idiosyncrasy supporting liver injury [1].

The circumstances under which liver injury occurs have been divided into (1) toxicologic, including: (i) occupational: routine exposure or accidental, (ii) domestic: accidental or suicidal exposure, ingestion of contaminated food, recreational drug use, e.g., euphorogenic substances, (iii) environmental: pollution, natural hepatotoxins, and (2) pharmaceutical: (i) iatrogenic, and (ii) self-medication [1].

The focus of this chapter is drug-induced liver injury (DILI). The most important intervention in DILI cases is to identify the agent and to discontinue its use. Rechallenge should not be done because of the risk of inducing a worse reaction than the first one, including liver failure. Livertox.NIH.gov is a search database with extremely valuable information, which should be accessed to evaluate a patient in whom DILI is being considered [2].

DILI is the injurious effect to the liver by an agent, natural or produced [3], exhibited by an increase in the SA of the liver associated enzymes, alanine and aspartate aminotransferases (ALT and AST), and alkaline phosphatase (AP) activities, which can be accompanied by hyperbilirubinemia and hepatic synthetic dysfunction, including acute liver failure (ALF) [4].

# Risk Factors for Dili

## Genetics

Individualization of treatment based on comprehensive new generation sequencing (NGS) genotyping data provides the opportunity to prescribe effective and safe medications to individuals according to their genetic predisposition to efficacy and side effects, i.e. the prescribed drug should be chosen according to the patient's probability of benefit and their susceptibility to developing side effects [5]. Accordingly, the inclusion of pharmacogenetics is of great importance in drug development. Pharmacogenetics is a field in evolution that will lead to a decrease in adverse reactions to drugs, as a genetic predisposition is proposed in cases of idiosyncratic DILI, and support for this idea has been provided.

A study of cultured T cells provided the immunological basis for flucloxacillin-induced liver injury. Flucloxacillin-responsive CD4+ and CD8+ T cells in patients with DILI from this medication were identified. Naive CD45RA + CD8+ T cells expressing HLA-B*57:01 from normal volunteers were activated with flucloxacillin when dendritic cells presented the agent antigen. The production of interferon gamma, T helper (Th) 2 cytokines, perforin, granzyme B, and FasL was reported in association with T-cell clones' exposure expressing CCR4 and CCR9 that migrated towards CCL17 and CCL 25 in response to stimulation by the drug. The activation of CD8+ clones with flucloxacillin was restricted by HLA-B*57:01 and related to HLA-B*58:01 and dependent on antigen processing. Additional reactivity to β-lactam antibiotics, including oxacillin, cloxacillin, and dicloxacillin, was documented by the clones [6].

A genetic predisposition to flucloxacillin-induced DILI was confirmed by a genome-wide association study (GWAS) in 51 cases with this condition versus 282 control samples. The study documented an association peak in the major histocompatibility complex (MHC) region with the strongest association noted for rs2395029[G], a marker in complete linkage disequilibrium with HLA-B*5701 [7].

Amoxicillin-clavulanate induced DILI has been significantly associated with the DRB1*1501-DRB5*0101-DQB1*0602 haplotype [8]. A genetic predisposition for amoxicillin-clavulanate induced DILI was confirmed and expanded by a GWAS study that included 822,927 single nucleotide polymorphism (SNP) markers from 201 white subjects in Europe and the United States versus 532 well-matched control subjects. The main finding was with an HLA class II SNP (rs9274407, $P = 4.8 \times 10(-14)$), which correlated with rs3135388, a tag SNP of HLA-DRB1*1501-DQB1*0602 [9].

The absence of HLA-DQA1*0102 and the presence of HLA-DQB1*0201 were independent risk factors for DILI in a group of 56 patients from 346 who developed DILI in association with antituberculous therapy with isoniazid, rifampicin, and pyrazinamide and ethambutol and streptomycin from North India [10, 11].

Genetic susceptibility to DILI from diclofenac has been reported in association with rs17036170 upstream of the gene peroxisome proliferator-activated receptor gamma (*PPARG*), which participates in lipid metabolism [12] and with rs7574865, near the signal transducer and activator of transcription 4 gene (*STAT4*). The latter has been implicated in autoimmune diseases [13, 14].

Idiosyncratic drug reactions also concern metabolic pathways of detoxification and hence the genetics behind drug metabolism. In this regard, studies have explored associations with the cytochrome p450 family because of its role in phase I drug metabolism [15], UDP-glucuronosyltransferases, the role of which is glucuronidation to end the biological actions of drugs and to facilitate the renal excretion of lipophilic medications [16].

N-acetyltransferases, which are drug-metabolizing enzymes that acetylate drugs and carcinogens [17], and glutathione S-transferases, the function of which includes to catalyzing the conjugation of electrophilic substrates to glutathione and protection of cells from peroxidation [18].

Susceptibility genes identified in association with DILI in the context of drug metabolism include: (i) in the cytochrome p450 group, *CYP2E1* for isoniazid [19] and *CYP2C9* for bosentan, (ii) the UDP-glucuronosyltransferases *UGT2B7* for diclofenac [20], (iii) the N-acetyltransferases *NAT2* for isoniazid [21], and in the glutathione S-transferases, *GSTM1* for troglitazone [22] and *GSTT1* for amoxicillin-clavulanate [23].

A GWAS included 55 subjects from India and 70 European with DILI and 1199 Indian and 10,397 European controls. The study found a significance for the *HLA-B\*52:01* and the rs117491755 in *ASTN2*, which was found in Europeans. The *NAT2\*5* frequency was lower in DILI cases than in controls. *NAT2\*6* and *NAT2\*7* were the most common genes, homozygotes for *NAT2\*6* or *NAT2\*7* or both, the more common in cases than in the control group. These results were interpreted to suggest that the HLA genotype makes a small contribution to DILI from anti-tuberculosis medications. An impact from NAT2 was documented when the metabolic effect of *NAT2\*5* and *NAT2\*6* and *NAT2\*7* was taken into consideration [24].

Transport proteins may be involved in DILI because of their function in uptake of drugs into the hepatocyte and biliary excretion of metabolites [25]. In this context, the C-24 T variant of *ABCC2*, which codes for the multidrug resistance protein 2 (MRP2) [26], was identified in association with DILI from diclofenac [20], and the ABCB1, which codes for P-glycoprotein [27], with DILI from nevirapine [28].

A genetic predisposition to DILI from certain drugs has been confirmed; therefore, it is important to determine if an individual is at risk for DILI before initiating treatment with a given drug. The use of drugs at high risk for DILI should be avoided if other options are available, in the author's opinion. In clinical practice, it may not be feasible to check genetic predisposition to DILI from certain drugs; however, there is precedent for the inclusion of HLA typing prior to prescribing abacavir to treat HIV. In this regard, "100% of those who develop it [hypersensitivity reaction] are positive for HLA-B\*57:01," which has resulted in the recommendation by drug regulators worldwide for genotyping for HLA-B\*57:01 prior to prescribing this drug [29]. Amoxicillin/clavulanate induced DILI has been significantly associated with the HLA class II antigen DRB1\*1501-DRB5\*0101-DQB1\*0602 haplotype [8]. Accordingly, an alternative medication can be used to avoid a devastating DILI, which can result in ductopenia and tremendous suffering from pruritus, and other complications from hepatobiliary disease. HLA-B\*1502 has been reported more frequently in patients who develop Stevens–Johnson's syndrome in association with carbamazepine; thus, alternative anticonvulsants can be prescribed. Clearly, significant efforts to facilitate testing for genetic predisposition, including clinical availability from commercial laboratories and pricing, must be made.

A search for studies on the subject of epigenetics, a phenomenon that may predispose to hepatotoxicity, and DILI did not yield any results; however, this is an area of research that will provide valuable information and will improve patient care when used in the clinical arena [5].

## Age

The capacity to metabolize medications may be impaired with age, and hence, may predispose individuals to DILI. However, in an observational study of 899 patients considered to have DILI, the age of at least 65 years was not associated with increased mortality or liver transplantation [30]. A similar distribution in gender and age was documented in a study from Spain that included 603 cases of DILI, with a peak distribution in the 40 to 49 and 60 to 69 age groups, with no reported cases in the 20 to 29 years aged group. Patients at least 60 years old accounted for 46% of cases, with a significant majority being men; however, fulminant liver failure and liver transplantation were more common in women than in men. The proportion of cholestatic liver injury increased with age [31], a finding similar to the study from the United States [30]. In contrast, a prospective study from Iceland that included 96 patients with DILI, excluding acetaminophen induced toxicity, documented the highest incidence in the group 80 to 106 years of age, i.e. 41 per 100,000 inhabitants. The mean prescription rate increased with age, and it was the highest for this group [32]. These findings have suggested that an increase in the number of medications in the elderly may be implicated in DILI risk [32, 33].

Isoniazid hepatotoxicity from a sample of 3377 patients was studied from a database of patients treated from 1996 to 2003 in a public health department clinic in the United States. Classified per 1000 individuals and according to age group, 4.40 events were reported in the 25 to 34 years group, 8.54 in the 35 to 49 years, and 20.83 for those at least 50 years old [34]. In contrast, the use of valproic acid as part of antiseizure therapy was associated with a marked increase, 1:600, in fatal hepatotoxicity in patients younger than 2 years of age [35]. Other risk factors included developmental delay and metabolic disorders [35].

In regards to isoniazid, a predominance of cholestatic liver injury occurs in the elderly, which differs from the typical hepatocellular injury associated with this drug, which happens more frequently in people over the age of 35, and that dramatically increases after age 50 [34].

## Gender

The studies from Spain, Iceland, and the United States did not support an increase in the incidence of DILI in women versus men [30–32]; however, it is noted that women tend to be more susceptible than men to DILI of the autoimmune type, which may be a reflection of the increased risk of some autoimmune liver diseases in this gender, including autoimmune hepatitis and primary biliary cholangitis [36, 37].

## Race and Ethnicity

The daily use of four grams of acetaminophen in a controlled study documented that Hispanic American subjects had a 1.9 relative risk (RR) (95% confidence interval (CI), 1.1–3.33) versus non-Hispanic subjects of exhibiting an increase in serum activity of ALT. There was no difference in the peak and trough or area under the drug curve levels between the subjects who exhibited versus those who did not exhibit an increase in serum ALT activity. The findings suggested that drug metabolism alone may not have been related to ALT activity increases, and perhaps, the ethnicity determined the increase in ALT activity. Racial characteristics of the Hispanic subjects were not reported; thus, it is unclear whether the ALT phenomenon was related to ethnicity, race, or both [38].

Idiosyncratic DILI was reported in association with increased morbidity and mortality in a study that included 144 African American versus 841 non-Hispanic white patients. Trimethoprim/sulfamethoxazole, methyldopa, and phenytoin were more injurious in African American than in non-Hispanic white subjects. The severity of DILI was worse in African American patients, who had more skin reactions, were hospitalized more often, underwent more liver transplantations, and had more liver related deaths 6 months post DILI than the non-Hispanic white subjects [39].

A meta-analysis of pharmacogenetic studies of drug-metabolizing enzyme polymorphisms that included 2225 patients and 4906 control subjects revealed an association between drug-induced liver injury from anti-tuberculosis drugs and CYP2E1*1A in East Asians when the data were stratified by ethnicity [40].

## Alcohol

The effect of alcohol on toxicity has been documented for substances that include acetaminophen, cocaine, halothane, and isoniazid, on which it has a marked enhancement, with a moderate enhancement for others, including vitamin A and methotrexate [41].

## Pregnancy

Pregnancy is included as a variable in causality assessment scales; however, there is no evidence that pregnancy per se increases the risk of DILI; however, some drugs used in pregnancy, including methyldopa, hydralazine, and propylthiouracil used to treat specific comorbidities can cause DILI; thus the clinician must be aware of their association with liver injury.

## Comorbidities

Risk factors for nonalcoholic fatty liver disease may be associated with steatosis and steatohepatitis from medications. In this regard, tamoxifen was associated with an increased risk for nonalcoholic steatohepatitis in patients with high serum triglyceride and fasting blood sugar concentrations, and low high density lipoprotein. Tamoxifen related injury was not associated with hypertension, obesity, and overweight state in a study from Iran [42]. These results contrast with those from a prospective randomized, double blind, placebo controlled trial from Italy in which tamoxifen was associated with an increased risk to develop nonalcoholic steatohepatitis only in overweight and obese women with characteristics of the metabolic syndrome [43].

Methotrexate is another drug that has received much attention regarding its therapeutic benefits and its risk for hepatotoxicity. In this regard, a record review from patients listed from 1987 to 2011 for liver transplantation with the Organ Procurement and Transplantation Network because of liver disease from methotrexate was conducted [44]. The study reported a low (0.07%) proportion of adult patients listed or transplanted for methotrexate induced liver disease, with Caucasian, middle-aged women with diabetes being significantly present in the group. These characteristics did not differ from the group listed for nonalcoholic steatohepatitis except for the race [44]. The results also indicated that a common pathway might underlie the pathogenesis of nonalcoholic steatohepatitis and methotrexate induced liver injury when it happens. However, the results cannot be interpreted to suggest that methotrexate increases the risk of toxicity in patients at risk for nonalcoholic steatohepatitis [44]. Although a slight deviation from the discussion of comorbidities as risk factors for DILI, it is worth noting that the authors cite a request for additional data regarding methotrexate induced hepatotoxicity [44], which might have been exaggerated for a drug that has important beneficial effects [45]. The authors add that their work fulfills that request and conclude that methotrexate induced hepatotoxicity is rare [44]. However, the EASLD (European Association for the Study of Liver Diseases) Clinical Practice Guidelines: Drug-induced liver injury state "components of the metabolic syndrome should be considered risk factors for the occurrence and the degree of DAFL [drug-induced fatty liver disease] in patients treated with tamoxifen and methotrexate" [33].

## Chronic Liver Disease

Baseline increased activity of aminotransferases and coinfection with the hepatitis C virus were identified as risk factors for DILI in association with antiretroviral drugs, from a retrospective review of data from 8851 patients enrolled in 16 Adult AIDS Clinical Trial Group studies from 1989 to 1999 [46].

In a study that included 371 patients with HIV infection, 24.5% of the patients diagnosed with tuberculosis had underlying liver disease, comprised of acute and chronic viral hepatitis, alcoholic hepatitis, "other hepatitis," and chronic liver disease, which was diagnosed at baseline or during anti-tuberculosis treatment. Increased serum AST and ALT activities occurred in 31.2% of the episodes of positive tuberculosis diagnosis during the first month of treatment, with the most common increases being twice the upper limits of normal (ULN) in half of the patients. However, five and ten times the ULN values were also documented. This study's relevance is that patients with HIV and tuberculosis may also have chronic liver disease, suggesting that liver profile monitoring during treatment is important [47].

Hepatitis C was also identified as a risk factor for DILI in association with anti-tuberculosis drugs, as documented from a retrospective study of 128 patients. Coinfection with hepatitis B and C was also identified as a risk factor for DILI as were increased age and baseline abnormality of the liver panel [48].

From a prospective study that examined the outcomes of 899 patients with DILI, it was reported that the severity of the liver injury was greater in patients with liver disease and that DILI was associated with a significant increase in mortality of 10.8% over those without preexisting liver disease. The most common drug associated with DILI in patients with preexisting liver disease was azithromycin [30].

## *Drug Dependent Risk Factors*

Medication dose contributes to liver injury, with greater than 50 mg per dose associated with an increased risk for DILI. For example, acetaminophen at a single dose greater than 7.5 g is related to acute liver toxicity. However, idiosyncratic DILI is characterized by a lack of clear dose dependency [49]; nevertheless, it is now considered that idiosyncratic DILI may also be related to dosage.

Among prescription medicines from pharmacy databases in the United States, a statistically significant relationship was observed between daily doses of oral medications and liver failure reports, liver transplantation, and death from DILI [50]. Recorded by the Swedish Adverse Drug Reactions Advisory Committee, 9% of all DILI cases were in the category of less than 10 mg per day, 14.2% in the 11–49 mg per day, and 77% in the at least 50 mg per day group, with an associated death or liver transplantation in 2%, 9.4%, and 13.2%, respective to the categories [50].

## *Drug Metabolism*

Drug metabolism can generate metabolites that react with intracellular substances that alter cellular function and provoke injury [51]. Some of the drugs documented to cause reactive metabolites include acetaminophen, tamoxifen, isoniazid, and carbamazepine [52].

Hepatic metabolism greater than 50% was defined as high for a study that explored the relationship between metabolism and DILI [53]. It was reported that drugs with high hepatic metabolism were associated with a significant increased frequency of high ALT activity, liver failure, and DILI associated with death [53].

## Lipophilicity

Lipophilicity is a chemical compound's ability to dissolve in fats, oils, lipids, and non-polar solvents. Highly lipophilic drugs have an increased ability to cause toxicity. The combination of lipophilicity and daily dose, known as the rule-of-two, is considered an indication of a drug's hepatotoxic potential [54]. In this regard, high lipophilicity may facilitate an increase in the drug uptake by the hepatocyte [54]. The Ro2 analysis is a model that may identify the hepatotoxicity potential of drugs in the development process [55, 56].

## Drug Interactions

It is not infrequent for patients with DILI to be taking multiple medications. The exercise of reviewing each medication's start date and the first day of documented abnormalities, clinical or laboratory, is fundamental, and it may take more than the 20 to 30 minutes allowed to see patients in many clinics. The identification of DILI culprits has been greatly facilitated by the creation of the LiverToxNIH.gov website [2]. The readers of this book must learn that unless a vigorous medication reconciliation, which may involve reviewing the medication bottles, calls to the pharmacy, and communication with other members of the health care team is done, the drug involved will not be identified, and the opportunity to discontinue it will be missed.

The mechanism of hepatotoxicity in drug interactions may be related to the ability of some agents to induce the cytochrome p450 family of enzymes, such as rifampicin, which, when coadministered with isoniazid, increases the odds of DILI [57], and carbamazepine and phenytoin, with valproic acid [58].

## Mitochondrial Toxicity

Drugs that decrease mitochondrial number and function are associated with fatty liver, including liver failure. The mechanism of this type of liver injury may result from increased production of reactive oxygen species, impaired mitochondrial permeability transition, altered mitochondrial respiration, mitochondrial DNA damage, or inhibition of beta-oxidation of fatty acids [59].

This category of hepatotoxic drugs includes fialuridine, a nucleoside analogue [60], thiazolidinediones, fibrates, cholesterol lowering drugs, antidepressants of the serotonin reuptake inhibitors type, serotonin antagonists used for nausea treatment, pain medications (NSAIDs), some antibiotics including fluoroquinolones and macrolides, kinase inhibitors and anthracyclins, anticancer drugs [61], and most of the reverse transcriptase inhibitors used in the treatment of HIV, which act by the inhibition of human DNA polymerase gamma [62].

## *Inhibition of Hepatobiliary Transporters*

Hepatobiliary transporters regulate the uptake of substances into the hepatocyte and the export of endobiotic and xenobiotics to prevent their intracellular accumulation, which can be toxic. The bile salt export protein (BSEP) is located on the hepatocyte's canalicular domain and removes monovalent, conjugated bile salts from those cells. An association between the pharmacological interference with BSEP function and DILI has been hypothesized [63].

The role of BSEP in DILI has been described for several drugs, including glitazones [64], some antiretrovirals agents [65], and endothelin antagonists [66]. In vitro models that test the function of BSEP have been suggested for inclusion in the development of drugs to identify potential toxic agents prior to the human testing phase [63].

## Epidemiology

Four hundred and sixty-one DILI cases were confirmed from 1994 to 2004 in Spain's cooperative network [67]. Antimicrobials were the most common type of drugs, with amoxicillin-clavulanate comprising 12.8% of the cases [67].

A prospective study conducted in Iceland from 2010 to 2011 included 96 subjects with DILI. The crude annual incidence was reported as 19.1 (95% confidence interval [CI], 15.4–23.3) cases per 100,000 inhabitants, 56% being women, with a median age of 55 years. Seventy-five percent was caused by prescription medications and 16% by dietary supplements. Again, the most common drug involved in DILI was amoxicillin-clavulanate, in 22% of the cases, with diclofenac in 6%, and azathioprine, infliximab, and nitrofurantoin in 4% [32].

The Drug-Induced Liver Injury Network from the United States provided a subgroup analysis of its prospectively collected data on DILI beginning in 2004 with patients followed for 6 months. From 1257, causality was assessed in 1091, with 899 being confirmed as definite, highly likely, or probable DILI. Azithromycin was significantly more common in patients with liver disease, 6.7%, versus those without liver disease, 1.5% [30].

It is essential to identify vitamins, minerals, dietary elements, food components, natural herbs, herbal preparations, and synthetic compounds taken to supplement the diet as possible culprits in the approach to a patient with liver injury. A report including these substances documented the DILI cases proportion from 7% in 2004 to 2005 to 20% in 2013–2014, with bodybuilding supplements as a cause of liver injury from 2% to 6% over the same period [68].

## Approach to a Patient with Suspected Drug-Induced Liver Injury

DILI is part of the differential diagnosis of a patient with an abnormal liver profile. It is a diagnosis of exclusion; thus, other causes of liver disease must be excluded before attributing liver disease to a drug, without the workup being an impediment to a rapid diagnosis [2].

A detailed medication history including those prescribed, over the counter and herbal supplements, and illicit drugs and alcohol is very important. In addition, serology for acute or chronic viral hepatitis A, B, C, and E [69], autoimmune markers, and serum concentration of immunoglobulins, ceruloplasmin, and alpha 1 antitrypsin, and iron studies comprise the laboratory investigation in a patient with liver disease, including DILI [70]. Ischemic hepatitis is a complication not infrequently identified in hospitalized patients [71]. In addition, hepatic manifestation of extra-hepatic diseases has to be considered in the differential diagnosis [72, 73].

The information required from the history in the approach to a patient with liver disease from DILI is: (1) time to onset or latency, i.e., challenge, which is the time from the first dose of the agent to the onset of liver injury, (2) time to recovery, i.e., dechallenge, (3) injury pattern and clinical phenotype, (4) exclusion of other causes of liver disease, (5) known information about a drug being the cause of liver injury, i.e., likelihood, and (6) response to reexposure, accidental or intentional, i.e., rechallenge, which is *not done intentionally.*

The time to onset can be established from the time the drug was prescribed to the time the first symptom or sign of liver injury is experienced or exhibited, e.g., fatigue, jaundice, or choluria, because the time to the first abnormal liver test cannot be identified unless the patient is being monitored with blood work [2, 74, 75].

The time to recovery is when the medication is stopped to the time the liver injury is resolved. In general, the resolution starts on discontinuation of the drug with notable decreases in liver associated enzyme activity within a week of discontinuing the agent; however, prolonged DILI can occur, which requires continuity of care to document resolution [2, 74, 75].

The pattern of liver injury, i.e., the pattern of the liver profile, or the clinical phenotype, may be typical and consistent with what has been reported in the literature, hence the importance of search databases, e.g., LiverToxNIH.gov and communication with pharmacists [2, 74, 75].

The exercise through which efforts are made to identify the DILI agent is called *causality assessment*. The instruments used in the causality assessment process for hepatotoxicity are the Roussel Uclaf Causality Assessment Method (RUCAM) [76] and its modification, Maria and Victorino (M & V) system [77]. Expert opinion is the best method to arrive at a diagnosis of DILI [78]; however, as it requires the participation of several clinicians, it may not be practical in some settings if an immediate opinion is necessary, but it is undoubtedly worthwhile to seek it as soon as possible.

In the context of clinical trials, and clinical work, possible hepatotoxicity by laboratory criteria is defined as [79]:

1. minimally abnormal serum test results, *which signify a warning*:

    (a) AST or ALT above the ULN and up to three times the ULN, *or,*
    (b) alkaline phosphatase up to 1.5 the ULN, *or,*
    (c) bilirubin up to two times the ULN, which "signify a warning" and,

2. markedly abnormal serum test results, which are an indication for immediate action, i.e., discontinuation of the drug and clinical follow up:

    (a) AST or ALT more than three times the ULN, *or,*
    (b) alkaline phosphatase more than 1.5 the ULN, *or,*
    (c) bilirubin more than two times the ULN.

Causes of liver disease must be excluded as the drug is discontinued, as already stated.

Mortality can be high when DILI is associated with hepatocellular injury and jaundice [1]. The early identification of the high potential for a bad outcome with this type of DILI phenotype is fundamental in clinical trials and clinical medicine. This observation is known as Hy's rule, after the master of hepatotoxicity, Dr. Hyman J. Zimmerman, who recorded it [1, 80]. Severe hepatocellular injury, reflected by increased activity of serum transaminases, can overwhelm the liver's capacity to function, e.g., to handle bilirubin, which is reflected by hyperbilirubinemia and is associated with a ten to 50 percent mortality from ALF from DILI [1]. The Food and Drug Administration has incorporated Hy's rule in their drug approval process, and it modified the term Hy's rule to Hy's Law [80, 81].

Hy's Law has been reexamined. The R value is a number that predicts the development of ALF from DILI [80, 81]. The development of the new R value, i.e., nR, has been published. Data recorded between 1994 and 2012 from 777 subjects with 805 episodes of DILI were examined regarding the peak in serum ALT activity and bilirubin concentration. Thirty-two of the 771 patients developed ALF. The independent high risk factors to develop ALF were female gender, high serum bilirubin concentration, and serum AST to ALT activities ratio (AST: ALT). Comparative analyses with total bilirubin greater than two times the ULN, and either serum ALT activity greater than three times the ULN, an R value of ALT times the ULN divided by SA of alkaline phosphatase times the ULN of at least five were included as variables versus an nR, which was calculated by the inclusion of whichever transaminase activity was the highest, ALT or AST, divided by SA of alkaline phosphatase times the ULN of at least five. At diagnosis, the R and the nR identified patients who developed ALF, with 67% and 63% specificity. The serum ALT activity and the nR model provided a 90% specificity for the development of ALF versus the R model, the sensitivity of which was 83%. The height of the serum alkaline phosphatase activity was similar between the group of patients who developed and those who did not develop ALF. An algorithm comprised of SA of AST greater than 17.3 times the upper limit of normal, a serum total bilirubin concentration of 6.6 times the ULN, and an AST: ALT activity ratio greater than 1.5 identified patients who developed ALF with a specificity and sensitivity of 82% and 80%, respectively. The use of this relatively new paradigm further facilitates the identification of patients who are at risk for ALF. It alerts the clinician to provide support measures to patients and vigilant follow up for timely evaluation for liver transplantation [82].

A study that included 250 patients with suspected DILI evaluated the causality assessment by the use of a structured expert opinion process versus the Roussel Uclaf causality assessment method. Detailed clinical and laboratory data from patients with suspected DILI were distributed to expert committee members who reviewed, adjudicated, and completed a RUCAM scale. For 187 cases associated with a single agent, there was an initial complete agreement for 50 cases (27%) within the expert opinion process, and for 34 (19%) with a five-category RUCAM scale, which was not significantly different. The two methods exhibited a modest correlation with each other. It was noted that the RUCAM method decreased the causality towards less probable than the expert opinion. Importantly, the RUCAM approach substantially shifted the causality likelihood towards lower probabilities than the DILI expert opinion process. The results were interpreted to suggest that the expert opinion process produced higher agreement rates and likelihood scores than the RUCAM scale. However, the authors noted a substantial interobserver variability in both methods [78].

The availability of the LiverTox.NIH.gov website has revolutionized and improved the approach to a patient with suspected DILI [2]. We access it in our clinic sessions to identify the likely agent in possible DILI cases and generate a discussion between at least two clinicians to develop an expert opinion.

## Clinical Manifestations

Patients with DILI may be asymptomatic or have fatigue, pruritus, or both, depending on the pattern of liver injury [2, 74, 75].

Physical examination may be normal and may reveal scleral icterus and spider angiomata, especially in chronic DILI cases. If chronic, patients may have hepatomegaly, splenomegaly, and ascites, as a sign of decompensation. In sinusoidal obstruction syndrome (SOS), tender hepatomegaly and ascites are typical, and jaundice can be present. Liver masses are usually identified by radiographic studies, especially adenomata, which tend not to be palpable. Malignant tumors can present with palpable liver masses and their complications (Table 14.2).

**Table 14.2** Clinical phenotypes of drug-induced liver injury [2]

| Clinical Phenotype | Typical agents | Latency | Clinical manifestations | Type of liver profile | Liver histology | Duration of liver injury/ prognosis |
|---|---|---|---|---|---|---|
| Acute hepatic necrosis | acetaminophen aspirin niacin intravenous amiodarone terbutaline | One to fourteen days | Nausea, vomiting, abdominal pain, and altered mental status, somnolence and coma jaundice systemic involvement (e.g., renal, bone marrow, lung) | Hepatocellular | Centrilobular necrosis, little lobular lymphocytic infiltration, minimal or no fibrosis or cholestasis | It can be fatal or associated with rapid recovery |
| Acute hepatitis | isoniazid, pyrazinamide, disulfiram, fenofibrate, ephedra greater celandine, green tea | Two to 24 weeks | Prodrome: inappetence fatigue nausea, jaundice, choluria | Hepatocellular | Hepatocellular necrosis, lobular disarray. lymphocytic infiltration, minimal or no fibrosis | Two to four weeks |
| 1) Cholestatic 2) mixed hepatitis | 1) amoxicillin/ clavulanate, sulfonylureas rifampin, penicillins, cephalosporins, methimazole 2) phenytoin, carbamapezine, iamotrigine sulfonamide, macrolide antibiotics, enalapril | 1) 2 to 24 weeks 2) 4–24 weeks | Pruritus and jaundice | 1) Cholestatic with modest hepatocellular features and bilirubin >2 mg/dl 2) Cholestatic and hepatocellular | 1) intrahepatic cholestasis with some inflammatory cells but mild to moderate focal hepatocellular necrosis 2) intrahepatic cholestasis with inflammatory cells and moderate to severe hepatocellular necrosis. | Short or prolonged. Liver associated enzymes may decrease by 50% over four to twelve weeks |

(continued)

**Table 14.2** (continued)

| Clinical Phenotype | Typical agents | Latency | Clinical manifestations | Type of liver profile | Liver histology | Duration of liver injury/prognosis |
|---|---|---|---|---|---|---|
| Increase SA of liver associated enzymes without hyperbilirubine-mia (anicteric hepatitis or anicteric cholestatic hepatitis) | isoniazid antiretroviral agents methotrexate, tacrine, aspirin, acetaminophen | 2 to 48 weeks. | Usually asymptomatic No jaundice | Bilirubin <2.5 mg/dL | ☐ see acute and chronic hepatitis phenotypes | Spontaneous decrease of AST and ALT SA into the normal range (i.e.. adaptation) or in association with the decrease or discontinuation of agent within 4 weeks. |
| Pure and bland cholestasis | estrogens and anabolic steroids, azathioprine, mercaptopurine | 4 to 24 weeks | Pruritus and jaundice | Variable increases in AP and ALT SA Bilirubin >2.5 mg/dl | Intrahepatic cholestasis with minimal inflammation or hepatocellular necrosis. | Slow recovery, over 4 weeks |
| Acute fatty liver with lactic acidosis | fialuridine [a] zidovudine, didanosine, stavudine, tetracycline intravenous linezolid | 7–28 days | Prodrome from 1–4 weeks. Shortness of breath and weakness are experienced when lactic acidosis appears, followed by stupor and coma. Jaundice is mild. | Increase in serum lactate, Increase in AST and ALT over 2x ULN | Microvesicular steatosis | Fatal |

| | | | | |
|---|---|---|---|---|
| Fatty liver (AKA nonalcoholic fatty liver disease) | methotrexate, tamoxifen | 3 to 12 months to years | Absent or non-specific for liver disease | Mild increase in AST and ALT SA | Steatosis, ballooning hepatocyte degeneration | Resolution or decrease in SA of liver associated enzymes over time after discontinuation of agent |
| Chronic hepatitis | Isoniazid, propylthiouracil, nitrofurantoin, minocylcine, fibrates, statins, hydralazine and methyldopa | Weeks or months | Absent or non-specific symptoms including fatigue | Hepatocellular or cholestatic of at least 6 months duration. Autoantibodies may be present | Portal inflammation, spotty lobular inflammation and necrosis, interface hepatitis, and portal fibrosis. | Chronic or slow resolution of acute injury |
| Sinusoidal obstruction syndrome | Chemotherapeutic agents including busulfan, vinca alkaloids, cyclophosphamide, melphalan, carmustine thiotepa, dacarbazine, carboplatin, cisplatin, and oxaliplatin | Acute: 1 to 3 weeks Subacute or chronic: Months and years | Typical manifestation is 1) Tender hepatomegaly, 2) sudden weight gain (>2% of body weight) From fluid retention, and ascites | Increase in AST and ALT SA and bilirubin concentration | Acute: Dilation of sinusoids and extravasation of red blood cells into the space of Disse. Subacute: Collagen deposition in sinusoids and small hepatic veins with further congestion, centrolobular necrosis, and apparent occlusion of hepatic venules. Chronic: Extensive collagenization of sinusoids and venules [107] | Can be severe and lead to acute liver failure. Patients can recover, they can also progress to cirrhosis and its complications |

(continued)

**Table 14.2** (continued)

| Clinical Phenotype | Typical agents | Latency | Clinical manifestations | Type of liver profile | Liver histology | Duration of liver injury/ prognosis |
|---|---|---|---|---|---|---|
| Nodular regenerative hyperplasia | Azathioprine, thioguanine, mercaptopurine, didanosine, stavudine, isoplatin, vitamin A | 1 to 6 years; occasionally within 6 months | Fatigue and symptoms of liver disease and hepatic synthetic dysfunction | Mild increase in AST and ALT SA | Regenerative nodules with minimal or no fibrosis | Complications of portal hypertension |
| Liver tumors and cancer | Estrogens, Thorotrast [b], Androgenic steroids | Chronic intake of agents | Liver mass: Adenomata, Angiosarcoma | Liver profile may be normal or cholestatic, from SOL | Characteristic of the type of tumor | Depending on the type of tumor and stage. |
| Immunoallergic hepatitis | sulfonamides, penicillins, macrolides, fluoroquinolones, nevirapine, efavirenz, allopurinol, or aromatic anticonvulsants. | Short, within 8 weeks, but as short as 1 to 2 days, especially with reexposure | Fever, arthralgias, rash, eosinophilia. DRESS syndrome (drug reaction with eosinophilia and systemic symptoms) can be associated with this type of hepatitis | Mixed or cholestatic pattern with increased AST and ALT and AP SA. Eosinophilia. | Hepatocellular necrosis and hepatic eosinophils | Cholestatic forms may evolve into vanishing bile duct syndrome |

| | | | | | | |
|---|---|---|---|---|---|---|
| Autoimmune hepatitis | methyldopa nitrofurantoin minocycline hydralazine fenofibrate alpha and beta interferon, infliximab, and etanercept NSAIDs, azathioprine, and herbals supplements | 2 months to years | Hepatocellular | Hepatocellular pattern, high serum [IgG] and autoimmune markers. Usually resolves in association with discontinuation of the agent | Hepatocellular necrosis with plasma cells and interface hepatitis | Discontinuation of the agent tends to be associated with resolution of the hepatitis over a month. Treatment with corticosteroids tends to be effective. Absence of relapse upon discontinuation of corticosteroids supports the diagnosis of drug-induced autoimmune hepatitis [108] |
| Immune-mediated hepatitis | Checkpoint inhibitors including nivolumab and Atezolizumab [86] | One to three months | Fatigue and pruritus. May be associated with systemic manifestations | Hepatocellular and mixed | Focal or confluent necrosis associated with lymphocytic (i.e., activated T cells) [85] | Discontinuation of the agent and intravenous steroids with oral tapering over 30 days |

(continued)

**Table 14.2** (continued)

| Clinical Phenotype | Typical agents | Latency | Clinical manifestations | Type of liver profile | Liver histology | Duration of liver injury/ prognosis |
|---|---|---|---|---|---|---|
| Granulomatous hepatitis | allopurinol carbamazepine methyldopa phenytoin quinidine sulphonamides etanercept [109] kratom [110] | Undetermined; 4 to 24 weeks documented for some drugs | Asymptomatic or fatigue and pruritus in cases of acute injury | Mixed or cholestatic | Noncaseous granulomata with eosinophils in early phases, especially in association with plasma cells on continuous exposure to the agent [84] | Recovery tends to follow drug withdrawal [111] |
| Acute liver failure | diclofenac isoniazid troglitazone telithromycin | Days to up to 6 months | Prodrome of fatigue and inappetence, jaundice, and choluria, and altered mental status | Predominantly hepatocellular, modest cholestasis, and synthetic dysfunction □ | Confluent hepatocellular necrosis with marked inflammatory activity, or without inflammation in the case of acetaminophen, cocaine, 3,4-methylenedioxy-methylamphetamine (MDMA) [112] | May be fatal and require liver transplantation NAC associated with improved transplant free survival |
| Vanishing bile duct syndrome | amoxicillin-clavulanate, NSAIDs sulfonamides aromatic anticonvulsants | | Pruritus | Cholestatic pattern and accompanied features of cholestasis including hyperlipidemia in chronicity | Bile duct injury and hepatocellular damage in early stages. Ductopenia and bile ductular proliferation. Cirrhosis in late stages [112]. | May resolve. Ductopenia and biliary cirrhosis and liver failure may develop. |

| Cirrhosis | methyldopa amiodarone valproate methotrexate | Considered from chronic (i.e., years) exposure to an agent probably from ongoing hepatitis or steatosis | Fatigue, pruritus, sarcopenia, complications of end-stage liver disease | Modest increase AST, ALT, and AP SA. Thrombocytopenia, from splenomegaly a reflection of portal hypertension | Nodules | Complications of cirrhosis |
|---|---|---|---|---|---|---|

Latency: the time from initiation of agent to onset of clinical manifestations

*ALT* alanine amino transferase, *AST* aspartate amino transferase, *SA* serum activity, *AP* alkaline phosphatase, *GGTP* gamma glutamyl transpeptidase, *ULN* upper limits of normal, *AKA* also known as, *NSAIDs* nonsteroidal anti-inflammatory drugs, *SOL* space occupying lesions

Hepatocellular pattern refers to the predominance of elevation of SA of AST and ALT

Cholestatic pattern refers to the predominance of elevation of SA of AP and GGTP

☐ no robust information available

☐ coagulopathy and low albumin

ᵃ: not in use

ᵇ: contrast agent for radiographic studies not in use

# Laboratory Exams

The pattern of liver injury has been classified as hepatocellular, cholestatic, or mixed hepatocellular and cholestatic. The R ratio is used to examine the probability of the type of liver injury, but it is not an exact determinant; it is clinical judgment and a good history that form the basis for a diagnosis of DILI. The R ratio is calculated as multiples of the upper limit of normal (ULN) for the given enzyme. The clinical phenotypes of DILI are shown in Table 14.2.

Hepatocellular injury is defined as an SA of ALT and AST, respectively more than ten times the ULN, with modest increases in SA of AP and gamma glutamyl transpeptidase (GGTP). An R ratio of ALT to AP of at least five defines the hepatocellular type of injury (Table 14.2).

Cholestatic liver injury is characterized by increased SA of AP and GGTP with minimal or modest increases of ALT and AST SAs. An R ratio of ALT to AP up to 2 defines cholestatic liver injury. The bilirubin may be high (Table 14.2).

Two types of DILI require particular attention because of their distinct features: granulomatous hepatitis and DILI secondary to immunotherapy, including checkpoint inhibitors.

Granulomatous hepatitis was reported as the least common type of histological injury pattern of DILI, 2.6%, in a retrospective study comprised of thirty-eight cases [83]. Granulomatous hepatitis has been reported in 5 to 10% of liver biopsy samples, with tuberculosis and sarcoidosis being considered the most common causes. A retrospective review documented 6% of cases of granulomatous hepatitis from 1500 cases obtained over ten years, with 29% of the cases being attributed to medications as a cause, including antihypertensive, antirheumatic, anticonvulsant, and antimicrobial agents [84] (Table 14.2).

DILI secondary to immunotherapy has emerged as a unique complication in the treatment of patients with cancer with this relatively new therapy of checkpoint inhibitors [86] and with other immunomodulators [85], including nivolumab [85, 86] (Table 14.2).

The most common pattern of DILI is a mixed liver profile, with hepatocellular and cholestatic features. The R ratio is between 2 and 5 (Table 14.2).

# Imaging Studies

A liver sonogram provides information on the liver architecture, including fat deposition, blood flow, space occupying lesions, and aspects of biliary obstruction, including intra and extrahepatic. The addition of Doppler studies increases the information regarding blood flow [2].

Computed tomography and magnetic resonance imaging (MRI) add information regarding the hepatic parenchyma and liver masses' characterization. The MRI is an excellent test to examine the intra and extrahepatic bile ducts, including strictures and dilatations [2].

## Liver Histology

A liver biopsy is not fundamental in the diagnosis of DILI, but it can help in the presence of comorbidities, confounding factors, and uncertain diagnosis. The decision to do a liver biopsy should always be individualized according to the risks versus benefits of the information from the procedure. The findings of liver histology versus the type of liver injury are reported in Table 14.2.

The histological findings associated with mild or moderate liver injury are granulomata and eosinophils, in contrast to neutrophil infiltration, marked necrosis and fibrosis, marked cholestasis in association with bile ductular proliferation, portal venopathy, and microvesicular steatosis, which are associated with severe liver injury, liver transplantation, or death [33].

## Natural History

DILI can present with acute liver failure (ALF) [2, 87]; accordingly, extreme efforts must be made to identify the drug and discontinue it. ALF is the rapid onset of hepatic synthetic dysfunction and hepatic encephalopathy in the absence of prior liver disease [88]. ALF is associated with high morbidity and mortality [88].

A sixteen-year prospective study of ALF from the United States from 1998 to 2013 enrolled 2070 patients, 69% of whom were women. DILI was the cause of ALF in 57.1%, 46.3% of which was due to acetaminophen hepatotoxicity, mostly due to accidental overdose, and 10.8% to other agents. Three notable observations were made from that study: admission to the intensive care unit increased, the use of N-acetylcysteine was not limited to acetaminophen induced ALF, and there was an increase in transplant-free survival and a decrease in liver transplantation listings for all causes of ALF, being statistically significant for ALF from acetaminophen induced DILI and other DILI cases [87].

Twenty-eight patients with a mean age of 55 years, 18 (62%) of whom were women comprised 5.7 of the 493 cases of idiosyncratic DILI reported to the Spanish registry. This group exhibited chronic changes on follow up of up to 20 months. Their liver panel was still abnormal at 3 months after discontinuing the drug associated with DILI for the hepatocellular phenotype of DILI, or more than 6 months after a cholestatic and mixed pattern of injury [89]. The most common drug classes implicated in the DILI event associated with chronicity were cardiovascular, 28.5%, and central nervous system agents, 25%, compared to their proportions in the whole DILI database, 9.8%, and 13%, respectively [89]. The most common drugs associated with DILI were amoxicillin-clavulanate, bentazepam, atorvastatin, and captopril. Nine percent of the patients with cholestatic and mixed DILI progressed to chronicity versus the 4% of hepatocellular cases, which significantly differed. Three of the patients with hepatocellular injury progressed to cirrhosis and two to chronic hepatitis. One with cholestatic and mixed injury progressed to cirrhosis, and three had documented bile duct lesions on liver histology. These data suggested that although cholestatic and mixed DILI are associated with chronicity more commonly than the hepatocellular type, the progression of the latter is of increased severity, i.e. cirrhosis [89].

A group of 59 patients, with a median age of 62 years (range 42–71) and a mean follow up of 48 weeks (range 26–96) post the DILI event, were evaluated in a clinic in Sweden. Prior to the DILI episode, nine patients had chronic liver disease from which progression was not documented on follow up. Three of the 50 (6%) without chronic liver disease had persistently abnormal liver panel not explained by another liver disease; they had been exposed to nitrofurantoin, clindamycin, and flucloxacillin, with the last two drugs having been associated with hyperbilirubinemia during the DILI occurrence. The diagnoses made de novo in patients who continued to have abnormal liver tests were nonalcoholic fatty liver disease in three and alcoholic liver disease in one. These results were interpreted to suggest that chronic liver abnormalities are uncommon long term in patients who recover from DILI [90]. However, another follow-up study from the same group reported outcomes in patients who had experienced DILI in association with hyperbilirubinemia to the Swedish Adverse Drug Reaction Advisory Committee from 1970 to 2004. This group of patients had survived the DILI event and could be linked to the Swedish Hospital Discharge and Cause of Death Registries. From the accessed group comprised of 685 patients, 23 (3.4%) had been hospitalized for liver disease, and 5 had liver related mortality, in whom the duration of treatment with the DILI implicated agent had been prolonged, 135 days, compared to those in whom liver related morbidity and mortality were not documented, 53 days, both significantly different. Autoimmune hepatitis was diagnosed in five of the 23 patients (22%) after a mean of 5.8 years of the DILI episode. Thus, although not common, liver disease with important detrimental consequences can develop after DILI in association with jaundice. A role of DILI in the triggering of subsequent hepatic complications was considered [91].

Most DILI cases from checkpoint inhibitors are reported to resolve after the triggering agent's discontinuation and treatment with steroids. Deaths have been reported in patients who have DILI in association with systemic complications and in whom there was a delay in treatment with steroids [85]. The guidelines from the EASLD provide recommendations on the management of immune-mediated liver injury from this type of drug [33].

The reintroduction of an agent after documented DILI, i.e., rechallenge, is controversial [33]. In cases of nonessential medications, this practice should be avoided.

In the context of cancer therapy, when the drug's benefits outweigh its risk for causing DILI, the expertise from internists, hepatogastroenterologists, and oncologists in concert with the will of the patient and information from the pharmaceutical companies is required. In the context of clinical trials, the advisory board should be involved. As pharmaco-oncology is fortunately an area of continuous growth, updated guidelines and the LiverToxNIH.gov website should be a frequently accessed recourse [2].

## Associated Conditions

The most common organs involved in the drug rash with eosinophilia and systemic symptoms (DRESS syndrome) is the liver and the skin, thus being part of the DILI spectrum and associated with substantial morbidity [92]. Removal of the implicated agent and steroids is the standard treatment [93]

## Treatment

The treatment of DILI is the *immediate discontinuation* of the suspected agent, providing supportive care, managing symptoms of pruritus, and evaluating for liver transplantation in liver failure cases, thus requiring close communication with a liver transplant center and early referral.

Acetaminophen overdose is treated with oral charcoal to prevent its absorption when the ingestion is documented three to four hours before the presentation. N-acetylcysteine is a modified amino acid [88], which has been extended as a treatment for ALF from causes other than acetaminophen toxicity [87]. Cysteine has antioxidant activity and is required to synthesize glutathione, an essential intracellular antioxidant, protecting against free radicals and other intracellular toxins such as intermediates of drug metabolism. Glutathione is depleted in patients with acetaminophen overdose leading to the formation of toxic adducts of acetaminophen metabolites with essential intracellular molecules [94].

In the context of ALF, the use of steroids is not the standard, including ALF from DILI; however, EASLD guidelines on DILI state: "in idiosyncratic DILI, routine use of corticosteroids treatment may not be substantiated" [33], which may leave room for their use. In a retrospective study that included 361 patients with ALF, 131 of whom had ALF from DILI, steroids were associated with what was considered a marginal beneficial effect on spontaneous survival, 35% versus 23%, but the effect was not sustained after multivariable analysis of the data [95]. The use of steroids and ursodeoxycholic acid in a group of ten patients with severe DILI was reported to decrease the SA of transaminases and bilirubin concentration by half within two weeks of treatment. Steroid therapy was tapered, and ursodeoxycholic acid was continued for several weeks [96].

Cholestyramine binds anions in the small bowel. It decreases the enterohepatic circulation of compounds, including bile acids, increasing their fecal excretion [97]. It is reported on the LiverToxNIH website that leflunomide induced DILI should be treated with cholestyramine to enhance drug clearance [98], in addition to the discontinuation of the drug.

Valproic acid treatment can be associated with hepatotoxicity [99]. Carnitine is essential in the beta-oxidation of fatty acids. Carnitine depletion is associated with impaired transport of long-chain fatty acids into the mitochondrial matrix, leading to decreased β-oxidation, acetyl-CoA, and ATP production. A decrease in β-oxidation can change the metabolism of valproic acid towards predominantly peroxisomal ω-oxidation, which is associated with an increase in the production of ω-oxidation products, including 4-en-valproic acid, a metabolite that is incriminated in valproic acid induced hepatotoxicity. The intravenous administration of carnitine is recommended for patients with valproic acid induced DILI [99, 100]

The use of N-acetylcysteine has been extended to all forms of DILI [94].

The treatment of DILI of the autoimmune phenotype is steroids, either at presentation or if a resolution is not noted within one to two weeks of diagnosis after discontinuation of the drug or if there is any evidence of hepatic synthetic dysfunction [101]. The treatment duration has not been confirmed in controlled studies; however, treatment has been suggested in doses of 20 to 60 mg orally per day to be decreased in association with improvement for three to 6 months and vigilant follow up. DILI of the autoimmune hepatitis phenotype tends not to relapse at least in a follow up of a few years after discontinuation of steroids, which supports the diagnosis of this phenotype [102].

## Prevention of Drug-Induced Liver Injury

Prevention of DILI requires vigilant monitoring to identify early liver injury and to discontinue the agent involved. Idiosyncratic DILI cannot be prevented [103]. Information about the likelihood of a drug or classes of drugs to cause DILI is very useful and can help build a DILI surveillance schedule during treatment. Knowledge regarding the documented latency to DILI in association with a newly prescribed drug reported to cause liver injury is an excellent practice to incorporate for the clinician to establish a monitoring schedule. In patients with liver disease, the author monitors liver tests two weeks after initiation of any therapy, and subsequently, in an individualized manner, depending on the drug and the patient.

The American Thoracic Society has provided guidelines to detect hepatotoxicity. However, the frequency of monitoring has not been established. Every two to four weeks at the start with spaced out testing subsequently was suggested. Its recommendation is that "Treatment should be interrupted and …. a modified or alternative regimen used for those with ALT elevation more than three times the upper limit of normal (ULN) in the presence of hepatitis symptoms and/or jaundice, or five times the ULN in the absence of symptoms" [104].

The importance of accessing the NIHLiverTox.gov website [2] and the recently upgraded Drug-induced liver injury severity and toxicity list cannot be overemphasized [105]. A genetic, cellular, organoid, and human-scale evidence testing platform to identify drugs associated with DILI has been developed [106]. Its use in drug development and clinical trials may facilitate the production of safe medications.

# References

1. Zimmerman HJ. Drug-induced liver injury. In: Zimmerman HJ, editor. Hepatotoxicity: the adverse effects of drugs and other chemicals on the liver; 1999. p. 427–56.
2. NIH. LiverTox: clinical and research information on drug-induced liver injury [Internet]. Bethesda (MD): National Institute of Diabetes and Digestive and Kidney Diseases; 2012-. Clinical Course and Diagnosis of Drug Induced Liver Disease. [Updated 2019 May 4]. Available from: https://www.ncbi.nlm.nih.gov/books/NBK548733/ 2019 [cited 2021 1/04/2021]. Available from: http://www.ncbi.nlm.nih.gov/books/NBK548733/.
3. Francis P, Navarro VJ. Drug induced hepatotoxicity. StatPearls. Treasure Island FL: © 2020, StatPearls Publishing LLC; 2020.
4. Hayashi PH, Fontana RJ. Clinical features, diagnosis, and natural history of drug-induced liver injury. Semin Liver Dis. 2014 May;34(2):134–44.
5. Lauschke VM, Zhou Y, Ingelman-Sundberg M. Novel genetic and epigenetic factors of importance for inter-individual differences in drug disposition, response and toxicity. Pharmacol Ther. 2019 May;197:122–52.
6. Monshi MM, Faulkner L, Gibson A, Jenkins RE, Farrell J, Earnshaw CJ, et al. Human leukocyte antigen (HLA)-B*57:01-restricted activation of drug-specific T cells provides the immunological basis for flucloxacillin-induced liver injury. Hepatology (Baltimore, Md). 2013 Feb;57(2):727–39.
7. Daly AK, Donaldson PT, Bhatnagar P, Shen Y, Pe'er I, Floratos A, et al. HLA-B*5701 genotype is a major determinant of drug-induced liver injury due to flucloxacillin. Nat Genet. 2009 Jul;41(7):816–9.
8. Hautekeete ML, Horsmans Y, Van Waeyenberge C, Demanet C, Henrion J, Verbist L, et al. HLA association of amoxicillin-clavulanate--induced hepatitis. Gastroenterology. 1999 Nov;117(5):1181–6.
9. Lucena MI, Molokhia M, Shen Y, Urban TJ, Aithal GP, Andrade RJ, et al. Susceptibility to amoxicillin-clavulanate-induced liver injury is influenced by multiple HLA class I and II alleles. Gastroenterology. 2011 Jul;141(1):338–47.
10. Sharma SK, Balamurugan A, Saha PK, Pandey RM, Mehra NK. Evaluation of clinical and immunogenetic risk factors for the development of hepatotoxicity during antituberculosis treatment. Am J Respir Crit Care Med. 2002 Oct 1;166(7):916–9.
11. Urban TJ, Daly AK, Aithal GP. Genetic basis of drug-induced liver injury: present and future. Semin Liver Dis. 2014 May;34(2):123–33.
12. Ahmadian M, Suh JM, Hah N, Liddle C, Atkins AR, Downes M, et al. PPARγ signaling and metabolism: the good, the bad and the future. Nat Med. 2013 May;19(5):557–66.
13. Ceccarelli F, Agmon-Levin N, Perricone C. Genetic factors of autoimmune diseases 2017. J Immunol Res. 2017;2017:2789242.
14. Urban TJ, Shen Y, Stolz A, Chalasani N, Fontana RJ, Rochon J, et al. Limited contribution of common genetic variants to risk for liver injury due to a variety of drugs. Pharmacogenet Genomics. 2012 Nov;22(11):784–95.

15. Danielson PB. The cytochrome P450 superfamily: biochemistry, evolution and drug metabolism in humans. Curr Drug Metab. 2002 Dec;3(6):561–97.

16. Rowland A, Miners JO, Mackenzie PI. The UDP-glucuronosyltransferases: their role in drug metabolism and detoxification. Int J Biochem Cell Biol. 2013 Jun;45(6):1121–32.

17. Sim E, Abuhammad A, Ryan A. Arylamine N-acetyltransferases: from drug metabolism and pharmacogenetics to drug discovery. Br J Pharmacol. 2014 Jun;171(11):2705–25.

18. Sheehan D, Meade G, Foley VM, Dowd CA. Structure, function and evolution of glutathione transferases: implications for classification of non-mammalian members of an ancient enzyme superfamily. Biochem J. 2001 Nov 15;360(Pt 1):1–16.

19. Huang YS, Chern HD, Su WJ, Wu JC, Chang SC, Chiang CH, et al. Cytochrome P450 2E1 genotype and the susceptibility to antituberculosis drug-induced hepatitis. Hepatology (Baltimore, Md). 2003 Apr;37(4):924–30.

20. Daly AK, Aithal GP, Leathart JB, Swainsbury RA, Dang TS, Day CP. Genetic susceptibility to diclofenac-induced hepatotoxicity: contribution of UGT2B7, CYP2C8, and ABCC2 genotypes. Gastroenterology. 2007 Jan;132(1):272–81.

21. Chan SL, Chua APG, Aminkeng F, Chee CBE, Jin S, Loh M, et al. Association and clinical utility of NAT2 in the prediction of isoniazid-induced liver injury in Singaporean patients. PLoS One. 2017;12(10):e0186200.

22. Watanabe I, Tomita A, Shimizu M, Sugawara M, Yasumo H, Koishi R, et al. A study to survey susceptible genetic factors responsible for troglitazone-associated hepatotoxicity in Japanese patients with type 2 diabetes mellitus. Clin Pharmacol Ther. 2003 May;73(5):435–55.

23. Lucena MI, Andrade RJ, Martínez C, Ulzurrun E, García-Martín E, Borraz Y, et al. Glutathione S-transferase m1 and t1 null genotypes increase susceptibility to idiosyncratic drug-induced liver injury. Hepatology (Baltimore, Md). 2008 Aug;48(2):588–96.

24. Nicoletti P, Devarbhavi H, Goel A, Venkatesan R, Eapen CE, Grove J, et al. Genetic risk factors in drug-induced liver injury due to isoniazid-containing Antituberculosis drug regimens. Clin Pharmacol Ther. 2020 Nov 1;

25. Patel M, Taskar KS, Zamek-Gliszczynski MJ. Importance of hepatic transporters in clinical disposition of drugs and their metabolites. J Clin Pharmacol. 2016 Jul;56(Suppl 7):S23–39.

26. Taniguchi K, Wada M, Kohno K, Nakamura T, Kawabe T, Kawakami M, et al. A human canalicular multispecific organic anion transporter (cMOAT) gene is overexpressed in cisplatin-resistant human cancer cell lines with decreased drug accumulation. Cancer Res. 1996 Sep 15;56(18):4124–9.

27. Hodges LM, Markova SM, Chinn LW, Gow JM, Kroetz DL, Klein TE, et al. Very important pharmacogene summary: ABCB1 (MDR1, P-glycoprotein). Pharmacogenet Genomics. 2011 Mar;21(3):152–61.

28. Haas DW, Bartlett JA, Andersen JW, Sanne I, Wilkinson GR, Hinkle J, et al. Pharmacogenetics of nevirapine-associated hepatotoxicity: an adult AIDS Clinical Trials Group collaboration. Clin Infect Dis. 2006 Sep 15;43(6):783.

29. Daly AK. Human leukocyte antigen (HLA) pharmacogenomic tests: potential and pitfalls. Curr Drug Metab. 2014 Feb;15(2):196–201.

30. Chalasani N, Bonkovsky HL, Fontana R, Lee W, Stolz A, Talwalkar J, et al. Features and outcomes of 899 patients with drug-induced liver injury: the DILIN prospective study. Gastroenterology. 2015 Jun;148(7):1340–52 e7.

31. Lucena MI, Andrade RJ, Kaplowitz N, García-Cortes M, Fernández MC, Romero-Gomez M, et al. Phenotypic characterization of idiosyncratic drug-induced liver injury: the influence of age and sex. Hepatology (Baltimore, Md). 2009 Jun;49(6):2001–9.

32. Björnsson ES, Bergmann OM, Björnsson HK, Kvaran RB, Olafsson S. Incidence, presentation, and outcomes in patients with drug-induced liver injury in the general population of Iceland. Gastroenterology. 2013;144(7):1419–25. 25 e1-3; quiz e19-20

33. EASLD. EASL clinical practice guidelines: drug-induced liver injury. J Hepatol. 2019 Jun;70(6):1222–61.

34. Fountain FF, Tolley E, Chrisman CR, Self TH. Isoniazid hepatotoxicity associated with treatment of latent tuberculosis infection: a 7-year evaluation from a public health tuberculosis clinic. Chest. 2005 Jul;128(1):116–23.
35. Bryant AE 3rd, Dreifuss FE. Valproic acid hepatic fatalities. III. U.S. experience since 1986. Neurology. 1996 Feb;46(2):465–9.
36. Floreani A, Restrepo-Jiménez P, Secchi MF, De Martin S, Leung PSC, Krawitt E, et al. Etiopathogenesis of autoimmune hepatitis. J Autoimmun. 2018 Dec;95:133–43.
37. Lleo A, Wang GQ, Gershwin ME, Hirschfield GM. Primary biliary cholangitis. Lancet (London, England). 2020 Dec 12;396(10266):1915–26.
38. Watkins PB, Kaplowitz N, Slattery JT, Colonese CR, Colucci SV, Stewart PW, et al. Aminotransferase elevations in healthy adults receiving 4 grams of acetaminophen daily: a randomized controlled trial. JAMA. 2006 Jul 5;296(1):87–93.
39. Chalasani N, Reddy KRK, Fontana RJ, Barnhart H, Gu J, Hayashi PH, et al. Idiosyncratic drug induced liver injury in African-Americans is associated with greater morbidity and mortality compared to Caucasians. Am J Gastroenterol. 2017 Sep;112(9):1382–8.
40. Cai Y, Yi J, Zhou C, Shen X. Pharmacogenetic study of drug-metabolising enzyme polymorphisms on the risk of anti-tuberculosis drug-induced liver injury: a meta-analysis. PLoS One. 2012;7(10):e47769.
41. Zimmerman HJ. Hepatotoxic effects of ethanol. Hepatotoxicity: the adverse effects of drugs and other chemicals on the liver; 1999. p. 147–75.
42. Akhondi-Meybodi M, Mortazavy-Zadah MR, Hashemian Z, Moaiedi M. Incidence and risk factors for non-alcoholic steatohepatitis in females treated with tamoxifen for breast cancer. Arab J Gastroenterol. 2011 Mar;12(1):34–6.
43. Bruno S, Maisonneuve P, Castellana P, Rotmensz N, Rossi S, Maggioni M, et al. Incidence and risk factors for non-alcoholic steatohepatitis: prospective study of 5408 women enrolled in Italian tamoxifen chemoprevention trial. BMJ (Clin Res ed). 2005 Apr 23;330(7497):932.
44. Dawwas MF, Aithal GP. End-stage methotrexate-related liver disease is rare and associated with features of the metabolic syndrome. Aliment Pharmacol Ther. 2014 Oct;40(8):938–48.
45. Kaplan MM. Methotrexate hepatotoxicity and the premature reporting of mark Twain's death: both greatly exaggerated. Hepatology (Baltimore, Md). 1990 Oct;12(4 Pt 1):784–6.
46. Servoss JC, Kitch DW, Andersen JW, Reisler RB, Chung RT, Robbins GK. Predictors of antiretroviral-related hepatotoxicity in the adult AIDS clinical trial group (1989-1999). J Acquir Immune Defic Syndr. 2006 Nov 1;43(3):320–3.
47. Dworkin MS, Adams MR, Cohn DL, Davidson AJ, Buskin S, Horwitch C, et al. Factors that complicate the treatment of tuberculosis in HIV-infected patients. J Acquir Immune Defic Syndr. 2005 Aug 1;39(4):464–70.
48. Kim WS, Lee SS, Lee CM, Kim HJ, Ha CY, Kim HJ, et al. Hepatitis C and not hepatitis B virus is a risk factor for anti-tuberculosis drug induced liver injury. BMC Infect Dis. 2016 Feb 1;16:50.
49. Kullak-Ublick GA, Andrade RJ, Merz M, End P, Benesic A, Gerbes AL, et al. Drug-induced liver injury: recent advances in diagnosis and risk assessment. Gut. 2017 Jun;66(6):1154–64.
50. Lammert C, Einarsson S, Saha C, Niklasson A, Bjornsson E, Chalasani N. Relationship between daily dose of oral medications and idiosyncratic drug-induced liver injury: search for signals. Hepatology (Baltimore, Md). 2008 Jun;47(6):2003–9.
51. Park BK, Boobis A, Clarke S, Goldring CE, Jones D, Kenna JG, et al. Managing the challenge of chemically reactive metabolites in drug development. Nat Rev Drug Discov. 2011 Apr;10(4):292–306.
52. Srivastava A, Maggs JL, Antoine DJ, Williams DP, Smith DA, Park BK. Role of reactive metabolites in drug-induced hepatotoxicity. Handb Exp Pharmacol. 2010;196:165–94.
53. Lammert C, Bjornsson E, Niklasson A, Chalasani N. Oral medications with significant hepatic metabolism at higher risk for hepatic adverse events. Hepatology (Baltimore, Md). 2010 Feb;51(2):615–20.

54. Chen M, Borlak J, Tong W. High lipophilicity and high daily dose of oral medications are associated with significant risk for drug-induced liver injury. Hepatology (Baltimore, Md). 2013 Jul;58(1):388–96.

55. Mishra P, Chen M. Direct-acting antivirals for chronic hepatitis C: can drug properties signal potential for liver injury? Gastroenterology. 2017 May;152(6):1270–4.

56. Weng Z, Wang K, Li H, Shi Q. A comprehensive study of the association between drug hepatotoxicity and daily dose, liver metabolism, and lipophilicity using 975 oral medications. Oncotarget. 2015 Jul 10;6(19):17031–8.

57. Steele MA, Burk RF, DesPrez RM. Toxic hepatitis with isoniazid and rifampin. A Meta-Analysis Chest. 1991 Feb;99(2):465–71.

58. Gopaul S, Farrell K, Abbott F. Effects of age and polytherapy, risk factors of valproic acid (VPA) hepatotoxicity, on the excretion of thiol conjugates of (E)-2,4-diene VPA in people with epilepsy taking VPA. Epilepsia. 2003 Mar;44(3):322–8.

59. Vuda M, Kamath A. Drug induced mitochondrial dysfunction: mechanisms and adverse clinical consequences. Mitochondrion. 2016 Nov;31:63–74.

60. McKenzie R, Fried MW, Sallie R, Conjeevaram H, Di Bisceglie AM, Park Y, et al. Hepatic failure and lactic acidosis due to fialuridine (FIAU), an investigational nucleoside analogue for chronic hepatitis B. N Engl J Med. 1995 Oct 26;333(17):1099–105.

61. Will Y, Dykens J. Mitochondrial toxicity assessment in industry--a decade of technology development and insight. Expert Opin Drug Metab Toxicol. 2014 Aug;10(8):1061–7.

62. Montessori V, Harris M, Montaner JS. Hepatotoxicity of nucleoside reverse transcriptase inhibitors. Semin Liver Dis. 2003 May;23(2):167–72.

63. Morgan RE, Trauner M, van Staden CJ, Lee PH, Ramachandran B, Eschenberg M, et al. Interference with bile salt export pump function is a susceptibility factor for human liver injury in drug development. Toxicological Sci. 2010 Dec;118(2):485–500.

64. Kostrubsky SE, Strom SC, Kalgutkar AS, Kulkarni S, Atherton J, Mireles R, et al. Inhibition of hepatobiliary transport as a predictive method for clinical hepatotoxicity of nefazodone. Toxicological Sci. 2006 Apr;90(2):451–9.

65. McRae MP, Lowe CM, Tian X, Bourdet DL, Ho RH, Leake BF, et al. Ritonavir, saquinavir, and efavirenz, but not nevirapine, inhibit bile acid transport in human and rat hepatocytes. J Pharmacol Exp Ther. 2006 Sep;318(3):1068–75.

66. Fattinger K, Funk C, Pantze M, Weber C, Reichen J, Stieger B, et al. The endothelin antagonist bosentan inhibits the canalicular bile salt export pump: a potential mechanism for hepatic adverse reactions. Clin Pharmacol Ther. 2001 Apr;69(4):223–31.

67. Andrade RJ, Lucena MI, Fernández MC, Pelaez G, Pachkoria K, García-Ruiz E, et al. Drug-induced liver injury: an analysis of 461 incidences submitted to the Spanish registry over a 10-year period. Gastroenterology. 2005 Aug;129(2):512–21.

68. Navarro VJ, Khan I, Björnsson E, Seeff LB, Serrano J, Hoofnagle JH. Liver injury from herbal and dietary supplements. Hepatology (Baltimore, Md). 2017 Jan;65(1):363–73.

69. Davern TJ, Chalasani N, Fontana RJ, Hayashi PH, Protiva P, Kleiner DE, et al. Acute hepatitis E infection accounts for some cases of suspected drug-induced liver injury. Gastroenterology. 2011 Nov;141(5):1665–72 e1-9.

70. Teschke R, Danan G. Drug induced liver injury with analysis of alternative causes as confounding variables. Br J Clin Pharmacol. 2018 Jul;84(7):1467–77.

71. Waseem N, Chen PH. Hypoxic hepatitis: a review and clinical update. J Clin Transl Hepatol. 2016 Sep 28;4(3):263–8.

72. Frech TM, Mar D. Gastrointestinal and hepatic disease in systemic sclerosis. Rheum Dis Clin N Am. 2018 Feb;44(1):15–28.

73. Correale M, Tricarico L, Leopizzi A, Mallardi A, Mazzeo P, Tucci S, et al. Liver disease and heart failure. Panminerva Med. 2020 Mar;62(1):26–37.

74. Garcia-Cortes M, Robles-Diaz M, Stephens C, Ortega-Alonso A, Lucena MI, Andrade RJ. Drug induced liver injury: an update. Arch Toxicol. 2020 Oct;94(10):3381–407.

75. Sandhu N, Navarro V. Drug-induced liver injury in GI practice. Hepatology Comm. 2020 May;4(5):631–45.
76. Danan G, Benichou C. Causality assessment of adverse reactions to drugs--I. a novel method based on the conclusions of international consensus meetings: application to drug-induced liver injuries. J Clin Epidemiol. 1993 Nov;46(11):1323–30.
77. Maria VA, Victorino RM. Development and validation of a clinical scale for the diagnosis of drug-induced hepatitis. Hepatology (Baltimore, Md). 1997 Sep;26(3):664–9.
78. Rockey DC, Seeff LB, Rochon J, Freston J, Chalasani N, Bonacini M, et al. Causality assessment in drug-induced liver injury using a structured expert opinion process: comparison to the Roussel-Uclaf causality assessment method. Hepatology (Baltimore, Md). 2010 Jun;51(6):2117–26.
79. NIH. In: Charles Sprecher Davidson CML, Earl C. Chamberlayne, editor. Guidelines for detection of hepatotoxicity due to drugs and chemicals: NIH publication 79–313. U.S. Dept of Health, Education, and Welfare, Public Health Service, National Institutes of Health; 1979; 1979.
80. Reuben A. Hy's law. Hepatology (Baltimore, Md). 2004 Feb;39(2):574–8.
81. Administration FD. Guidance for industry. Premarketing Clinical, Evaluation: Drug-Induced Liver Injury; 2009.
82. Robles-Diaz M, Lucena MI, Kaplowitz N, Stephens C, Medina-Cáliz I, González-Jimenez A, et al. Use of Hy's law and a new composite algorithm to predict acute liver failure in patients with drug-induced liver injury. Gastroenterology. 2014 Jul;147(1):109–18 e5.
83. Siddique AS, Siddique O, Einstein M, Urtasun-Sotil E, Ligato S. Drug and herbal/dietary supplements-induced liver injury: a tertiary care center experience. World J Hepatol. 2020 May 27;12(5):207–19.
84. McMaster KR 3rd, Hennigar GR. Drug-induced granulomatous hepatitis. Laboratory Investigation. 1981 Jan;44(1):61–73.
85. NIH. Nivolumab 2016. Available from: LiverTox: clinical and research information on drug-induced liver injury [Internet]. Bethesda (MD): National Institute of Diabetes and Digestive and Kidney Diseases; 2012-. Nivolumab. [Updated 2016 May 1]. Available from: https://www.ncbi.nlm.nih.gov/books/NBK548206/.
86. NIH. Atezolizumab 2016. Available from: LiverTox: clinical and research information on drug-induced liver injury [Internet]. Bethesda (MD): National Institute of Diabetes and Digestive and Kidney Diseases; 2012-. Atezolizumab. [Updated 2016 Dec 6]. Available from: https://www.ncbi.nlm.nih.gov/books/NBK548858/.
87. Reuben A, Tillman H, Fontana RJ, Davern T, McGuire B, Stravitz RT, et al. Outcomes in adults with acute liver failure between 1998 and 2013: an observational cohort study. Ann Intern Med. 2016 Jun 7;164(11):724–32.
88. Polson J, Lee WM. AASLD position paper: the management of acute liver failure. Hepatology (Baltimore, Md). 2005 May;41(5):1179–97.
89. Andrade RJ, Lucena MI, Kaplowitz N, García-Muṇoz B, Borraz Y, Pachkoria K, et al. Outcome of acute idiosyncratic drug-induced liver injury: long-term follow-up in a hepatotoxicity registry. Hepatology (Baltimore, Md). 2006 Dec;44(6):1581–8.
90. Björnsson E, Kalaitzakis E, Av Klinteberg V, Alem N, Olsson R. Long-term follow-up of patients with mild to moderate drug-induced liver injury. Aliment Pharmacol Ther. 2007 Jul 1;26(1):79–85.
91. Björnsson E, Davidsdottir L. The long-term follow-up after idiosyncratic drug-induced liver injury with jaundice. J Hepatol. 2009 Mar;50(3):511–7.
92. Isaacs M, Cardones AR, Rahnama-Moghadam S. DRESS syndrome: clinical myths and pearls. Cutis. 2018 Nov;102(5):322–6.
93. Martínez-Cabriales SA, Rodríguez-Bolaños F, Shear NH. Drug reaction with eosinophilia and systemic symptoms (DReSS): how far have we come? Am J Clin Dermatol. 2019 Apr;20(2):217–36.

94. NIH. Acetylcysteine 2016. Available from: LiverTox: clinical and research information on drug-induced liver injury [Internet]. Bethesda (MD): National Institute of Diabetes and Digestive and Kidney Diseases; 2012-. Acetylcysteine. [Updated 2016 Nov 7]. Available from: https://www.ncbi.nlm.nih.gov/books/NBK548401/.
95. Karkhanis J, Verna EC, Chang MS, Stravitz RT, Schilsky M, Lee WM, et al. Steroid use in acute liver failure. Hepatology (Baltimore, Md). 2014 Feb;59(2):612–21.
96. Wree A, Dechêne A, Herzer K, Hilgard P, Syn WK, Gerken G, et al. Steroid and ursodes-oxycholic acid combination therapy in severe drug-induced liver injury. Digestion. 2011;84(1):54–9.
97. Thompson WG. Cholestyramine. Can Med Assoc J. 1971 Feb 20;104(4):305–9.
98. NIH. Leflunomide 2019. Available from: LiverTox: clinical and research information on drug-induced liver injury [Internet]. Bethesda (MD): National Institute of Diabetes and Digestive and Kidney Diseases; 2012-. Leflunomide. [Updated 2019 Apr 15]. Available from: https://www.ncbi.nlm.nih.gov/books/NBK548725/.
99. Lheureux PE, Penaloza A, Zahir S, Gris M. Science review: carnitine in the treatment of valproic acid-induced toxicity–what is the evidence? Crit Care. 2005 Oct 5;9(5):431–40.
100. NIH. Valproate 2020. Available from: LiverTox: clinical and research information on drug-induced liver injury [Internet]. Bethesda (MD): National Institute of Diabetes and Digestive and Kidney Diseases; 2012-. Valproate. [Updated 2020 Jul 31]. Available from: https://www.ncbi.nlm.nih.gov/books/NBK548284/.
101. Castiella A, Zapata E, Lucena MI, Andrade RJ. Drug-induced autoimmune liver disease: A diagnostic dilemma of an increasingly reported disease. World J Hepatol. 2014;6(4):160–8.
102. Björnsson ES, Bergmann O, Jonasson JG, Grondal G, Gudbjornsson B, Olafsson S. Drug-induced autoimmune hepatitis: response to corticosteroids and lack of relapse after cessation of steroids. Clin Gastroenterol Hepatol. 2017 Oct;15(10):1635–6.
103. Chen M, Borlak J, Tong W. Predicting idiosyncratic drug-induced liver injury: some recent advances. Expert Rev Gastroenterol Hepatol. 2014 Sep;8(7):721–3.
104. Saukkonen JJ, Cohn DL, Jasmer RM, Schenker S, Jereb JA, Nolan CM, et al. An official ATS statement: hepatotoxicity of antituberculosis therapy. Am J Respir Crit Care Med. 2006 Oct 15;174(8):935–52.
105. Thakkar S, Li T, Liu Z, Wu L, Roberts R, Tong W. Drug-induced liver injury severity and toxicity (DILIst): binary classification of 1279 drugs by human hepatotoxicity. Drug Discov Today. 2020 Jan;25(1):201–8.
106. Koido M, Kawakami E, Fukumura J, Noguchi Y, Ohori M, Nio Y, et al. Polygenic architecture informs potential vulnerability to drug-induced liver injury. Nat Med. 2020 Oct;26(10):1541–8.
107. DeLeve LD, Shulman HM, McDonald GB. Toxic injury to hepatic sinusoids: sinusoidal obstruction syndrome (veno-occlusive disease). Semin Liver Dis. 2002;22(1):27–42.
108. Czaja AJ. Drug-induced autoimmune-like hepatitis. Dig Dis Sci. 2011;56(4):958–76.
109. Peixoto A, Martins Rocha T, Santos-Antunes J, Aguiar F, Bernardes M, Vaz C, et al. Etanercept-induced granulomatous hepatitis as a rare cause of abnormal liver tests. Acta Gastroenterol Belg. 2019;82(1):93–5.
110. Aldyab M, Ells PF, Bui R, Chapman TD, Lee H. Kratom-Induced Cholestatic Liver Injury Mimicking Anti-Mitochondrial Antibody-Negative Primary Biliary Cholangitis: A Case Report and Review of Literature. Gastroenterology Res. 2019;12(4):211–5.
111. Ishak KG, Zimmerman HJ. Drug-induced and toxic granulomatous hepatitis. Baillieres Clin Gastroenterol. 1988;2(2):463–80.
112. Ramachandran R, Kakar S. Histological patterns in drug-induced liver disease. J Clin Pathol. 2009;62(6):481–92.

# Chapter 15
# Complications of Liver Disease

Nora V. Bergasa

## Pruritus

The pruritus or itch of liver disease is considered to be secondary to cholestasis. Cholestasis is defined as impaired secretion of bile [1]. Cholestasis is a complication of all types of liver diseases; however, pruritus is more prevalent in conditions primarily due to cholangiopathies, where cholestasis can be profound.

The etiology of the pruritus of cholestasis is unknown. The ideas that have prevailed concern the accumulation of bile acids and increased opioidergic tone [2]. A role of autotaxin and lysophosphatidic acid in the pruritus of cholestasis has been proposed [2].

Pruritus is always annoying. The pruritus of cholestasis can be mild, without major interference with regular activities, moderate, prompting patients to seek therapeutic intervention, and severe and intractable, leading to sleep deprivation. The pruritus of cholestasis is not readily relieved by scratching; this characteristic stimulates the patients to scratch with abrasive objects such as forks, knives, and hairbrushes. It can be generalized or localized to particular parts of the body, particularly the palms of the hands and the soles of the feet where the symptom is often first perceived. The perception of pruritus of cholestasis varies considerably among patients, and it does not appear to correlate with serum biochemical parameters of liver disease. This form of pruritus can be persistent or intermittent. The perception of pruritus may be influenced by various factors, such as changes in mood and distractions. It can be exacerbated by normal physiologic changes such as the premenstrual state in women; therefore, it is essential to obtain this information during the clinical interview.

N. V. Bergasa (✉)
Department of Medicine, H+H/Metropolitan, New York, NY, USA

New York Medical College, Valhalla, NY, USA

Hepatology, H+H/Woodhull, Brooklyn, NY, USA

N. V. Bergasa (ed.), *Clinical Cases in Hepatology*,
https://doi.org/10.1007/978-1-4471-4715-2_15

The treatment of pruritus secondary to cholestasis can be classified according to the presumed antipruritic mechanism of the intervention.

Specific treatment of liver disease associated with cure should resolve the pruritus because cholestasis would decrease or disappear. For example, in cases of pruritus from biliary obstruction, e.g., common duct stone, the removal of the obstruction is associated with the relief of pruritus. However, cholestasis from liver inflammation and ductopenia from cholangiopathies including primary biliary cholangitis (PBC), primary sclerosing cholangitis (PSC), and cholestasis from congenital conditions are chronic and can be associated with intermittent or chronic pruritus in a substantial proportion of patients; thus, specific treatments for pruritus are necessary, in the absence of a cure of the primary liver disease. Treatments of pruritus have evolved based on what is believed to be its cause. Often, however, there is no clear rationale supporting the use of certain interventions. In addition, the exclusive use of subjective methodology to assess the effect of therapeutic interventions on pruritus makes it difficult to interpret data from clinical studies, including those that are placebo-controlled, as the placebo effect is strong.

Pruritus is a perception, and, as a perception, it cannot be directly measured; in contrast, scratching activity, the behavioral manifestation of pruritus, can be recorded independently from gross body movements. Thus, the inclusion of behavioral methodology in clinical trials of pruritus offers the opportunity to obtain objective, analyzable data, and it should be part of the design of clinical studies.

The development of effective treatments for pruritus is desperately needed. In this chapter, some of the interventions used to treat the pruritus of cholestasis are described according to their presumed aim.

## *Therapies that Aim at the Removal of the Pruritogenic Substances(s) from the Body*

Cholestyramine is a nonabsorbable resin used to treat hypercholesterolemia [3]. It is believed that the pruritogenic substances or cofactors to the pruritogens are made in the liver and excreted in bile, and as a result of cholestasis, accumulate in tissues. The presumed aim of resins, which also include colestipol and colesevelam, is to increase the excretion of pruritogen(s) in feces, that may include bile acids; however, many patients with pruritus from cholestasis who report relief on cholestyramine at the start of treatment report recurrence of pruritus after some time on the medication. This observation tends to suggest some tolerance to the drug, which may be a form of receptor-mediated tachyphylaxis.

In a single-blind, open-label, placebo-controlled crossover trial of 6–32 months duration cholestyramine at doses between 3.3 and 12 g orally per day was associated with relief of pruritus in 23 of 27 patients as compared to an observational control group that did not receive cholestyramine, but that received norethandrolone or no treatment [4]. There is a clinical consensus supporting that the administration of cholestyramine is associated with the amelioration of pruritus in many patients with cholestasis, including patients with PBC [4, 5]. The maximum recommended dose of cholestyramine is 16 g per day, 4 g per dose. In patients with the gallbladder in situ, there is a rationale to administer the resins immediately before and after breakfast because it is inferred that the pruritogen(s) is excreted in bile and that it accumulates in the gallbladder during the overnight fast; extra doses with lunch and dinner may be added if there is no satisfactory effect with the first two doses. In general, cholestyramine is well tolerated, although some patients report bloating, constipation, and diarrhea. It is recommended that other prescribed medications be taken at least 2 hours apart from the resins, as they can interfere with the absorption of other drugs. The administration of cholestyramine interferes with the absorption of fat-soluble vitamins, which are malabsorbed in cholestasis; thus, assessing for deficiencies of these vitamins and coagulation profile, a reflection of vitamin K deficiency (i.e., prothrombin time) is prudent during long-term treatment with cholestyramine.

In a meta-analysis that addressed the efficacy and safety of bile acid-binding agents [6], the inclusion criteria of the identified studies were described as heterogeneous, not allowing for combination and proper analysis of the data [6].

GSK2330672 is a selective inhibitor of human ileal bile acid transporter (IBAT), preventing the enterohepatic circulation of bile acids. GSK2330672 was studied in 22 patients with pruritus from PBC in a phase 2a, double-blind, randomized, placebo-controlled, crossover study. The drug was reported to be associated with a significant decrease in baseline "itch scores" of $-57\%$ (95% Confidence Interval (CI), $-73$ to $-42$, $p < 0.0001$), a $-31\%$ ($-42$ to $-20$, $p < 0.0001$) decreased in the itch domain of the PBC 40 questionnaire, suggestive of improvement, and a $-35\%$ ($-45$ to $-25$, $p < 0.0001$) decrease in the 5-D itch scale, which includes findings in physical examination pertinent to excoriations from scratching. There was a significant reduction in the serum total bile acid concentrations in association with the drug. Diarrhea was reported as a limiting factor in the long-term use of this medication [7]. Odevixibat is a drug reported to be associated with a decrease in pruritus in children with progressive familial intrahepatic cholestasis, recently approved for this clinical indication [8].

Invasive procedures have been used to treat patients with intractable pruritus. A transient relief from pruritus has been reported in association with anion adsorption and plasma separation [9], and the extracorporeal liver support systems Prometheus ™ and MARS ™ [10–14]. These interventions may never be submitted to controlled clinical trials because of their nature; however, the tremendous need to provide relief to patients with severe pruritus supports the use of this type of intervention by experienced operators in a controlled environment. The placebo effect of these interventions may be substantial and the relief provided temporary [11].

Reports of relief of the pruritus have also been published in association with nasobiliary drainage [15], partial internal diversion of bile in patients with progressive familial intrahepatic cholestasis [16] (see above), and partial external diversion of bile [17, 18] and ileal diversion in children with cholestasis [19], in whom an improvement in quality of life was also reported.

## Antibiotics

Rifampicin is an antibiotic, and an enzyme inducer reported to increase 2 hr. post prandial serum levels of bile acids in patients with cirrhosis of the liver [20]. A study that assessed the enzyme-inducing effect of rifampicin in patients with liver disease reported an improvement in their pruritus [21]. Rifampicin has been studied to treat pruritus in patients with PBC in several clinical studies, none of which had comparable designs [22–24]. One double-blind, randomized placebo-controlled crossover study of 4 weeks duration studied the effect of rifampicin at doses of 150 mg by mouth twice a day for patients with serum bilirubin greater than 3 mg/dl, and 150 mg three times a day for patients with serum bilirubin lower than 3 mg /dl in nine patients with PBC. Rifampicin was reported to be associated with a significant decrease in the 7-day aggregated visual analog score for pruritus [22]. In one study, rifampicin was reported to be more effective than phenobarbital in inducing amelioration of pruritus [23]. Two published meta-analyses have reported that rifampicin administration is associated with relief of pruritus in cholestasis [6, 25] and that in short term, the side effects were not major and disappeared after discontinuation of the drug. Side effects of rifampicin, however, remain a serious concern [23, 26] as cases of hepatitis and hepatic failure have been associated with rifampicin administration over periods longer than reported in some publications [22–24]; therefore, if rifampicin is prescribed, close and regular follow-up of blood tests, including liver panel, is necessary.

The mechanism of the reported antipruritic effect of rifampicin is unknown. Rifampicin is an agonist ligand of the pregnane X receptor, the stimulation of which induces drug-metabolizing enzymes and transporters [27]; thus, rifampicin administration may result in the relief of pruritus by stimulating the intrahepatic metabolizing pathways, leading to the metabolism and excretion of substances, including the pruritogen(s). In addition, it may have opiate antagonist activity [28].

## Changes in Neurotransmission

### Opiate Antagonists

The pharmacological increase in opioidergic tone, e.g., after the intrathecal administration of morphine in clinical medicine, is associated with pruritus [29, 30]. This type of pruritus is prevented and ameliorated by opiate antagonists, suggesting an opioid-receptor mediated effect [31, 32]. There is also evidence to suggest that in cholestasis, there is an increased opioidergic tone [33]; thus, this altered neurotransmission may mediate the pruritus. If increased opioidergic tone mediates the pruritus of cholestasis, opiate antagonist drugs such as naloxone should decrease the pruritus and its behavioral manifestation, scratching activity. The effect of intravenous naloxone infusions on hourly scratching activity was studied in a double-blind, randomized placebo-controlled, crossover study of four consecutive days duration in 29 patients with cholestasis and pruritus, 19 of whom had PBC [34]. Naloxone infusions at a dose of 0.2 micrograms per kg per min preceded by 0.4 mg intravenous bolus were associated with a significant 34% decrease in the geometric mean of hourly scratching activity compared to placebo infusions [34]. The results of other controlled clinical trials [35–42], some of which included behavioral methodology (i.e., recording of scratching activity) [34, 36, 39, 40] have also revealed that the administration of naloxone [36], and the opiate antagonists nalmefene [35, 39, 40], and naltrexone [37, 38, 41, 42], is associated with an amelioration of the pruritus in patients with cholestasis. These results support the hypothesis that endogenous opioids mediate, at least in part, the pruritus of cholestasis. A publication of a meta-analysis reported that opiate antagonists significantly reduced the pruritus of cholestasis [6]. Although there are concerns on the use of meta-analyses to derive strong conclusions on therapeutic interventions because of the heterogeneity of clinical studies, the rationale to use this type of drug and the results from several clinical studies from different parts of the world support the use of this type of medication to treat pruritus in patients with PBC [38, 39, 40–42].

The limiting factor on the use of opiate antagonists for the treatment of the pruritus of cholestasis is the opioid withdrawal-like reaction that can be experienced by patients with cholestasis after the intake of opiate antagonists [35, 36, 34, 40]. Naltrexone at a dose of 50 mg orally per day [38] was associated with an improvement in the visual analog score for pruritus; however, 50 mg may be a high dose to start treatment because of the potential risk of an opioid withdrawal-like reaction; thus, a lower dose can be given by cutting the tablet in four and taking a quarter (12.5 mg) every day to be increased by a quarter every 3–7 days, until the pruritus is ameliorated. Doses of 250 mg of naltrexone per day have been required to control pruritus in some patients [43]. Alternatively, the protocol implemented in a randomized double-blind placebo-controlled study that included 29 patients with cholestasis and pruritus can be followed [34]. Patients can be admitted to the hospital for intravenous infusions of naloxone, at a dose of 0.2 micrograms/kg/min, a dose associated with opiate antagonist effect, in 250 or 500 cc of a suitable intravenous solution, preceded by an intravenous bolus administration of 0.4 mg [34] for 48 hours followed by the introduction of oral naltrexone and discontinuation of the infusion. The opiate withdrawal-like reaction can be characterized by abdominal pain, high blood pressure, tachycardia, goose bumps, nightmares, depersonalization, or by a feeling of not being right. It is not possible to predict who will develop an opiate-withdrawal like reaction. Clinical experience has suggested that patients who have severe pruritus may have a higher opioidergic tone and may be at risk for a more severe reaction; these patients may benefit from the initiation of ultralow naloxone infusions in the hospital, even at lower doses than those stated above (e.g., 0.002 micrograms/kg/min) [44] to be gradually increased as described above. The dose should not be increased if signs of an opiate-withdrawal like syndrome develop; in general, the drug can be held or maintained at the same dose, as the reaction tends to subside spontaneously [39, 40]. Hepatotoxicity is not common [45], but it has been reported [46]; thus, follow-up of the comprehensive metabolic panel is recommended. In patients with decompensated liver disease, naltrexone metabolites can accumulate in the body [47]; therefore, reducing the dose is necessary. As liver disease progresses, pruritus tends to cease; thus, the need to use naltrexone in decompensated liver disease is not common [48].

Naloxone nasal spray is now available as an emergency treatment of opiate overdose in the community [49]. NARCAN Nasal Spray is supplied as a single-dose intranasal spray containing 2 or 4 mg of naloxone hydrochloride in 0.1 mL [49]. This preparation could be used as an alternative to treat the pruritus of cholestasis in a properly designed protocol (Sunny Patel, MD, 2019, unpublished personal communication, with permission).

The use of nalfurafine, a kappa-agonist drug, was reported to ameliorate the pruritus of cholestasis [50]; this result provides support for the role of the endogenous opioid system in the pruritus of cholestasis, as follows: (i) the stimulation of the mu receptor is associated with scratching behavior in laboratory animals [51, 52] and pruritus in human beings [29, 30], (ii) the stimulation of the kappa receptor prevents the pruritogenic and the scratching producing effect from the stimulation of the mu receptor [51, 52]. In this context, butorphanol is an antagonist at the mu opioid receptor and an agonist at the kappa receptor [53]. In a patient with intractable pruritus from liver disease secondary to chronic hepatitis C, butorphanol in nasal spray form (1 mg per application) was associated with prolonged relief of pruritus [54]. It was subsequently reported that butorphanol was associated with pruritus relief in a series of patients with PBC [55]. The potential addiction to butorphanol, initially considered low [56], is important [57]; thus, the use of this drug to treat the pruritus of cholestasis has to be considered carefully, e.g., short courses. Anecdotal reports on the use of codeine, an agonist at the mu opioid receptor [58], and buprenorphine, an agonist at the mu receptor, and an antagonist at the kappa receptor [59] in association with amelioration of the pruritus of cholestasis have been published. These reports have to be reconciled with the effects of butorphanol in regards to its receptor preference.

### Serotonin Antagonists

The serotonin system participates in the neurotransmission of nociceptive stimuli [60], the rationale provided to study ondansetron, a serotonin antagonist at the type 3 receptor, to treat pruritus in cholestasis. In addition, ondansetron has been reported to ameliorate pruritus associated with the administration of opiates [61]. Ondansetron was reported to decrease the pruritus associated with cholestasis in studies that used subjective methodology only [62–65]; however, studies that incorporated behavioral methodology have not confirmed an antipruritic effect of ondansetron in cholestasis [66, 67].

## Antidepressants

Antidepressants, including selective serotonin reuptake inhibitors [68–70] and mirtazapine, a noradrenergic and serotonergic related antidepressant, have been reported to have antipruritic effects [71–73].

Sertraline, a selective serotonin reuptake inhibitor, was reported to be associated with pruritus relief in patients with PBC [74, 75]. Sertraline was evaluated in a controlled study which consisted of a dose-finding open-label first phase of 21 patients, followed by the second phase, in which 12 patients with liver disease, including PBC, participated in a randomized placebo-controlled cross over design. At doses associated with relief of pruritus (75–100 mg) in the first phase of the study, this drug was reported to decrease the pruritus and its cutaneous consequences, i.e., scratch marks as measured by a visual analog scale and by a physical examination in the second phase [75]. Eight of twenty-one subjects associated the use of sertraline with mood stability, and those who met the criteria for depression at baseline improved on sertraline; however, it was reported that the decrease in the visual analog score for pruritus was independent of the improvement in depression [75].

## Potential Regulation of a 24-Hour Rhythm of Scratching Behavior

The expression of a 24-hour rhythm in scratching behavior displayed by some patients with cholestasis and pruritus suggested that this behavior may be under circadian control. It provided the rationale to study the effect of bright-light phototherapy indirectly reflected toward eyes in patients with chronic liver disease and pruritus in a pilot study [76]. Bright-light phototherapy was associated with marked suppression of outbursts of scratching over the day. However, after 8 weeks of treatment, the hourly scratching activity was not significantly different from the baseline value [76]. It was suggested that this type of light therapy could be used in combination with other antipruritic interventions, but controlled studies to test this idea have not been conducted.

## Drugs to Treat the Liver Disease

Ursodeoxycholic acid, a treatment approved for PBC, has not been consistently found to decrease the pruritus of cholestasis [2].

Fibrates are being studied to treat cholestatic liver disease including PBC and PSC. Bezafibrate is a peroxisome proliferator-activated receptor (PPAR) agonist reported in association with relief of pruritus. The effect may be from the salutary effects of this type of drug on the disease itself, as interpreted by the investigators [77].

Bezafibrate at doses of 400 mg per day in combination with ursodeoxycholic acid in patients with PBC was reported to be associated with decrease or disappearance of pruritus as measured by the visual analog and the 5-D scale after a period of treatment of 38 months [78]. Alone, also at a dose of 400 mg per day, bezafibrate was associated with relief of pruritus measured by a visual analog and the 5-D scales, in patients with cholestasis, in a double-blind randomized, placebo-controlled trial of 21 days duration. The improvement was interpreted to have resulted from a decrease in liver injury [77].

Other interventions have been reported to decrease the sensation of pruritus as assessed by various subjective methods in controlled studies, uncontrolled observations, and case series and reports in patients with liver disease, including hepatic enzyme inducers flumecinol [79] and phenobarbital [23], the antibiotic metronidazole [80], antioxidants [81], androgens [82], phototherapy to the skin [83], the anesthetic propofol [84, 85], dronabinol, an agonist at the cannabinoid receptor B1 [86], lidocaine [87], S-adenosylmethionine [88], methotrexate [89], and tacrolimus [90].

In the context of the exclusive use of the subjective methodology in studies of pruritus, in a randomized, double-blind placebo-controlled trial of the drug gabapentin, the placebo intervention was associated with almost complete suppression of scratching behavior and a decrease in the visual analog score for pruritus, in contrast to the active drug, which seemed to worsen pruritus and its behavioral consequence, scratching [91]. These results emphasize the uncertainty in interpreting the outcomes of any intervention to treat pruritus in studies that use subjective methodology only and the importance of including behavioral methodology to record scratching in clinical trials of pruritus [91].

Erythema and edema, the classic findings of histamine-mediated pruritus, are absent from the skin of patients with liver disease and pruritus. Antihistamine drugs do not appear to have any specific antipruritic effect in patients with cholestasis. Still, some patients report relief on this type of medication [92], which may result from its sedative properties. Sedation mediated by antihistamines may help patients sleep, which is often interrupted in patients with pruritus; however, the dryness of mucous membranes associated with this type of drug may limit its use in patients with PBC and sicca symptoms.

Patients with severe pruritus are at risk for depression and suicidal ideations and actions. The patients may require hospital admission for parenteral administration of medications, including opiate antagonists. Intractable pruritus can be an indication for liver transplantation. As pruritus can be intermittent, the decision to perform a liver transplant has to be weighed against the complications of that procedure. However, patients with pruritus of cholestasis suffer tremendously; accordingly, liver transplantation should be considered as an alternative.

The management of patients with pruritus includes skincare to identify any primary pruritic skin lesions; the use of soaps for sensitive skin may help.

A guidance to treat patients with pruritus from cholestasis is provided in Table 15.1.

**Table 15.1** Treatment of patients with the pruritus of cholestasis

Skin care

Cholestyramine 4 g before and after breakfast;
add 4 g at lunch and dinner, if necessary, not to exceed 16 g per day

Relief

Yes

No relief

\* The combination of these drugs in the treatment of pruritus has not been studied. Medication reconciliation is required prior to the initiation of any form of therapy

Continue therapy; Check coagulation profile periodically

\*Opiate antagonists

\*Rifampicin

\*Sertraline

- Naloxone,  0.4 mg by intravenous bolus immediately followed by intravenous infusions of naloxone (0.2 micrograms per kg/minute) (33).Dose can be increased gradually (e.g. every 4 hours) to 0.8 micrograms per kg/minute
- After 12 to 24 hours of infusion therapy start oral naltrexone, 12.5 mg (a quarter of a tablet), once a day for 3 days.
- Increase dose of naltrexone by 12.5 mg per day , if the patient has not experienced relief of the pruritus,  to 50 mg per day
- Higher doses than 50 mg in divided doses have been used (42).

- 150 mg orally, twice a day, if serumbilirubin >3 mg/dl or 150 mg orally three time a day if serum bilirubin <3 mg/dl (21).

- Check liver profile two and four weeks after starting the medication, and at least monthly thereafter.  If changes in liver profile suggest hepatotoxicity, stop rifampicin

- 75 mg orally daily, to be increased to 100 mg daily (74).

- Naltrexone can be started without a leading phase of naloxone infusions, 12.5 mg (a quarter of a tablet), once a day for 3 days
- Increase dose of naltrexone by 12.5 mg per day , if the patient has not experienced relief of the pruritus,  to 50 mg per day
- If the patient experiences any signs of opiate withdrawal like reaction, the dose can be maintained at the prior dose for a day or two with subsequentincrease, until relief of pruritus is attained
- Check blood work after the initiation of naltrexone

Patients not responsive to treatments above
- Refer to other options to treat pruritus in text.
- Refer patient for liver transplant evaluation
- Consider MARS$^{TM}$ therapy

Explore clinical trial options

# Fatigue

In a study of patients with cholestasis, most of whom had PBC, a decrease in fatigue, as assessed by a visual analog scale, was reported after administering the opiate antagonist nalmefene [35]. This result may suggest that increased opioidergic tone may contribute to the fatigue of PBC [33]; however, the effect of opiate antagonists on fatigue has not been studied in controlled clinical trials.

The use of antioxidants was not confirmed to be associated with an improvement in fatigue as assessed by the Fisk Fatigue Severity Score in a double-blind, randomized placebo-controlled study [81].

The mechanism that supports the stimulant effect of modafinil used to treat narcolepsy is unknown; however, it was reported to decrease fatigue in a case series of patients with PBC [93]. Patients with PBC were reported to sleep during the day significantly more than a control group, as assessed with sleep monitors [94]. These findings were provided as a rationale to the study of modafinil at doses from 100 to 200 mg in an open-label trial of 8 weeks duration in 21 patients with PBC and excessive daytime sleepiness [95]. The degree of daytime sleep correlated with fatigue severity, assessed by the PBC-40, a disease-specific health-related quality of life measure [95]. Modafinil was associated with a significant improvement in the fatigue domain score compared to baseline, as assessed by the PBC-40; in addition, modafinil was associated with a significant decrease in daytime somnolence [95].

Aerobic training increases maximal work capacity, which leads to a reduction in the percentage of total capacity required for activities of daily living. This reduction is associated with decreased fatigue. During an 8-week structured exercise program, aerobic training was associated with decreased fatigue as assessed with validated fatigue questionnaires in three patients with chronic hepatitis C [96]. These preliminary results support the conduct of studies of aerobic training for the treatment of fatigue secondary to PBC.

There are no specific therapies for the treatment of fatigue in liver disease.

# Portal Hypertension

Cirrhosis is defined as a change in liver architecture to a nodular structure [97]. It is a diagnosis of histology [97]. Efforts to obtain information on the status of the liver by noninvasive techniques are vigorous, including scores such as FIB-4, fibrosure, APRI, magnetic resonance imaging (MRI) elastography, the interpretation of the liver shape via computed tomography (CT) scan and sonogram, and transient elastography because liver biopsy is an invasive procedure not devoid of complications [98, 99].

Portal hypertension is defined as an increase in portal venous pressure. It is a complication of cirrhosis from any etiology and relatively severe liver injury in the absence of cirrhosis, e.g., alcoholic hepatitis. Portal hypertension is classified as prehepatic, intrahepatic, and post hepatic [100]. The liver diseases included in this book are associated with intrahepatic portal hypertension. Noncirrhotic portal hypertension is an entity characterized by portal hypertension in the absence of liver disease; however, cirrhosis is the most common cause of portal hypertension [100, 101].

The normal pressure gradient between the portal vein and the vena cava is 1–5 mmHg; complications from portal hypertension tend to arise when the gradient increases to at least 10. The portal pressure gradient results from the relationship between portal blood flow and the vascular resistance against which the blood must flow; accordingly, portal pressure increases due to an increase in the blood flow, an increase in resistance, or a combination of both [101]. The causes of the increased resistance include the existence of obstacles to blood flow, e.g., fibrosis and nodule formation, and a functional resistance resulting from the contraction of resident cells, including hepatic stellate cells and vascular smooth muscle. In portal hypertension, there is an intrahepatic deficiency of nitric oxide, mostly due to a decrease in the release of eNOs and increased oxidative stress, which leads to enhanced scavenging due to increased oxidative stress [102, 103]. The marked arteriolar vasodilatation that characterizes the vasculature of the organs that drain into the portal vein, i.e., the splanchnic circulation, results from excess in nitric oxide, as well as altered production of prostacyclin, carbon monoxide, endocannabinoids, glucagon, and by angiogenesis, mediated by vascular endothelial growth factor (VEGF) and platelet-derived growth factor (PDGF) [101, 104, 105]. The paradox of decreased nitric oxide inside the liver and increased nitric oxide in the splanchnic vasculature mediates the pathogenesis of portal hypertension [106].

Diversion of blood flow from the liver to the systemic circulation is sustained via collaterals that form from the vascular connections that close after embryological development, and include gastroesophageal varices; in addition, angiogenesis mediated by VEGF and PDGF contribute to a collateral circulation through which a substantial proportion of the blood volume circulates in cirrhosis and advanced portal hypertension [101, 104, 105].

Guidelines for the screening and management of portal hypertension and its complications are available from several medical societies and are updated regularly, consistent with the evolution of information and changes in practice; the reader is referred to them for guidance [107].

Upper gastrointestinal endoscopy (EGD) has been recommended to screen for gastroesophageal varices at the time a diagnosis of cirrhosis is made [108]; however, with the advent of transient elastography, it is considered that patients with liver stiffness less than 20 kilopascals and a platelet count greater than $150,000/mm^3$ do not require a screening EGD at diagnosis because the probability of having high-risk varices is less than 5% [107]. For all other patients, EGD is recommended at the time of diagnosis of cirrhosis [107].

If varices are not found, a repeat endoscopy is recommended in 2 years. In patients in whom the driving cause of the liver disease has been removed, i.e., cure of hepatitis C virus infection, abstinence from alcohol in liver disease from alcohol, the procedure can be repeated in 3 years [107].

Nonselective beta-blockers, carvedilol, or variceal ligation are recommended to prevent the index bleed in patients with large varices defined as an estimated diameter greater than 5 mm; the experience of the endoscopist and patient's preference should be considered in deciding how to proceed [107]. Pharmacological therapy may be preferred over endoscopic variceal ligation in patients with large varices not associated with high bleeding [109]. The dose of nonselective beta-blocker, e.g., propranolol, nadolol, with the dose adjusted to what is maximally tolerated, is recommended, with a target of a heart rate of 60 [109]; carvedilol can be prescribed to patients who cannot tolerate nonselective beta-blockers. Patients intolerable to pharmacological therapy should be managed with variceal ligation to eradication [107].

Patients identified as having high-risk (for bleeding) varices, e.g., red wale sign [110], should be started on beta-blockers in tandem with banding, as the eradication of varices does not decrease portal pressure, and thus, the risk remains. The use of endoscopic variceal ligation is also recommended to prevent the index bleed in patients with cirrhosis, Child's class B and C; however, the guidelines suggest that the decision regarding what intervention to use be considered in the context of local expertise [109, 107]. If this option is taken, variceal ligation should be repeated every 2 weeks, depending on the tolerance of the endoscopist and stability of the patients, e.g., post banding ulcers, until eradication is documented, followed by

**Fig. 15.1** Contrast enhanced computed tomography on a 45 year old man with cirrhosis and portal hypertension showing a nodular liver (thin black arrow), ascites (white large arrow), gastroesophageal varices (small white arrow), and splenomegaly (small black arrow)

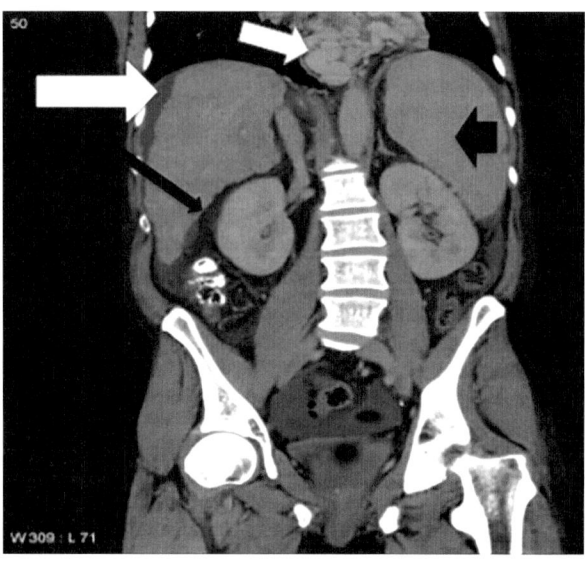

surveillance upper endoscopy 1–3 months after eradication, and every 6–12 months subsequently.

Gastroesophageal varices develop from connections between short gastric and coronary veins and the esophageal, azygos, and intercostal veins (Fig. 15.1); rectal and ectopic varices may also develop. Bleeding from gastroesophageal varices is one of the complications from cirrhosis and portal hypertension that changes the course of a patient's life, i.e., it is one of the events that define decompensation of liver disease and is associated with a mortality that ranges between 15–20%. Patients who survive an index bleed have a high probability of rebleeding and death. At 1–2 years, the probability of rebleeding is 63%, and that of dying in association with such is 33% [111]. Thus, prevention of subsequent bleeding is pivotal in the management of patients with gastroesophageal varices and should be implemented [112].

The recommendations on the management of suspected variceal bleeding include fluid resuscitation and blood transfusions, as necessary, a 7-day course of antibiotic therapy with ceftriaxone, the drug recommended at present, 1 g intravenously every 24 hours, and pharmacological therapy to decrease portal pressure with intravenous infusions of octreotide, an analog of somatostatin [107, 112, 113]. Upper endoscopy within 12 hours of presentation to determine the source of bleeding is recommended in cases where there is room for resuscitation. If not, endoscopy should be performed as soon as possible [107, 112, 113] after appropriate protection of the airway via endotracheal intubation. If the bleed is considered variceal in origin, endoscopic therapy with variceal ligation or sclerotherapy should be provided [109]. The use of proton pump inhibitors during acute variceal bleeding seems controversial. Persistent or recurrent variceal bleeding in spite of combined pharmacological and endoscopic therapy should be managed with the placement of a transjugular intrahepatic portosystemic shunt (TIPS). Balloon tamponade is recommended as a temporary measure prior to endoscopic management or TIPS placement [109]. The recommendations to manage bleeding from gastric varices include sealing the varices with adhesive substances, where available, variceal ligation, and balloon-occluded retrograde transvenous obliteration (BRTO) [114]. TIPS placement is recommended for patients in whom the bleeding does not cease despite pharmacological and endoscopic therapy [109].

## Ascites

Ascites is the accumulation of fluid in the abdominal cavity. The pathophysiology of ascites concerns the splanchnic vasodilatation that characterizes portal hypertension, i.e., hyperdynamic circulation, and that leads to a decrease in effective arterial blood volume [115], which leads to activation of vasoconstrictor systems, the renin–aldosterone system, and of antidiuretic hormone, which results in sodium and fluid retention [115]. Splanchnic vasodilatation is due to an excess of nitric oxide (NO) [106]. As disease progresses, impaired excretion of free water ensues, and cardiac output, which initially increases, decreases likely secondary to a form of cirrhotic cardiomyopathy, further decreasing organ perfusion, all of which results in further fluid and sodium retention.

Ascites results from portal hypertension in 80% of the cases. In patients with liver disease, portal hypertension is a sine qua non for the formation of ascites. Ascites tends to develop at a rate of 5–10% per year, with 60% of patients with cirrhosis having ascites after 10 years of diagnosis [116]. The survival of patients after the development of ascites was reported to be from 45% to 82% at 1 year, and 22% to 52% at 5 years [117]; thus, ascites is recognized as a defining complication in the natural history of cirrhosis, i.e., from compensated to decompensated state [117, 118], and an indication for referral to liver transplantation when clinically detected [119].

In portal hypertension secondary to cirrhosis, there is an increase in blood volume and lymph formation, which overwhelms the intrahepatic lymphatic ducts, resulting in the pouring of lymph from the liver's surface into the abdominal cavity, i.e., ascites [120]. Ascites is a complication of conditions that lead to sinusoidal portal hypertension, including thrombosis of hepatic veins, sinusoidal obstruction syndrome or venoocclusive disease, severe alcoholic hepatitis, and cirrhosis; it is unusual to have ascites formation in cases in which the obstruction to blood flow is presinusoidal, e.g., schistosomiasis, congenital hepatic fibrosis, idiopathic portal hypertension (i.e., noncirrhotic). In cases in which the block to blood flow is outside the liver, ascites occurs when there is repercussion on the sinusoids to cause increased pressure, such as in right-sided congestive heart failure, constrictive pericarditis, and obstruction of the inferior vena cava, e.g., by congenital webs but, it does not occur when the obstruction is in the splenic or portal veins.

The hepatic sinusoids flow from their origin in their portal tract to the central veins; they are lined by endothelial cells, Kupffer cells, and hepatic stellate cells, the latter found in the space of Disse, between the sinusoids and the hepatocytes. Hepatic sinusoids are histologically unique because of the absence of a basement membrane and the presence of fenestrae, i.e., pores of approximately 100–500 nm in diameter through which microvilli of hepatocytes can be appreciated by electron microscopy, and which make them permeable to proteins that circulate in the blood through the sinusoids. It is suggested that the fluid within the space of Disse in communication with the liver interstitial space enters the lymphatics channels present in the portal tracts and the central veins as hepatic lymph. As there is permeability via the sinusoids, the protein concentration in plasma and fluid within the space of Disse is almost identical, e.g., 95% homogeneity [121]. The hepatic lymph drains out of the liver via vessels from the hepatic hilum to the thoracic duct.

The direct consequence of increased sinusoidal pressure and ascites can be appreciated by the marked increase in lymph production from portal hypertension, i.e., lymph production increases by 60% for every millimeter increase in portal pressure [122]. It has been demonstrated in experimental models of sinusoidal hypertension from venous obstruction that there is a marked increase in lymph flow via the hepatic and thoracic ducts (e.g., 8–9 liters per day), regardless of the presence or absence of ascites [123]. As the lymph cannot be contained within the channels, there is pouring of it from the liver's surface into the abdominal cavity; thus, ascites from sinusoidal portal hypertension is lymph [122, 124–126]. Intestinal permeability increases in advanced liver disease, thus providing a second source of fluid toward ascites accumulation [127, 128]. It is considered that hepatic and splanchnic lymph contributes to ascites.

In portal hypertension from cirrhosis, the permeability of the sinusoids dramatically decreases because of capillarization [129], with the marginal areas of regenerating nodules being irrigated by capillaries, although sinusoids remain in the center of the nodules; as a result of capillarization, the protein concentration of the draining lymph decreases to about 65% of that of plasma [130]. The hepatic sinusoids are completely impermeable to albumin in some patients [131].

Cirrhosis is a sodium avid state, which plays a fundamental role in the pathogenesis of ascites. Prior to ascites formation, sodium retention happens in the collecting tubules, and, in the late stages, in the proximal tubules [132]. Sodium is reabsorbed, followed by water, leading to the expansion of extracellular fluid volume and interstitial fluid. Patients with compensated cirrhosis do not retain sodium, but they exhibit abnormal sodium handling as evidenced by the inability to excrete an acute sodium loading [133, 134]. However, patients with cirrhosis and substantially high portal pressure retain sodium when exposed to mineralocorticoids, in contrast to noncirrhotic normal controls who develop transient sodium and water retention that subsides within a few days [135, 136].

Contributing to fluid overload and hyponatremia in cirrhotic patients with ascites is the impaired excretion of free water, which varies in degree among patients with cirrhosis, portal hypertension, and ascites [137, 138].

Characterization of ascites, which can be made with a few milliliters of fluid, e.g., 20 ml, is fundamental in managing patients with this complication. Serum protein concentration and portal pressure determine the ascitic fluid protein concentration in patients with chronic liver disease.

A seminal study in patients with chronic liver disease provided information now established as the gold standard to confirm ascites as a complication of portal hypertension [139]. In 56 patients with chronic liver disease, the ascites and serum concentrations of albumin and globulin and transhepatic portal pressure were simultaneously measured to reveal that the mean concentration of albumin in ascites was $1.04 \pm 0.73$ gm/dl and that of globulin $1.31 \pm 0.80$ gm/dl, with a total ascites protein concentration of $2.35 \pm 1.49$ gm/dl. In serum, the mean albumin concentration was $2.58 \pm 0.57$ gm/dl, and that of globulin $3.91 \pm 0.86$ gm/dl, with the total serum protein concentration of $6.49 \pm 1.30$ gm/dl. The serum to ascites albumin concentration gradient was $1.54 \pm 0.45$ gm/dl. The mean transhepatic portal pressure above the inferior vena cava was $14.5 \pm 4.3$ mm Hg. The serum to ascites albumin concentration gradient correlated strongly with the mean transhepatic portal pressure above the inferior vena cava ($r = 0.73, p < 0.0001$). The protein concentration in ascites correlated significantly with the serum albumin, serum globulin, and the mean transhepatic portal pressure above the inferior vena cava, although these variables did not correlate with each other. The additional analysis documented a high correlation of the protein in ascites with the serum albumin concentration after correction for serum globulin and serum to ascites albumin concentration gradient ($r = 0.97, p < 00001$), or transhepatic portal pressure above the inferior vena cava ($r = 0.90; p < 0.0001$). These data indicated that most of the variation in protein concentration in ascites in the study group was associated with serum protein and transhepatic portal pressure above the inferior vena cava, or serum ascites albumin concentration gradient. It was further documented that the difference between the groups of patients in whom the concentration of protein in ascites was $\leq 2.5$ vs. $\geq 2.5$ gm/dl was due to differences in serum albumin and serum globulin in combination with the serum to ascites albumin concentration gradient ($r = 0.808$), or transhepatic portal pressure above inferior vena cava ($r = 0.806$). The variables described could identify the low and high ascitic fluid protein groups in 96% and 93% of patients, respectively. These data were interpreted to indicate that the serum to ascites albumin concentration gradient is associated with the degree of portal hypertension and that the difference in the concentration of protein in ascites among patients with chronic liver disease is related to variations in portal pressure and serum protein concentration [139].

The use of the serum albumin ascites gradient (SAAG), i.e., the subtraction of the albumin concentration in the fluid from that of the serum, has been established as the method to identify ascites from portal hypertension when the difference is $\geq 1.1$ g/dl, as documented in a study that included 901 paired samples of ascites and serum in which portal hypertension was accurately identified in 96.7% of cases [140].

The difference between the serum albumin and the ascites albumin originates from the fact that, as a result of the capillarization of the hepatic sinusoids in cirrhosis, the intimate connection between the blood that circulates through the sinusoids and that of the space of Disse is lost; thus, there is a difference in concentration of albumin (vide supra).

To perform a paracenthesis, the author prefers the linea alba, approximately 2 cm below the umbilicus, as the site to enter the peritoneal cavity to obtain ascites fluid. The bladder should be empty. We avoid the left quadrant of the abdomen because of splenomegaly; the spleen can be punctured inadvertently. With the advent of point of care sonogram and the collaboration with interventional radiology, the best areas to puncture can be identified. The techniques for the procedure are established [141].

Ascites from portal hypertension tends to be clear and straw colored. The necessary tests in the characterization of ascites from portal hypertension include ascites concentration of protein and albumin obtained simultaneously from ascites and serum, and protein to calculate the SAAG; it is possible to use serum data from the immediate periprocedure days. Total white blood cell count and differential, and ascites culture is included as the exclusion of infection is fundamental in the management of patients with ascites. In this regard, in patients with cirrhosis and ascites, if the fluid protein concentration is <1.5 g/dL in association with a serum creatinine ≥1.2 mg/dL, a blood urea nitrogen level ≥ 25 mg/dL, or a serum sodium ≤130 mEq/L, or liver failure, as per a Child–Pugh score ≥ 9 and a bilirubin ≥3 mg/dL prophylaxis with antibiotics to prevent SBP (e.g., quinolones) is indicated whether patients are hospitalized or not.

Ascites has been graded as grade 1 when it is only detectable by sonogram, grade 2, characterized by abdominal distension, and grade 3, associated with marked abdominal distension [142].

The management of ascites concerns treating the cause of liver disease, e.g., alcohol abstinence in liver disease from alcohol use, viral hepatitis, and sodium restriction in combination with diuretics. Sodium consumption is limited to 80–120 mmol/day. In our clinic, we recommend no salt added and no food consumed from a bag or can, i.e., freshly prepared food ideally. This recommendation is a challenge faced by patients with difficult social circumstances, e.g., homelessness, and shelter dwellers; thus, an effort to provide education in consultation with a dietitian is fundamental. The treatment of grade 1 ascites has not been studied in clinical trials; however, it seems reasonable to limit sodium intake and avoid drugs that can enhance sodium retention, e.g., nonsteroidal anti-inflammatory drugs (NSAIDs). Although salt restriction and spironolactone, an aldosterone antagonist, can be used in the initial management of ascites, limited response to this single diuretic therapy and hyperkalemia limit this therapy. Thus, the addition of a loop diuretic, e.g., furosemide, is favored [143–145]. Spironolactone is a once-a-day drug that can be started at a dose of 50 mg, in combination with furosemide, at 20 mg per day. The aim is to induce a weight loss not to exceed 1 lb. per day in patients without peripheral edema and two pounds per day in patients with edema [146]. The dose can be increased not sooner than 72 hours after the initiation of therapy. We favor a slow increase in the dose of diuretics not sooner than every seven days, during weekly evaluations in the clinic with results of serum electrolytes, blood urea nitrogen, and creatinine. The published guidelines recommend doses of spironolactone and furosemide to be 100 mg and 40 mg, respectively, to be increased to 200 mg and 80 mg, respectively, and 400 mg and 160 mg, respectively, the maximum doses recommended [144]. The clinician should be able to titrate the doses according to tolerability and response to therapy. It is pivotal that sodium intake is limited; thus, the measurement of urine excretion of sodium helps to confirm adherence to sodium restriction and response to diuretics, which should help to adjust doses. In this regard, a 24-hour urine collection is useful but cumbersome to complete; thus, a random spot urine sodium concentration greater than the potassium concentration is reported to correlate with the 24-hour sodium excretion. When the ratio is greater than one, there should be a fluid loss, with an increase in the ratio indicating an increase in urine sodium excretion and thus water, which follows sodium [147]. Diuretics' side effects include intravascular volume depletion and electrolyte imbalance, leading to renal insufficiency and hepatic encephalopathy [146]. In cases of hyponatremia within a range of 120–125 mmol/L, it is recommended that diuretics be discontinued [145]. After ascites is satisfactorily mobilized, i.e., conversion to grade 1 [148], diuretic doses should be decreased to the lowest possible to keep maximum diuresis.

The initial treatment of grade 3 ascites is large volume paracentesis, defined as the removal of at least 5 liters of ascites per session [144], in association with intravenous infusions of albumin, 8 g/L removed, to prevent post paracentesis circulatory dysfunction [149–151]; diuretic therapy is prescribed according to tolerability and renal function [152].

Refractory ascites is defined as that which cannot be mobilized in association with sodium restriction and maximal doses of diuretics or that recur within 4 weeks of removal [142, 148]. Two categories have been further defined: (1) diuretic resistant ascites: "… that cannot be mobilized or the early recurrence of which cannot be prevented because of lack of response to dietary sodium restriction and intensive diuretic therapy," and (2) "… that cannot be mobilized or the early recurrence of which cannot be prevented because of the development of diuretic-induced complications that preclude the use of effective diuretic dosage" [148]. Diagnostic criteria for refractory ascites include lack of response to sodium restriction and diuretic therapy alone after at least 1 week of therapy with maximum doses (see above), i.e., weight loss of fewer than 2 lbs. per day, recurrence of ascites to grades 2 or 3 within 4 weeks of mobilization, and complications from diuretics, i.e., hepatic encephalopathy in the absence of a precipitating factor, renal insufficiency with doubling of serum creatinine to more than 2 mg/dl in patients who are responding to diuretics, hyponatremia to serum sodium to <125, and hypokalemia of <3 meq/L or hyperkalemia to >6 meq/L. Patients with refractory ascites can be managed with large-volume paracentesis. Diuretic treatment should be discontinued in patients with refractory ascites unless natriuresis exceeds 30 mmol per day [144, 145].

A transjugular intrahepatic peritoneal shunt (TIPS) shunts blood from an intrahepatic portal branch to a hepatic vein; it decreases portal pressure, and improves effective arterial volume after the first 4–6 weeks of insertion, with subsequent diuresis [153]. Recurrence of ascites is lower in association with TIPS than with diuretic therapy [153]. Complications from TIPS include hepatic encephalopathy, occlusion of the graft itself, hemolysis, and liver failure; thus, their use must be individualized [145] and in collaboration with a liver transplant center, in our view.

The absolute contraindications for TIPS are elevated right or left heart pressures, heart failure or severe cardiac valvular insufficiency, rapidly progressive liver failure, severe or uncontrolled hepatic encephalopathy, uncontrolled systemic infection or sepsis, unrelieved biliary obstruction, polycystic liver disease, extensive primary or metastatic hepatic malignancy, and severe, uncorrectable coagulopathy [154].

Patients who cannot have TIPS can be managed with midodrine, an alpha 1 adrenergic agonist associated with improved systemic perfusion and renal function. At a dose of 7.5 mg orally three times a day in combination with diuretics, midodrine was associated with a significant increase in natriuresis, urine volume, mean arterial pressure, and decrease in plasma renin activity after one month of treatment, and a significant increase in cardiac output and peripheral vascular resistance at 3 months of therapy, with reported mortality significantly higher in the group that received diuretics alone, in a randomized controlled trial that included 20 patients in each arm [155].

Nonsteroidal anti-inflammatory drugs (NSAIDs) block prostaglandins, which are endogenous vasodilators; thus, NSAIDs in patients with cirrhosis should not be used as they induce sodium retention and ascites formation. The use of angiotensin-converting enzyme (ACE) inhibitors should be avoided in patients with ascites as they will block the endogenous vasoconstriction that develops to maintain renal blood flow. Nephrotoxic drugs should be avoided.

The Alfapump® transfers ascites to the urinary bladder for elimination. It has been documented to remove ascites effectively and be associated with improved quality of life; bacterial infections and electrolyte imbalance were documented as the most serious side effects. The use of this device may become an alternative to the management of patients who require large volume paracentesis (LVP) [156].

# Hepatic Hydrothorax

Hepatic hydrothorax is fluid in the thoracic cavity in patients with decompensated liver disease from the escape of ascites into the chest, most commonly in the right side, via rents in the diaphragm and facilitated by the negative pressure in association with inspiration in patients without pulmonary or cardiac disease [157]. The fluid is transudate with a serum to pleural fluid albumin gradient >1.1 g/dl. Peritoneal scintigraphy can be performed to confirm the fluid trajectory. It can be complicated by empyema [157]. The prognosis of patients who develop hepatic hydrothorax is poor, with survival reduced to 8–12 months; thus, patients should be evaluated for liver transplantation [157].

Treatment of hepatic hydrothorax is diuretics and sodium restriction. The use of chest tubes is contraindicated. TIPS can be used as temporalizing therapy. In patients who cannot have liver transplantation, pleurodesis is an option; however, the complication rate is high. Repair of well-defined diaphragmatic defects via thoracoscopy has been reported [158].

# Hyponatremia

Patients who develop hypovolemic hyponatremia, usually secondary to diuretics, require volume repletion with normal saline. Patients with hypervolemic hyponatremia require the restriction of fluids to 1–2 liters, as tolerated. The threshold at which treatment is necessary varies, usually being between 120 and 125 meq/L [144], although 130 meq/L has also been cited [145].

# Bacterial Infections

Patients with cirrhosis are vulnerable to infections from an impaired immune system, dysbiosis, and bacterial translocation [159–161]. Subtle signs of infection must be sought in the evaluation of patients with liver disease.

# Spontaneous Bacterial Peritonitis

Spontaneous bacterial peritonitis (SBP) is infected ascites without an identified intraabdominal focus of infection [162]. The pathogenesis of this condition includes bacterial translocation, a phenomenon that concerns the migration of bacteria from the intestinal lumen to the mesenteric lymph nodes from where they infect ascites hematogenously [160, 163], increased intestinal permeability, and bacterial overgrowth. It is usually monomicrobial, with Escherichia coli being the most common bacteria; the presence of more than one organism or fungi or anaerobes tends to suggest a secondary source.

The clinical presentation of SBP includes fever and abdominal pain, but a subtle deterioration of hepatic, renal, and mental status is a clue to the diagnosis. Patients who undergo paracentesis, whether diagnostic or therapeutic, should have SBP excluded (see above).

A total neutrophil count in ascites of at least 250 cells is diagnostic of SBP. Ascites fluid should be inoculated directly into culture bottles at the bedside. Complete blood count and blood cultures should also be done simultaneously, prior to antibiotic administration, which should be started liberally based on clinical suspicion; cefotaxime, 2 g every 8 hours intravenously, is the treatment of choice for 5–7 days, in association with albumin 1.5 mg/kg by infusion on day one and 1 mg/kg on day three of treatment. A repeat ascites analysis 48 hours post initiation of therapy is recommended to confirm the efficacy of therapy; if the results do not suggest a successful response to treatment, i.e., a decrease in the total polymorphonuclear cell count, secondary bacterial peritonitis should be suspected, and studies to exclude it should be done [145]. Prompt administration of antibiotics has been documented as the most important predictor of survival [164]. The probability of SBP in hospitalized patients with liver disease is 20% [165]; thus, careful follow up of patients with liver disease and ascites who did not have SBP at hospitalization is critical, i.e., paracentesis should be repeated, and antibiotics administered, according to the clinical situation. Patients who are on beta-blockers should have these discontinued if they develop SBP [166].

After the first episode of SBP, prophylaxis with ciprofloxacin, 500 mg orally per day is recommended; an alternative to this medication is daily, double strength trimethoprim-sulfamethoxazole [144].

## Renal Insufficiency

The impairment of renal function is detrimental to the survival of patients with cirrhosis. Decompensated liver disease complicated by renal insufficiency portends poor survival, characterizing the last stages of liver dysfunction.

Patients with cirrhosis may have *chronic kidney disease* in association with comorbidities including diabetes and hypertension, or from intrinsic disease including IgA nephropathy and glomerulonephritis secondary to chronic viral hepatitis. *Chronic kidney disease* is defined as a glomerular filtration rate (GFR) of <60 ml/min per 1.73 m2 *for more than 3 months*. Acute kidney disease is defined as a decrease in GFR of <60 ml/min per 1.73 m2, or a reduction in GFR by at least 35%, or an increase in serum creatinine by at least 50%, *all three for less than 3 months*. Acute kidney injury (AKI) is defined by renal impairment of short duration; specifically, the increase in serum creatinine by more than 0.3 mg/dl within 48 hours, or an increase in serum creatinine by 50%, documented or presumed to have occurred in the 7 days prior to the measure [167]. The stages of AKI are: (1) an increase in serum creatinine to ≥0.3 mg/dl, or by ≥1.5- to two-fold from baseline, with 1a including patients in whom serum creatinine did not exceed 1.5 mg/dL, and whose mortality is similar to that of patients without AKI, and 1b, including patients whose serum creatinine increased beyond 1.5 mg /dl, whose short term mortality may be comparable that of patients who have not developed AKI [168], (2) an increase in serum creatinine to two- to threefold from baseline, and (3) an increase in serum creatinine by more than threefold from baseline, or a serum creatinine ≥4 mg/dl with an acute rise of ≥0.3 mg/dl or dialysis initiation [167].

Precipitating factors of AKI must be identified rapidly to address them quickly. In this regard, dehydration from the use of diuretics, infection, gastrointestinal bleeding, and NSAIDs use are common precipitating factors of AKI in patients with cirrhosis. AKI in patients with cirrhosis is associated with poor prognosis with a reported survival of 2–30% in hospitalized patients with this complication [169].

The management of AKI includes discontinuation of diuretics and any drugs contributing to renal impairment. Beta-blockers should be discontinued, although there are differences of opinion regarding this matter [144, 145]. Volume repletion with crystalloids, as appropriate, and, in cases of gastrointestinal bleeding, blood transfusions to keep the hemoglobin between 7 and 9 g/dl [170]. In patients with tense ascites, paracentesis should be performed in association with albumin infusions at doses of 8 g/liter removed [149–151, 171], which has been reported to be associated with improvement in renal function. Patients with ascites should receive albumin infusions in the same manner done during LVP in the absence of AKI. Based on the consensus published in 2007 [172] and on the recommendations from the European Association for the Study of Liver Disease [145], when AKI does not have an identifiable cause(s), its stage is greater than 1a, or it is associated with infection, patients should receive 20% albumin infusions at a dose of 1 g/kg of body weight for two consecutive days up to 100 g total.

Traditionally the terminology of acute renal insufficiency, now acute kidney injury, has been pre renal, associated with decreased renal perfusion due to dehydration, renal, due to intrinsic renal disease including acute tubular necrosis, glomerulonephritis, and interstitial nephritis, and post-renal, secondary to obstruction, which may be of sufficient magnitude to lead to hydronephrosis. All types of AKI can develop in patients with cirrhosis; the use of biomarkers to identify the type of AKI is being proposed, with urinary neutrophil gelatinase-associated lipocalin (NGAL) and interleukin 18 being reported to differentiate patients with acute tubular necrosis from other types of renal impairment [173].

## Hepatorenal Syndrome

Hepatorenal syndrome (HRS) is a complication unique to patients with decompensated liver disease and is associated with a poor prognosis. HRS happens in the context of altered hemodynamics secondary to portal hypertension characterized by profound systemic vasodilatation accentuated in the splanchnic circulation mediated, at least in part, by excessive production of nitric oxide (NO), and which results in ineffective arterial volume, i.e., relative hypovolemia, and the activation of the neurohumoral systems of rescue including the renin–angiotensin–aldosterone system, the sympathetic nervous system, and non-osmotic release of antidiuretic hormone. In cirrhosis, at first, there is an increase in sodium and water retention in response to the relative hypovolemia, which results in increased intravascular volume and increased cardiac output. However, as cirrhosis progresses, there is increased vasodilatation, with further activation of vasoconstrictive systems, leading to vasoconstriction and decreases in renal blood flow [174, 175] and deterioration of cardiac function, i.e., high output heart failure, as the heart cannot keep up with perfusion demands, further contributing to renal hypoperfusion and dysfunction [148, 176, 177]. HRS has traditionally been considered to be caused by extrarenal factors that cause functional renal failure. This interpretation has been supported by the improved or normalized renal function in patients with HRS after liver transplantation, suggesting that it was the liver and the hemodynamic complications of portal hypertension that perpetuated the renal dysfunction [178], and by the suggested normality of renal histology in patients with HRS. However, there is a paucity of data in this regard; thus, the idea of HRS as being only functional is being reconsidered [145]. In this context, it is being suggested that the pathogenesis of HRS be considered under the light of recent data documenting the role of inflammation and microvascular dysfunction on mitochondrial function and the effect of profound cholestasis on renal function [179, 180].

## Muscle Cramps

Sixty-seven percent of subjects in a study comprised of 101 patients with cirrhosis experienced muscle cramps [181]. An electromyogram of a muscle during a cramp was reported to reveal involuntary repetitive firing of motor unit action potentials at high rates up to 150 per second, producing a sustained muscle contraction [181]. Patients with cramps were reported to have had significantly lower serum albumin concentrations than those without cramps. Cramps were associated with impaired quality of life. The etiology of muscle cramps, including those in patients with cirrhosis, is unknown.

Treatments used to treat muscle cramps in patients with cirrhosis include albumin infusions [182], based on the hypothesis that decreased effective arterial volume is increased by albumin, thus improving perfusion, and baclofen, which, in a randomized, placebo-controlled study was associated with the disappearance of muscle cramps at 3 months of treatment, at a dose of 30 mg per day (e.g., 10 mg three times a day) [183].

## Hepatic Encephalopathy

Hepatic encephalopathy (HE) is a reversible neuropsychiatric behavioral complication of cirrhosis, acute liver failure, and chronic portosystemic shunting, characterized by inhibitory neurotransmission. Pathological brain findings similar to those found in patients with congenital hyperammonemia resulting from inherited defects of urea cycle enzymes, i.e., Alzheimer's type II astrocytosis, have been described in HE [184–187].

HE is detrimental to patients with survival significantly decreased in those continuing to have this complication at one year after its first episode [188, 189].

The pathogenesis of HE is unknown. Hyperammonemia in association with increased GABAergic neurotransmission, which is inhibitory, in relationship to neurosteroids is considered to contribute to the pathogenesis of this complication of liver disease [190–196].

Nitrogen, which is ingested in food, is converted to ammonia. NH4+ is the form in which ammonia exists in human beings in physiological conditions and is produced by transamination followed by deamination of biogenic amines and amino groups of nitrogenous bases such as purine and pyrimidine, and from the effect of intestinal bacterial through the action of urease on urea [197–199]. The concentration of ammonia in the portal system is significantly higher than that of the systemic circulation. Through the urea cycle, the liver converts ammonia to urea by combining it with ornithine, bicarbonate, and aspartate, and is excreted as urea through the kidneys, which are instrumental in ammonia metabolism [199].

In liver disease or portosystemic shunting, the uptake of ammonia by the liver is decreased; thus, it circulates at high concentrations systemically. The brain lacks the urea cycle. In the brain, ammonia's clearance concerns its combination with glutamate to form glutamine in the cortical Alzheimer's type II astrocyte. The excess of glutamine results in astrocytes' swelling, associated with impaired intercellular communication and neurotransmission [184, 196].

There is a proposed relationship between ammonia and GABA-ergic neurotransmission in the pathogenesis of HE. Ammonia in the brain is associated with the upregulation of the peripheral type of benzodiazepine receptors on the astrocyte mitochondrial membrane, which results in the formation of neurosteroids, which increase GABAergic neurotransmission via GABA A receptors [193–196]. Improvement of patients with HE, albeit of short duration, in association with flumazenil, a GABA A receptor antagonist, supports the hypothesis of increased GABA ergic tone contributing to HE [200].

Other theories proposed to explain HE include altered serotonin neurotransmission, false neurotransmitters, inflammation, manganese neurotoxicity, and gut dysbiosis [201, 202]. In addition, genetic susceptibility has been reported in patients with cirrhosis and HE; specifically, glutaminase TACC and CACC haplotypes were reported as risks for the development of overt HE [203].

HE has been classified as type A in acute liver failure cases, type B when associated with portosystemic shunts in the absence of liver disease, and C when associated with cirrhosis, portal hypertension, and portosystemic shunting. Type C HE has been further classified as episodic, persistent, and minimal [186, 204]. HE can be episodic, usually triggered by commonly identified precipitating factors (see below), recurrent, when bouts occur in intervals of at least 6 months, and persistent when behavioral manifestations are always present, with superimposed relapses of overt HE. HE has also been classified according to the existence of precipitating factors, i.e., nonprecipitated and precipitated.

Clinically, patients may have covert HE or may be in a coma. The exclusion of causes of encephalopathy and altered mental status beyond liver disease is part of the assessment of patients with liver disease and includes acute head injury, remote subdural hematoma, and space-occupying lesions, which require radiological tests [186]. The West Haven classification of HE grades it from 0 to 4 with 0 exhibiting no clinical findings; (1) including decreased attention span, sleep alterations, and the presence or absence of asterixis; (2) including lethargy, disorientation to time, amnesia related to recent events, and asterixis; (3) including somnolence, confusion, disorientation to place with asterixis tending to be absent; and (4) characterized by coma. Family members can help to identify findings of HE in patients with covert HE, which include subtle personality changes. Changes in sleep patterns are typical of HE, with patients being awake at night and sleepy during the day [186].

In evaluating patients with HE, it is essential to review medications and eliminate sedatives, especially benzodiazepines, which lead to increased gabaergic neurotransmission. The physical examination of a patient with HE is characterized by minimal attention span and constructional apraxia. Completion of the number connection test is delayed [205]; this test can be given in the clinic and provides an objective evaluation against which to assess the effect of treatment. Asterixis is a typical finding of HE (see above). Electroencephalogram shows the typical triphasic sharp and slow waves of HE [206], with a predominance of theta activity (slowing) as the degree of HE progresses [207]. The interpretation of EEG requires expertise, and it is a desirable tool to incorporate as a measure in clinical trials of HE.

The treatment of HE includes the identification of precipitating factors and their reversal. The precipitating factors tend to be dehydration, gastrointestinal bleeding, infections, sedative use, and electrolyte imbalance. In this context, hypokalemia is notorious for causing HE because it is associated with an increase in ammonia genesis and decreased urinary ammonia excretion; hypokalemia (an acidosis) stimulates glutamine uptake and the expression of ammoniagenic enzymes in the proximal tubule, thus increasing ammonia concentration in blood [208], changes that appear to contribute to HE in patients with impaired liver function.

The pharmacological therapy of HE includes lactulose, a nonabsorbable disaccharide, considered the first line of treatment, although debate remains regarding the robustness of the data derived from clinical studies [186, 209]. The rationale for the use of lactulose [210] includes: (i) absence of specific disaccharidase on the microvillus membrane of enterocytes in the human small bowel, allowing lactulose to enter the colon. In the colon, lactulose (and lactitol, also used in HE's management outside the United States) is catabolized by the colonic bacteria to short-chain fatty acids, including lactic and acetic acids, which results in a decrease in pH of the stool to approximately 5. The acidic milieu propitiates the formation of $NH4+$, which is nonabsorbable, from $NH3+$, which gets trapped in the colon, thus decreasing the concentration of ammonia in the blood; the importance of an acidic colonic environment in the management of HE has been documented in clinical studies [211], (ii) increased incorporation of ammonia by bacteria for synthesis of nitrogen compounds, (iii) change in colonic flora from urease producing bacteria, which contribute to ammonia production, to non-urease producing *Lactobacillus* species [212], and (iv) cathartic properties that result in a decrease in time available for ammonia to be absorbed from the colon [213]; the value of catharsis in the management of HE has been reported in clinical studies that included other agents [214].

In acute HE, in patients who can swallow, a dose of 30 ml of lactulose is administered every hour until diarrhea occurs and then tapered to 2–3 times a day to cause 2–3 soft bowel movements, targeted to the improvement of symptoms, i.e., avoidance of an excessive number of bowel movements stands to reason. Lactulose can be administered by enemas if necessary [210].

The rationale to use antibiotics to treat patients with HE is to decrease the number of bacteria that contribute to ammonia production; neomycin, metronidazole, and vancomycin have been studied [210]. Rifaximin is a nonabsorbable antibiotic that changes the gut microbiota toward a less encephalopathogenic mix than the endogenous flora; it is approved for the treatment of HE at a dose of 550 mg orally twice a day, at which dose the drug was documented to decrease the risk of overt HE recurrence in adult subjects. It is used in combination with lactulose, the dose of which can be changed to suit the patient's convenience while still offering clinical improvement [215, 216].

Other treatments that have been used in HE include sodium benzoate, zinc, branched chain amino acids, and probiotics [186].

HE has a profound negative impact on the lives of patients with liver disease. Liver transplantation (LT) is a therapeutic alternative for patients with decompensated liver disease as per established criteria [186]. In cases of HE from portosystemic shunts, their closure is indicated prior to referral for LT or at the time of surgery [186].

## Cardiomyopathy

Cardiac dysfunction may be present in as many as 50% of patients who undergo liver transplantation for end-stage liver disease [217].

Cirrhotic cardiomyopathy was defined as: (i) systolic dysfunction with a resting ejection fraction of less than 55% associated with a blunted increase in cardiac output in response to exercise or pharmacological stimulation; (ii) diastolic dysfunction with an early diastolic atrial filling ratio less than 1.0 (corrected to age), deceleration time greater than 200 milliseconds, and prolonged isovolumetric relaxation time greater than 80 milliseconds; (iii) with supporting criteria that include electrophysiological abnormalities, e.g., prolonged QT, abnormal chronotropic response, electromechanical uncoupling, enlarged left atrium, increased myocardial mass, increased brain natriuretic peptide, and pro-peptide, and increased troponin I [218]. Right ventricular dysfunction is also involved [219].

The heart function is best evaluated by echocardiogram in patients with cirrhosis.

The treatment of cirrhotic cardiomyopathy concerns the improvement of left ventricular function done with sodium restriction, diuretics, and afterload reduction, except in advanced disease because of profound peripheral vasodilation intrinsic to the hemodynamic milieu of portal hypertension [220].

Cardiac alterations in cirrhosis are reported to be reversed after liver transplantation [220].

## Hepatopulmonary Syndrome

The hepatopulmonary syndrome (HPS) is a complication of cirrhosis and portal hypertension characterized by abnormal arterial oxygenation through ventilation-perfusion mismatch that results from intrapulmonary vascular dilatation [221]. The clinical manifestations of HPS include dyspnea, and platypnea, defined as shortness of breath on sitting up and improved on lying down. The characteristic physical findings are orthodeoxia, defined as hypoxemia exacerbated in the upright position, digital clubbing, and cyanosis.

The mechanism that leads to pulmonary vasodilation is considered to be multi-factorial from data derived mostly from animal studies, and include: (i) endothelin-1, which is increased in cirrhosis and portal hypertension stimulates pulmonary endothelial nitric oxide synthase (eNOS), which results in increased production of nitric oxide (NO), the most potent endogenous vasodilator [222–224]; (ii) bacterial translocation, which is a feature of portal hypertension and which is associated with accumulation of macrophages, triggers production of inflammatory cytokines, including tumor necrosis factor (TNF) alpha, which leads to an increase in the production of inducible nitric oxide synthase (iNOS) [225, 226]; (iii) an increase in macrophage-induced heme oxygenase-1 (HO-1) increases the production of carbon monoxide, a pulmonary vasodilator [227]; and (iv) pulmonary angiogenesis mediated by macrophages and increased in TNF-alpha stimulates production of vascular endothelial growth factor (VEGF) [104, 228]. As portal hypertension is characterized by a hyperdynamic circulation, the rapidity with which mixed venous blood circulates through the capillaries, which normally measure 8–15 μm and can be as dilated as 100 μm in diameter, does not allow for appropriate gas exchange because oxygen has to travel a longer distance from the alveolus to the center of the dilated vessels, as interpreted from animal studies [224], thus causing a ventilation-perfusion mismatch, resulting in arterial hypooxygenation and high alveolar-arterial gradient [229], worsened by the right to left shunts (venous to arterial) from arterio-venous shunts [230]. The diagnosis of HPS is made by excluding primary cardio-pulmonary disease and by identifying gas exchange alterations. Oxygen saturation of less than 96% by pulse oximeter should trigger the exclusion of HPS. This test is reported to have a sensitivity of 100% and a specificity of 88% in patients with a partial pressure of oxygen (PaO2) of less than 70% [231, 232]. A contrast bubble echocardiogram is the initial recommended diagnostic test; it is done by administering agitated normal saline while doing a transthoracic echocardiogram. The bubbles opacify the right ventricle from where they are transported to the lungs via the pulmonary circulation where they are absorbed; in the presence of a right to left shunt, bubbles immediately appear in the left ventricle, i.e., early shunting; however, in the presence of intrapulmonary shunt, as in hepatopulmonary syndrome, bubbles appear in the left atrium three cardiac cycles after the administration of agitated saline, i.e., delayed shunting thus supporting the diagnosis of HPS.

Another diagnostic modality is the use of radionuclide lung perfusion scanning. Intravenously injected technetium-labeled macroaggregated 20-micron albumin (Tc-99 m MAA) normally gets trapped almost completely within the pulmonary capillary bed. In HPS, the Tc-99 m MAA particles pass through the dilated pulmonary capillaries and enter the systemic circulation, being trapped in the capillaries of the brain, kidneys, and other organs. Normally less than 6% of Tc-99 m MAA particles bypass the lung to lodge themselves into the capillaries of other organs [233, 234].

Two findings have been reported from pulmonary angiography in HPS, type 1, characterized by the diffuse spongiform appearance of pulmonary vessels in the arterial phase, and type 2, small arteriovenous communications; however, it is not recommended as a screening test as it is invasive and not sensitive for the diagnosis of HPS.

The treatment of HPS depends on its severity. For patients with mild or moderate HPS, defined as A-a gradient ≥ to 15 mmHg, with a PaO2 ± 80 mmHg, or A-a gradient ≥ to 15 mmHg, PaO2 ≥ 60 mmHg and < 80 mmHg, respectively, clinical follow up, including pulse oximetry every six months, is recommended. Oxygen supplementation is not recommended unless hypoxemia occurs during exercise (e.g., 6-minute walk test) or sleep. Patients with severe HPS, defined as A-a gradient ≥ to 15 mmHg with a PaO2 ≥ 50 mmHg and < 60 mmHg, and for patients with very severe HPS, defined as <50 mmHg or patients with a PaO2 < 300 mmHg while breathing 100% oxygen [221] should be evaluated for liver transplantation, which is reported to be associated with improvement in symptoms of HPS and oxygenation over the first year post surgery [235, 236].

Investigational therapies have included TIPS [237] and embolization in patients with large shunts [238, 239]. A study that explored the use of garlic, which contains allium sativum, which decreases the production of nitric oxide, documented an increase in baseline arterial oxygen concentration by 25%, as compared to an increase by 7% as compared to placebo, prescribed in a randomized fashion [240].

## Portopulmonary Hypertension

Portopulmonary hypertension (PoPH) is defined as the coexistence of portal hypertension and pulmonary arterial hypertension regardless of cirrhosis [241], in the absence of volume overload or intrinsic cardiopulmonary disease. It was reported to be present in 6% of liver transplant candidates [242]. From a registry that included 637 patients with PoPH, 57% had compensated cirrhosis [243]. A genetic predisposition to develop PoPH has been explored with reported multiple single nucleotide polymorphisms in the genes that code for estrogen receptor 1, aromatase, phosphodiesterase 5, angiopoietin 1, and calcium-binding protein A4 [242].

The clinical manifestations of PoPH include dyspnea, fatigue, syncope, orthopnea, and peripheral edema [244]. Many patients are asymptomatic. On physical exam, jugular vein distension, a loud $P_2$, or a murmur suggestive of tricuspid insufficiency may be appreciated, with leg edema out of proportion to ascites in advanced cases. Hypoxemia is not common.

Histologically, the pulmonary vasculature displays proliferation of the intima, with media hypertrophy, fibrosis, and thrombosis leading to thickened arterial walls and impaired blood flow, which result in increased pulmonary vascular resistance [245, 246]. The mediators of such changes are unknown. It is considered that a disequilibrium between vasoconstrictor and vasodilator substances contributes to the pathogenesis of PoPH, and they include thromboxane A2, interleukin-1, interleukin-6, angiotensin-1, glucagon, serotonin, and ET-1A [247–250].

A Doppler transthoracic echocardiogram can be used to screen for PoPH; if a systolic pulmonary arterial pressure greater than 40 mmHg is identified [244], direct measurement of pulmonary pressures is done by right heart catheterization [251]. A mean pulmonary artery pressure greater than 25 mmHg in association with a pulmonary capillary wedge pressure less than 15 mmHg is diagnostic of PoPH. In addition, a transpulmonary gradient greater than 10 mmHg and a high pulmonary vascular resistance are used to differentiate pulmonary arterial hypertension from pulmonary venous hypertension from the hyperdynamic circulation and hypervolemia of portal hypertension [244].

Patients with PoPH should be referred to centers with expertise in this condition. Drugs that have been used to treat PoPH have been taken from the experience with primary pulmonary hypertension [252]; however, calcium channel blockers and anticoagulation are not recommended for PoPH. The therapies that have been tried in PoPH include endothelin receptor antagonists, e.g., bosentan, which can be associated with hepatitis, thus, follow-up for possible liver injury is necessary, and macitentan, which, in a multicenter, randomized, double-blind, placebo-controlled, phase 4 trial was documented to decrease pulmonary vascular resistance, significantly, without hepatotoxicity [253], phosphodiesterase inhibitors, e.g., sildenafil, prostacyclin analogs, e.g., epoprostenol, vasopressin analogs, e.g., terlipressin, and tyrosine kinase inhibitors, e.g., imatinib have been considered.

The use of beta-blockers to prevent variceal bleed in patients with PoPH is not recommended because of the effect on cardiovascular hemodynamics [254].

Liver transplantation is not an option in patients with severe pulmonary hypertension because of high operative and perioperative mortality from cardiovascular complications [253]. Patients with pulmonary arterial pressure are less than 35 mmHg are considered for liver transplantation.

## Fat Malabsorption

Fat malabsorption may be a complication of cholestasis, but the degree of steatorrhea is modest, with over 70% of the ingested fat being absorbed [255]; important fat malabsorption in patients with cholestasis, including that from PBC, can be treated with the administration of medium-chain triglycerides [255]. There is literature on an association between PBC and celiac disease [256, 257]; thus, in patients with PBC and findings suggestive of malabsorption of fat or deficiencies in elements such as magnesium and iron, celiac disease should be excluded and specific treatment, i.e., gluten-free diet, recommended.

# Vitamin Deficiencies

Retinol provides vitamin A from animal sources and beta carotene from plant sources. Retinol-binding protein regulates the uptake of retinol by intestinal cells. The absorption of beta-carotene depends on the availability of bile acids in the small intestine. In addition to poor absorption secondary to bile acid deficiency, decreased availability of retinol-binding protein, which results from chronic hepatobiliary disease, contributes to vitamin A deficiency because of the impaired release of the vitamin from liver stores [258]. Enhanced urinary clearance of retinol due to deficiency in transthyretin, a thyroxine-binding globulin to which retinol-binding globulin is bound in the circulation, may also occur. Zinc is necessary for the activation of retinol to a photochemical compound; in addition, the hepatic secretion of retinol-binding protein depends on zinc; thus, it is necessary to check zinc levels and correct a deficiency if present [259]. Oral doses of 25,000 international units (IU) per day [260] to 30,000 IU three times a week [261] have been recommended for vitamin A supplementation. Vitamin A can be toxic to the liver and other organs; accordingly, it must be supplemented not to exceed what is considered normal levels, administered under supervision, and intermittently [259].

Endogenous production is the most important source of vitamin D. The metabolism of vitamin D has been reported to be normal, at least in patients with PBC [262]. These facts have suggested that poor exposure to sunlight in a debilitated chronically ill patient may be the main cause of vitamin D deficiency in cholestasis. Vitamin D, parathyroid hormone, and calcitonin regulate plasma calcium and phosphorus homeostasis; thus, these elements may be abnormal in cases of vitamin D deficiency. Doses that have been recommended for vitamin D supplementation include 400–4000 IU orally per day [263], or 50,000 IU orally three times a week [261]. Prolonged supplementation of vitamin D can lead to hypercalcemia and soft tissue calcifications, although these are not common complications [264, 265].

The main vitamin E sources are the naturally occurring tocopherols, which require micellar solubilization for absorption; thus, deficiency is a complication of conditions associated with cholestasis. Vitamin E inhibits the oxidation of unsaturated fatty acids, prevents lipid peroxidation, and is a scavenger of free radicals. Vitamin E deficiency manifests itself with a neurological syndrome characterized by peripheral neuropathy, cerebellar degeneration, and abnormal eye movements, i.e., reverse internuclear ophthalmoplegia. Retinal degeneration has been ascribed to vitamin E and A deficiencies alone or combined. In children, the complications of vitamin E deficiency are more severe than in adults with cholestasis [266]. Recommendations to treat deficiency of vitamin E include 100 mg twice a day [261] or 10 to 25 IU/kg/day [267].

Vitamins K1 and K2 require micellar solubilization for absorption in the small intestine. The forms that contribute to vitamin K activity are K1 or phytonadione, found in most vegetables, and K2, a series of menaquinones, formed by

**Table 15.2** Selected regimens for vitamin supplementation in patients with cholestasis and vitamin deficiencies

| Deficient vitamin | Preparation | Dose/mode of administration/frequency |
|---|---|---|
| A | Vitamin A | 30,000 IU/orally / three times per week [261]. |
| D | Cholecalciferol | 50,000 IU/ orally/ three times a week [261]. |
| E | tocopherol | 100 mg twice a day [261] |
| K | $K_1$ | 1–10 mg/ SC/ daily for three consecutive days or monthly[a] [268]. |

[a]for patients who have chronic cholestasis

Gram-positive bacteria in the intestine. Other compounds that have vitamin K activity are structurally related to menadione (K3) [268]. Vitamin K deficiency may present with coagulopathy, as measured by prolonged prothrombin time secondary to deficiency of vitamin K-dependent clotting factors, or it may be subclinical [269]. Coagulopathy from vitamin K deficiency resolves upon administration of the vitamin, which can be given subcutaneously at doses of 1–10 mg of vitamin K1 daily for three consecutive days. In patients with chronic cholestasis, vitamin K deficiency may be prevented by monthly administration of 10 mg of vitamin K subcutaneously [268]. The intramuscular administration of vitamin K, or any other medication, is contraindicated in patients with coagulopathy because of the risk of intramuscular hemorrhage. If the coagulopathy results from hepatocellular failure, it will not resolve in association with vitamin K administration.

It is important to supplement vitamin deficiencies as documented by blood levels and replace them, as required [270]. Periodic checkups of serum vitamin levels to provide sufficient but not excessive amounts can guide vitamin supplementation, in general. Selected recommended regimes to supplement vitamins when there is deficiency are listed in Table 15.2.

# Gynecomastia

Gynecomastia is a physical finding in men with cirrhosis. In control subjects, gynecomastia was reported in 55% of the group versus 44% of men with cirrhosis. The total estrogen-free testosterone ratio and the estradiol-free testosterone ratio was similar between the patients with cirrhosis and those without, results interpreted to suggest factors other than estrogen contribute to the pathogenesis of gynecomastia in cirrhosis, or that there may be an increase in the sensitivity to estrogens in breast tissue in cirrhosis [271].

# Cholelithiasis

The prevalence of cholelithiasis in patients with cirrhosis is higher than that of the general population [272] and reported as 25–30% [273]. There are specific recommendations for the management of gallstones associated with symptoms, which will not be reviewed in this section; however, it is important to know that in patients with cirrhosis from any cause, gallbladder surgery carries important risks for complications that must be considered in collaboration with hepatobiliary surgeons, if surgery is being considered [274–276].

# Malnutrition

The prevalence of malnutrition and sarcopenia was reported as 23 to 60% from a recent review [277]. Malnutrition can be profound in patients with end stage liver disease and is associated with a negative impact on the quality of life, and decreased survival including over the post liver transplant period [278]. It is recommended that patients with cirrhosis ingest 35 to 40 kcal/kg of body weight, with 1 to 1.5 g/kg of protein, preferably plant and dairy based. Six to eight meal "events" have been recommended, with snacks between breakfast, and lunch, and lunch and dinner [279, 280]. We emphasize on a night snack, e.g., hard-boiled egg, especially in hospitalized patients to avoid a prolonged overnight fasting. In patients with decompensated liver disease, branched chained amino acid and leucine enriched amino acid supplements are suggested. Patients who cannot have adequate oral intake, episodic enteral nutrition is recommended [280]. Early referral to the nutritionist is part of the care of patients with liver disease.

**Acknowledgments** The author acknowledges Dr. Anatole Sladen for having contributed the Figure.

# References

1. Reichen J, Simon F. Cholestasis. In: Arias IMJW, Popper H, Schachter D, Schafritz DA, editors. The liver: biology and pathobilogy. 2nd ed. New York: Raven Press; 1988. p. 1105–24.
2. Bergasa NV. Pruritus of cholestasis. In: Carstens E, Akiyama T, editors. Itch: mechanisms and treatment. Frontiers in neuroscience. Boca Raton (FL); 2014.
3. Ast M, Frishman WH. Bile acid sequestrants. J Clin Pharmacol. 1990 Feb;30(2):99–106.
4. Datta DV, Sherlock S. Cholestyramine for long term relief of the pruritus complicating intrahepatic cholestasis. Gastroenterology. 1966 Mar;50(3):323–32.
5. Van Itallie TB, Hashim SA, Crampton RS, Tennent DM. The treatment of pruritus and hypercholesteremia of primary biliary cirrhosis with cholestyramine. N Engl J Med. 1961 Sep 7;265:469–74.

6. Tandon P, Rowe BH, Vandermeer B, Bain VG. The efficacy and safety of bile acid binding agents, opioid antagonists, or rifampin in the treatment of cholestasis-associated pruritus. Am J Gastroenterol. 2007 Jul;102(7):1528–36.

7. Hegade VS, Kendrick SFW, Dobbins RL, Miller SR, Thompson D, Richards D, Dukes GE, Corrigan M, Oude-Elferink RPJ, Beuers U, Hirschfield GM, Jones DE. Effect of ileal bile acid transporter inhibitor GSK2330672 on pruritus in primary biliary cholangitis: a double-blind, randomised, placebo-controlled, crossover, phase 2a study. Lancet. 2017;389(10074):1114–23.

8. Deeks ED. Odevixibat: first approval. Drugs 2021; https://doi.org/10.1007/s40265-021-01594-y.

9. Pusl T, Denk GU, Parhofer KG, Beuers U. Plasma separation and anion adsorption transiently relieve intractable pruritus in primary biliary cirrhosis. J Hepatol. 2006 Dec;45(6): 887–91.

10. Sturm E, Franssen CF, Gouw A, Boverhof R, De Knegt RJ, et al. Extracorporal albumin dialysis (MARS) improves cholestasis and normalizes low apo A-I levels in a patient with benign recurrent intrahepatic cholestasis (BRIC). Liver. 2002;22(Suppl 2):72–5.

11. Doria C, Mandala L, Smith J, Vitale CH, Lauro A, Gruttadauria S, et al. Effect of molecular adsorbent recirculating system in hepatitis C virus-related intractable pruritus. Liver Transpl. 2003 Apr;9(4):437–43.

12. Pares A, Cisneros L, Salmeron JM, Caballeria L, Mas A, Torras A, et al. Extracorporeal albumin dialysis: a procedure for prolonged relief of intractable pruritus in patients with primary biliary cirrhosis. Am J Gastroenterol. 2004 Jun;99(6):1105–10.

13. Acevedo Ribo M, Moreno Planas JM, Sanz Moreno C, Rubio Gonzalez EE, Rubio Gonzalez E, Boullosa Grana E, et al. Therapy of intractable pruritus with MARS. Transplant Proc. 2005 Apr;37(3):1480–1.

14. Pares A, Herrera M, Aviles J, Sanz M, Mas A. Treatment of resistant pruritus from cholestasis with albumin dialysis: combined analysis of patients from three centers. J Hepatol. 2010 Aug;53(2):307–12.

15. Beuers U, Gerken G, Pusl T. Biliary drainage transiently relieves intractable pruritus in primary biliary cirrhosis. Hepatology. 2006 Jul;44(1):280–1.

16. Gun F, Erginel B, Durmaz O, Sokucu S, Salman T, Celik A. An outstanding non-transplant surgical intervention in progressive familial intrahepatic cholestasis: partial internal biliary diversion. Pediatr Surg Int. 2010 Aug;26(8):831–4.

17. Whitington P, Whitington G. Partial external diversion of bile for the treatment of intractable pruritus associated with intrahepatic cholestasis. Gastroenterology. 1988;95:130–6.

18. Schukfeh N, Metzelder ML, Petersen C, Reismann M, Pfister ED, Ure BM, et al. Normalization of serum bile acids after partial external biliary diversion indicates an excellent long-term outcome in children with progressive familial intrahepatic cholestasis. J Pediatr Surg. 2012 Mar;47(3):501–5.

19. Ng VL, Ryckman FC, Porta G, Miura IK, de Carvalho E, Servidoni MF, et al. Long-term outcome after partial external biliary diversion for intractable pruritus in patients with intrahepatic cholestasis. J Pediatr Gastroenterol Nutr. 2000;30(2):152–6.

20. Galeazzi R, Lorenzini I, Orlandi F. Rifampicin-induced elevation of serum bile acids in man. Dig Dis Sci. 1980 Feb;25(2):108–12.

21. Hoensch HP, Balzer K, Dylewizc P, Kirch W, Goebell H, Ohnhaus EE. Effect of rifampicin treatment on hepatic drug metabolism and serum bile acids in patients with primary biliary cirrhosis. Eur J Clin Pharmacol. 1985;28(4):475–7.

22. Ghent CN, Carruthers SG. Treatment of pruritus in primary biliary cirrhosis with rifampin. Results of a double-blind, crossover, randomized trial. Gastroenterology. 1988;94(2):488–93.

23. Bachs L, Parés A, Elena M, Piera C, Rodés J. Comparison of rifampicin with phenobarbitone for treatment of pruritus in biliary cirrhosis. Lancet. 1989;1(8638):574–6.

24. Podesta A, Lopez P, Terg R, Villamil F, Flores D, Mastai R, et al. Treatment of pruritus of primary biliary cirrhosis with rifampin. Digestive Dis Sci. 1991;36(2):216–20.

25. Khurana S, Singh P. Rifampin is safe for treatment of pruritus due to chronic cholestasis: a meta-analysis of prospective randomized-controlled trials. Liver Int. 2006 Oct;26(8):943–8.
26. Prince MI, Burt AD, Jones DE. Hepatitis and liver dysfunction with rifampicin therapy for pruritus in primary biliary cirrhosis. Gut. 2002;50(3):436–9.
27. Tirona RG, Kim RB. Nuclear receptors and drug disposition gene regulation. J Pharm Sci. 2005 Jun;94(6):1169–86.
28. Kreek MJ, Garfield JW, Gutjahr CL, Giusti LM. Rifampin-induced methadone withdrawal. N Engl J Med. 1976 May 13;294(20):1104–6.
29. Ballantyne JC, Loach AB, Carr DB. Itching after epidural and spinal opiates. Pain. 1988;33(2):149–60.
30. Ballantyne JC, Loach AB, Carr DB. The incidence of pruritus after epidural morphine. Anaesthesia. 1989;44(10):863.
31. Dailey PA, Brookshire GL, Shnider SM, Abboud TK, Kotelko DM, Noueihid R, et al. The effects of naloxone associated with the intrathecal use of morphine in labor. Anesth Analg. 1985;64(7):658–66.
32. Abbound TK, Lee K, Zhu J, Reyes A, Afrasiabi A, Mantilla M, et al. Prophylactic oral naltrexone with intrathecal morphine for cesarean section: effects on adverse reactions and analgesia. Anesth Analg. 1990;71(4):367–70.
33. Bergasa NV, Jones EA. The pruritus of cholestasis: potential pathogenic and therapeutic implications of opioids. Gastroenterology. 1995;108(5):1582–8.
34. Bergasa NV, Alling DW, Talbot TL, Swain MG, Yurdaydin C, Turner ML, et al. Effects of naloxone infusions in patients with the pruritus of cholestasis. A double-blind, randomized, controlled trial. Ann Intern Med. 1995 Aug 1;123(3):161–7.
35. Thornton JR, Losowsky MS. Opioid peptides and primary biliary cirrhosis. Br Med J. 1988;297(6662):1501–4.
36. Bergasa NV, Talbot TL, Alling DW, Schmitt JM, Walker EC, Baker BL, et al. A controlled trial of naloxone infusions for the pruritus of chronic cholestasis. Gastroenterology. 1992;102(2):544–9.
37. Carson KL, Tran TT, Cotton P, Sharara AI, Hunt CM. Pilot study of the use of naltrexone to treat the severe pruritus of cholestatic liver disease. Am J Gastroenterol. 1996;91:1022–3.
38. Wolfhagen FHJ, Sternieri E, Hop WCJ, Vitale G, Bertolotti M, van Buuren HR. Oral naltrexone treatment for cholestatic pruritus: a double-blind, placebo-controlled study. Gastroenterology. 1997;113(4):1264–9.
39. Bergasa NV, Schmitt JM, Talbot TL, Alling DW, Swain MG, Turner ML, et al. Open-label trial of oral nalmefene therapy for the pruritus of cholestasis. Hepatology. 1998 Mar;27(3):679–84.
40. Bergasa NV, Alling DW, Talbot TL, Wells MC, Jones EA. Oral nalmefene therapy reduces scratching activity due to the pruritus of cholestasis: a controlled study. J Am Acad Dermatol. 1999 Sep;41(3 Pt 1):431–4.
41. Terg R, Coronel E, Sorda J, Munoz AE, Findor J. Efficacy and safety of oral naltrexone treatment for pruritus of cholestasis, a crossover, double blind, placebo-controlled study. J Hepatol. 2002;37(6):717–22.
42. Mansour-Ghanaei F, Taheri A, Froutan H, Ghofrani H, Nasiri-Toosi M, Bagherzadeh AH, et al. Effect of oral naltrexone on pruritus in cholestatic patients. World J Gastroenterol. 2006 Feb 21;12(7):1125–8.
43. Neuberger J, Jones EA. Liver transplantation for intractable pruritus is contraindicated before an adequate trial of opiate antagonist therapy. Eur J Gastroenterol Hepatol. 2001;13(11):1393–4.
44. Jones EA, Dekker LR. Florid opioid withdrawal-like reaction precipitated by naltrexone in a patient with chronic cholestasis. Gastroenterology. 2000;118(2):431–2.
45. Krystal JH, Cramer JA, Krol WF, Kirk GF, Ra R. Naltrexone in the treatment of alcohol dependence. N Engl J Med. 2001;345:1734–9.
46. Mitchell JE. Naltrexone and hepatotoxicity. Lancet. 1986;i:1215.

47. Bertolotti M, Ferrari A, Vitale G, Stefani M, Trenti T, Loria P, et al. Effect of liver cirrhosis on the systemic availability of naltrexone in humans. J Hepatol. 1997;27:505–11.
48. Lloyd-Thomas HG, Sherlock S. Testosterone therapy for the pruritus of obstructive jaundice. Br Med J. 1952 Dec 13;2(4797):1289–91.
49. NARCAN® Nasal Spray [prescribing information]. Plymouth Meeting PAP, Inc.; 2020. 2020 [cited 2020 December 8th, 2020]. Available from: http://www.narcannasalspray.
50. Kamimura K, Yokoo T, Kamimura H, Sakamaki A, Abe S, Tsuchiya A, et al. Long-term efficacy and safety of nalfurafine hydrochloride on pruritus in chronic liver disease patients: patient-reported outcome based analyses. PLoS One. 2017;12(6):e0178991.
51. Ko MC, Lee H, Song MS, Sobczyk-Kojiro K, Mosberg HI, Kishioka S, et al. Activation of kappa-opioid receptors inhibits pruritus evoked by subcutaneous or intrathecal administration of morphine in monkeys. J Pharmacol Exp Ther. 2003 Apr;305(1):173–9.
52. Ko MC, Song MS, Edwards T, Lee H, Naughton NN. The role of central mu opioid receptors in opioid-induced itch in primates. J Pharmacol Exp Ther. 2004 Jul;310(1): 169–76.
53. Reisine T. Pasternak. Opioid analgesics and antagonists. In: Molinoff PB, Ruddon RW, editors. The Pharmacologica basis of therapeutics. 9th ed. New York: McGraw-Hill; 1996. p. 521–55.
54. Yosipovitch G, Stander S. Meeting report of the 3rd international workshop for the study of itch. J Invest Dermatol. 2006 Sep;126(9):1928–30.
55. Dawn AG, Yosipovitch G. Butorphanol for treatment of intractable pruritus. J Am Acad Dermatol. 2006 Mar;54(3):527–31.
56. Stehling LC, Zauder HL. Double-blind comparison of butorphanol tartrate and meperidine hydrochloride in balanced anaesthesia. J Int Med Res. 1978;6(5):384–7.
57. Fisher MA, Glass S. Butorphanol (Stadol): a study in problems of current drug information and control. Neurology. 1997 May;48(5):1156–60.
58. Zylicz Z, Krajnik M. Codeine for pruritus in primary billiary cirrhosis. Lancet. 1999 Mar 6;353(9155):813.
59. Zylicz Z, Krajnik M. Codeine for pruritus in primary billiary cirrhosis [letter]. Lancet. 1999;353(9155):813.
60. Richardson BP. Serotonin and nociception. Annals of the New York Academy of Sci. 1990;600:511–20.
61. Kjellberg F, Tramer MR. Pharmacological control of opioid-induced pruritus: a quantitative systematic review of randomized trials. Eur J Anaesthesiol. 2001;18(6):346–57.
62. Raderer M, Muller C, Scheithauer W. Ondansetron for pruritus due to cholestasis. N Engl J Med. 1994;21:1540.
63. Schworer H, Ramadori G. Improvement of cholestatic pruritus by ondansetron. Lancet. 1993;341:1277.
64. Muller C, Pongratz S, Pidlich J, Penner E, Kaider A, Schemper M, et al. Treatment of pruritus in chronic liver disease with the 5-hydroxytryptamine receptor type 3 antagonist ondansetron: a randomized, placebo-controlled, double-blind cross-over trial. Eur J Gastroenterol Hepatol. 1998;10:865–70.
65. Schworer H, Hartmann H, Ramadori G. Relief of cholestatic pruritus by a novel class of drugs: 5- hydroxytryptamine type 3 (5-HT3) receptor antagonists: effectiveness of ondansetron. Pain. 1995;61(1):33–7.
66. O'Donohue JW, Pereira SP, Ashdown AC, Haigh CG, Wilkinson JR, Williams R. A controlled trial of ondansetron in the pruritus of cholestasis. Aliment Pharmacol Ther. 2005 Apr 15;21(8):1041–5.
67. Jones EA, Molenaar HA, Oosting J. Ondansetron and pruritus in chronic liver disease: a controlled study. Hepato-Gastroenterology. 2007 Jun;54(76):1196–9.
68. Diehn F, Tefferi A. Pruritus in polycythaemia vera: prevalence, laboratory correlates and management. Br J Haematol. 2001;115:619–21.
69. Zylicz Z, Krajnik M, Sorge AA, Costantini M. Paroxetine in the treatment of severe non-dermatological pruritus: a randomized, controlled trial. J Pain Symptom Manag. 2003 Dec;26(6):1105–12.

70. Zylicz Z, Smits C, Krajnik M. Paroxetine for pruritus in advanced cancer. J Pain Symptom Manag. 1998 Aug;16(2):121–4.
71. Nutt D. Mirtazapine: pharmacology in relation to adverse effects. Acta Psychiatr Scand Suppl. 1997;391:31–7.
72. Davis MP, Frandsen JL, Walsh D, Andresen S, Taylor S. Mirtazapine for pruritus. J Pain Symptom Manag. 2003 Mar;25(3):288–91.
73. Hundley JL, G. Y. Mirtazapine for reducing nocturnal itch in patients with chronic pruritus: a pilot study. J Am Acad Dermatol. 2004;50:889–91.
74. Browning J, Combes B, Mayo MJ. Long-term efficacy of sertraline as a treatment for cholestatic pruritus in patients with primary biliary cirrhosis. Am J Gastroenterol. 2003;98(12):2736–41.
75. Mayo MJ, Handem I, Saldana S, Jacobe H, Getachew Y, Rush AJ. Sertraline as a first-line treatment for cholestatic pruritus. Hepatology. 2007 Mar;45(3):666–74.
76. Bergasa NV, Link MJ, Keogh M, Yaroslavsky G, Rosenthal RN, McGee M. Pilot study of bright-light therapy reflected toward the eyes for the pruritus of chronic liver disease. Am J Gastroenterol. 2001;96(5):1563–70.
77. De Vries E, Bolier R, van Buuren H, Beueres U. Fibrates for itch (FITCH) in Fibrosing Cholangiopathies: a double-blind, randomized, placebo-controlled trial (n press). Gastroenterology. 2020; Epub October 05, 2020
78. Reig A, Sesé P, Parés A. Effects of Bezafibrate on outcome and pruritus in primary biliary cholangitis with suboptimal Ursodeoxycholic acid response. Am J Gastroenterol. 2018;113(1):49–55.
79. Turner IB, Rawlins MD, Wood P, James OF. Flumecinol for the treatment of pruritus associated with primary biliary cirrhosis. Aliment Pharmacol Ther. 1994;8(3):337–42.
80. Berg CL, Gollan JL. Primary biliary cirrhosis: new therapeutic directions. Scand J Gastroenterol Suppl. 1992;192:43–9.
81. Watson JP, Jones DE, James OF, Cann PA, Bramble MG. Case report: oral antioxidant therapy for the treatment of primary biliary cirrhosis: a pilot study. J Gastroenterol Hepatol. 1999;14(10):1034–40.
82. Walt R, Daneshmend T, Fellows I. Effect of stanozolol on itching in primary biliary cirrhosis. Br Med J. 1988;296:607.
83. Hanid MA, Levi AJ. Phototherapy for pruritus in primary biliary cirrhosis [letter]. Lancet. 1980;2(8193):530.
84. Borgeat A, Wilder-Smith OHG, Mentha G. Subhypnotic doses of propofol relieve pruritus associated with liver disese. Gastroenterlogy. 1993;104:244–7.
85. Borgeat A, Wilder-Smith O, Saiah M, Rifat K. Subhypnotic doses of propofol relieve pruritus induced by epidural and intrathecal morphine. Anesthesiology. 1992;76:510–2.
86. Neff GW, O'Brien CB, Reddy KR, Bergasa NV, Regev A, Molina E, et al. Preliminary observation with dronabinol in patients with intractable pruritus secondary to cholestatic liver disease. Am J Gastroenterol. 2002 Aug;97(8):2117–9.
87. Villamil AG, Bandi JC, Galdame OA, Gerona S, Gadano AC. Efficacy of lidocaine in the treatment of pruritus in patients with chronic cholestatic liver diseases. Am J Med. 2005 Oct;118(10):1160–3.
88. Frezza M, Centini G, Cammareri G, Le Grazie C, Di Padova C. S-adenosylmethionine for the treatment of intrahepatic cholestasis of pregnancy. Results of a controlled clinical trial. Hepatogastroenterology. 1990;37 Suppl 2:122–5.
89. Babatin MA, Sanai FM, Swain MG. Methotrexate therapy for the symptomatic treatment of primary biliary cirrhosis patients, who are biochemical incomplete responders to ursodeoxycholic acid therapy. Aliment Pharmacol Ther. 2006 Sep 1;24(5):813–20.
90. Aguilar-Bernier M, Bassas-Vila J, Sanz-Munoz C, Miranda-Romero A. Successful treatment of pruritus with topical tacrolimus in a patient with primary biliary cirrhosis. Br J Dermatol. 2005 Apr;152(4):808–9.
91. Bergasa NV, McGee M, Ginsburg IH, Engler D. Gabapentin in patients with the pruritus of cholestasis: a double-blind, randomized, placebo-controlled trial. Hepatology. 2006 Nov;44(5):1317–23.

92. Rishe E, Azarm A, Bergasa NV. Itch in primary biliary cirrhosis: a patients' perspective. Acta Derm Venereol. 2008;88(1):34–7.

93. Kaplan MM, Gershwin ME. Primary biliary cirrhosis. N Engl J Med. 2005 Sep 22;353(12):1261–73.

94. Newton JL, Gibson GJ, Tomlinson M, Wilton K, Jones D. Fatigue in primary biliary cirrhosis is associated with excessive daytime somnolence. Hepatology. 2006 Jul;44(1):91–8.

95. Jones D, Newton JL. An open study of modafinil for the treatment of daytime somnolence and fatigue in primary biliary cirrhosis. Aliment Pharmacol Ther. 2007;25(4):471–6.

96. Bergasa NV, Mehlman J, Bir K. Aerobic exercise: a potential therapeutic intervention for patients with liver disease. Med Hypotheses. 2004;62(6):935–41.

97. Schuppan D, Afdhal NH. Liver cirrhosis. Lancet. 2008 Mar 8;371(9615):838–51.

98. Thampanitchawong P, Piratvisuth T. Liver biopsy:complications and risk factors. World J Gastroenterol. 1999 Aug;5(4):301–4.

99. Bravo AA, Sheth SG, Chopra S. Liver biopsy. N Engl J Med. 2001 Feb 15;344(7):495–500.

100. Berzigotti A, Seijo S, Reverter E, Bosch J. Assessing portal hypertension in liver diseases. Expert Rev Gastroenterol Hepatol. 2013 Feb;7(2):141–55.

101. Bosch J, Abraldes JG, Berzigotti A, Garcia-Pagan JC. Portal hypertension and gastrointestinal bleeding. Semin Liver Dis. 2008 Feb;28(1):3–25.

102. Gracia-Sancho J, Lavina B, Rodriguez-Vilarrupla A, Garcia-Caldero H, Fernandez M, Bosch J, et al. Increased oxidative stress in cirrhotic rat livers: a potential mechanism contributing to reduced nitric oxide bioavailability. Hepatology. 2008 Apr;47(4):1248–56.

103. Iwakiri Y, Groszmann RJ. Vascular endothelial dysfunction in cirrhosis. J Hepatol. 2007 May;46(5):927–34.

104. Bosch J. Vascular deterioration in cirrhosis: the big picture. J Clin Gastroenterol. 2007 Nov-Dec;41(Suppl 3):S247–53.

105. Bosch J, Iwakiri Y. The portal hypertension syndrome: etiology, classification, relevance, and animal models. Hepatol Int. 2018 Feb;12(Suppl 1):1–10.

106. Wiest R, Groszmann RJ. The paradox of nitric oxide in cirrhosis and portal hypertension: too much, not enough. Hepatology. 2002 Feb;35(2):478–91.

107. Garcia-Tsao G, Abraldes JG, Berzigotti A, Bosch J. Portal hypertensive bleeding in cirrhosis: risk stratification, diagnosis, and management: 2016 practice guidance by the American association for the study of liver diseases. Hepatology. 2017 Jan;65(1):310–35.

108. Garcia-Tsao G, Sanyal AJ, Grace ND, Carey W. Practice guidelines Committee of the American Association for the study of liver D, practice parameters Committee of the American College of G. prevention and management of gastroesophageal varices and variceal hemorrhage in cirrhosis. Hepatology. 2007 Sep;46(3):922–38.

109. Garcia-Tsao G, Sanyal AJ, Grace ND, Carey W. Prevention and management of gastroesophageal varices and variceal hemorrhage in cirrhosis. Hepatology. 2007 Sep;46(3):922–38.

110. North Italian Endoscopic Club for the S, Treatment of Esophageal V. Prediction of the first variceal hemorrhage in patients with cirrhosis of the liver and esophageal varices. A prospective multicenter study. N Engl J Med. 1988 Oct 13;319(15):983–9.

111. D'Amico G, Pagliaro L, Bosch J. Pharmacological treatment of portal hypertension: an evidence-based approach. Semin Liver Dis. 1999;19(4):475–505.

112. de Franchis R, Baveno VF. Revising consensus in portal hypertension: report of the Baveno V consensus workshop on methodology of diagnosis and therapy in portal hypertension. J Hepatol. 2010 Oct;53(4):762–8.

113. Boregowda U, Umapathy C, Halim N, Desai M, Nanjappa A, Arekapudi S, et al. Update on the management of gastrointestinal varices. World J Gastrointest Pharmacol Ther. 2019 Jan 21;10(1):1–21.

114. Lee SJ, Kim SU, Kim MD, Kim YH, Kim GM, Park SI, et al. Comparison of treatment outcomes between balloon-occluded retrograde transvenous obliteration and transjugular intrahepatic portosystemic shunt for gastric variceal bleeding hemostasis. J Gastroenterol Hepatol. 2017 Aug;32(8):1487–94.

115. Schrier RW, Arroyo V, Bernardi M, Epstein M, Henriksen JH, Rodes J. Peripheral arterial vasodilation hypothesis: a proposal for the initiation of renal sodium and water retention in cirrhosis. Hepatology. 1988 Sep-Oct;8(5):1151–7.

116. Gines P, Quintero E, Arroyo V, Teres J, Bruguera M, Rimola A, et al. Compensated cirrhosis: natural history and prognostic factors. Hepatology. 1987 Jan-Feb;7(1):122–8.

117. Guevara M, Uriz J, Ginès P. Prognosis in patients with cirrhosis and ascites. In: AV GP, Rodés J, Schrier R, editors. Ascites and renal dysfunction in liver disease: pathogenesis, diagnosis and treatment. MA, USA: Malden: Blackwell; 2005. p. 260–70.

118. Planas R, Montoliu S, Balleste B, Rivera M, Miquel M, Masnou H, et al. Natural history of patients hospitalized for management of cirrhotic ascites. Clin Gastroenterol Hepatol. 2006 Nov;4(11):1385–94.

119. Biselli M, Dall'Agata M, Gramenzi A, Gitto S, Liberati C, Brodosi L, et al. A new prognostic model to predict dropout from the waiting list in cirrhotic candidates for liver transplantation with MELD score <18. Liver Int. 2015 Jan;35(1):184–91.

120. Witte MH, Dumont AE, Cole WR, Witte CL, Kintner K. Lymph circulation in hepatic cirrhosis: effect of portacaval shunt. Ann Intern Med. 1969 Feb;70(2):303–10.

121. Witte CL, Witte MH, Dumont AE, Frist J, Cole WR. Lymph protein in hepatic cirrhosis and experimental hepatic and portal venous hypertension. Ann Surg. 1968 Oct;168(4):567–77.

122. Laine GA, Hall JT, Laine SH, Granger J. Transsinusoidal fluid dynamics in canine liver during venous hypertension. Circ Res. 1979 Sep;45(3):317–23.

123. Witte MH, Witte CL, Dumont AE. Progress in liver disease: physiological factors involved in the causation of cirrhotic ascites. Gastroenterology. 1971 Nov;61(5):742–50.

124. Brauer RW, Holloway RJ, Leong GF. Changes in liver function and structure due to experimental passive congestion under controlled hepatic vein pressures. Am J Phys. 1959 Sep;197:681–92.

125. Granger DN, Miller T, Allen R, Parker RE, Parker JC, Taylor AE. Permselectivity of cat blood-lymph barrier to endogenous macromolecules. Gastroenterology. 1979 Jul;77(1):103–9.

126. Granger HJ, Laine GA. Consecutive barriers to movement of water and solutes across the liver sinusoids. Physiologist. 1980 Feb;23(1):83–5.

127. Witte CL, Witte MH, Cole WR, Chung YC, Bleisch VR, Dumont AE. Dual origin of ascites in hepatic cirrhosis. Surg Gynecol Obstet. 1969 Nov;129(5):1027–33.

128. Witte MH, Witte CL, Dumont AE. Estimated net transcapillary water and protein flux in the liver and intestine of patients with portal hypertension from hepatic cirrhosis. Gastroenterology. 1981 Feb;80(2):265–72.

129. Schaffner F, Poper H. Capillarization of hepatic sinusoids in man. Gastroenterology. 1963 Mar;44:239–42.

130. Dumont AE, Witte CL, Witte MH. Protein content of liver lymph in patients with portal hypertension secondary to hepatic cirrhosis. Lymphology. 1975 Dec;8(4):111–3.

131. Huet PM, Goresky CA, Villeneuve JP, Marleau D, Lough JO. Assessment of liver microcirculation in human cirrhosis. J Clin Invest. 1982 Dec;70(6):1234–44.

132. Fernandez-Llama P, Gines P, Schrier RW. Pathogenesis of sodium retention in cirrhosis: the arterial vasodilation hypothesis of ascites formation. In: Ginès P, Rodés J, Schrier R, editors. Ascites and renal dysfunction in liver disease: pathogenesis, diagnosis and treatment. MA, USA: Malden: Blackwell; 2005. p. 201–13.

133. Caregaro L, Lauro S, Angeli P, Merkel C, Gatta A. Renal water and sodium handling in compensated liver cirrhosis: mechanism of the impaired natriuresis after saline loading. Eur J Clin Investig. 1985 Dec;15(6):360–4.

134. Wood LJ, Massie D, McLean AJ, Dudley FJ. Renal sodium retention in cirrhosis: tubular site and relation to hepatic dysfunction. Hepatology. 1988 Jul-Aug;8(4):831–6.

135. Denison EK, Lieberman FL, Reynolds TB. 9- -fluorohydrocortisone induced ascites in alcoholic liver disease. Gastroenterology. 1971 Oct;61(4):497–503.

136. Wilkinson SP, Jowett TP, Slater JD, Arroyo V, Moodie H, Williams R. Renal sodium retention in cirrhosis: relation to aldosterone and nephron site. Clin Sci. 1979 Feb;56(2):169–77.

137. Arroyo V, Rodes J, Gutierrez-Lizarraga MA, Revert L. Prognostic value of spontaneous hyponatremia in cirrhosis with ascites. Am J Dig Dis. 1976 Mar;21(3):249–56.

138. Gines P, Berl T, Bernardi M, Bichet DG, Hamon G, Jimenez W, et al. Hyponatremia in cirrhosis: from pathogenesis to treatment. Hepatology. 1998 Sep;28(3):851–64.

139. Hoefs JC. Serum protein concentration and portal pressure determine the ascitic fluid protein concentration in patients with chronic liver disease. J Lab Clin Med. 1983 Aug;102(2):260–73.

140. Runyon BA, Montano AA, Akriviadis EA, Antillon MR, Irving MA, McHutchison JG. The serum-ascites albumin gradient is superior to the exudate-transudate concept in the differential diagnosis of ascites. Ann Intern Med. 1992 Aug 1;117(3):215–20.

141. Thomsen TW, Shaffer RW, White B, Setnik GS. Videos in clinical medicine. Paracentesis. N Engl J Med. 2006 Nov 9;355(19):e21.

142. Moore KP, Wong F, Gines P, Bernardi M, Ochs A, Salerno F, et al. The management of ascites in cirrhosis: report on the consensus conference of the international Ascites Club. Hepatology. 2003 Jul;38(1):258–66.

143. Stanley MM, Ochi S, Lee KK, Nemchausky BA, Greenlee HB, Allen JI, et al. Peritoneovenous shunting as compared with medical treatment in patients with alcoholic cirrhosis and massive ascites. Veterans administration cooperative study on treatment of alcoholic cirrhosis with Ascites. N Engl J Med. 1989 Dec 14;321(24):1632–8.

144. Runyon BA. Introduction to the revised American Association for the Study of Liver Diseases practice guideline management of adult patients with ascites due to cirrhosis 2012. Hepatology. 2013 Apr;57(4):1651–3.

145. European Association for the Study of the Liver. Electronic address eee, European Association for the Study of the L. EASL clinical practice guidelines for the management of patients with decompensated cirrhosis. J Hepatol. 2018 Aug;69(2):406–60.

146. Pockros PJ, Reynolds TB. Rapid diuresis in patients with ascites from chronic liver disease: the importance of peripheral edema. Gastroenterology. 1986 Jun;90(6):1827–33.

147. El-Bokl MA, Senousy BE, El-Karmouty KZ, Mohammed Iel K, Mohammed SM, Shabana SS, et al. Spot urinary sodium for assessing dietary sodium restriction in cirrhotic ascites. World J Gastroenterol. 2009 Aug 7;15(29):3631–5.

148. Arroyo V, Gines P, Gerbes AL, Dudley FJ, Gentilini P, Laffi G, et al. Definition and diagnostic criteria of refractory ascites and hepatorenal syndrome in cirrhosis. Int Ascites Club Hepatol. 1996 Jan;23(1):164–76.

149. Salerno F, Badalamenti S, Incerti P, Tempini S, Restelli B, Bruno S, et al. Repeated paracentesis and i.v. albumin infusion to treat 'tense' ascites in cirrhotic patients. A safe alternative therapy. J Hepatol. 1987 Aug;5(1):102–8.

150. Gines P, Arroyo V, Quintero E, Planas R, Bory F, Cabrera J, et al. Comparison of paracentesis and diuretics in the treatment of cirrhotics with tense ascites. Results of a randomized study. Gastroenterology. 1987 Aug;93(2):234–41.

151. Moreau R, Valla DC, Durand-Zaleski I, Bronowicki JP, Durand F, Chaput JC, et al. Comparison of outcome in patients with cirrhosis and ascites following treatment with albumin or a synthetic colloid: a randomised controlled pilot trail. Liver Int. 2006 Feb;26(1):46–54.

152. Fernandez-Esparrach G, Guevara M, Sort P, Pardo A, Jimenez W, Gines P, et al. Diuretic requirements after therapeutic paracentesis in non-azotemic patients with cirrhosis. A randomized double-blind trial of spironolactone versus placebo. J Hepatol. 1997 Mar;26(3): 614–20.

153. Rossle M, Ochs A, Gulberg V, Siegerstetter V, Holl J, Deibert P, et al. A comparison of paracentesis and transjugular intrahepatic portosystemic shunting in patients with ascites. N Engl J Med. 2000 Jun 8;342(23):1701–7.

154. Dariushnia SR, Haskal ZJ, Midia M, Saiter CK, Nikolic B. Quality improvement guidelines for Transjugular intrahepatic portosystemic. J Vasc Interv Radiol. 2016;27(1):1–7.

155. Singh V, Dhungana SP, Singh B, Vijayverghia R, Nain CK, Sharma N, Bhalla A, Gupta PK. Midodrine in patients with cirrhosis and refractory or recurrent ascites: a randomized pilot study. J Hepatol. 2012;56:348–54.

156. Wong F, Bendel E, Sniderman K, Frederick T, Haskal ZJ, Sanyal A, et al. Improvement in quality of life and decrease in large volume paracentesis requirements with the automated low flow Ascites pump. Liver Transpl. 2020 Jan 30;

157. Garbuzenko DV, Arefyev NO. Hepatic hydrothorax: an update and review of the literature. World J Hepatol. 2017 Nov 8;9(31):1197–204.

158. Huang PM, Kuo SW, Chen JS, Lee JM. Thoracoscopic mesh repair of diaphragmatic defects in hepatic hydrothorax: a 10-year experience. Ann Thorac Surg. 2016 May;101(5):1921–7.

159. Wasmuth HE, Kunz D, Yagmur E, Timmer-Stranghoner A, Vidacek D, Siewert E, et al. Patients with acute on chronic liver failure display "sepsis-like" immune paralysis. J Hepatol. 2005 Feb;42(2):195–201.

160. Wiest R, Garcia-Tsao G. Bacterial translocation (BT) in cirrhosis. Hepatology. 2005 Mar;41(3):422–33.

161. Mookerjee RP, Stadlbauer V, Lidder S, Wright GA, Hodges SJ, Davies NA, et al. Neutrophil dysfunction in alcoholic hepatitis superimposed on cirrhosis is reversible and predicts the outcome. Hepatology. 2007 Sep;46(3):831–40.

162. Such J, Runyon BA. Spontaneous bacterial peritonitis. Clin Infect Dis. 1998;27(4):669–74. quiz 75-6

163. Bellot P, Frances R, Such J. Pathological bacterial translocation in cirrhosis: pathophysiology, diagnosis and clinical implications. Liver Int. 2013 Jan;33(1):31–9.

164. Kumar A, Roberts D, Wood KE, Light B, Parrillo JE, Sharma S, et al. Duration of hypotension before initiation of effective antimicrobial therapy is the critical determinant of survival in human septic shock. Crit Care Med. 2006 Jun;34(6):1589–96.

165. Garcia-Tsao G. Spontaneous bacterial peritonitis. Gastroenterol Clin N Am. 1992 Mar;21(1):257–75.

166. Mandorfer M, Bota S, Schwabl P, Bucsics T, Pfisterer N, Kruzik M, et al. Nonselective beta blockers increase risk for hepatorenal syndrome and death in patients with cirrhosis and spontaneous bacterial peritonitis. Gastroenterology. 2014 Jun;146(7):1680–90 e1.

167. Angeli P, Gines P, Wong F, Bernardi M, Boyer TD, Gerbes A, et al. Diagnosis and management of acute kidney injury in patients with cirrhosis: revised consensus recommendations of the International Club of Ascites. Gut. 2015 Apr;64(4):531–7.

168. Piano S, Rosi S, Maresio G, Fasolato S, Cavallin M, Romano A, et al. Evaluation of the acute kidney injury network criteria in hospitalized patients with cirrhosis and ascites. J Hepatol. 2013 Sep;59(3):482–9.

169. Belcher JM, Garcia-Tsao G, Sanyal AJ, Bhogal H, Lim JK, Ansari N, et al. Association of AKI with mortality and complications in hospitalized patients with cirrhosis. Hepatology. 2013 Feb;57(2):753–62.

170. Nadim MK, Durand F, Kellum JA, Levitsky J, O'Leary JG, Karvellas CJ, et al. Management of the critically ill patient with cirrhosis: a multidisciplinary perspective. J Hepatol. 2016 Mar;64(3):717–35.

171. Umgelter A, Reindl W, Wagner KS, Franzen M, Stock K, Schmid RM, et al. Effects of plasma expansion with albumin and paracentesis on haemodynamics and kidney function in critically ill cirrhotic patients with tense ascites and hepatorenal syndrome: a prospective uncontrolled trial. Crit Care. 2008;12(1):R4.

172. Salerno F, Gerbes A, Gines P, Wong F, Arroyo V. Diagnosis, prevention and treatment of hepatorenal syndrome in cirrhosis. Gut. 2007 Sep;56(9):1310–8.

173. Puthumana J, Ariza X, Belcher JM, Graupera I, Gines P, Parikh CR. Urine interleukin 18 and Lipocalin 2 are biomarkers of acute tubular necrosis in patients with cirrhosis: a systematic review and meta-analysis. Clin Gastroenterol Hepatol. 2017 Jul;15(7):1003–13 e3.

174. Schrier R, Arroyo V, Bernardi M, Epstein M, Henriksen J, Rodés J. Peripheral arterial vasodilation hypothesis: a proposal for the initiationof renal sodium andwater retention in cirrhosis. Hepatology. 1988;8:1151–7.

175. Ring-Larsen H. Renal blood flow in cirrhosis: relation to systemic and portal haemodynamics and liver function. Scand J Clin Lab Invest. 1977 Nov;37(7):635–42.

176. Cohn JN. Renal hemodynamic alterations in liver disease. Perspect Nephrol Hypertens. 1976;3:255–34.
177. Iwakiri Y, Groszmann RJ. The hyperdynamic circulation of chronic liver diseases: from the patient to the molecule. Hepatology. 2006 Feb;43(2 Suppl 1):S121–31.
178. Wong F, Leung W, Al Beshir M, Marquez M, Renner EL. Outcomes of patients with cirrhosis and hepatorenal syndrome type 1 treated with liver transplantation. Liver Transpl. 2015 Mar;21(3):300–7.
179. Szeto HH, Liu S, Soong Y, Seshan SV, Cohen-Gould L, Manichev V, et al. Mitochondria protection after acute ischemia prevents prolonged upregulation of IL-1beta and IL-18 and arrests CKD. J Am Soc Nephrol. 2017 May;28(5):1437–49.
180. van Slambrouck CM, Salem F, Meehan SM, Chang A. Bile cast nephropathy is a common pathologic finding for kidney injury associated with severe liver dysfunction. Kidney Int. 2013 Jul;84(1):192–7.
181. Chatrath H, Liangpunsakul S, Ghabril M, Otte J, Chalasani N, Vuppalanchi R. Prevalence and morbidity associated with muscle cramps in patients with cirrhosis. Am J Med. 2012 Oct;125(10):1019–25.
182. Angeli P, Albino G, Carraro P, Dalla Pria M, Merkel C, Caregaro L, et al. Cirrhosis and muscle cramps: evidence of a causal relationship. Hepatology. 1996 Feb;23(2):264–73.
183. Elfert AA, Abo Ali L, Soliman S, Zakaria S, Shehab El-Din I, Elkhalawany W, et al. Randomized placebo-controlled study of baclofen in the treatment of muscle cramps in patients with liver cirrhosis. Eur J Gastroenterol Hepatol. 2016 Nov;28(11):1280–4.
184. Butterworth RF, Giguere JF, Michaud J, Lavoie J, Layrargues GP. Ammonia: key factor in the pathogenesis of hepatic encephalopathy. Neurochem Pathol. 1987 Feb-Apr;6(1–2):1–12.
185. Norenberg MD. Astrocytic-ammonia interactions in hepatic encephalopathy. Semin Liver Dis. 1996 Aug;16(3):245–53.
186. Vilstrup H, Amodio P, Bajaj J, Cordoba J, Ferenci P, Mullen KD, et al. Hepatic encephalopathy in chronic liver disease: 2014 practice guideline by the American Association for the Study of Liver Diseases and the European Association for the Study of the liver. Hepatology. 2014 Aug;60(2):715–35.
187. Jayakumar AR, Norenberg MD. Hyperammonemia in hepatic encephalopathy. J Clin Exp Hepatol. 2018 Sep;8(3):272–80.
188. Bustamante J, Rimola A, Ventura PJ, Navasa M, Cirera I, Reggiardo V, et al. Prognostic significance of hepatic encephalopathy in patients with cirrhosis. J Hepatol. 1999 May;30(5):890–5.
189. Riggio O, Efrati C, Catalano C, Pediconi F, Mecarelli O, Accornero N, et al. High prevalence of spontaneous portal-systemic shunts in persistent hepatic encephalopathy: a case-control study. Hepatology. 2005 Nov;42(5):1158–65.
190. Schafer DF, Jones EA. Hepatic encephalopathy and the gamma-aminobutyric-acid neurotransmitter system. Lancet. 1982 Jan 2;1(8262):18–20.
191. Basile AS, Jones EA, Skolnick P. The pathogenesis and treatment of hepatic encephalopathy: evidence for the involvement of benzodiazepine receptor ligands. Pharmacol Rev. 1991 Mar;43(1):27–71.
192. Basile AS, Harrison PM, Hughes RD, Gu ZQ, Pannell L, McKinney A, et al. Relationship between plasma benzodiazepine receptor ligand concentrations and severity of hepatic encephalopathy. Hepatology. 1994 Jan;19(1):112–21.
193. Basile AS, Jones EA. Ammonia and GABA-ergic neurotransmission: interrelated factors in the pathogenesis of hepatic encephalopathy. Hepatology. 1997 Jun;25(6):1303–5.
194. Norenberg MD. Astroglial dysfunction in hepatic encephalopathy. Metab Brain Dis. 1998 Dec;13(4):319–35.
195. Bender AS, Norenberg MD. Effect of benzodiazepines and neurosteroids on ammonia-induced swelling in cultured astrocytes. J Neurosci Res. 1998 Dec 1;54(5):673–80.
196. Butterworth RF. Neurosteroids in hepatic encephalopathy: novel insights and new therapeutic opportunities. J Steroid Biochem Mol Biol. 2016 Jun;160:94–7.
197. Cordoba J, Blei AT. Treatment of hepatic encephalopathy. Am J Gastroenterol. 1997 Sep;92(9):1429–39.
198. Mohiuddin SSKD. Biochemistry, ammonia. Treasure Island: Florida; 2019.

199. Walker V. Ammonia metabolism and hyperammonemic disorders. Adv Clin Chem. 2014;67:73–150.
200. Als-Nielsen B, Gluud LL, Gluud C. Benzodiazepine receptor antagonists for hepatic encephalopathy. Cochrane Database Syst Rev. 2004;2:CD002798.
201. Wijdicks EF. Hepatic encephalopathy. N Engl J Med. 2016 Oct 27;375(17):1660–70.
202. Ahluwalia V, Betrapally NS, Hylemon PB, White MB, Gillevet PM, Unser AB, et al. Impaired gut-liver-brain Axis in patients with cirrhosis. Sci Rep. 2016 May 26;6:26800.
203. Romero-Gomez M, Jover M, Del Campo JA, Royo JL, Hoyas E, Galan JJ, et al. Variations in the promoter region of the glutaminase gene and the development of hepatic encephalopathy in patients with cirrhosis: a cohort study. Ann Intern Med. 2010 Sep 7;153(5):281–8.
204. Ferenci P, Lockwood A, Mullen K, Tarter R, Weissenborn K, Blei AT. Hepatic encephalopathy--definition, nomenclature, diagnosis, and quantification: final report of the working party at the 11th world congresses of gastroenterology, Vienna, 1998. Hepatology. 2002 Mar;35(3):716–21.
205. Weissenborn K, Ruckert N, Hecker H, Manns MP. The number connection tests a and B: interindividual variability and use for the assessment of early hepatic encephalopathy. J Hepatol. 1998 Apr;28(4):646–53.
206. Parsons-Smith BG, Summerskill WH, Dawson AM, Sherlock S. The electroencephalograph in liver disease. Lancet. 1957 Nov 2;273(7001):867–71.
207. Amodio P, Montagnese S. Clinical neurophysiology of hepatic encephalopathy. J Clin Exp Hepatol. 2015 Mar;5(Suppl 1):S60–8.
208. Han KH. Mechanisms of the effects of acidosis and hypokalemia on renal ammonia metabolism. Electrolyte & Blood Pressure: E & BP. 2011 Dec;9(2):45–9.
209. Shehata HH, Elfert AA, Abdin AA, Soliman SM, Elkhouly RA, Hawash NI, et al. Randomized controlled trial of polyethylene glycol versus lactulose for the treatment of overt hepatic encephalopathy. Eur J Gastroenterol Hepatol. 2018 Dec;30(12):1476–81.
210. Ferenci P. Treatment options for hepatic encephalopathy: a review. Serminars Liver Dis. 2007;27(S2):10–7.
211. Uribe M, Campollo O, Vargas F, Ravelli GP, Mundo F, Zapata L, et al. Acidifying enemas (lactitol and lactose) vs. nonacidifying enemas (tap water) to treat acute portal-systemic encephalopathy: a double-blind, randomized clinical trial. Hepatology. 1987 Jul-Aug;7(4):639–43.
212. Riggio O, Varriale M, Testore GP, Di Rosa R, Di Rosa E, Merli M, et al. Effect of lactitol and lactulose administration on the fecal flora in cirrhotic patients. J Clin Gastroenterol. 1990 Aug;12(4):433–6.
213. Portalatin M, Winstead N. Medical management of constipation. Clin Colon Rectal Surg. 2012 Mar;25(1):12–9.
214. Rahimi RS, Singal AG, Cuthbert JA, Rockey DC. Lactulose vs polyethylene glycol 3350--electrolyte solution for treatment of overt hepatic encephalopathy: the HELP randomized clinical trial. JAMA Intern Med. 2014 Nov;174(11):1727–33.
215. Bass NM, Mullen KD, Sanyal A, Poordad F, Neff G, Leevy CB, et al. Rifaximin treatment in hepatic encephalopathy. N Engl J Med. 2010 Mar 25;362(12):1071–81.
216. Sharma BC, Sharma P, Lunia MK, Srivastava S, Goyal R, Sarin SK. A randomized, double-blind, controlled trial comparing rifaximin plus lactulose with lactulose alone in treatment of overt hepatic encephalopathy. Am J Gastroenterol. 2013 Sep;108(9):1458–63.
217. Zardi EM, Abbate A, Zardi DM, Dobrina A, Margiotta D, Van Tassell BW, et al. Cirrhotic cardiomyopathy. J Am Coll Cardiol. 2010 Aug 10;56(7):539–49.
218. Wiese S, Hove JD, Bendtsen F, Moller S. Cirrhotic cardiomyopathy: pathogenesis and clinical relevance. Nat Rev Gastroenterol Hepatol. 2014 Mar;11(3):177–86.
219. Chen Y, Chan AC, Chan SC, Chok SH, Sharr W, Fung J, et al. A detailed evaluation of cardiac function in cirrhotic patients and its alteration with or without liver transplantation. J Cardiol. 2016 Feb;67(2):140–6.
220. Moller S, Hove JD, Dixen U, Bendtsen F. New insights into cirrhotic cardiomyopathy. Int J Cardiol. 2013 Aug 20;167(4):1101–8.
221. Rodriguez-Roisin R, Krowka MJ, Herve P, Fallon MB, Committee ERSTFP-HVDS. Pulmonary-hepatic vascular disorders (PHD). Eur Respir J. 2004 Nov;24(5):861–80.

222. Cremona G, Higenbottam TW, Mayoral V, Alexander G, Demoncheaux E, Borland C, et al. Elevated exhaled nitric oxide in patients with hepatopulmonary syndrome. Eur Respir J. 1995 Nov;8(11):1883–5.

223. Zhang M, Luo B, Chen SJ, Abrams GA, Fallon MB. Endothelin-1 stimulation of endothelial nitric oxide synthase in the pathogenesis of hepatopulmonary syndrome. Am J Phys. 1999 Nov;277(5):G944–52.

224. Katsuta Y, Zhang XJ, Ohsuga M, Akimoto T, Komeichi H, Shimizu S, et al. Arterial hypoxemia and intrapulmonary vasodilatation in rat models of portal hypertension. J Gastroenterol. 2005 Aug;40(8):811–9.

225. Nunes H, Lebrec D, Mazmanian M, Capron F, Heller J, Tazi KA, et al. Role of nitric oxide in hepatopulmonary syndrome in cirrhotic rats. Am J Respir Crit Care Med. 2001 Sep 1;164(5):879–85.

226. Zhang HY, Han DW, Wang XG, Zhao YC, Zhou X, Zhao HZ. Experimental study on the role of endotoxin in the development of hepatopulmonary syndrome. World J Gastroenterol. 2005 Jan 28;11(4):567–72.

227. Arguedas MR, Drake BB, Kapoor A, Fallon MB. Carboxyhemoglobin levels in cirrhotic patients with and without hepatopulmonary syndrome. Gastroenterology. 2005 Feb;128(2):328–33.

228. Liu L, Liu N, Zhao Z, Liu J, Feng Y, Jiang H, et al. TNF-alpha neutralization improves experimental hepatopulmonary syndrome in rats. Liver Int. 2012 Jul;32(6):1018–26.

229. Rodriguez-Roisin R, Roca J, Agusti AG, Mastai R, Wagner PD, Bosch J. Gas exchange and pulmonary vascular reactivity in patients with liver cirrhosis. Am Rev Respir Dis. 1987 May;135(5):1085–92.

230. Berthelot P, Walker JG, Sherlock S, Reid L. Arterial changes in the lungs in cirrhosis of the liver--lung spider nevi. N Engl J Med. 1966 Feb 10;274(6):291–8.

231. Abrams GA, Sanders MK, Fallon MB. Utility of pulse oximetry in the detection of arterial hypoxemia in liver transplant candidates. Liver Transpl. 2002 Apr;8(4):391–6.

232. Arguedas MR, Singh H, Faulk DK, Fallon MB. Utility of pulse oximetry screening for hepatopulmonary syndrome. Clin Gastroenterol Hepatol. 2007 Jun;5(6):749–54.

233. Wolfe JD, Tashkin DP, Holly FE, Brachman MB, Genovesi MG. Hypoxemia of cirrhosis: detection of abnormal small pulmonary vascular channels by a quantitative radionuclide method. Am J Med. 1977 Nov;63(5):746–54.

234. Abrams GA, Nanda NC, Dubovsky EV, Krowka MJ, Fallon MB. Use of macroaggregated albumin lung perfusion scan to diagnose hepatopulmonary syndrome: a new approach. Gastroenterology. 1998 Feb;114(2):305–10.

235. Eriksson LS, Soderman C, Ericzon BG, Eleborg L, Wahren J, Hedenstierna G. Normalization of ventilation/perfusion relationships after liver transplantation in patients with decompensated cirrhosis: evidence for a hepatopulmonary syndrome. Hepatology. 1990 Dec;12(6):1350–7.

236. Gupta S, Castel H, Rao RV, Picard M, Lilly L, Faughnan ME, et al. Improved survival after liver transplantation in patients with hepatopulmonary syndrome. Am J Transplant. 2010 Feb;10(2):354–63.

237. Chevallier P, Novelli L, Motamedi JP, Hastier P, Brunner P, Bruneton JN. Hepatopulmonary syndrome successfully treated with transjugular intrahepatic portosystemic shunt: a three-year follow-up. J Vascular Int Radiol: JVIR. 2004 Jun;15(6):647–8.

238. Tsauo J, Weng N, Ma H, Jiang M, Zhao H, Li X. Role of Transjugular intrahepatic portosystemic shunts in the Management of Hepatopulmonary Syndrome: a systemic literature review. J Vascular Int Radiol: JVIR. 2015 Sep;26(9):1266–71.

239. Grady K, Gowda S, Kingah P, Soubani AO. Coil embolization of pulmonary arteries as a palliative treatment of diffuse type I hepatopulmonary syndrome. Respir Care. 2015 Feb;60(2):e20–5.

240. De BK, Dutta D, Pal SK, Gangopadhyay S, Das Baksi S, Pani A. The role of garlic in hepatopulmonary syndrome: a randomized controlled trial. Can J Gastroenterol. 2010 Mar;24(3):183–8.

241. Savale L, Watherald J, Sitbon O. Portopulmonary hypertension. Semin Respir Crit Care Med. 2017 Oct;38(5):651–61.
242. Roberts KE, Fallon MB, Krowka MJ, Brown RS, Trotter JF, Peter I, et al. Genetic risk factors for portopulmonary hypertension in patients with advanced liver disease. Am J Respir Crit Care Med. 2009 May 1;179(9):835–42.
243. Savale L, Guimas M, Ebstein N, Fertin M, Jevnikar M, Renard S, et al. Portopulmonary hypertension in the current era of pulmonary hypertension management. J Hepatol. 2020 Mar;4
244. Pilatis ND, Jacobs LE, Rerkpattanapipat P, Kotler MN, Owen A, Manzarbeitia C, et al. Clinical predictors of pulmonary hypertension in patients undergoing liver transplant evaluation. Liver Transpl. 2000 Jan;6(1):85–91.
245. Krowka MJ, Edwards WD. A spectrum of pulmonary vascular pathology in portopulmonary hypertension. Liver Transpl. 2000 Mar;6(2):241–2.
246. Pietra GG, Capron F, Stewart S, Leone O, Humbert M, Robbins IM, et al. Pathologic assessment of vasculopathies in pulmonary hypertension. J Am Coll Cardiol. 2004 Jun 16;43(12 Suppl S):25S–32S.
247. Giaid A, Saleh D. Reduced expression of endothelial nitric oxide synthase in the lungs of patients with pulmonary hypertension. N Engl J Med. 1995 Jul 27;333(4):214–21.
248. Rubens C, Ewert R, Halank M, Wensel R, Orzechowski HD, Schultheiss HP, et al. Big endothelin-1 and endothelin-1 plasma levels are correlated with the severity of primary pulmonary hypertension. Chest. 2001 Nov;120(5):1562–9.
249. Maruyama T, Ohsaki K, Shimoda S, Kaji Y, Harada M. Thromboxane-dependent portopulmonary hypertension. Am J Med. 2005 Jan;118(1):93–4.
250. Pellicelli AM, Barbaro G, Puoti C, Guarascio P, Lusi EA, Bellis L, et al. Plasma cytokines and portopulmonary hypertension in patients with cirrhosis waiting for orthotopic liver transplantation. Angiology. 2010 Nov;61(8):802–6.
251. Colle IO, Moreau R, Godinho E, Belghiti J, Ettori F, Cohen-Solal A, et al. Diagnosis of portopulmonary hypertension in candidates for liver transplantation: a prospective study. Hepatology. 2003 Feb;37(2):401–9.
252. Krowka MJ. Treatment of Portopulmonary hypertension with Macitentan in patients with cirrhosis. Gastroenterol Hepatol. 2019;15(2):108–10.
253. Stibon O, Bosch J, Cottreel E, Csonka D, de Groote P, Hoeper MM, Kim NH, Martin N, Savale L, Krowka M. Macitentan for the treatment of portopulmonary hypertension (PORTICO): a multicentre, randomised, double-blind, placebo-controlled, phase 4 trial. Lancet. 2019;7(7):594–604.
254. Provencher S, Herve P, Jais X, Lebrec D, Humbert M, Simonneau G, Sitbon O. Deleterious effects of beta-blockers on exercise capacity and hemodynamics in patients with portopulmonary hypertension. Gastroenterology. 2006;130(1):120–6.
255. G-P RE, Reixach M, Cuso E, Rodes J. Fat digestion and exocrine pancreatic function in primary biliary cirrhosis. Gastroenteorlogy. 1984;1984(1):180–7.
256. Logan RF, Ferguson A, Finlayson ND, Weir DG. Primary biliary cirrhosis and coeliac disease: an association? Lancet. 1978;1(8058):230–3.
257. Fidler HM, Butler P, Burroughs AK, McIntyre N, Bunn C, McMorrow M, Walmsley R, Dooley J. Co-screening for primary biliary cirrhosis and coeliac disease: a study of relative prevalences. Gut. 1998;43(2):300.
258. Kanai M, Raz A, Goodman DS. Retinol-binding protein: the transport protein for vitamin a in human plasma. J Clin Invest. 1968;47(9):2025–44.
259. Russell RM. The vitamin a spectrum: from deficiency to toxicity. Am J Clin Nutr. 2000 Apr;71(4):878–84.
260. Walt RP, Kemp CM, Lyness L, Bird AC, Sherlock S. Vitamin a treatment for night blindness in primary biliary cirrhosis. Br Med J. 1984;288(6423):1020–31.
261. Angulo P, Lindor KD. Primary biliary cirrhosis and primary sclerosing cholangitis. Clin Liver Dis. 1999 Aug;3(3):529–70.
262. Danielsson A, Lorentzon R, Larsson SE. Intestinal absorption and 25-hydroxylation of vitamin D in patients with primary biliary cirrhosis. Scand J Gastroenterol. 1982;17:349–55.

263. Davies M, Mawer EB, Klass HJ, Lumb GA, Berry JL, Warnes TW. Vitamin D deficiency, osteomalacia, and primary biliary cirrhosis. Response to orally administered vitamin D3. Dig Dis Sci. 1983;28(2):145–53.
264. Reichel H, Koeffler HP, Norman AW. The role of the vitamin D endocrine system in health and disease. N Engl J Med. 1989 Apr 13;320(15):980–91.
265. Marinaccio M, Pinto V, Sambati GS, Papandrea D, De Veteris M. Uncomplicated pregnancy in patients with unrecognized primary biliary cirrhosis. Minerva Ginecol. 1992;44(5):273–6.
266. Elias E, Muller DP, Scott J. Association of spinocerebellar disorders with cystic fibrosis or chronic childhood cholestasis and very low serum vitamin E. Lancet. 1981;2(8259):1319–21.
267. Sokol RJ. Fat-soluble vitamins and their importance in patients with cholestatic liver diseases. Gastroenterol Clin N Am. 1994 Dec;23(4):673–705.
268. Suttie JW. Recent advances in hepatic vitamin K metabolism and function. Hepatology. 1987 Mar-Apr;7(2):367–76.
269. Kowdley KV, Emond MJ, Sadowski JA, Kaplan MM. Plasma vitamin K1 level is decreased in primary biliary cirrhosis. Am J Gastroenterol. 1997;92(11):2059–61.
270. Kaplan MM, Elta GH, Furie B, Sadowski JA, Russell RM. Fat-soluble vitamin nutriture in primary biliary cirrhosis. Gastroenterology. 1988 Sep;95(3):787–92.
271. Cavanaugh J, Niewoehner CB, Nuttall FQ. Gynecomastia and cirrhosis of the liver. Arch Intern Med. 1990;150(3):563–5.
272. Acalovschi M, Badea R, Dumitrascu D, Varga C. Prevalence of gallstones in liver cirrhosis: a sonographic survey. Am J Gastroenterol. 1988 Sep;83(9):954–6.
273. Acalovschi M. Gallstones in patients with liver cirrhosis: incidence, etiology, clinical and therapeutical aspects. World J Gastroenterol. 2014 Jun 21;20(23):7277–85.
274. Aranha GV, Sontag SJ, Greenlee HB. Cholecystectomy in cirrhotic patients: a formidable operation. Am J Surg. 1982 Jan;143(1):55–60.
275. Cucchiaro G, Watters CR, Rossitch JC, Meyers WC. Deaths from gallstones. Incidence and associated clinical factors. Ann Surg. 1989 Feb;209(2):149–51.
276. Laurence JM, Tran PD, Richardson AJ, Pleass HC, Lam VW. Laparoscopic or open cholecystectomy in cirrhosis: a systematic review of outcomes and meta-analysis of randomized trials. HPB (Oxford). 2012 Mar;14(3):153–61.
277. Bunchorntavakul C, Reddy KR. Review article: malnutrition/sarcopenia and frailty in patients with cirrhosis. Aliment Pharmacol Ther. 2020;51(1):64–77.
278. Hammad A, Kaido T, Aliyev V, Mandato C, Uemoto S. Nutritional Therapy in Liver Transplantation. Nutrients 2017;9(10):1126.
279. Moss O. Nutrition Priorities: Diet Recommendations in Liver Cirrhosis. Clin Liver Dis (Hoboken). 2019;14(4):146–8.
280. European Association for the Study of the Liver. Electronic address eee, European Association for the Study of the L. EASL Clinical Practice Guidelines on nutrition in chronic liver disease. J Hepatol. 2019;70(1):172–93.

# Index

Printed by Printforce, the Netherlands